ESSENTIALS OF
Family Medicine

SEVENTH EDITION

ESSENTIALS OF
Family Medicine

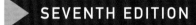
SEVENTH EDITION

Mindy A. Smith, MD, MS

Clinical Professor
Department of Family Medicine
Michigan State University
East Lansing, Michigan
Honorary Associate
Department of Family Medicine and Community Health
University of Wisconsin School of Medicine and Public Health
Madison, Wisconsin

Sarina Schrager, MD, MS

Professor (CHS)
Department of Family Medicine and Community Health
University of Wisconsin School of Medicine and Public Health
Madison, Wisconsin

Vince WinklerPrins, MD, FAAFP

Assistant Vice President for Student Health
Georgetown University
Washington, DC

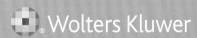 Wolters Kluwer

Philadelphia • Baltimore • New York • London
Buenos Aires • Hong Kong • Sydney • Tokyo

Acquisitions Editors: Matt Hauber
Development Editor: Andrew Hall (freelance), Andrea Vosburgh (in-house)
Editorial Coordinator: Alexis Pozonsky
Marketing Manager: Mike McMahon
Production Project Manager: Barton Dudlick
Design Coordinator: Steve Druding
Manufacturing Coordinator: Margie Orzech
Prepress Vendor: Aptara, Inc.

7th edition

Library of Congress Cataloging-in-Publication Data

Names: Smith, Mindy A., editor. | Schrager, Sarina B., editor. |
  WinklerPrins, Vince, editor.
Title: Essentials of family medicine / [edited by] Mindy A Smith, Sarina
  Schrager, Vince WinklerPrins.
Description: Seventh edition. | Philadelphia : Wolters Kluwer, [2019] |
  Includes bibliographical references and index.
Identifiers: LCCN 2017060691 | ISBN 9781496364975 (paperback)
Subjects: | MESH: Family Practice
Classification: LCC RC46 | NLM WB 110 | DDC 616—dc23 LC record available at https://lccn.loc.gov/2017060691

To the many students, residents, fellows, and faculty who I have been honored to learn from and teach; and to my daughter, Jenny, and partner, Ted.

—M.S.

I would like to thank my family.

—S.S.

In thanks to my wife, Antoinette WinklerPrins

—V.W.P.

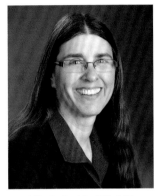

Mindy Smith, MD, MS

Mindy Smith, MD, MS is a Clinical Professor in the Department of Family Medicine at Michigan State University College of Human Medicine and an Honorary Associate in the Department of Family Medicine and Community Health at the University of Wisconsin School of Medicine and Public Health. She serves as an Associate Medical Editor of the American Academy of Family Physician *FP Essentials*™ and Deputy Editor of *Essential Evidence Plus*. She has published hundreds of book chapters and peer-reviewed publications and edited dozens of monographs and 12 books. Teaching and writing are two of her passions and she is privileged to do both.

Sarina Schrager, MD, MS is a Professor in the University of Wisconsin Department of Family Medicine and Public Health. She joined the faculty in 1996. Her areas of focus include faculty development, women's health, and shared decision making. She has two teenaged boys and when not working, enjoys being a soccer mom and hockey mom.

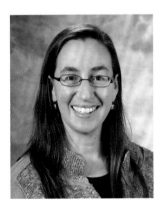

Sarina Schrager, MD, MS

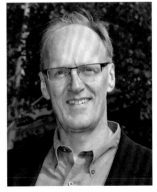

Vince WinklerPrins, MD, FAAFP

Vince WinklerPrins, MD, FAAFP is the Assistant Vice President for Student Health at Georgetown University. He has been the director of medical student education and Family Medicine clerkship director at both Georgetown University School of Medicine and Michigan State University's College of Human Medicine. He is a hopeless generalist, bicyclist, and proud father of two boys.

Elana R. Bannerman, MD

Primary Care Sports Medicine Fellow
Department of Family Medicine
University of Massachusetts
Worcester, Massachusetts

Jensena Carlson, MD

Assistant Professor
Department of Family Medicine and
    Community Health
University of Wisconsin School of Medicine
    and Public Health
Madison, Wisconsin

Jennifer G. Chang, MD

Assistant Professor
Department of Family Medicine
Uniformed Services University of the Health
    Sciences
Bethesda, Maryland

Beth Choby, MD, FAAFP

Associate Professor
Director—Kaplan Center for Clinical Skills
Co-Director—Principles of Clinical Medicine
Department of Medical Education
University of Tennessee College of Medicine
Memphis, Tennessee

Molly Cohen-Osher, MD, MMedEd

Family Medicine Clerkship Director & Director
    of Medical Student Education
Assistant Professor
Department of Family Medicine and
    Department of Medical Sciences &
    Education
Boston University School of Medicine
Boston, Massachusetts

Amy C. Denham, MD, MPH

Associate Professor
Department of Family Medicine
University of North Carolina at Chapel Hill
Chapel Hill, North Carolina

Mark H. Ebell, MD, MS

Professor
College of Public Health
University of Georgia
Athens, Georgia

Nancy C. Elder, MD, MSPH

Professor
Department of Family and Community
    Medicine
University of Cincinnati College of Medicine
Cincinnati, Ohio

Radha Ramana Murthy Gokula, MD, CMD

Clinical Associate Professor
Department of Family Medicine
University of Toledo
Toledo, Ohio

Adrienne Hampton, MD

Assistant Professor
Department of Family Medicine and
    Community Health
University of Wisconsin School of Medicine
    and Public Health
Madison, Wisconsin

Cynthia Haq, MD

Professor and Chair, Department of Family
    Medicine University of California, Irvine
University of Wisconsin School of Medicine
    and Public Health
Madison, Wisconsin

Ronni Hayon, MD

Assistant Professor
Department of Family Medicine and
    Community Health
University of Wisconsin School of Medicine
    and Public Health
Madison, Wisconsin

Miriam Hoffman, MD

Associate Dean of Medical Education
Associate Professor of Family Medicine
Seton Hall—Hackensack Meridian School of
Medicine
South Orange, New Jersey

Patrick A. Huffer, MD

Assistant Director
Marquette Family Medicine Residency
Program
Marquette, Michigan

Miranda M. Huffman, MD

Associate Professor
Community and Family Medicine Department
University of Missouri—Kansas City
Kansas City, Missouri

Robert Jackman, MD

Assistant Professor of Family Medicine
Associate Program Director and Medical
Director of the Cascades East Family
Practice Residency Program
Oregon Health and Science University
Portland, Oregon

Yumi Shitama Jarris, MD

Professor
Department of Family Medicine
Assistant Dean for Population Health and
Prevention
Georgetown University School of Medicine
Washington, DC

Alexander Kaysin, MD, MPH

Assistant Professor
Department of Family Medicine
University of North Carolina at Chapel Hill
Chapel Hill, North Carolina

Kjersti Knox, MD

Clinical Adjunct Assistant Professor,
Department of Family Medicine and
Community Health
University of Wisconsin School of Medicine
and Public Health
Madison, Wisconsin
Aurora Family Medicine Residency Program
Aurora UW Medical Group
Milwaukee, Wisconsin

Kenneth W. Lin, MD, MPH

Associate Professor of Family Medicine
Director of the Robert L. Phillips, Jr., Health
Policy Fellowship
Associate Deputy Editor of *American Family
Physician* journal
Georgetown University School of Medicine
Washington, DC

Andrea Ildiko Martonffy, MD

Associate Professor (CHS)
Department of Family Medicine and
Community Health
University of Wisconsin School of Medicine
and Public Health
Madison, Wisconsin

Coral Matus, MD, FAAFP

Assistant Professor
Department of Family Medicine
University of Toledo
Toledo, Ohio

Ganesh Merugu, MD

Assistant Professor
Department of Family Medicine
University of Toledo
Toledo, Ohio

Radu Moisa, MD

Assistant Professor
Department of Family Medicine
Oregon Health and Science University
Klamath Falls, Oregon

Donald E. Nease, Jr., MD

Green-Edelman Chair for Practice-Based
Research
Associate Professor and Vice Chair for
Research
Department of Family Medicine
University of Colorado School of Medicine
Aurora, Colorado

Mary B. Noel, MPH, PhD, RD

Professor
Department of Family Medicine
Michigan State University College of Human
Medicine
East Lansing, Michigan

Cristen P. Page, MD, MPH

William B. Aycock Distinguished Professor
and Chair
Department of Family Medicine
University of North Carolina at Chapel Hill
Chapel Hill, North Carolina

Linda Prine, MD

Professor
Department of Family and Community
Medicine
Icahn School of Medicine at Mount Sinai
Mount Sinai Downtown & Harlem Family
Medicine Residency
Women's Health Director and Fellowship
Director
Institute for Family Health
New York, New York

Alex J. Reed, PsyD, MPH

Assistant Professor
Department of Family Medicine
University of Colorado School of Medicine
Aurora, Colorado

Sarina Schrager, MD, MS

Professor (CHS)
Department of Family Medicine and
Community Health
University of Wisconsin School of Medicine
and Public Health
Madison, Wisconsin

H. Russell Searight, PhD, MPH

Professor
Department of Psychology
Lake Superior State University
Sault Ste. Marie, Michigan

Allen F. Shaughnessy, PharmD, MMedEd

Director
Master Teacher Fellowship
Professor
Department of Family Medicine
Tufts University School of Medicine
Boston, Massachusetts

Kimberly Sikule, MD

Primary Care Sports Medicine Fellow
Department of Family Medicine
University of Massachusetts
Worcester, Massachusetts

Martha A. Simmons, MD

Assistant Professor
Department of Family and Community
Medicine
Icahn School of Medicine at Mount Sinai
Harlem Residency in Family Medicine
The Institute for Family Health
New York, New York

David C. Slawson, MD

Director of Information Sciences
B. Lewis Barnett, Jr., Professor of Family
Medicine
University of Virginia Health System
Charlottesville, Virginia

Philip D. Sloane, MD, MPH

Elizabeth and Oscar Goodwin Distinguished
Professor
Department of Family Medicine
University of North Carolina at Chapel Hill
Chapel Hill, North Carolina

Mindy A. Smith, MD, MS

Clinical Professor
Department of Family Medicine
College of Human Medicine
Michigan State University
East Lansing, Michigan

Linda Speer, MD

Professor
Department of Family Medicine
University of Toledo
Toledo, Ohio

J. Herbert Stevenson, MD

Director of Sports Medicine
Director Sports Medicine Fellowship Program
Associate Professor
Department of Family and Community
  Medicine
Joint Appointment University of Massachusetts
  Department of Orthopedics
University of Massachusetts Medical School
Worcester, Massachusetts

Arianna Sundick, MD

General Practitioner
Te Taiwhenua o Heretaunga
Hastings, New Zealand

Margaret E. Thompson, MD

Associate Professor
Department of Family Medicine
Michigan State University College of Human
  Medicine
East Lansing, Michigan

Richard P. Usatine, MD

Distinguished Teaching Professor
Professor of Family and Community Medicine
Professor of Dermatology and Cutaneous
  Surgery
Medical Director, Student Faculty
  Collaborative Clinics
Center for Medical Humanities and Ethics
University of Texas Health Science Center at
  San Antonio
San Antonio, Texas

Anthony J. Viera, MD, MPH

Professor
Department of Family Medicine
University of North Carolina at Chapel Hill
Chapel Hill, North Carolina

Adam J. Zolotor, MD, DrPH

Associate Professor
Department of Family Medicine
University of North Carolina at Chapel Hill
Chapel Hill, North Carolina

During the development of this book, our panel of student editors/advisers included Daniel McCorry, Joseph Brodine, and Racheli Schoenberg, who were fourth-year medical students at Georgetown University School of Medicine; and Lindsey Anderson, Nate Baggett, and Brian Eby, who were fourth-year medical students at the University of Wisconsin School of Medicine. These students reviewed all of the chapter outlines and draft book chapters, providing invaluable input that helped the senior medical editors stay focused and keep material relevant to what students need to know.

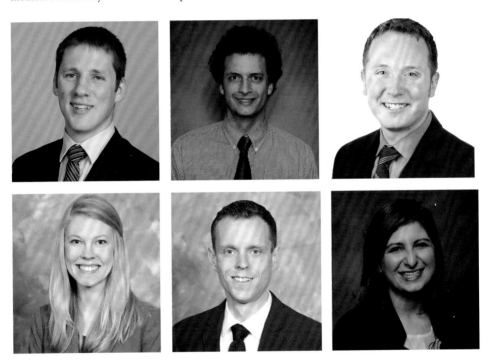

To Our Teachers and Learners

Why this book? Basically, it is because we were starting with something good. *Essentials of Family Medicine* has been a staple of family medicine training for 30 years, given its focus on preventive care and common ambulatory care problems. In addition to routine updating, this book has evolved through six editions, adding greater amounts of evidence-based content, a more streamlined format, and greater learner accessibility through use of algorithms and tables—these features will continue. We also attract excellent authors and have an outstanding editorial team. Finally, we provide learners with test questions for shelf and board exam preparation.

We strongly believe that textbooks are still relevant for providing essential background information (see Chapter 3). Concurrently, we recognize that foreground questions require up-to-the-minute information, best obtained by continually updated sources. We therefore set out on a somewhat different course for this 7th edition—emphasizing the how questions (e.g., How do I best approach a patient? How do I engage a patient in behavior change? How do I assess a patient with a health problem?) and not as much on the what questions (e.g., What is the best drug to use for X? What is the best test for Y). While we answer the "what to dos" for the most common acute, chronic, dermatologic, and musculoskeletal conditions that a student is likely to see on family medicine and other ambulatory care rotations, we reinforce the habits that you have already acquired in medical school—using online, regularly updated secondary data sources and guidelines.

Why this approach? We realized that, in our current information-rich environment, we needed to create something that offered guidance to focus learning. We needed to be more streamlined, keeping the essential aspects of providing ambulatory-based medical care while providing instructions on how to synthesize medical information, work within a healthcare team, approach patients of different ages, prevent medical and medication errors, and support behavior change. We are also aware that most of our learners are millennials—computer savvy, accepting of diversity, and attracted to teamwork and community building; they are also used to getting information quickly and concisely. To help us with this aspect, we assembled a team of fourth-year medical students to serve as our advisors. Our students were involved in the whole process of creating this book—commenting on chapter outlines, suggesting resources, and reviewing finished chapters for content, presentation, and relevance.

What's in this book? We present what we consider the essentials of family medicine in 24 chapters. We conceptualized these as falling into aspects of **direct care, context, and community** that are vital to medical student's education.

Direct Care: The practice of family medicine is about the patient. Our offices need to be empowering and safe environments. We created two new chapters: one on approaches to behavior change and one on patient safety. We present chapters on information mastery, preventive care; care specific to men, woman, and children, including pregnancy care and care of elderly patients; the most common acute and chronic problems; nutrition; common skin problems; chronic pain; common psychosocial problems; and addiction.

Context: The context of care, in relation to health and illness, is also important—this includes the patient within their family (chapters on relationship issues and family violence) and within their larger communities (chapters on the U.S. healthcare system and population health). Chapter 2 introduces the concepts of health equity and the social determinants of health.

Community: We practice medicine as part of a wider community in which we and our patients live. In addition to understanding social determinants of health, we, as physicians, have an opportunity to influence and move our communities toward healthier living and social justice for its members. Chapter 24 not only presents information on how students can engage within their practices and communities, but how to care for yourself and build professional support.

We welcome our teachers and learners to use this resource to enhance the learning experience that is Family Medicine, to better serve our patients, and to participate more fully in creating powerful, equitable, and evidence and value-based places for healing.

Mindy A. Smith
Sarina Schrager
Vince WinklerPrins

Contents

About the Editors   vii
Contributors   ix
The Student Advisory Group   xiii
Preface   xv

1. Primary Care and the Evolving United States Healthcare System 1
   PHILIP D. SLOANE, MD, MPH; CRISTEN P. PAGE, MD, MPH

2. Population Health 15
   YUMI SHITAMA JARRIS, MD; KENNETH W. LIN, MD, MPH

3. Information Mastery 27
   MOLLY COHEN-OSHER, MD, MMEDED; DAVID C. SLAWSON, MD;
   MARK H. EBELL, MD, MS; ALLEN F. SHAUGHNESSY, PHARMD, MMEDED

4. Working in an Ambulatory Care Office 45
   MIRANDA M. HUFFMAN, MD

5. Behavior Change 60
   H. RUSSELL SEARIGHT, PHD, MPH

6. Patient Safety in Primary Care 73
   NANCY C. ELDER, MD, MSPH

7. Overview of Prevention and Screening 85
   ANTHONY J. VIERA, MD, MPH; ALEXANDER KAYSIN, MD, MPH

8. Prenatal Care 98
   BETH CHOBY, MD, FAAFP

9. The Pediatric Well-Child Check 119
   ANDREA ILDIKO MARTONFFY, MD; JENSENA CARLSON, MD

10. Care for the Aging Patient 137
    RADHA RAMANA MURTHY GOKULA, MD, CMD; GANESH MERUGU, MD

11. Acute Problems: Approach and Treatment 161
    MINDY A. SMITH, MD, MS; PATRICK A. HUFFER, MD; SARINA SCHRAGER, MD, MS

12. Approach to Common Chronic Problems 229
    SARINA SCHRAGER, MD, MS; MINDY A. SMITH, MD, MS; PATRICK A. HUFFER, MD

13. Weight Management and Nutrition 291
    MARGARET E. THOMPSON, MD; MARY B. NOEL, MPH, PHD, RD

14. Contraception 308
    MARTHA A. SIMMONS, MD; LINDA PRINE, MD

15. Women's Health Care 321
    CORAL MATUS, MD, FAAFP; LINDA SPEER, MD

16. Men's Health Care 335
    JENNIFER G. CHANG, MD

17. Musculoskeletal Problems 354
    ELANA R. BANNERMAN, MD; KIMBERLY SIKULE, MD; J. HERBERT STEVENSON, MD

18. Sexuality and Relationship Issues 381
    RONNI HAYON, MD; ADRIENNE HAMPTON, MD

19. Skin Problems 392
    RICHARD P. USATINE, MD

20. Chronic Pain 409
    ROBERT JACKMAN, MD; RADU MOISA, MD

21. Family Violence 426
    AMY C. DENHAM, MD, MPH; ADAM J. ZOLOTOR, MD, DRPH

22. Common Psychosocial Problems 440
    ALEX J. REED, PSYD, MPH; DONALD E. NEASE, JR., MD

23. Substance Use Disorders 453
    H. RUSSELL SEARIGIIT, PIID, MPII

24. Community Engagement, Health Equity, and Advocacy 468
    KJERSTI KNOX, MD; ARIANNA SUNDICK, MD; CYNTHIA HAQ, MD

Index   481

Primary Care and the Evolving United States Healthcare System

KEY POINTS

1 ▶ Family medicine principles include prompt access to care, coordination with empowerment, care within the patient's context, care continuity, population management, resource stewardship, prevention focus, and wise use of evidence.

2 ▶ Well-functioning healthcare systems have high performing primary care practices mirroring the principles of family medicine.

3 ▶ The United States is ranked below most industrialized nations in healthcare indicators but spends more per capita on healthcare. Despite improvements, many health disparities persist.

4 ▶ Quality improvement is a central feature of quality care and includes identification of priorities, benchmarks and measurable outcomes, monitoring, establishment of quality improvement goals, and regular reporting.

5 ▶ The quadruple aim—simultaneously optimizing patient experience, quality outcomes, provider experience, and value—is now considered the cornerstone of healthcare reform.

The McCauley Family in 2005

Ten years ago, Sara McCauley had an initial prenatal visit with Dr. Carol Collins. Sara was noticeably overweight (BMI 53) and accompanied by her husband Herb, their 3-year-old son Ethan, and 9-month-old Anna. She was referred by a nurse in the local emergency department (ED) where she'd presented 2 weeks earlier with a positive pregnancy test. The ED staff referred to the family as "frequent flyers" because they appeared almost every month for such problems as otitis media, skin rashes, diarrhea, and upper respiratory infections. The children had recently been approved for Medicaid and the ED nurse hoped that the more comprehensive care provided at a family medicine clinic might be an improvement over the limited services they'd been receiving through sporadic visits to the local health department and urgent care center.

During the pregnancy, Dr. Collins provided Sara's prenatal care and also got to know the entire family. She learned that Sara held a steady job as a bookkeeper for a local furniture company and was the family's primary breadwinner because Herb, a high school dropout with a learning disability and attention deficit disorder, had never been able to hold down a steady job. Sara's employment provided her with health insurance, but she could not afford the cost of covering the rest of her family; so when Medicaid expansion provided that option for her family, Sara had enrolled. They lived in a mobile home and often housed friends and extended family members on the couch or floor during times of transition.

This pregnancy was Sara's sixth. In addition to Ethan and Anna, she had seven-year-old twin boys and had suffered two miscarriages. The twins, Andy and Eric, were in second grade and the teacher had sent several notes home about Eric's disruptive behavior in class. Andy was at the 98th percentile in weight for his age. Sara and Herb had low health and nutritional literacy; not realizing, for example, that their smoking in the home might be contributing to Ethan's recurrent ear infections. Figure 1.1 is a genogram of the McCauley family from that time period.

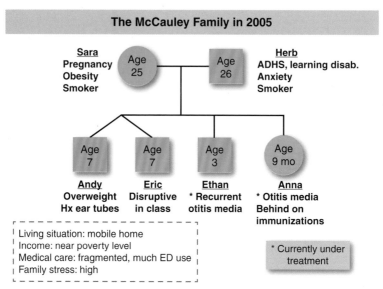

Figure 1.1 ▶ Genogram of the McCauley family. (Sources for constructing genograms include www.genpro.com and www.genogramanalytics.com.)

HEALTHCARE ORGANIZATION AND THE ROLE OF PRIMARY CARE

The McCauley family illustrates many of the issues facing today's healthcare providers, administrators, and policy makers in the United States. These include:

▶ Chronic medical problems

▶ Acute medical conditions

▶ Unhealthy habits and lifestyle choices

▶ Mental health issues

▶ Poverty/limited economic resources

▶ Low health literacy

▶ Inconsistent health insurance coverage

▶ Lack of consistent or coordinated healthcare

Looking at this array of medical, psychosocial, and economic issues presented by the McCauley in 2005 exemplifies why improving health status can be so challenging.

Yet other industrialized, wealthy nations have been able to address the breadth of health-related factors better than the United States.[1] In fact, the United States is ranked below practically every other industrialized, wealthy nation in the world in healthcare indicators such as life expectancy and infant mortality (Table 1.1), in spite of our spending the most money per capita on healthcare.[2-4]

As shown in the table, the United States has the highest healthcare and pharmaceutical spending per capita and the highest proportion of GDP spent on healthcare. However, health benefits are not commensurate with cost, as many of the other nations have better societal health outcomes. For example, the United States has the lowest reported life

Table 1.1 ▶ Comparison of Healthcare Systems in Selected Developed Nations

Measure	United States	Canada	France	Germany	Switzerland	Japan	Australia
Population Health Outcomes							
Life expectancy at birth[d]	78.8	81.5[c]	82.3	80.9	82.9	83.4	82.2
Infant mortality per 1,000 live births[d]	6.1[c]	4.8[c]	3.6	3.3	3.9	2.1	3.6
Prevalence of obesity (BMI > 30)	35.3%	25.8%	14.5%[b]	23.6%	10.3%[b]	3.7%	28.3%[c]
Percent of population age 65+	14.1	15.2	17.7	21.1	17.3	25.1	14.4
Percent of population age 65+ with two or more chronic conditions	68%	56%	43%	49%	44%		54%
Care Provision							
Number of physicians per 1,000 individuals	2.56	2.48[b]	3.10	4.05	4.04	2.29[b]	3.39
Average hospital length of stay (days)	5.4[c]	7.6[b]	5.7[b]	7.7	5.9	17.2	4.8[b]
Percent of primary care practices that review clinical outcomes data	52%	23%	43%	44%	9%		35%
Mean number of prescription medications per adult	2.2	1.8	1.5	1.6	1.3		1.4
Healthcare Costs							
Total spending per capita[a]	$9,086	$4,569	$4,361	$4,920	$6,325	$3,713	$4,115[b]
Percent of GDP spent on healthcare	17.1%	10.7%	11.6%	11.2%	11.1%	10.2%	9.4%[b]
Out of pocket spending per capita[a]	$1,074	$623	$277	$649	$1,630	$503[b]	$771[b]
Amount spent on drugs per capita[a]	$1,034	$761	$622	$678	$696	$756[b]	$509[b]
Public Opinion							
Percent of adults for whom cost is a barrier to care	37%	13%	18%	15%	13%		16%
Percent of public feeling health system needs to be restructured	27%	8%	11%	10%	7%		9%

Unless otherwise indicated, all statistics are from 2013.
[a]US dollars, adjusted for cost of living difference.
[b]2012 data.
[c]2011 data.
[d]2015 data.

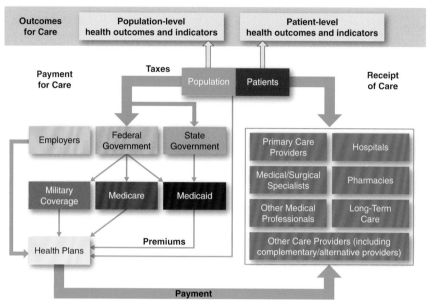

Figure 1.2 ▶ Diagram of the US healthcare system.

expectancy, highest infant mortality rate, and highest obesity prevalence. In addition, the US public reports higher levels of discontent with their healthcare system than their counterparts in other nations.

The reasons for this are complex but in large measures reflect America's wide disparities in a variety of factors that influence health, most notably personal health habits and behaviors, income, education, healthcare access and provision, and housing and neighborhood quality and safety (Chapter 24).[2,5,6] Many of these factors are remediable and examples from other countries can inform policies to improve school and family nutrition, maternity leave, subsidized childcare, education systems including low-cost or free access to college, better work hours, and better pay.

It can be argued that the United States historically has a health nonsystem rather than a health system, due to its fragmented and often incomplete insurance coverage, lack of integration across health settings, and emphasis on acute care and procedures rather than prevention and chronic disease management.[7] In the recent decades, however, particularly since passage of the Affordable Care Act, increased attention has been paid to chronic disease management, prevention, and transitions across settings, such that the United States is looking more like a health system than in previous decades. Still, as is illustrated graphically in Figure 1.2, US healthcare remains a rather confusing and a suboptimally functioning network of payment programs and provider types.

As shown in this model of the US healthcare system, there are three main elements:

1. Payment of care through a complex system of governmental and private health insurance providers
2. Provision of care by a wide range of settings and providers, which until recently operated and were paid autonomously, with little coordination
3. Health outcomes at the population and individual patient level

The result is much variation in access and insurance coverage, considerable duplication of services in some sectors (such as MRI scanners), and woefully inadequate service provision in other sectors (such as mental health), with the overall result being much variation in individual health outcomes, leading to lower-than-optimal population health outcomes. The Triple Aim (improving patient care experience, reducing cost, improving population health) seeks to align these three elements so that each performs optimally.[8]

The role of formal health services (such as prenatal care, access to specialists, and child-hood immunizations) in promoting health disparities appears to be modest compared to other factors, such as psychosocial variables and living environment.[9] This is in large measure because many of America's poorest individuals have one of America's best health insurance programs—Medicaid. The comprehensiveness and lack of out-of-pocket costs associated with Medicaid provides important and valuable access to healthcare for indigent Americans. Many families, however, like the McCauley family, do not qualify for Medicaid and lack of insurance provided through jobs and limited income make health insurance unaffordable. In addition, since formal healthcare is not enough, a well-functioning health system must reach beyond the "medical" to address the other factors that affect health (Chapter 24). Within medical practice, this can be most effectively done at the primary care level.

ROLE OF PRIMARY CARE

Primary care clinicians are held accountable for attending to the broad healthcare needs of their respective communities, and thus serve as the cornerstone to medical society. Primary care physicians (PCPs) include those in family medicine, general internal medicine, pediatrics, and in some cases gynecology—but PCPs have the same responsibility: to utilize patient-centered medical care to address a large majority of the personal health needs of their patients.[10,11]

To address the variety of problems exemplified by the McCauley family, primary care practices must employ an interdisciplinary team to deliver integrated healthcare services, something that remains a challenge in today's health system. In addition, PCPs are tasked with coordination of care involving, but not limited to, referrals to other medical specialists as needed.[12]

Since primary care is such a crucial component of the US healthcare framework, it is important to delineate the characteristics of "high-performing primary care." These include engaged leadership, data-driven improvement, a sense of responsibility for a panel of patients, team-based care, patient–team partnership, continuity of care, comprehensiveness, care coordination, and prompt access to care. Because the success of PCPs requires close patient relationships, continuity of care is clearly an influential aspect of quality primary care. Continuity of care relies on successful use of a care team to complement the PCP and to achieve comprehensiveness and care coordination, so as to provide care that is inclusive enough to address a significant portion, if not all, of a patient's needs.[11]

The McCauley Family in 2014

During the subsequent 9 years, Dr. Collins and her office staff helped the McCauley family through numerous transitions. Sara's pregnancy was successfully managed with the delivery of a healthy 8-pound girl whom they named Caroline. Two years later their sixth child, Charlotte was born. By this time, Dr. Collins' relationship with Sara and Herb had developed enough trust, so that she was able to educate them about how medications work, including birth control, to the point where Sara decided an intrauterine device would help them achieve their family planning goals.

Visits to the ED have become rare. The children are getting their immunizations on schedule rather than, as happened with the twins, needing a series of urgent "catch-up" appointments before enrolling in kindergarten.

Sara is still obese and now has diabetes and hypertension, both managed with oral medications that she takes regularly. Herb is on disability, sees a mental health counselor regularly, and takes a selective serotonin reuptake inhibitor for his anxiety. He is better able to care for the children. Both Sara and Herb still smoke, but now they do so on the front porch, which has helped to reduce the number of ear infections experienced by their last two children.

PRINCIPLES OF FAMILY MEDICINE

The principles of good primary care are embodied in the principles of family medicine as displayed in Table 1.2.

QUALITY MONITORING IN FAMILY MEDICINE

To help family medicine practices better promote and monitor the health status of their patients, the field has embraced the need to regularly monitor, track, and report how well patients are doing. To date, this quality monitoring has focused on preventive care and chronic disease management, as these are important cornerstones of primary care. In addition, many practices monitor how well they are addressing some of the other principles of family medicine, such as continuity of care and access to care.

Figure 1.3 provides examples of some typical elements of quality monitoring, as carried out by the Family Medicine Center at the University of North Carolina at Chapel Hill. Performance on these measures is reported on a monthly basis not just to practice managers but to all providers, including the nursing staff. National benchmarks are available for some of these measures, and practices often set annual improvement goals on key measures that are foci of quality improvement efforts. Practice-based monitoring of diabetes could be used to identify Sara's elevated blood pressure readings or A1c level to trigger intensified therapy. In this manner, family medicine and other primary care practices seek to continually improve the processes and outcomes of care.

ENHANCING THE US HEALTHCARE SYSTEM: THE TRIPLE AND QUADRUPLE AIM

In the pursuit of enhancing the US healthcare system, the Institute for Healthcare and Improvement (www.ihi.org) developed a novel, three-pronged framework known as the "Triple Aim." The approach involves optimization in three major cruxes of the system: **patient experience, per capita cost,** and **population health**.[8]

Although presented as three discrete aims, the triple aim delineates goals which are interconnected, with a crucial role of primary care in the achievement of all three. Studies on primary care not only delineate its beneficial impact on each of these goals but also how the aims are mutually reliant on each other.[17–19]

Despite an array of studies promulgating the positive effects of the Triple Aim, the Triple Aim still may have shortcomings. In particular, it does not include the health and well-being

Table 1.2 ▸ Key Principles of Family Medicine Practice

Principle	Description	Comments
Access to care	Care is organized so that each patient's problems can be addressed in a timely manner	Enhanced through open access,[a] online scheduling, 24-hour call service, telemedicine, and secure email correspondence
Coordination with empowerment	Patients are guided through health and illness in a manner that fosters empowerment, self-care, and community support	Being aware of available services, advising about and making appropriate referrals, collecting and interpreting outside tests and specialist visits, ensuring comprehension and advocating self-care and informed choice
Care in lifecycle and family context	Illness and preventive care is provided in the context of the human life cycle and family relationships	Understanding and providing guidance that is consonant with each patient's life context (e.g., age, work and home life, health, culture)
Care continuity	Personal and team continuity of care is provided across and between settings, over time	Favorable outcomes demonstrated[13,14]; promotes fuller, more satisfying patient relationships[15]; enhanced by using a comprehensive, shared medical record and small healthcare teams
Population management	Focus is not just at the individual level but at the practice and population level, using data systems to guide outreach and quality of care	Requires access and attention to information systems that provide data about patient panels, and steps for conducting outreach (see Chapter 2)
Community focus	Focus on the most prevalent and pressing problems within their practice communities and adapt practice to address those needs	Being aware of pressing health problems in the local community, adapting work and scope of practice to those needs (e.g., incorporating testing or providers not otherwise available), volunteering (Chapter 24)
Resource stewardship	Responsibility for managing each patient optimally in the context of social justice and population health	Contain healthcare costs through practice of prevention, test ordering (does a test influence management?), making referrals, advising patients
Prevention	All visits considered as opportunities for preventive healthcare	Some visits are focused on prevention such as prenatal care, adult and well-child examinations, pre-employment and sports physicals (Chapter 7)
Wise use of evidence	The medical provider knows and uses scientific evidence while recognizing the subjective and individual aspects of illness and health	Uses available literature to guide practice (Chapter 3); integrates different kinds of evidence, depending on logic; clinical intuition; and knowledge of the patient, family, and community to arrive at the best decisions

[a]A system that keeps slots open for same day appointments, uses telephone protocols to triage patients by urgency of need, and organizes schedules to correspond with consumer demand.[16]

of health professionals—and if health professionals are stressed, overworked, and consequently burn out or relocate, the entire health service delivery system will suffer. Therefore, many healthcare leaders are stressing the need to expand the quality improvement framework by adding a quadruple aim—to enhance the quality of work life in healthcare providers.[20]

A

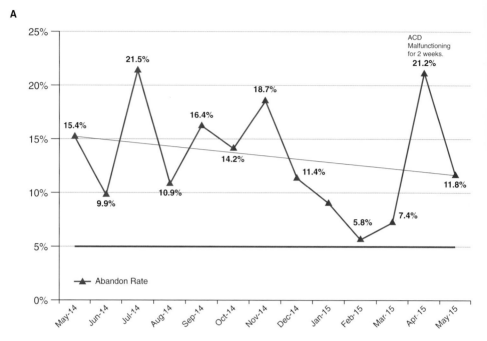

B

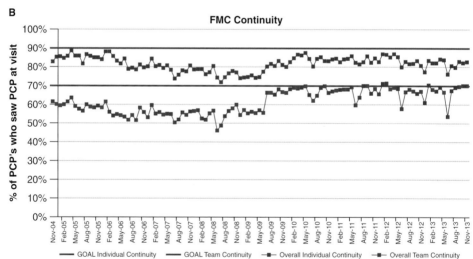

Figure 1.3 ▶ Graphs generated by the Family Medicine Center at the University of North Carolina to track performance on selected principles of family medicine, as part of quality monitoring and improvement activities. **A.** Access to care, measured using the rate at which telephone callers hang up, often because operators respond too slowly (abandonment). Goal is <10% abandonment. Note that the goal has been difficult to achieve. The trend has been in the right direction, but in April an equipment malfunction for 2 weeks led to temporary worsening. **B.** Continuity of care, measured as the proportion of patient visits with their primary care provider (*blue line*) and the primary provider's team (*red line*). Because many providers are part-time (including residents), the practice's goal is 70% provider continuity and 90% team continuity. Graph shows gradual improvement over several years. (*continued*)

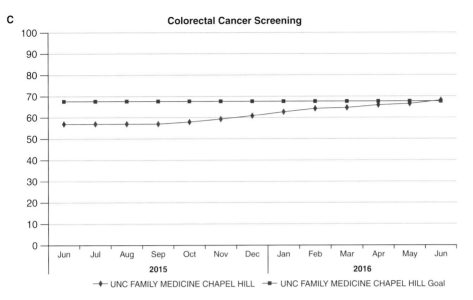

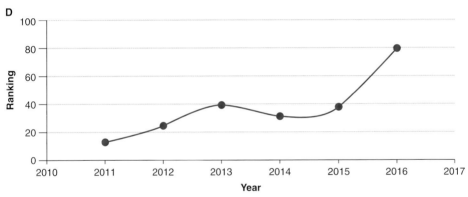

Figure 1.3 ▶ *Continued.* **C.** Prevention, in this case measured using the rate of colorectal cancer screening. By focusing on this indicator as a practice goal, rates were able to achieve target levels. **D.** Patient satisfaction, based on survey reports by an external agency contracted to provide feedback to the practice. Shows increasing satisfaction relative to other clinics. Patient satisfaction is a good global measure, as it reflects practice performance on multiple principles of quality care. (From Department of Family Medicine, University of North Carolina at Chapel Hill. Quality improvement graphics, 2016. Unpublished. Provided courtesy of Tommy Koonce, MD, Medical Director, UNC Family Medicine Center, Chapel Hill, North Carolina.)

The McCauley Family in 2017: The Family's Physician Reflects on Over a Decade of Care

"Every family physician has patients and families like the McCauleys. The problems they face are chronic, endemic, and inter-related. They present with a range of economic, social, psychological, and medical issues."

"You empathize with the challenges they face and do what you can, hoping to make a positive difference. You bend your schedule, knowing, for example, that they have an old, unreliable car. Or that, due to lack of organizational skills, they may phone at the last minute, perhaps about a school health form that needs completion. Or that, if you don't fit them in,

Herb's anxiety may precipitate an ER visit and from that a series of unnecessary tests and very possibly an inappropriate prescription. You and your practice staff put in extra, uncompensated time trying to arrange services, because otherwise they'd be unable to negotiate our complex healthcare system to get what they need."

"What impact have I had over the past 10 years with this family? In many respects you might say not much. They still cram into a double-wide with four small bedrooms, still have a broken-down car, and still have trouble making ends meet. The twins—now age 20 years—remain at home and are in and out of temporary jobs. Herb remains on disability for mental health reasons. Sara's BMI is still 43 and she's beginning to develop symptomatic arthritis in her knees."

"But the family is still together, Sara's diabetes and hypertension are fairly well controlled, and the children's preventive services have been up-to-date for over a decade. The parents smoke less and periodically quit for months at a time. The younger children are healthier and on track to be more successful in school. And through it all they've had an anchor—a primary care physician who will listen, help them access needed services, and advise them from a more informed and optimistic perspective. For me, this is the great privilege of being a family physician—to share in the journey of my patient's lives."

THE FUTURE ROLE OF PRIMARY CARE AND FAMILY MEDICINE IN US HEALTHCARE

Health policy experts have noted that United States is suffering from a shortage of PCPs, and that the need for primary care is expected to mushroom in the coming decade.[21–23] Behind this concern is an aging population and an increasing awareness that a strong primary care system can better contain costs and produce superior outcomes than specialist-dominated healthcare.[20,24]

Because of these issues, implementation of the Affordable Care Act has included provisions aimed at making primary care more attractive, including expansion of scholarship and loan forgiveness programs and bonuses for family physicians, internists, geriatricians, nurse practitioners, and physician assistants engaged in primary care practice. Yet interest in family medicine as a residency choice has not increased in response to the needs and incentives provided. So it is worth looking objectively at family medicine as a career to find out what is appealing and unappealing to students, what options it can and will provide, and whether, and to what extent, family physicians who have entered the field are satisfied.

Who Enters Family Medicine and Why?

There is no single background, motivation, or personality type that defines a family physician; however, research has shown that certain characteristics are more common in medical students who enter family medicine and other primary care disciplines than in those who choose specialties. Students entering primary care tend to:

▶ Value people skills over technical skills

▶ Express greater concern about addressing societal problems

▶ Desire variety in their work

▶ Be married or in a long-term relationship

▶ Come from a nonprofessional family

▶ Have a history of volunteer work in a developing nation

▶ Desire a shorter residency

▶ Lack interest in scientific research

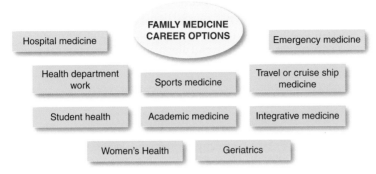

Figure 1.4 ▶ Career options for physicians considering practicing family medicine.

In contrast, students who enter specialties tend to value science and technical skills over interpersonal skills, prefer a more limited scope of practice, desire prestige within the medical profession, and aspire to have higher incomes relative to other specialties and/or relative to the number of hours worked.[25–27]

The issue of compensation is controversial. Many feel that the low incomes of family physicians and other primary care specialties is an important driver, or at least a modifier, of student career choice.[28] According to Medscape's April, 2015 report on physician compensation by specialty, the average family physician made $195,000 annually, second lowest after pediatrics ($189,000). Most lucrative were the procedure-focused specialties of orthopedics ($421,000), cardiology ($376,000), gastroenterology ($370,000), anesthesiology ($358,000), plastic surgery ($354,000), and radiology ($351,000).[29]

So, yes, compared to other specialties, and especially in the context of the six-figure student loan debts carried by many medical school graduates, family physician incomes are modest. However, outside medical circles, one gets very little sympathy from complaints about "low" primary care compensation, considering that the median household income in the United States is $56,516.[30] As a result, policy initiatives to reduce disparities in physician incomes have tended to focus more on reducing pay for specialists than on markedly increasing compensation for primary care.

Career Options in Primary Care and Family Medicine

For physicians entering family medicine, the career options are much more varied than in any other medical field. Just a few of the areas of medicine occupied to a large extent by family medicine graduates are rural primary care practice, inner-city and/or health center practices, and suburban office care. Other options within family medicine are shown in Figure 1.4.

Because of their people skills and breadth of training, family physicians often gravitate to leadership positions in health departments, insurance plans, and managed care organizations. Part time positions are common, too, and it is not unusual to limit one's practice to one area, such as outpatient practice. Consequently, family physicians can have multiple different "careers" over their working lifetime without having to change their specialty, and physicians with young families can work part time if they desire.

How Satisfied are Family Physicians?

Evidence suggests that overall, they are about in the middle. Across the specialties, differences in satisfaction are modest and appear to be largely independent of income, as some of the most lucrative specialties tend to be the least satisfied.[31,32] Among practicing family physicians, overall career satisfaction is positively associated with satisfaction in choice of medicine overall as a career, satisfaction with one's workplace, ability to practice with a sense of service and altruism, and training that was broad and in-depth.[33]

QUESTIONS

1. Compared with Canada, France, Germany, Switzerland, Japan, and Australia, which one of the following is true of the United States healthcare system?
   A. Life expectancy is highest.
   B. Infant mortality is lowest.
   C. Number of physicians per 1,000 individuals is highest.
   D. Percent of primary care practices reviewing clinical outcomes data is lowest.
   E. Total spending per Capita is highest.

2. Elements of the United States HealthCare System include a complex system of insurance providers, provision of care in a wide range of settings, and population and individual patient health outcomes. Which one of the following is a result of these elements?
   A. Considerable duplication of services.
   B. Health insurance coverage for nearly all Americans.
   C. Access to care for nearly all Americans.
   D. Population health outcomes that are optimal, although individual health outcomes are compromised.

3. Which one of the following is true of care by primary care physicians in the United States?
   A. Primary care physicians are exclusively family physicians.
   B. Primary care physicians utilize patient-centered medical care to address a large majority of their patient's health needs.
   C. Primary care physicians require the patient to be accountable for preventive care.
   D. Primary care physicians offer referrals rather than interdisciplinary team care.
   E. Primary care physician groups rarely provide care continuity.

4. Elements of care quality monitoring, such as delivery of preventive care and chronic disease benchmarks, are routinely conducted by many Family Medicine physicians.
   A. True.
   B. False.

5. Which one of the following is most true about students entering the discipline of Family Medicine?
   A. They are mostly single.
   B. They tend to be highly interested in performing scientific research.
   C. They often have a history of volunteer work in a developing nation.
   D. They disproportionately come from professional families.
   E. There are no characteristics more common in medical students who enter family medicine.

ANSWERS

Question 1: The correct answer is E.

As shown in Table 1.1, the United States has the highest healthcare and pharmaceutical spending per capita and the highest proportion of GDP spent on healthcare. However, health benefits are not commensurate with cost, as many of the other nations have better societal health outcomes. For example, the United States has the lowest reported life expectancy, highest infant mortality rate, and highest obesity prevalence.

Question 2: The correct answer is A.

The result is much variation in access and insurance coverage, considerable duplication of services in some sectors (such as MRI scanners), and woefully inadequate service provision in other sectors (such as mental health), with the overall result being much variation in individual health outcomes, leading to lower-than-optimal population health outcomes.

Question 3: The correct answer is B.

Primary care physicians (PCPs) include those in family medicine, general internal medicine, pediatrics and in some cases gynecology—but PCPs have the same responsibility: to utilize patient-centered medical care to address a large majority of the personal health needs of their patients. As shown in Table 1.2, key principles of Family Medicine practice include care continuity and coordination.

Question 4: The correct answer is A.

To help family medicine practices better promote and monitor the health status of their patients, the field has embraced the need to regularly monitor, track, and report how well patients are doing. To date, this quality monitoring has focused on preventive care and chronic disease management, as these are important cornerstones of primary care. In addition, many practices monitor how well they are addressing some of the other principles of family medicine, such as continuity of care and access to care.

Question 5: The correct answer is C.

Research has shown that certain characteristics are more common in medical students who enter family medicine and other primary care disciplines than in those who choose specialties. These include a tendency to value people skills over technical skills, express greater concern about addressing societal problems, desire variety in their work, be married or in a long-term relationship, come from a nonprofessional family, and have a history of volunteer work in a developing nation.

REFERENCES

1. Ginsburg JA, Doherty RB, Ralston JF Jr, et al. Achieving a high-performance health care system with universal access: what the United States can learn from other countries. *Ann Intern Med.* 2008;148: 55–75.
2. Avendano M, Kawachi I. Why do Americans have shorter life expectancy and worse health than do people in other high-income countries? *Annu Rev Public Health.* 2014;35:307–325.
3. Mossialos E, Djordjevic A, Osborn R, Sarnak D. *International Profiles of Health Care Systems.* The Commonwealth Fund; 2017. Available from: http://www.commonwealthfund.org/publications/fund-reports/2017/may/international-profiles
4. Squires D, Anderson C. *U.S. Health Care from a Global Perspective: Spending, Use of Services, Prices, and Health in 13 Countries.* New York, NY: The Commonwealth Fund; 2015. Available from: http://www.commonwealthfund.org/publications/issue-briefs/2015/oct/us-health-care-from-a-global-perspective

5. Chen A, Oster E, Williams H. Why is infant mortality higher in the US than in Europe? *Am Econ J Econ Policy.* 2016;8(2):89–124.
6. Murray CJ, Kulkarni S, Ezzati M. Eight Americas: new perspectives on U.S. health disparities. *Am J Prev Med.* 2005;29(5 suppl 1):4–10.
7. Sloane PD, Warshaw GA, Potter JF, et al. Principles of primary care of older adults. In: *Primary Care Geriatrics.* 5th ed. Chicago: Mosby-Yearbook; 2014.
8. Berwick DM, Nolan TW, Whittington J. The triple aim: care, health, and cost. *Health Affairs.* 2008;27(3):759–769.
9. Asch SM, Kerr EA, Keesey J, et al. Who is at greatest risk for receiving poor-quality health care? *N Engl J Med.* 2006;354(11):1147–1156.
10. Sloane PD, Green L, Newton WP, et al. Primary care and the evolving U.S. health care system. In: Sloane PD, Slatt L, Ebell M, Viera A, Power D, Smith M, eds. *Essentials of Family Medicine.* 6th ed. Baltimore, MD: Lippincott, Williams & Wilkins; 2011:3–11.
11. Phillips RL Jr, Bazemore AW. Primary care and why it matters for US health system reform. *Health Aff (Millwood).* 2010;29(5):806–810.
12. Bodenheimer T, Ghorob A, Willard-Grace R, et al. The 10 building blocks of high-performing primary care. *Ann Fam Med.* 2014;12(2):166–171.
13. Cabana MD, Jee SH. Does continuity of care improve patient outcomes? *J Fam Pract.* 2004;53(12):974–980.
14. Saultz JW, Albedaiwi W. Interpersonal continuity of care and patient satisfaction: a critical review. *Ann Fam Med.* 2004;2(5):445–451.
15. Hall MN. Continuity: a central principle of primary care. *J Grad Med Educ.* 2016;8(4):615–616.
16. Parente DH, Pinto MB, Barber JC. A pre post comparison of service operational efficiency and patient satisfaction under open access scheduling. *Health Care Management Rev.* 2005;30(3):220–228.
17. Bodenheimer TS, Smith MD. Primary care: proposed solutions to the physician shortage without training more physicians. *Health Affairs.* 2013;32(11):1881–1886.
18. Nielsen M, Gibson L, Buelt L, et al. *The Patient-Centered Medical Home's Impact on Cost and Quality: Annual Review of Evidence, 2014–2015.* Washington, DC: Patient-Centered Primary Care Collaborative; 2017. Available from: https://www.milbank.org/publications/the-patient-centered-primary-care-collaborative-releases-5th-annual-evidence-report/
19. Shi L. The impact of primary care: a focused review. *Scientifica (Cairo).* 2012;2012:432892.
20. Bodenheimer T, Sinsky C. From triple to quadruple aim: care of the patient requires care of the provider. *Ann Fam Med.* 2014;12(6):573–576.
21. Fodeman J, Factor P. Solutions to the primary care physician shortage. *Am J Med.* 2015;128(8):800–801.
22. Phillips RL Jr, Bazemore AM, Peterson LE. Effectiveness over efficiency: underestimating the primary care physician shortage. *Med Care.* 2014;52(2):97–98.
23. AAMC predicts significant primary care physician shortage by 2025. *Am Fam Physician.* 2015;91(7):425.
24. Starfield B, Shi LY, Macinko J. Contribution of primary care to health systems and health. *Milbank Q.* 2005;83(3):457–502.
25. Newton DA, Grayson MS, Whitley TW. What predicts medical student career choice? *J Gen Intern Med.* 1998;13(3):200–203.
26. Scott I, Gowans M, Wright B, et al. Determinants of choosing a career in family medicine. *CMAJ.* 2011;183(1):E1–E8.
27. Senf JH, Campos-Outcalt D, Kutob R. Factors related to the choice of family medicine: a reassessment and literature review. *J Am Board Fam Pract.* 2003;16(6):502–512.
28. Phillips J. The impact of debt on young family physicians: unanswered questions with critical implications. *J Am Board Fam Med.* 2016;29(2):177–179.
29. *Medscape Physician Compensation Report* 2015. Available at: http://www.medscape.com/features/slideshow/compensation/2015/public/overview#page=2. Accessed October 2016.
30. Proctor BD, Semega JL, Kollar MA. *Income and poverty in the United States, 2015.* Washington: United States Census Bureau; 2016. Available from: http://www.census.gov/content/dam/Census/library/publications/2016/demo/p60-256.pdf. Downloaded October 28, 2016.
31. Leigh JP, Tancredi DJ, Kravitz RL. Physician career satisfaction within specialties. *BMC Health Serv Res.* 2009;9:166.
32. Kearns M. *Which specialty produces the happiest doctors?* Medical Practice Insider; 2015. Available from: http://www.medicalpracticeinsider.com/news/which-specialty-produces-happiest-doctors. Accessed October 2016.
33. Young R, Webb A, Lackan N, et al. Family medicine residency educational characteristics and career satisfaction in recent graduates. *Fam Med.* 2008;40(7):484–491.

Population Health

KEY POINTS

1 ▶ Poor health outcomes and increased cost are driving a national initiative to improve population health.

2 ▶ To improve health, we must broaden healthcare beyond the medical setting to improve the controllable social determinants of health-socioeconomic factors, the physical environment, health behaviors, access, and care quality.

3 ▶ Students can contribute to better health for their patients by assessing the social determinants of health, incorporating population health data, identifying community health needs, and considering interventions from all levels of the social ecologic model.

4 ▶ Policy interventions have the greatest impact on population health.

WHAT DETERMINES HEALTH?

The United States spends more on healthcare than any other developed country, yet we lag behind most Organization for Economic Cooperation and Development countries in nearly every important international health outcome measurement (Chapter 1).[1,2] For the first time in our history, we are raising children who may live sicker, shorter lives than their parents.[3] Why are we not healthier and what can we do to create opportunities for all of our patients to live longer, healthier lives?

POPULATION HEALTH

Population health refers to the health outcomes of a group of individuals, including the distribution of such outcomes within the group. The field of population health includes health outcomes, patterns of health determinants, and policies and interventions that link these two.[4]

The defined population depends on the where one sits in the system. For a provider or medical practice, the population will be their patient panel. For a hospital, it will be those living in their service area. For an insurer, it will be the enrollees in their health plan. For a city, county, or state health department, it will be all the people living in the geopolitical jurisdiction. However, it is critical to remember that the population does not only include patients seeking care, but also those who do not, healthy or unhealthy, for whatever reason.[5]

To improve population health, we must address the health inequities of the sub-populations in greatest need. **Health equity** is "when every person has the opportunity to attain his or her full health potential and no one is disadvantaged from achieving this potential because of social position or other socially determined circumstances"

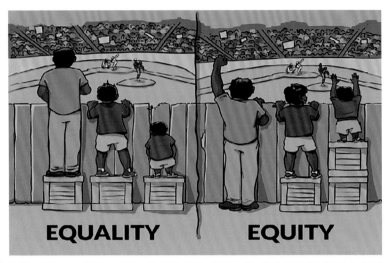

Figure 2.1 ▸ The difference between equality and equity. (Image Credit: *Interaction Institute for Social Change* | *Artist: Angus Maguire* (interactioninstitute.org and madewithangus.com)).

(https://www.cdc.gov/chronicdisease/healthequity/). It is not enough to distribute resources equally; to improve population health and eliminate health disparities, we must focus resources on the areas of greatest need (Fig. 2.1). Health equity is discussed in detail in Chapter 24.

Health disparities refer to differences in the health status of different groups of people. Health disparities "adversely affect groups who have systematically experienced greater obstacles to health based on their racial or ethnic group; religion; socioeconomic status; gender; age; mental health; cognitive, sensory, or physical disability; sexual orientation or gender identity; geographic location; or other characteristics historically linked to discrimination or exclusion."[6] Institutionalized racism and discriminatory practices against vulnerable groups contribute to unequal access to quality education, housing, employment, and medical care, which in turn contribute to poorer health outcomes.[7]

Two cousins, Tom and Bob were raised and live in the District of Columbia. Both have type 2 diabetes, have health insurance, and receive regular medical care. Washington, D.C. is divided into eight geopolitical areas called "wards." Tom lives in Ward 8 and Bob lives in Ward 2. Adults who live in Ward 8 have almost five times the diabetes mortality rate than those who live in Ward 2. The difference in life expectancies between Ward 2 and Ward 8 can be as high as 15 years. What factors may lead to these differences in health? (Fig. 2.2)

Social determinants are strongly linked to health outcomes:

▸ College graduates can expect to live at least 5 years longer than those who have not completed high school.

▸ Poor Americans are greater than three times as likely as upper middle-class Americans to suffer physical limitations from a chronic illness.

▸ People with middle incomes are less healthy and can expect to live shorter lives than those with higher incomes, even when they are insured (RWJF, Commission to Build a Healthier America, 2009).

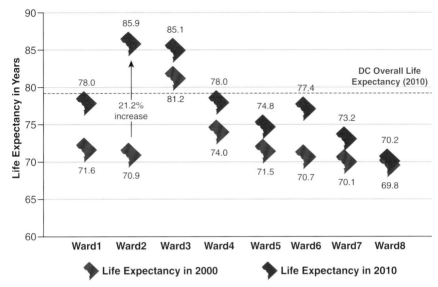

Figure 2.2 ▶ Life expectancy by birth by ward, 2000–2010. (From *District of Columbia Community Health Needs Assessment*, Vol 1, p 17, revised Mar 15, 2013. *Data Management and Analysis Division, Center for Policy, Planning, and Evaluation*, DX Department of Health. https://doh.dc.gov/sites/default/files/dc/sites/doh/page_content/attachments/2nd%20Draft%20CHNA%20(v4%202)%2006%2004%20 2013%20-%20Vol%201.pdf.)

To view an entertaining video that illustrates how your zip code is more important than your genetic code in determining how long you live, see https://www.youtube.com/watch?v=mhzUC-F-Q8c. The California Endowment is a private health foundation with a mission to expand access and improve health in underserved communities in CA. The video elaborates on the pathways through which social determinants shape health and further explains the gradients in health. Although focused on California, the same situation occurs in most of the United States. In the case of the two cousins, Tom's ward has few grocery stores and he must take a bus to get to one. His neighborhood is unsafe for outdoor exercise. If we counsel Tom in the same manner as Bob—providing advice to eat more fresh foods, limit his fast food intake and exercise more—we will likely have far less success in helping Tom achieve optimal diabetes control.

STUDENT ACTIVITY

Using the County Health Rankings and Roadmaps Interactive website: http://www.countyhealthrankings.org/

▶ Select the community in which you live. Compare the health ranking to other counties in your state.

▶ Which counties in your state have the lowest health outcomes ranking? Which of the social determinants (from health behaviors, clinical care, social and economic factors, or the physical environment) contribute most to poor health?

▶ What interventions might target the problems?

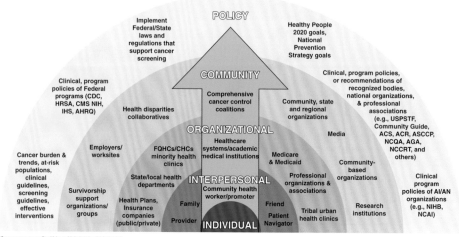

Figure 2.3 ▶ CDC Adaption of the social ecologic model for colorectal cancer prevention. (http://www.cdc.gov/cancer/crccp/sem.htm)

A POPULATION HEALTH APPROACH TO PATIENTS

When caring for patients in the clinic setting, students can address population health in each step of the SOAP note process.

▶ **Subjective**—Take a history that includes the social determinants of health.

▶ **Objective**—Incorporate population health and community level data.

▶ **Assessment**—Expand the assessment to include the social determinants of health and a Community Health Needs Assessment (see below).

▶ **Plan**—Consider interventions from all levels of the social ecologic model (Fig. 2.3): individual, interpersonal, organizational, community, and policy. Interventions from multiple levels will have the greatest influence on health. For Tom, the care plan may need to include assistance in identifying places to grocery shop on his way home from work and exercise opportunities with local gyms or through work.

Subjective: A Social Determinants History

In addition to taking a "traditional" social history that includes health behaviors like tobacco, alcohol, and drug use; diet; exercise; and sexual history, ask about social and economic factors like education and employment and environmental factors, like exposure to mold and air pollutants, access to transportation and housing, and community safety (Chapter 24). The Health Leads Screening Toolkit questionnaire (available for free download and use at https://healthleadsusa.org/resources/tools/) provides questions about social needs that may be affecting your patient's health. Examples of the questions from this tool are bulleted below. WellRx is another example of an 11-question instrument to screen for social needs experienced by patients in the office setting.[8]

▶ In the last 12 months, did you ever eat less than you felt you should because there was not enough money for food?

▶ Are you worried that in the next 2 months, you may not have stable housing?

▶ In the last 12 months, have you ever had to go without healthcare because you did not have a way to get there?

The office case manager screens Tom for social determinants of health and learns that he recently lost his job and has not been filling his medications. He has been living on friends' couches since he was evicted from his apartment for not being able to pay the rent. The case manager begins work with Tom to seek unemployment income and apply for Medicaid. She notifies his family physician who obtains a 3-month supply of medication for him through the pharmaceutical company patient assistance program. Without exploring the patient's life in context, these issues might not have been identified until his health deteriorated.

Objective: Incorporate Population Health Data

Practice–Level Population Health Data

Healthcare delivery is transforming from a fee-for-service to a value-based care model to improve the patient experience, reduce the cost of care, and improve population health.[9] The electronic health record (EHR) can be used to support population health management functions such as[10]:

▶ Subpopulation identification

▶ Identification of care gaps

▶ Patient engagement

▶ Care management and care coordination

▶ Outcomes measurement

A patient registry can identify subpopulations of patients who have "gaps in care," including those who need preventive care, those overdue for care or who do not meet management goals, those who may benefit from risk reduction, or those who have not followed up after reminders. The EHR should be able to generate a list based on diagnostic codes, lab results, medications, or other codified data. This list can be narrowed down by subpopulations to identify those in greatest need, for example, patients with diabetes with hemoglobin A1C levels over 9% or patients with asthma who are refilling their rescue inhalers too frequently. These data can then generate notifications to prompt patients to make appointments or alert staff of patient care needs. These data can be used to track performance measures, a critical component of value-based reimbursement. More and more practices have these data available to help focus on patients with the greatest need.

Practice level data: The diabetic registry in your office shows that Tom's hemoglobin A1C increased from 8.3% to 9.5%. You, the family physician, now understand that this occurred when he lost his job and stopped filling his prescriptions. Had you not conducted earlier screening, this change would have triggered an outreach to Tom and an opportunity to assist him with medications and accessing services. You set up a follow-up visit for Tom.

Community-Level Population Health Data

The population (patient panel) in a typical family medicine practice will be a subset of the populations of the city, county, or healthcare system, and may have different types of needs. In order to help practices identify community resources available to their patients, the American Academy of Family Physicians developed a mapping tool called the Community Health Resource Navigator (http://www.aafp.org/patient-care/social-determinants-of-health/chrn.html). This tool graphically illustrates community-level statistics such as age-adjusted morbidity and mortality from acute and chronic conditions, smoking and obesity prevalence, percentage of adults who do not meet physical activity recommendations, median household income, and unemployment rate. It also allows practices to identify resources such as farmer's markets, grocery stores, parks and public gymnasiums, and recreational areas. In Tom's case, community level data demonstrates that there are no grocery stores within one mile from his home, few parks and public gymnasiums, the crime rate is high, and there is a lack of affordable housing options. Some EHRs are beginning to integrate social determinants data.[11,12]

Assessment: Expand to Include Social Determinants of Health and a Community Health Needs Assessment

Practices can apply the Community Health Needs Assessment (CHNA) process to identify population health priorities and coordinate with community agencies regarding interventions.

Community Health Needs Assessments

The Affordable Care Act requires not-for-profit hospitals and healthcare systems to work with public health agencies and other organizations to perform CHNAs at least every 3 years, and to create implementation strategies to address identified needs. CHNAs should identify existing healthcare resources and prioritize community health needs.

The first step in the CHNA process is constructing a population health profile that includes a set of outcome measures that is limited but comprehensive, coherent, significant, and measurable over time. Once the profile has been created, its measures can be compared to state or national benchmarks based on publicly available data sources (e.g., the Robert Wood Johnson Foundation's County Health Rankings at http://www.countyhealthrankings.org/) in order to prioritize specific areas in need of improvement.

Improving the health of a community is a shared responsibility and therefore requires shared accountability. For each identified outcome, all parties with a stake in a healthy community should use a set of agreed-on performance indicators to ensure accountability. Table 2.1 shows a sample performance indicator set for tobacco use and tobacco-related complications.

Based on your case manager's notes, you add patient's intentional underdosing of medication regimen due to financial hardship (ICD 10 code Z91.120), unemployment (ICD 10 code Z56.0), and inadequate housing (ICD 10 code Z59.1) to Tom's problem list, in addition to diabetes.

From the hospital's community health needs assessment, you learn that homelessness is a major problem in Tom's community. Realizing that helping others like Tom locate and keep affordable housing is a good way to prevent health problems, you learn more about the scope of the homelessness problem in your own community and what is being done to address it.

Table 2.1 ► Sample Performance Indicator Set for Tobacco and Health

Indicator	Accountability
Deaths from tobacco-related conditions	Shared community responsibility
Smoking-related residential fires	Shared community responsibility
Prevalence of smoking in adults	Shared community responsibility
Initiation of smoking among youth	Shared community responsibility
Ordinances to control environmental tobacco smoke	City council
Local enforcement of laws on tobacco sales to youth	Shopkeepers, police
Tobacco use prevention in school curricula	School board
Counseling and interventions by health providers	Healthcare providers
Availability of cessation programs	Local organizations
Health insurance coverage for cessation program	Health plans, employers

From Stoto MA. Population health measurement: applying performance measurement concepts in population health settings. *EGEMS (Wash DC).* 2015;2(4):1132 (Table 5); Available from: https://www.ncbi.nlm.nih.gov/pmc/articles/PMC4438103/

Plan: Consider Interventions From All Levels of the Social Ecologic Model

Individual care—Provide appropriate preventive care, behavioral, and clinical interventions (Chapters 5, 7, 12, 13).

► Interpersonal—Engage friends, family, care coordinators, and/or community health workers.

► Organizational—Involve healthcare plans, health departments, academic medical centers, accountable care organizations (ACOs) in shared responsibility for improving population health.

► Community—Link patients to a wide range of community services through a social worker, care coordinator, or online resources (https://www.auntbertha.com/). Become involved in community engagement and advocacy (Chapter 24).

► Policy—Advocate for local, state, and federal policies to improve health.

At the follow-up visit with Tom, he informs you that he received his medication in the mail and appreciates the help of your case manager. You link Tom with a community social worker and employee assistance. You suggest a local homeless shelter and provide him with a list of community agencies that offer rental assistance for low-income persons.

Tom's previous employer did not offer health insurance, but due to his income level he purchased subsidized private insurance through his state's health insurance marketplace. When Tom lost his job, he could no longer afford the private plan premiums and has now enrolled in a Medicaid plan. It is fortunate for Tom that your office accepts Medicaid. When patients lose private insurance, they may need to find a new physician and appointments can be several months out.

NEGATIVE EFFECTS OF INSURANCE CHURNING ON POPULATION HEALTH

The Affordable Care Act lowered the US uninsured rate from 16% in 2010 to 9.1% in 2015 by expanding Medicaid eligibility and creating federal- and state-based health insurance marketplaces where adults without employer-based or other sources of health coverage could shop for tax-subsidized private plans. Since many lower-income persons have significant income fluctuations, changes in eligibility for public or subsidized insurance will cause changes in insurance coverage over time, known as "churning." A 2015 survey of low-income adults in Kentucky, Arkansas, and Texas found that 25% had changed coverage in the previous 12 months, and that "churning was associated with disruptions in physician care and medication adherence, increased emergency department use, and worsening self-reported quality of care and health status."[13]

The study authors suggested several policy options that could reduce churning or ameliorate its negative health consequences: 12-month continuous Medicaid eligibility for adults; a single state program covering both Medicaid-eligible and ineligible low-income persons; and increased use of multimarket plans (plans with the same provider network and benefit design on Medicaid and the health marketplaces).

POLICY INTERVENTIONS FOR IMPROVED POPULATION HEALTH

Hospitals and Accountable Care Organizations Investing in Communities

Working with community collaborators, a few hospitals and health systems across the United States have invested community benefit funds into improving social determinants of health such as food insecurity (ProMedica, Toledo, Ohio), affordable housing (Bon Secours, Marriottsville, Maryland), and health professions education (Children's Hospital of San Diego and University of Pittsburgh Medical Center). To encourage more hospitals to participate in "community building," the American Hospital Association has advocated that the Internal Revenue Service clarify that these types of community activities are as legitimate for tax-exempt hospitals as those that provide direct medical benefit "that in fact supporting things like stable housing or access to healthy food is supporting health."[14]

Motivated by financial incentives from the Centers for Medicare and Medicaid Services, ACOs (groups of doctors, hospitals, and other healthcare providers who work together to provide coordinated care to improve quality and reduce costs) are also expanding their scope outside of traditional medical care services to ensure that the populations for whom they are responsible remain healthy.[15] However, a recent national survey revealed a wide spectrum of population health approaches among ACOs, with 58% reporting that

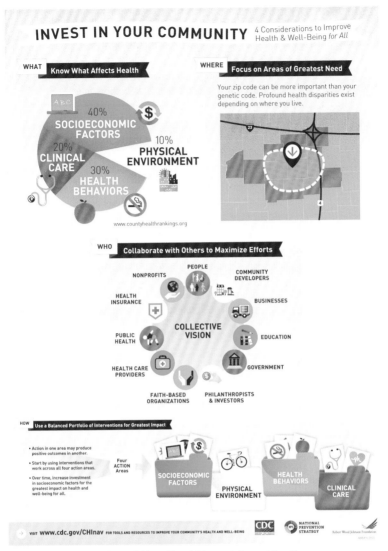

Source: https://www.cdc.gov/chinav/docs/chi_nav_infographic.pdf

they were working to improve health outcomes for the entire geographic area they served (including non-ACO participants) and only 37% devoting resources to improving health conditions within their communities (e.g., safety, access to healthy foods).[16]

Evidence-Based Community Interventions: What Works?

Well-intended community health interventions may flounder if their design is not based on strong evidence of effectiveness. The Centers for Disease Control and Prevention maintains a "Community Health Improvement Navigator" website (http://www.cdc.gov/chinav/) that provides resources, tools, Frequently Asked Questions, and a database of successful interventions for persons or organizations pursuing community health improvement.

Table 2.2 ▸ Selected Community Guide Topics and Recommendations

Topic	Recommendations
Cardiovascular disease	• Self-measured blood pressure monitoring interventions: *Recommended* • Interventions engaging community health workers: *Recommended* • Clinical decision-support systems: *Recommended* • Reducing out-of-pocket costs: *Recommended*
Excessive alcohol consumption	• Electronic screening and brief interventions: *Recommended* • Publicized sobriety checkpoint programs: *Recommended* • Privatization of retail alcohol sales: *Recommended against* • Responsible beverage service training: *Insufficient evidence*
Tobacco use and secondhand smoke exposure	• Comprehensive tobacco control programs: *Recommended* • Mass-reach health communication interventions: *Recommended* • Internet-based cessation interventions: *Insufficient evidence* • Interventions to increase the unit price for tobacco products: *Recommended* • Smoke-free policies: *Recommended*
Health equity	• School-based health centers: *Recommended* • Center-based early childhood education: *Recommended* • Out-of-school–time academic programs: *Recommended* • Full day kindergarten programs: *Recommended*

Data from: https://www.thecommunityguide.org/

Since 1996, the CDC has convened the Task Force on Community Preventive Services, a group of independent nonfederal experts in population-based and public health, to produce The Community Guide of evidence-based recommendations on population health interventions (https://www.thecommunityguide.org/). Recommendations (also called "findings") are based on systematic reviews of the supporting evidence for the effectiveness and economic impact of each intervention and graded as Recommended, Recommended Against, or Insufficient Evidence.[17]

The Community Guide includes recommendations on preventive strategies for specific health conditions such as asthma, cancer, cardiovascular disease, diabetes, and sexually-transmitted infections; risk factors for chronic diseases such as excessive alcohol consumption, obesity, and tobacco use; and social determinants such as health inequality, nutrition, and violence (Table 2.2).

Using the AAFP's Community Health Resource Navigator, you learn that the counties served by your practice have higher rates of homelessness than the state as a whole. You then turn to the CDC website to identify relevant evidence-based interventions. The Task Force on Community Preventive Services recommends tenant-based rental assistance (or voucher) programs that allow low-income families to live in safer and/or better resourced neighborhoods, based on a systematic review finding that these programs are associated with reduced crime and neighborhood social disorder. A randomized trial found that housing vouchers that allowed low-income families to move from high- to low-poverty areas led to lower body-mass index and glycated hemoglobin levels 10 to 15 years later.[18] Therefore, advocating for rental assistance policies will not only benefit individuals like Tom, but also improve the health of the community. You will learn more about health advocacy in Chapter 24.

QUESTIONS

1. Mario is a family physician trying to incorporate elements of population health thinking into his medical practice. He is attempting to define his patient population. What would be the best example of that for his purposes?
   A. All the people in the catchment area of his practice who are patients.
   B. All the people who live in the county.
   C. All the active patients in his practice, including those who might be patients but are not, for whatever reason.
   D. All the enrollees in the health plan that covers the majority of his patients.

2. Equity and Equality, for the purposes of population health, mean the same thing.
   A. True.
   B. False.

3. From this list, which factor most contributes to health outcomes?
   A. Your genetic code.
   B. Distance to closest hospital.
   C. Insurance copay amount.
   D. Your zip code.
   E. Medicaid versus commercial insurance.

4. Your rural community has significant substance use problems and, with input from community members who serve on your health center board, you decide that more work is needed to address alcohol problems. Using CDC's "The Community Guide" (https://www.thecommunityguide.org), which one of the following is recommended against in addressing excessive alcohol consumption?
   A. Maintaining limits on days of sale of alcohol.
   B. Privatization of retail alcohol sales.
   C. Electronic screening and brief interventions.
   D. Publicized sobriety check point programs.

ANSWERS

Question 1: The correct answer is C.
Population health refers to the health outcomes of a group of individuals, including the distribution of such outcomes within the group... For a provider or medical practice, the population will be their patient panel... However, it is critical to remember that the population does not only include patients seeking care, but also those who do not, healthy or unhealthy, for whatever reason.

Question 2: The correct answer is B.
Because healthcare disparities greatly contribute to differential health outcomes it is not enough to give the same to each population (equality). Instead, as shown in Figure 2.1, we must distribute services differentially, or equitably, to give those with the greatest need opportunities to improve their health outcomes.

Question 3: The correct answer is D.
Your zip code is a surrogate measure of social determinants of health and social determinants of health are the single biggest contributor to health outcomes, good or bad. The chapter

includes a video that illustrates how your zip code is more important than your genetic code in determining how long you live.

Question 4: The correct answer is B.

The Community Guide has a "What Works" Fact Sheet: Preventing Excessive Alcohol Consumption and within this are green, yellow and red community based recommendations. Privatization of retail alcohol outlets is recommended against.

REFERENCES

1. Health at a Glance 2017: OECD Indicators. 2017; available from: http://www.oecd-ilibrary.org/social-issues-migration-health/health-at-a-glance-2017_health_glance-2017-en

2. How does health spending in the US compare. 2015; Available from: http://www.oecd.org/unitedstates/Country-Note-UNITED STATES-OECD-Health-Statistics-2015.pdf. Accessed January 2017.

3. Beyond Health Care: New Directions to a Healthier America. 2009; Available from: http://www.commissiononhealth.org/PDF/779d4330-8328-4a21-b7a3-deb751dafaab/Beyond%20Health%20Care%20-%20New%20Directions%20to%20a%20Healthier%20America.pdf

4. Kindig D, Stoddart G. What is population health? *Am J Pub Health.* 2003;93(3):380–383.

5. Washington AE, Coye MJ, Boulware LE. Academic health systems' third curve: population health improvement. *JAMA.* 2016;315(5):459–460.

6. Disparities. 2016; Available from: https://www.healthypeople.gov/2020/about/foundation-health-measures/Disparities. Accessed January 2017.

7. Jones CP. Levels of racism: a theoretic framework and a gardener's tale. *Am J Pub Health.* 2000;90(8):1212–1215.

8. Page-Reeves J, Kaufman W, Bleecker M, et al. Addressing social determinants of health in a clinic setting: the WellRx pilot in Albuquerque, New Mexico. *J Am Board Fam Med.* 2016;29(3):414–418.

9. Berwick DM, Nolan TW, Whittington J. The triple aim: care, health, and cost. *Health Affairs.* 2008;27(3):759–769.

10. Population Health Management. A Roadmap for Provider-Based Automation in a New Era of Healthcare. 2012; Available from: http://www.exerciseismedicine.org/assets/page_documents/PHM%20Roadmap%20HL.pdf

11. Bazemore AW, Cottrell EK, Gold R, et al. "Community vital signs": incorporating geocoded social determinants into electronic records to promote patient and population health. *J Am Med Inform Assoc.* 2015;23(2):407–412.

12. Hughes LS, Phillips RL Jr, DeVoe JE, et al. Community vital signs: taking the pulse of the community while caring for patients. *J Am Board Fam Med.* 2016;29(3):419–422.

13. Sommers BD, Gourevitch R, Maylone B, et al. Insurance churning rates for low-income adults under health reform: lower than expected but still harmful for many. *Health Aff (Millwood).* 2016;35(10):1816–1824.

14. Hostetter MK. In Focus: Hospitals Invest in Building Stronger, Healthier Communities. The Commonwealth Fund, Transforming Care newsletter; Available from: http://www.commonwealthfund.org/publications/newsletters/transforming-care/2016/september/in-focus. Accessed January 2017.

15. Goldman LR, Kumanyika SK, Shah NR. Putting the health of communities and populations first. *JAMA.* 2016;316(16):1649–1650.

16. Performance evaluation: what is working in Accountable Care Organizations? Report #1: How ACOs are addressing population health. 2016; Available from: https://www.premierinc.com/wp-content/uploads/2016/10/What-Is-Working-In-ACOs-Report-10.16.pdf. Accessed January 2017.

17. Briss PA, Zaza S, Pappaioanou M, et al. Developing an evidence-based guide to community preventive services–methods. *Am J Prev Med.* 2000;18(1):35–43.

18. Ludwig J, Sanbonmatsu L, Gennetian L, et al. Neighborhoods, obesity, and diabetes—a randomized social experiment. *New Engl J Med.* 2011;365(16):1509–1519.

Information Mastery

KEY POINTS

1 ▶ Not all information resources are of equal value. In assessing information resources, consider the relevance and validity of the information provided, the work involved in answering your question, and the transparency of their processes.

2 ▶ Determine if the clinical questions you are generating are background or foreground questions. Match the question type to the best information resource for that question.

3 ▶ Familiarize yourself with different point-of-care resources to use in your work. Choose a few that you like best and develop a system to integrate new information into your practice.

4 ▶ Utilize the statistical tools, such as number needed to treat (NNT), that make research information most clinically relevant and useful to you and your patients.

5 ▶ Evidence-based medicine is a tool to support high-quality clinical practice. It is not a substitute for shared-decision making, but informs it.

The practice of evidence-based medicine (EBM) is a core feature of modern medicine. This approach involves "an acknowledgment that there is a hierarchy of evidence and that conclusions related to evidence from controlled experiments are accorded greater credibility than conclusion grounded in other sorts of evidence."[1]

An evidence-based approach means that the clinician has made the effort to identify the strongest, most valid data, can change his or her mind when the evidence supports a change in practice, and acknowledges when the evidence available for deciding is less than ideal. Sometimes we have high-quality evidence to support medical practices and sometimes we have relatively little useful information to help guide care. The goal is to know the strength of evidence available, to acknowledge that level of evidence when making decisions, and to use this information to help patients choose the best approaches given their own specific situation.

A major barrier to using the best available evidence to guide medical decisions during patient care is that most physicians have not been trained to do this quickly and effectively. Historically, EBM training focused on reading primary journal articles. With the amount of new data published daily, and the skill and time needed to critically appraise a single article, this approach to staying current is untenable. The total number of records in PubMed as of February 20th, 2017, was 26,935,290; in addition, the medical literature expands with the publication of 75 trials and 11 systematic reviews daily.[2]

With the concepts of Information Mastery, physicians are now utilizing resources that appraise, synthesize, and structure the medical literature into databases that are valid, reliable, and require little work to use. As such, clinicians can quickly identify and use the best available evidence in their practices. This chapter will provide the concepts and tools to ask and organize questions, identify resource types that are appropriate for answering different types of questions, and provide the concepts and skills to evaluate the usefulness of a resource. We also briefly review the most useful statistical tools for translating research information into clinically useful information.

PRACTICING MEDICINE IN THE INFORMATION AGE

The vast amounts of information out there—in the medical literature, on the internet, in the world—creates a challenge for finding the *best* information to inform your patient care.

> Mrs. Devon is a 68-year-old woman with longstanding knee degenerative joint disease. She has taken oral medications to manage her pain, but recently her symptoms have impacted her ability to do her usual activities. She wants something to help her pain. She has a friend with knee pain who was given a steroid injection, which really improved her friend's pain, but Mrs. Devon tells you she is afraid of needles, so she only wants an injection if you think it will work. How can you find the information you need to advise her?

You quickly search for the answer to your question and realize your results can go in one of two different directions:

1. You find one study that showed significant benefit with a steroid injection for the treatment of knee osteoarthritis; or you find one answer in an online resource you have used before.
2. You get hundreds of seemingly relevant results.

This dichotomy—between finding information *quickly but not systematically or reliably* and being *overwhelmed by the quantity of information* out there—is a central challenge to practicing medicine in the information age. To provide the highest quality patient care, you must be able to match your specific clinical question with the best information resource for answering that question. To do this, you will need the knowledge and skills to:

▶ Quickly find the best available evidence.

▶ Identify useful information resources to assist with information acquisition.

▶ Understand the strengths and limitations of different types of information resources.

▶ "Pull back the curtain" to figure out if a resource is transparent, reliable, and valid, and determine the type of questions for which the resource is most appropriate.

INFORMATION MANAGEMENT

To manage information effectively you will typically go through these steps:

1. Generate a question.
2. Identify the appropriate resource(s) to answer your question.
3. Find the information.
4. Apply what you learned.

BOX 3.1 BACKGROUND AND FOREGROUND QUESTIONS

Types of Questions

Background Questions	Foreground Questions
▶ Who, what, where, when, why, and how of anything, such as a disease or medication	▶ Ask for specific information needed to guide a clinical decision
▶ Examples: *What are the types of diagnoses that cause knew pain in adults? What are the medication classes for smoking cessation?*	▶ Example: *In patients who smoke, does bupropion or varenicline lead to better rates of smoking abstinence?*

You can generate a question from Mrs. Devon's situation. For example, you might ask: "In older adults with knee osteoarthritis, does intra-articular steroid injection, as compared to oral NSAIDS, decrease pain and improve function?"

To find the correct information resource to search for an answer to this question, you first need to know what type of question you are asking.

Background and Foreground Questions

Back ground questions give you the information you need to ask your foreground questions (Box 3.1). Foreground questions are the questions that come up during patient care that you need to answer to decide what to do for your patients (e.g., what is the best treatment to recommend?)

As you will see below, correctly categorizing your question is key to matching that question to the most appropriate information resource.

Finding Information Framework

The finding information framework (FIF), shown in Figure 3.1, is a tool that can help you:

▶ Correctly categorize your question.

▶ Understand different types of information resources.

▶ Match your question with the best information resource for that question.

To use the FIF begin at the top with your question. Is your medical question a background or foreground question? If it is a background question, is it a basic science or clinical question? If a clinical question, is it common or rare?

For new clinicians, it can be difficult to differentiate what topics are *Common* and which are *Rare/of Academic Interest*. Because the vast majority of questions can be answered quickly with Clinical Background and Point-of-Care Resources, we recommend starting with those resources first, and moving to the Literature Search Resources only if you do not find your answer.

INFORMATION MASTERY

Returning to the question we generated for Mrs. Devon:

"In older adults with knee osteoarthritis, does intra-articular steroid injection, as compared to oral NSAIDS, decrease pain and improve function?"

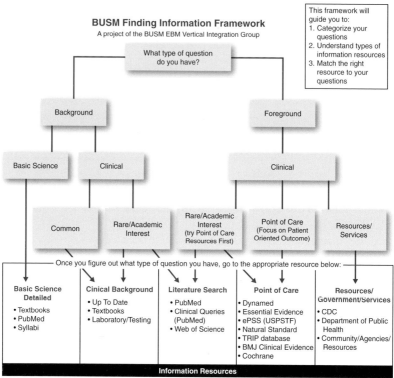

Figure 3.1 ▶ Finding information framework (FIF). (Redrawn from Boston University School of Medicine, BUSM Finding Information Framework; http://medlib.bu.edu/busm/fif/)

If you define this question using the FIF you see it is a Clinical Foreground Question. This brings us to the concept of **Information Mastery**—how to quickly and effectively find the best evidence-based answers to inform your clinical decisions in real time at the point-of-care. The best way to do this is to learn how to ask good clinical questions.

Structuring Clinical Foreground Questions

Clinical Foreground Questions are best structured using the PICO (pronounced *pee-koh*) format (Box 3.2).

Putting the PICO pieces together will give you your well-crafted clinical foreground question: "In older adults with knee osteoarthritis, does intra-articular steroid injection, as compared to oral NSAIDS, decrease pain and improve function?"

Patient-Oriented Evidence and Disease-Oriented Evidence

Another critical method for filtering information is to identify research studies that report patient-oriented outcomes.

▶ Patient-oriented evidence (POE) is evidence that measures *an outcome that patients care about* such as symptoms, morbidity, or mortality.

▶ Disease-oriented evidence (DOE) is evidence that measures *outcomes that are markers of disease* such as blood pressure, peak flow, bacteriologic cure, or serum creatinine.

BOX 3.2 PICO

P = Population

Use a population that is general enough so that you will find results (e.g., *older adults with knee osteoarthritis* and not *68-year-old African American women with osteoarthritis for 15 years*). Also, make your population specific enough to be applicable to your patient (e.g., *older adults with knee osteoarthritis* and not simply *adults*).

I = Intervention

The treatment, test, or other interventions you are considering (e.g., *intra-articular steroid injection*).

C = Comparison or Control group (e.g., *oral NSAIDs* or *physical therapy*).

O = Outcome

Your outcome should be patient-oriented (more on this below) (e.g., *reduce pain* or *improve function*).

Although DOE is crucial to clinical researchers, it does not always translate to clinical medicine. Disease-oriented information assumes a chain of causality that may look convincing, but links are often missing or broken when the topic is studied with patient-oriented outcomes.

For example, studies have shown that intensive glucose lowering can decrease hemoglobin A1c levels in patients with diabetes. This DOE has affected the way that we treat patients with diabetes by following a fairly convincing chain of causality—if intense glucose control lowers the A1c, it must help prolong life by decreasing myocardial infarctions, strokes, and renal failure. However, subsequent studies have shown that intensive glucose lowering does not decrease the POE of mortality and may increase mortality, in part from hypoglycemia.[3,4] Considering Mrs. Devon, we would not be particularly interested in studies demonstrating changes in inflammatory markers, synovial volume, or knee cartilage resulting from steroid injection (DOE), but would focus our search on pain and functional outcomes (POE).

Sometimes the DOE will align with the POE and sometimes the POE disproves a therapy that had been promising based on DOE. If the POE is particularly noteworthy or practice changing, we refer to it as Patient-Oriented Evidence that Matters (POEM). See Table 3.1 for more examples in which potentially promising DOE did not align with subsequent POE.

Table 3.1 ▶ Comparison of Disease-Oriented Evidence (DOE) with Patient-Oriented Evidence that Matters (POEM) for Common Conditions

Disease or Condition	Disease-Oriented Evidence (DOE)	Patient-Oriented Evidence (POE)
Antiarrhythmic medication following acute myocardial infarction[5]	Suppresses arrhythmias	Increases mortality
Sleeping infants on their stomach or side[6]	Anatomy and physiology suggest this will decrease aspiration	Increased risk of sudden infant death syndrome
Vitamin E to prevent heart disease[7]	Reduces levels of free radicals	No change in mortality
Hormone replacement therapy to prevent heart disease[8]	Reduced LDL cholesterol, increased HDL cholesterol	No decrease in cardiovascular or all-cause mortality and an increase in cardiovascular events
β-blockers for heart failure[9]	Reduced cardiac output	Reduced mortality in moderate to severe disease

How Many Questions Will You Have During Patient Care?

During a typical day of patient care, physicians generate about 15 to 20 clinical questions.[10] On average, physicians spend less than 2 minutes (!) looking up the answers to these questions while seeing patients, and studies have shown that approximately two-thirds of these questions go unanswered.[11] Although most physicians want to provide evidence-based care and to further their own understanding and abilities, there are many reasons that these questions are never answered. They include lack of time, lack of resources, lack of the ability to find the answer, or the physician's perception that there is no good answer to their clinical question.[12]

Further, when physicians do spend time looking up the answers to their clinical questions, they often use Google, e-textbooks, UpToDate, or talk to colleagues.[13,14] Although they may get their questions answered, search engines can take them to websites that do not necessarily contain valid or reliable information—e-textbooks are quickly outdated and colleagues are subject to their own biases.

Historically, when physicians were trained in EBM, they were instructed to use PubMed or a similar search engine to go to the primary literature to answer their questions. Given the number of studies related to any PICO question, and the skills needed to assess and synthesize a body of literature on a topic, this method is extremely time consuming, making it an unlikely source for a physician to find answers in real time. A central concept of information mastery involves using sources that give you the highest yield of relevant and valid information with the least amount of work. This is the concept of "usefulness."

DETERMINING USEFULNESS

A key concept of information mastery is recognizing that not all sources of information are equal—they differ regarding their usefulness.

$$\text{Usefulness of information} = \frac{\text{Relevance} \times \text{Validity}}{\text{Work}}$$

▶ *Relevance* refers to the applicability of information to your clinical practice or question.

▶ *Validity* refers to the extent to which the information is scientifically based and free of bias.

▶ *Work* refers to the time and energy required to answer the question.

Relevance

When determining relevance, consider whether the information is what you need to help decide for your specific patient. Three questions help you determine if information is POEM:

1. Is the information POE, such as symptoms, morbidity, or mortality?
2. Does the information matter to your practice? Is the problem/question common in your practice and is the intervention feasible?
3. If the information is true, would the findings require you to change the way you practice?

Validity

Assessing research validity is time-consuming and difficult without formal training and a great deal of practice. Several secondary sources have been created to evaluate the validity of studies and list evidence in a way that is transparent and easy to evaluate. Such sources are listed under point-of-care resources in the FIF such as DynaMed (http://www.dynamed.com/), Essential Evidence Plus (http://www.essentialevidenceplus.com/), and BMJ Clinical Evidence (http://clinicalevidence.bmj.com). These sources remove the time-consuming step of evaluating the validity of each study on your own.

Work

Work is the amount of time and effort required to find the answer to your question. The more work you must do, the less useful is that information resource. When you compare the time that you would need to spend searching for the answer to your question on PubMed (including the time needed to find the relevant articles, critically appraise all of the articles, critique and synthesize the body of information) to the amount of time needed to get an answer from an attending or colleague or using an online search engine, the amount of work is vastly different.

So why would you not always want to do something quick like call an expert or use an online search engine? To answer this, you need to look at the other parts of the usefulness equation: the relevance and the validity. If you used an online search engine to look for an answer for treatment of pediatric asthma and it brings you to a parent's blog that answers your specific question, finding the answer may have taken little work, but it has a good chance of not being scientifically valid. An e-textbook might have helpful information, but it could be outdated. See below about why talking to experts is not always the best approach. Remember that relevance and validity are multiplied: if the information is not valid, its usefulness is low.

You decide to take the time to answer the question about steroid injection and knee osteo-arthritis. Using PubMed, you find an older Cochrane review (2006) and many other articles and conclude that steroid injections likely provide short-term (2 to 3 weeks) pain relief similar to intra-articular nonsteroidal anti-inflammatory injections; effects are not as durable as use of hyaluronic acid. This process took about 15 minutes. You also check a secondary source that also concludes that steroid injection is effective for short-term (at least 1 week) pain reduction for knee osteoarthritis with a strength of evidence rating B (see later). This process took 3 minutes. You plan to discuss these options with Mrs. Devon at her follow-up appointment.

DIFFERENT RESOURCES ARE APPROPRIATE FOR DIFFERENT QUESTIONS

Mr. Walker is a 77-year-old man here for follow-up of hypertension diagnosed by your preceptor 2 months ago. He has been trying lifestyle modification since his last visit but has not started any medications yet. You review his record and notice that he has a history of postpolio syndrome. You also look at his vital signs before you enter in the room and note his BP is 160/94 mm Hg today. It was 155/92 mm Hg at his last visit, 2 months ago.

You generate a few questions from this case:

▶ What is postpolio syndrome?
▶ When do I need to start a patient on antihypertensive medications?

▸ For an adult patient with hypertension, is hydrochlorothiazide or a beta-blocker a better medication to reduce strokes and heart attacks?

Use the FIF to categorize these questions and to identify the most appropriate resources to answer your questions. You will notice that numerous resources are available, each with advantages and disadvantages. There is no one perfect information resource, although some will be better than others, depending on your question(s). This is often the case.

Resources for Background Questions

The first two questions that you generated for Mr. Walker, above, are background questions. Keeping in mind that background questions ask the *who, what, where, when, why,* and *how of something* (a pathway, a disease, a medication), you can think about background resources as textbook-like resources. They are resources you will read when you need to expand your background knowledge about a topic. See examples of background resources listed in Figure 3.1. These resources are not appropriate for making evidence-based decisions at the point of care.

While you certainly want your background resources to be valid, reliable, and easy to use, the structure of background resources can allow for somewhat less efficient reading than is required of a point-of-care resource. For example, it is not a problem to read paragraphs in a background resource while you are trying to wrap your brain around learning and understanding a disease. A point-of-care resource, however, would be better served with bulleted information for quick assessment of the bottom line.

In addition, while you want information in background resources to be as valid and reliable as possible, it is acceptable for background resources to use evidence that has a lower credibility, and sometimes lower transparency than what would be acceptable in clinically focused point-of-care resource used to try to answer foreground question. This is because background information is the foundation for understanding, and foreground information directly informs patient-care decisions. Table 3.2 reviews some categories of background resources.

Resources for Foreground Questions

The remaining question that you generated for Mr. Walker, "For an adult patient with hypertension, is hydrochlorothiazide or a beta-blocker a better medication to reduce strokes and heart attacks?" is a foreground question.

In the clinic setting, when you need to find information in real time to guide your patient care decisions, you need to quickly access the best information available. As you can see in the FIF, for most foreground questions, you should use secondary databases or *point-of-care resources*. Use the **usefulness equation** to evaluate and assess point-of-care resources.

The most useful resources grade the validity of an individual study and the strength of the evidence of a recommendation based on a body of research. These systems are important because they give you a quick way to judge the usefulness of the information you are reading, and the transparency of the information resource itself.

While many systems are used to rate and rank evidence, in 2004, a common taxonomy was developed that many journals and organizations have adopted (Table 3.3). It is called Strength of Recommendation Taxonomy (SORT) (http://www.aafp.org/afp/2004/0201/p548.html).[15]

Not all information resources use SORT but it and other evidence-ranking systems are very powerful tools in critiquing information and guiding clinical decision making.

Table 3.2 ▸ Categories of Background Resources

Background Resources	
Summary review articles (e.g., American Family Physician or New England Journal of Medicine review articles)	Effective tools for learning the overall structure, nature, and foundational content of a subject. It is important to understand why these types of articles are not useful for foreground point-of-care questions. Summary review articles cover a lot of ground, making in-depth discussion of individual points impossible. As a result, it is difficult to assess the validity of the information behind the conclusion, and bias, often unrecognized by the author, can creep into these reviews. Summary reviews may not be current, especially in rapidly changing areas of medicine. In addition, searching in a text-heavy article for an answer to a specific point-of-care question along with its supportive evidence takes a fair amount of work and time.
Textbooks/ e-textbooks	Can be thought of as collections of summary reviews. They usually present the bottom line and are sometimes hard to evaluate for validity. Poor efficiency of searching for information also increases the amount of work needed to use them.
Syllabi	Information resources that faculty compile for students. As such, their validity, transparency, and outdatedness can be hard to assess. As a student expanding your knowledge base in a subject, these can be very useful resources for achieving learning objectives in a course.

In addition to grading the evidence, the more useful point-of-care resources are transparent, meaning that they describe the process that they use to gather and synthesize the evidence, the inclusion and exclusion criterion for information, and any conflicts of interest with study sponsors (see below).

Given how important and also hard it is to effectively and efficiently answer clinical questions in real time, you need to have a cadre of reliable resources that you *understand*, *trust*, and *know how to use.*

Though the FIF provides a list of resources for answering clinical foreground questions, it is important to develop the skills you need to ascertain if an information resource is appropriate for the point-of-care. This is critical because foreground questions directly inform the care you provide to your patients. In addition, given that information and information resources themselves are changing and evolving daily, you need the knowledge and skills to be able to assess the resources you use.

To determine how reliable your resource is for foreground questions, you need to identify:

▸ What the resource is telling you.
▸ Where the resource got the information.

Table 3.3 ▸ Strength of Recommendation Taxonomy (SORT)

Strength of Recommendation	Basis for Recommendation
A	Consistent, good-quality patient-oriented evidence
B	Inconsistent or limited-quality patient-oriented evidence
C	Consensus, disease-oriented evidence, usual practice, expert opinion, or case series for studies of diagnosis, treatment, prevention, or screening.

▶ The quality (validity) of that information.

▶ How the resource critiqued and synthesized the information.

A good secondary database/point-of-care resource should have an easily accessible webpage clearly explaining how they:

▶ Survey the medical literature to ensure that they are up to date and complete.

▶ Assess the validity of the literature.

▶ Synthesize information.

A clear and easily accessible answer to those questions is a marker of an information resource's **transparency**. Without that transparency, you have no way of knowing if the information in that resource is valid, up to date, or complete. If you cannot quickly ascertain the answers to those three questions you should be cautious about using that resource to answer your clinical foreground questions.

EVIDENCE HAS A HIERARCHY

As physicians, we can fall into a false dichotomy asking ourselves –*is this information evidence based or not*? Assessing the evidence for a clinical practice is not a black/white, yes/no, either/or question. Rather, evidence falls onto a spectrum. Certain types of evidence are given higher credibility than others because they are better able to control for bias.[16] Figure 3.2 illustrates the hierarchy of evidence.

Below are explanations of some of the types of evidence on the hierarchy, in order from least quality to highest quality.

Pathophysiologic Reasoning

Pathophysiologic reasoning occurs when we use a marker for a disease and assume it to have a causal relationship to a patient-oriented outcome. Often, the pathophysiologic-reasoned linkage is proven to be correct; however, there are many examples when the patient-oriented outcome disproves pathophysiologic reasoning (Table 3.1). For example,

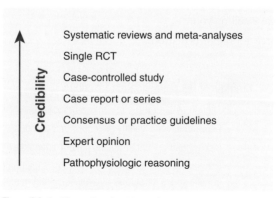

Figure 3.2 ▶ Hierarchy of evidence in clinical medicine.

pathophysiologic reasoning supported the use of hormone replacement therapy in women for decades. We reasoned that because women's rates of myocardial infarction increase when they go through menopause (as their estrogen levels drop), estrogen therapy would decrease mortality by decreasing rates of myocardial infarction. However, once subsequent patient-oriented data were collected and analyzed looking at outcomes such as venous thromboembolism and death, this was not the case.

Expert Opinion

We often turn to someone with greater experience and knowledge in a particular area when we have a question. Information from a content expert is subjective; even in narrowly focused specialties experts have a tough time agreeing.[17] The more expert the writer of a review article, the lower the methodologic rigor of the article.[18] The experts cannot be faulted for these discrepancies, for all of medicine has built-in imprecision, and the toughest areas are often the ones involving human interpretation. Furthermore, experts will often have diagnostic or therapeutic approaches based on belief, and for which evidence is not as strong as their opinion. All these issues make expert opinion questionable, though unquestionably at times quite useful.

Consensus or Practice Guidelines

The goal of practice guidelines (also called policies, consensus reports, or practice parameters) is to help clinicians improve the quality of care that they deliver and reduce inappropriate practice variation. Although some guidelines come from a careful synthesis of all available evidence, others are developed by simply polling selected experts for their consensus opinion. The latter may reduce variation in practice, but do not necessarily improve the quality of care. When evaluating a guideline, assess its usefulness using the same criteria you would for a point-of-care resource, especially validity, relevance, and transparency. The best use of clinical guidelines is as a suggestion to help govern most practice most of the time, and not as an inviolable protocol. One good resource to access a summary of clinical practice guidelines is the National Guideline Clearinghouse (https://www.guideline.gov/).

> You check the Eighth Joint National Commission evidence-based guideline on hypertension and find the answer to your second question: In the general population aged 60 years or older, initiate pharmacologic treatment at a systolic blood pressure of 150 mm Hg or higher or diastolic blood pressure of 90 mm Hg or higher and treat to a goal of lower than 150/90 mm Hg.[19] They recommend initial treatment with either a thiazide-type diuretic, calcium channel blocker, angiotensin-converting enzyme inhibitor, or angiotensin receptor blocker (see Chapter 12 for additional information on hypertension).

Systematic Reviews and Meta-Analyses

Systematic reviews and meta-analyses focus on only one or two clinical questions. A good systematic review has four steps:

1. Identification of one or two highly focused clinical questions.
2. An exhaustive search of the world's medical literature.
3. Evaluation of each article's quality, with inclusion of only those that meet quality criteria.

4. Synthesis of data
   a. Qualitative (a textual description of the bottom line)
   b. Quantitative (using specific statistical methods to combine the data from different studies into a single summary measure of effect, a technique called meta-analysis, which can only be done when the outcome measures from different studies are generally the same and their study designs are similar).

Systematic reviews and meta-analyses can be powerful tools because they have an increased ability to draw valid conclusions over single articles.

One of the best sources of this type of high-quality review is the Cochrane Library (http://www.cochranelibrary.com/) which includes the Cochrane Database of Systematic Reviews.

▶ Each review is aimed at answering a specific question.

▶ The methods used to identify all relevant research on this question are outlined in the review.

▶ Usually, only results of randomized controlled trials—the strongest form of clinical research—are used in the reviews.

Not Every Clinical Decision will have a Systematic Review to Guide You

While we strive for the most credible, POE as possible, not everything we do in clinical medicine has a systematic review, meta-analysis, or even a randomized trial to support it. That is why transparency and being able to quickly ascertain the evidence for a clinical practice is so important. We, and our patients, often assume there is highly credible evidence for a clinical practice because we are doing that clinical practice in our patient care! This circular thinking will prevent us from being lifelong learners. We need to always be asking questions, learning, and striving to improve our practice for the benefit of our patients. However, the lack of highly credible POE should not prevent you from treating your patients. It is reasonable to recommend a treatment for which there is little or no evidence to support it if you know and disclose the level of evidence.

A SYSTEMS-BASED APPROACH TO EVIDENCE-BASED MEDICINE

Keeping up with the Literature

In addition to having the skills to effectively search for the answers to your point-of-care questions when they arise, you need to have a system for keeping up with new information that would change your clinical practice. Given how much new information is published weekly, you need to have a filter to receive only information relevant to your practice. New important research with POEMs is being generated at a rapid pace, but unless you know that this new information exists, you would not know that there is a need to change your practice. Therefore, it is imperative that students and physicians develop a system to keep up with the POE that matters.

The most useful tools for this will "push out" this information to you (e.g., in a weekly email) and will be transparent, clearly describing their criterion for inclusion and exclusion, methods, and affiliations or conflicts of interest. E-mail services such as Daily InfoPOEMs from Essential Evidence Plus present information filtered for relevance and validity in bite-sized pieces (https://www.essentialevidenceplus.com/product/features_dailyip.cfm). DynaMed Topic Alerts will send e-mails when specific practice-relevant topics are updated with new evidence. This allows users to tailor their updates to specific topics and disciplines (https://help.ebsco.com/interfaces/DynaMed/DynaMed_User_Guide/set_up_alert_DynaMed_Topic). There are also podcasts to help stay current with POEMs such as the InfoPOEMs podcast (https://www.essentialevidenceplus.com/subscribe/netcast.cfm) and the American Family Physician Podcast (http://www.aafp.org/journals/afp/explore/podcast.html); both are free.

Clinical Practice Design

The knowledge and skills we have discussed thus far are applicable to the individual practicing physician. Today, physicians rarely practice alone, and even a small practice is itself a system. While individual physicians need to use information mastery to provide effective patient care, each clinical practice needs to develop systems to promote and support this as well. This includes using clinical decision support tools, which can be integrated into the Electronic Health Record, as well as clinical practice redesign (see Chapter 4: Working in an Ambulatory Care Office).

DECIPHERING RESEARCH

Reading an original research study can be enlightening, but for most clinical foreground questions that come up during patient care in any setting, original research articles are NOT the best sources of information to inform patient-care decisions. Occasionally you will need to use original research articles to answer your clinical questions and to do so you will need to understand and be familiar with commonly used concepts and terms so that you can effectively interpret and references these articles.

An explanation of study design and interpretation is part of most medical schools' preclinical curricula, and is beyond the scope of this chapter. An example of curricular materials with that content is: http://medicine.tufts.edu/Education/Academic-Departments/Clinical-Departments/Family-Medicine/Center-for-Information-Mastery/Teaching-Materials.

More useful statistical tools needed to translate clinical research into information useful for talking to patients and guiding clinical decisions include:

▶ **NNT and number needed to harm (NNH)**
The advantage of using NNT, NNH, or the graphic depiction of smiley faces (Fig. 3.3) is that it is easier to understand, especially when comparing different interventions.

NNT and NNH also facilitate communication with patients about risk and benefit. When the likelihood of an outcome is low, NNTs will be high. NNTs will decrease as either the likelihood of the outcome increases or as the benefit of the treatment increases. See http://www.thennt.com/ for NNT resources and information. Table 3.4 lists some NNTs and NNHs for various medical interventions.

For Mr. Walker, based on a Cochrane review, pharmacologic treatment of his hypertension with a thiazide diuretic would confer an absolute risk reduction in cerebrovascular mortality and morbidity of 2% (NNT = 50) and an absolute risk

Of 100 possible outcomes for you, 10 will involve experiencing a heart attack or stroke in 10 years without Statins, which is reduced to 8 out of 100 with Statins.

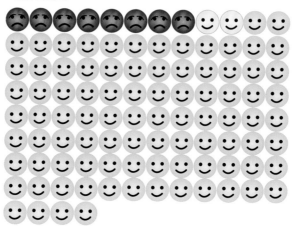

😞 Experience anyway

☺ Saved by Statins

☺ Avoided anyway

Figure 3.3 ▶ Number needed to treat (NNT) using graphic depiction. (With permission, from: Spiegelhalter DJ, Pearson M. 2,845 ways to spin the Risk. 2010. Available at: http://understandinguncertainty.org/node/233.)

Table 3.4 ▶ List of NNTs for Some Common Treatments

Therapy	Event Prevented	NNT	NNH
Blood pressure medicine for 5 years	Death	125	1:10 (medication side effects, stopping the drug)
Statin drugs for 5 years for HD prevention (no known HD)	Death	None were helped (no lives saved)	1:50 (develop diabetes) 1:10 (muscle damage)
Co-administration of probiotics with prescribed antibiotics	*Clostridium difficile* diarrhea	25	None were harmed
Thrombolytics for major heart attack (STEMI)	Death	43 (when given within 6 hours) 200 (given at 12–24 hours)	1:143 (major bleeding episode) 1:250 (hemorrhagic stroke)
Strength and balance training programs for preventing falls in the elderly	Fall prevention	11	None were harmed
Systemic steroids for acute COPD exacerbations	Prevented failed treatment	10	7 (adverse drug effects)

HD, heart disease; NNH, number needed to harm; NNT, number needed to treat; STEMI, ST elevation myocardial infarction.
Data from The NNT Group, 2010–2017: Quick summaries of evidence-based medicine; Available from: http://www.thennt.com/.

Table 3.5 ▶ Interpreting a Likelihood Ratio	
Likelihood Ratio	**Interpretation**
>10	Strong evidence to rule in disease
5–10	Moderate evidence to rule in disease
2–5	Weak evidence to rule in disease
0.5–2	No significant change in the likelihood of disease
0.2–0.5	Weak evidence to rule out disease
0.1–0.2	Moderate evidence to rule out disease
<0.1	Strong evidence to rule out disease

reduction in coronary heart disease mortality and morbidity of 1.0% (NNT = 100) over 4.5 years.[20]

▶ **Positive predictive value (PPV) and negative predictive value (NPV)**
PPVs and NPVs are more useful to clinicians than sensitivity and specificity because they reflect diagnostic test performance at different degrees of prevalence of disease (pretest probability). The PPV is the proportion of patients with a positive test who actually have disease, whereas the NPV is the proportion of patients with a negative test who are actually free of disease.
    Here are two useful YouTube videos:

- Sensitivity, specificity, and predictive values: https://www.youtube.com/watch?v=gkWNNrr5Tl8
- PPV and NPV: https://www.youtube.com/watch?v=NdKdocmuMY0

▶ **Likelihood ratios (LRs)**
The LR describes the degree that a positive or negative test result increases or decreases the likelihood of having a disease (Table 3.5). Every test has its own LR. An LR >1 indicates an increased likelihood of disease, whereas an LR <1 reduces the likelihood of disease. The further the LR is from 1, the more likely the test will signify the presence or absence of disease. LRs can be used to describe the accuracy of tests with multiple outcomes, such as a test that categorizes patients as low, moderate, high, and at very high risk. Here is a YouTube video explaining LR: https://www.youtube.com/watch?v=lnZTOoGc_F0.

USING INFORMATION TO CHANGE YOUR PRACTICE WITH CONFIDENCE

As a student or as a clinician, you should continuously reflect on your performance, learn to value the clinical questions that arise in daily practice, and make an effort to answer them with the best available evidence. The best physician asks more questions, not fewer.
    Develop a system for yourself to keep track of your clinical questions. Familiarize yourself with useful (high validity, reliability, and transparency; low work) resources that you feel comfortable using in order to answer your questions either during the point-of-care or soon after. Find high-quality tools and systems that help keep you up to date. Shape your clinical practice to promote and facilitate the finding and using of high-quality information to guide care.

While having the knowledge and skills to find the best evidence available for a clinical practice is critical to providing high-quality healthcare, the best evidence-based answer is only the starting point for a conversation with your patient. Shared-decision making must consider the individual patient's goals, values, and context (Chapter 5). Just as the answers to questions are not always black and white, using information to help our patients is a central art to the practice of medicine.

QUESTIONS

1. In reviewing the strength of evidence to support a clinical question that you derived after a patient care session today, you determine that the SORT level is C. How should you interpret this?
   A. The probability that the evidence is valid is very high.
   B. The probability that the evidence is relevant is very high.
   C. Consistent, good-quality patient-oriented evidence is available.
   D. Limited-quality patient-oriented evidence is available.
   E. Consensus, disease-oriented evidence, usual practice, expert opinion, or case series is available.

2. "The best way to lower blood pressure in a patient with hypertension is?" Is this a background or foreground question and why?
   A. It is a foreground question because it deals with a condition that is relevant to your patients.
   B. This is a foreground question because it is in the PICO format.
   C. This is a background question because it tries to answer a "who" question.
   D. This is a background question because it tries to answer a "what" question.
   E. This is a background question because it tries to answer a "why" question.

3. Please arrange Single RCT (1), Consensus/Practice Guidelines (2), Systematic reviews/ Meta-analyses (3), Expert Opinion (4), and Case Report/Series (5) in the correct order of evidence hierarchy from least to most credible.
   A. 1, 2, 3, 4, 5.
   B. 3, 2, 5, 4, 1.
   C. 5, 2, 4, 1, 3.
   D. 4, 2, 5, 1, 3.

4. You have a background clinical question of a common clinical problem. According to the Finding Information Framework, the best source of your answer is likely to be:
   A. Textbook.
   B. PubMed.
   C. DynaMed.
   D. TRIP Database.
   E. Web of Science.

5. The most useful and clinically relevant resources to aid in your clinical work are those that are:
   A. Valid.
   B. Inexpensive.
   C. High work.

D. Answer background questions.
E. Utilize expert opinion.

ANSWERS

Question 1: The correct answer is E.
While many systems are used to rate and rank evidence, in 2004, a common taxonomy was developed that many journals and organizations have adopted (Table 3.3). It is called Strength of Recommendation Taxonomy. Table 3.3 shows that SORT C is based on consensus, disease-oriented evidence, usual practice, expert opinion, or case series for studies of diagnosis, treatment, prevention, or screening.

Question 2: The correct answer is D.
Background questions answer who, what, where, why, and how of anything, such as a disease or a medication. Examples include "What are the types of diagnoses that cause knee pain in adults?" and "What are the medication classes for smoking cessation?"

Question 3: The correct answer is D.
The hierarchy of evidence is illustrated in Figure 3.2. Credibility increases from pathophysiologic reasoning, expert opinion, consensus or practice guidelines, case report or series, case-controlled study, single RCT, systematic reviews, and meta-analyses.

Question 4: The correct answer is A.
As shown in Figure 3.1, appropriate sources for answering background questions for common clinical problems are UpToDate, textbooks, or laboratory/testing.

Question 5: The correct answer is A.
A key concept of information mastery is recognizing that not all sources of information are equal—they differ regarding their usefulness. Usefulness is measured as relevance × validity divided by work.

REFERENCES

1. Hurwitz B. How does evidence based guidance influence determinations of medical negligence? *BMJ.* 2004; 329:1024–1028.
2. Bastian H, Glasziou P, Chalmers I. Seventy-five trials and eleven systematic reviews a day: how will we ever keep up? *PLoS Med.* 2010;7(9):e1000326. doi:10.1371/journal.pmed.1000326
3. Duckworth W, Abraira C, Moritz T, et al.; for the VADT Investigators. Glucose control and vascular complications in veterans with type 2 diabetes. *N Engl J Med.* 2009;360(2):129–139.
4. Gerstein HC, Miller ME, Byington RP; for the Action to Control Cardiovascular Risk in Diabetes (ACCORD) Study Group. Effects of intensive glucose lowering in type 2 diabetes. *N Engl J Med.* 2008;358: 2545–2559.
5. Echt DS, Liebson PR, Mitchell LB, et al. Mortality and morbidity in patients receiving encainide, flecainide, or placebo. *N Engl J Med.* 1991;324:781–788.
6. Dwyer T, Ponsonby A. Sudden infant death syndrome: after the "back to sleep" campaign. *Br Med J.* 1996; 313:180–181.
7. The HOPE Investigators. Vitamin E supplementation and cardiovascular events in high risk patients. *N Engl J Med.* 2000;342:154–160.
8. Writing Group for the Women's Health Initiative Investigators. Risks and benefits of estrogen plus progestin in healthy postmenopausal women. Principal results from the Women's Health Initiative randomized controlled trial. *JAMA.* 2002;288:321–333.

9. Heidenreich PA, Lee TT, Massie BM. Effect of beta-blockade on mortality in patients with heart failure: a meta-analysis of randomized controlled trials. *J Am Coll Cardiol.* 1997;30:27–34.

10. Covell DG, Uman GC, Manning PR. Information needs in office practice: are they being met? *Ann Intern Med.* 1985;103:596–599.

11. Ely JW, Osheroff JA, Ebell MH, et al. Analysis of questions asked by family doctors regarding patient care. *BMJ.* 1999;319(7206):358–361.

12. Ebell MH. Information at the point of care: answering clinical questions. *J Am Board Fam Pract.* 1999;i2(s):225–235.

13. Beck JB, Tieder JS. Electronic resources preferred by pediatric hospitalists for clinical care. *J Med Libr Assoc.* 2015;103(4):177–183.

14. Kosteniuk JG, Morgan DG, D'Arcy CK. Use and perceptions of information among family physicians: sources considered accessible, relevant, and reliable. *J Med Libr Assoc.* 2013;101(1):32–37.

15. Ebell MH, Siwek J, Weiss BD, et al. Strength of Recommendation Taxonomy (SORT): a patient-centered approach to grading evidence in the medical literature. *Am Fam Physician.* 2004;69(3):548–556.

16. Howick J, Chalmers I, Glasziou P, et al. "The 2011 Oxford CEBM Evidence Levels of Evidence (Introductory Document)." *OCEBM.* Available from: http://www.cebm.net/index.aspx?o=5653. Accessed March 2017.

17. Slawson DC, Shaughnessy AF. Obtaining useful information from expert based sources. *BMJ.* 1997;314: 947–949.

18. Oxman AD, Guyatt GH. The science of reviewing research. *Ann New York Acad Sci.* 1993;703(1):125–134.

19. James PA, Ooparil S, Carter BL, et al. 2014 evidence-based guideline for the management of high blood pressure in adults report from the panel members appointed to the Eighth Joint National Committee. *JAMA.* 2014;311(5):507–520.

20. Musini VM, Tejani AM, Bassett K, et al. Pharmacotherapy for hypertension in the elderly. *Cochrane Database Syst Rev.* 2009;(4):CD000028.

Working in an Ambulatory Care Office

KEY POINTS

1 ▶ Because each ambulatory care office functions differently, students should regularly ask questions and seek feedback to ensure they are meeting expectations.

2 ▶ Family physicians approach patients using the biopsychosocial model—a holistic model of medical care.

3 ▶ Ambulatory care offices optimize health by focusing on wellness and chronic disease management, as well as diagnosing and treating acute concerns.

4 ▶ Working in ambulatory care settings can provide opportunities for students to advance their history taking, physical examination, differential diagnosis, procedural and patient education skills and to learn about the process of care delivery.

You are working with Dr. Butler in his family medicine clinic. Before the day starts, Dr. Butler looks at his schedule for the day. He recommends that you see the following patients in the morning:

1. Priya Chaudhry, a 3-year-old coming in for a cough and fever.
2. Brian Clem, a 57-year-old man who is coming for follow-up for hypertension and chronic obstructive pulmonary disease (COPD).
3. Octavia Johnson, a 29-year-old woman who has scheduled a well-woman examination.
4. Frank Newton, a 78-year-old man who is coming in for removal of a lesion on his neck that is likely a basal cell carcinoma.

WHY AMBULATORY CARE?

Medical students have traditionally completed most of their training in a hospital setting, but a variety of factors have led to the incorporation of ambulatory care experiences into medical school.[1-3]

Patients today will receive most of their care in an ambulatory setting. In addition, most preventive care and chronic disease management occurs in outpatient clinics. Students may find learning in an ambulatory setting easier than in the hospital, as patients in an outpatient setting are generally well enough to speak for themselves and provide an accurate history. Patients are also more able to participate in physical examination techniques. Students also appreciate the opportunity to work one-on-one with a faculty member, often over several days to weeks.[4] Table 4.1 displays contrasts between inpatient and outpatient settings with respect to volume, patient types, and composition of the care team.

Table 4.1 ▶ Features of Inpatient versus Ambulatory Setting

Feature	Inpatient Setting	Ambulatory Setting
Patient volume	Low volume (students see 1–3 patients daily)	High volume (students may see 8–10 patients daily)
Patient types	Focus on acute illness, patients are potentially unresponsive or with altered mental status and more likely to be bedbound	Focus on wellness and chronic illnesses, patients are generally alert and oriented, and able to ambulate unassisted
Care team (will vary from site-to-site)	Attending physicians Residents Fellows Nurse practitioners Physician assistants Floor nurses Social workers Clinical pharmacists	Attending physicians Nurse practitioners Physician assistants Clinic nurses Medical assistants Patient educators Behavioral health specialists Social workers Clinical pharmacists Office managers

THINKING LIKE A PRIMARY CARE PHYSICIAN

Disease versus Illness

A disease is a defined biochemical abnormality,[5] such as a left lower lobe pneumonia due to *Streptococcus pneumoniae* identified on sputum culture or autoimmune thyroiditis with a suppressed thyroid stimulating hormone. Illness, on the other hand, is a patient-defined construct that incorporates their perception and their cultural experiences. Said another way, an illness is what a patient has on their way to the doctor, while a disease is what a patient has on their way home from the doctor.[6] While primary care physicians seek to arrive at a diagnosed disease using a group of signs and symptoms, they also consider the patient's illness experience.

Your first patient Priya's cough and fever (illness) is most likely due to a viral infection (disease). Her parent is likely concerned about a serious condition and may have gotten little sleep. Should your examination confirm your suspected diagnosis, you will need to add reassurance and perhaps a cough suppressant to help the child (and her parents) sleep.

A patient with community-acquired pneumonia may conceptualize their illness as a harbinger of death if their sister died from pneumonia. On the other hand, a patient with hyperthyroidism may believe the illness is minor and does not require treatment. Skilled primary care physicians recognize disparities between illness and disease and assist patients with resolving cognitive dissonance for their patients.

Biopsychosocial Model

The biopsychosocial approach to patient care recognizes that making a correct diagnosis and prescribing an effective treatment are only part of the physician's role. Physicians must also address the psychological effect of symptoms and diseases on the patient and their social network.[7,8] Patients are also affected by their psychological state and social environment. Primary care physicians must be in tune with how these interact to cause a disease state and potential for compliance with treatment recommendations. For example, if your second scheduled patient, Mr. Clem, has uncontrolled hypertension or is experiencing additional symptoms from his COPD, attention to psychosocial factors such as stress, occupational exposures, and cost issues in addition to medication adherence may uncover contributing factors.

Recommendations to provide care using the biopsychosocial approach include:

▶ Obtain a social history focusing on the patient's living situation, employment status, religious preferences, and support system in addition to substance use.

▶ Ask patients about their concerns and worries during history taking and while discussing a treatment plan.

▶ Consider costs of recommended evaluations and treatments (use GoodRx at https://www.goodrx.com/ to identify the most inexpensive pharmacy for a specific medication, or use Epocrates or UpToDate to compare costs of medications).

▶ Recognize that no conditions are purely psychological or purely biologic, and instead see how the two interact to present with various symptoms.

Physician–Patient Communication

While communication is important for all members of the healthcare team, the longitudinal relationship between a patient and their primary care physician makes strong interpersonal skills even more important. Because of the nature of primary care, your preceptor will often know a great deal about the patient's personal and family life. They likely care for other family members. Skills like empathic listening, humor, and therapeutic touch[9] are essential for ensuring good communication and promotion of wellness.

Primary care physicians use a variety of communication techniques to assist patients with managing their chronic diseases (Chapter 5).[10,11] Ambulatory clinics are also ideal settings to learn and practice shared decision making and motivational interviewing, especially in offices that utilize trained patient educators and behavioral health consultants. Your third scheduled patient, as a 29-year-old woman, may have contraceptive needs if in a heterosexual relationship—an ideal time to engage in shared decision making around the many contraceptive options.

Chronic Disease Management

Managing chronic diseases requires a team of people, with an active and engaged patient at the center.[12] Rather than focusing on making a diagnosis and prescribing a treatment, chronic disease management focuses on empowering a patient to adopt a healthy lifestyle and adhere to what is often a complicated regimen. For Mr. Clem, it is likely that cigarette smoking was an issue in the past and may continue to be a concern. He is also likely to have been prescribed at least several medications that may be difficult to remember to take regularly. For this reason, primary care physicians (and other members of the patient's healthcare team) are often required to function as coaches rather than instructors. Managing chronic diseases often involves work done outside of the examination room by the physician, nurses, pharmacists, and behavioral health specialists.

Table 4.2 ▸ Types of Bias Affecting Illness Scripts

Name of Bias	Description
Availability	Considering easily remembered diagnoses more likely, irrespective of prevalence
Base rate neglect	Pursuing "zebras"
Representativeness	Ignoring atypical features that are inconsistent with the favored diagnosis
Confirmation bias	Seeking data to confirm, rather than refute the initial hypothesis
Premature closure	Stopping the diagnostic process too soon

Differential Diagnosis of the Undifferentiated Complaint

Primary care physicians are often the first person to see a patient with a new symptom. There are two main strategies they use to arrive at a diagnosis: illness scripts and systematic differential diagnosis. Illness scripts are based on previous experiences with patients, allowing physicians to rapidly correlate signs and symptoms with a diagnosis.[13] However, bias can affect the accuracy of illness scripts and scripts require extensive experience (Table 4.2).[14]

Sample illness scripts:

▸ Pediatric patient with nighttime cough, history of eczema = asthma

▸ Obese patient with burning in feet, increased frequency of urination = diabetes

▸ Pleuritic chest pain in a pregnant woman who recently took a cross-country trip = pulmonary embolus

While developing illness scripts, students will benefit from using more systematic techniques to arrive at a differential diagnosis. These include algorithms and clinical decision support tools. Resources for differential diagnosis are found in Table 4.3.

Table 4.3 ▸ Resources for Differential Diagnosis

Online/Mobile Resources (subscription required, may be available through institution)
• BMJ Best Practices http://bestpractice.bmj.com/
• Diagnosaurus http://accessmedicine.mhmedical.com/diagnosaurus.aspx
• DynaMed http://www.dynamed.com/home/
• Epocrates http://www.epocrates.com/
• Essential Evidence Plus http://www.essentialevidenceplus.com/
• Isabel Dx http://www.isabelhealthcare.com/
• UpToDate http://uptodate.com
• VisualDx https://www.visualdx.com/

Textbooks
• 5-Minute Clinical Consult https://5minuteconsult.com/ (also available as app)
• Ferri's Clinical Advisor http://store.elsevier.com/Ferris-Clinical-Advisor-2017/Fred-Ferri/isbn-9780323280488/
• Symptom to Diagnosis http://www.langetextbooks.com/0071496130.php?c=home

Calibrating Yourself

Primary care physicians recognize that each patient encounter takes place in a specific context.[15] In addition to recognizing how the patient's perception of their illness and current mental state are influencing the patient, primary care physicians recognize that their current level of fatigue, emotional reserves, and attitude toward the patient will affect the patient visit.[16,17] Self-reflection activities and discussions with peers and mentors can help students and physicians alike learn to manage the difficult patient encounter effectively (Chapter 24).

FUNCTIONING WELL IN THE AMBULATORY CARE SETTING

For each educational experience, you should be familiar with the objectives of your experience and how you will be assessed. Plan to review the syllabus and any evaluation tools thoroughly before your first day.

When considering advice for success in any rotation, consider the source and their intentions. Rely more heavily on your rotation director and your supervising preceptor for recommendations on your performance than advice from peers or online resources.

In general, you should do the following:

▸ Arrive on time (or, better yet, early).

▸ Present yourself professionally in terms of appearance, language, and attitude to all members of the healthcare team, including the patient.

▸ Use your patients as a guide for your reading and plan to spend a significant amount of time outside of your clinical responsibilities learning about your patients.

▸ Ask for feedback frequently and respond accordingly.[18,19]

▸ Be respectful of the culture of the clinic and let their behavior be your guide; if in doubt on the acceptability of your behavior, ask, do not assume!

Your First Day

You should anticipate a general tour and an introduction to staff on your first day. Make note of the following:

▸ Location of extra medical equipment (e.g., blood pressure cuffs, tongue depressors)

▸ Function of equipment in the examination room (e.g., otoscope, examination room table)

▸ Examination room layout

▸ Locations of sinks and hand sanitizer

▸ The names and roles of office staff

▸ Patient and staff bathrooms

▸ Areas where you may eat and drink

▸ Areas where you may secure your personal belongings

Clarify with your preceptor their expectation of your role in the clinic, especially if there are other learners in the clinic who may have different responsibilities. As your time progresses, you may also ask to work with nonphysician members of the healthcare to get a sense of how everyone contributes to patient care.

Every Day

Share your goals for the day with the preceptor, then seek feedback on these goals at the end of the day. Review the daily schedule with your preceptor at the beginning of every day or half-day. Identify any patients who will help you focus on your goals and knowledge deficits. While Dr. Butler has identified four patients with a mix of acute, chronic, preventive, and procedural concerns, you may request to see a patient with diabetes rather than COPD if you feel less comfortable managing the former. Also identify patients your preceptor may prefer that you not see. Introduce yourself to whomever is rooming patients for the physician. Ask them to let patients know that they may see a student.

You should expect to have a mix of shadowing and seeing patients on your own, depending on your current level of training. Your physician will need to spend some time every day addressing patients' messages and returning phone calls. Use this time to read on patients you have seen or anticipate seeing later in the day.

Retaining a positive attitude and having a flexible response to each day will help ensure you and your preceptor have a good experience working together. As with most aspects of medical education, the quality of your experience in an ambulatory care clinic depends largely on the amount of effort you put into your education.

Case Presentations

When you see patients independently, you will need to present a summary of your history and physical examination, as well as your assessment and plan, to the physician. Depending on the preference of your preceptor, you may present in the room with the patient or in a separate area. You should ask your preceptor how they would like you to present as preferences for thoroughness and order can vary widely. SNAPPS is a mnemonic that may help with learner-centered presentations to preceptors (Box 4.1).[20]

Documentation

After seeing a patient, you should document your findings, assessment, and plan in the medical record. Most ambulatory care offices will have an electronic health record (EHR).

BOX 4.1 SNAPPS, A MNEMONIC FOR LEARNER-CENTERED MODEL OF CASE PRESENTATIONS TO PRECEPTORS IN THE OUTPATIENT SETTING

The learner will:

1. Summarize briefly the history and findings
2. Narrow the differential to two or three relevant possibilities
3. Analyze the differential by comparing and contrasting the possibilities
4. Probe the preceptor by asking questions about uncertainties, difficulties, or alternative approaches
5. Plan management for the patient's medical issues
6. Select a case-related issue for self-directed learning

From: Wolpaw TM, Wolpaw DR, Papp KK. SNAPPS: a learner-centered model for outpatient education. *Acad Med.* 2003;78(9):893–898.

This will vary from office to office, and may be different from the EHR you use in an inpatient setting. You may be asked to do training on the EHR, or learn on your own. You may or may not have your own sign-on to the EHR, although this is recommended by multiple national organizations.[21] While the physician may allow you to use their log-in to review the record, you should not be asked to document without signing your name or enter orders without the physician ultimately co-signing them.

While Medicare does not restrict students from documenting in the health record only the provider's history, physical exam and medical decision making can be used for billing purposes.

Depending on school and office policies, students may also be able to (and should!) do the following:

▸ Place orders to be co-signed by the physician.

▸ Reconcile the medication list with what the patient is actually taking.

▸ Update allergies.

▸ Function as a scribe when observing the physician taking a history or performing a physical examination.

▸ Add discharge instructions.

You may choose to practice documenting in the room with patient. Ensure you are fluent with the EHR first, then ensure that you integrate what you are seeing and doing on the EHR into your visit with the patient by explaining your actions to the patient and pointing to key elements you would like the patient to see.[24]

Making Yourself Indispensable

Your primary role in an ambulatory care clinic is to learn how to care for patients in the environment where patients are seen most frequently. Your preceptor will have more time to teach and you will have a greater diversity of learning experiences if you work to fulfill certain roles within the clinic. Your role may be predefined by your curriculum objectives or the office in which you are working. However, the more initiative you take to integrate yourself into the work of the clinic, the more opportunities you will have to learn and grow your skills.

Over time, you may assume a greater responsibility in many areas as shown in Table 4.4.

GENERAL APPROACH TO PATIENT CARE

In general, there will be four types of visits in an ambulatory care setting, represented by the four patients that you are scheduled to see. These are:

▸ Acute/sick visit

▸ Chronic disease follow-up visit

▸ Wellness visit

▸ Procedure visit

Table 4.4 ► Opportunities for Greater Student Responsibility

Patient Education	Patient Follow-up	Teaching	Disease Management
• Use a glucometer	• Call acutely ill patients 2 days later to assess progress	• Summarize a new guideline on a common problem	• Work on a practice improvement project to increase the number of patients receiving influenza vaccinations
• Use crutches or wrap a sprained ankle	• Contact patients who are overdue for recommended health screening	• Access an evidence-based resource to answer a clinical question	• Identify patients with type 2 diabetes who are overdue on monitoring and arrange a clinic visit
• Strategies for smoking cessation	• Use the EHR to message patients on new program or medication	• Provide a summary of a rare condition seen in clinic	• Scan requests for refills from pharmacies to determine if a refill is appropriate or if the patient needs an appointment
• Diet instruction	• Follow-up with patients recently discharged from a hospital	• Call the health department about needed vaccines and cost for a patient who is traveling internationally	• Identify patients who are having difficulty managing a chronic disease and connect them with resources
• Review postprocedure instructions and follow-up plans	• Review normal labs with patients you have previously seen in clinic	• Present the results of a quality improvement project to team members	
• Demonstrate rehabilitation exercises			
• Create a patient education handout			
• Provide written visit summaries			
• Help patients get to the blood draw station, radiology or the restroom			

Each visit requires a slightly different approach from the student. In addition, many patients present with elements from different visit types. For example, a patient who has scheduled a wellness visit may also want to address a new symptom. A patient scheduled for a diabetes follow-up may need to be referred for a mammogram.

Acute or Sick Visit

These are the types of visits students may be most comfortable with from previous education on history-taking. Patients have generally scheduled the appointment recently and want to

Table 4.5 ▶ OLD CARTS Mnemonic for Evaluation of New Pain Complaints

O	Onset	*When did it start? What was going on when the pain started?*
L	Location	*Use one finger to point to the pain.*
D	Duration	*How long did it last? Is it getting better/worse/staying the same?*
C	Character	*What kind of pain is it?*
A	Aggravating/Alleviating	*What makes it better? What makes it worse? What did you try to help?*
R	Radiation	*Does it go anyplace else?*
T	Timing	*How frequently does it occur?*
S	Severity	*On a scale of 1 to 10, how much does it bother you?*

focus on a couple of key concerns. Students should complete a focused history and physical examination relevant to the patient's chief complaint, then develop a differential diagnosis based on the patient's chief complaint (Chapter 11). For evaluating a new pain symptom for example, history taking can proceed using the mnemonic OLDCARTS (Table 4.5).

Prior to entering the examination room to see your first patient, you review the differential diagnosis for fever in pediatric patients. Three-year-old Priya has a 2-day history of cough and fever of 102.3°F. She is previously healthy. Mom has not tried any medications. Priya's brother had similar symptoms last week and was diagnosed with viral bronchitis. You complete an examination focused on the ears, nose, throat, and chest, then report your findings of a likely viral infection with Dr. Butler and recommend symptomatic treatment.

Chronic Disease Follow-up Visit

These are often the most common visits in a family medicine and internal medicine clinics. Chronic care requires a team and, depending on the office you are working in, much of the work in these visits may be provided by other members of the team.[25,26] Patients have a known diagnosis and are presenting for follow-up. These visits focus on the following:

▶ Disease control—Is the patient having new or worsening symptoms related to the underlying disease? Has the patient received recommended testing to monitor control?

▶ Development of complications—Has the patient developed symptoms that suggest complications from their underlying disease? Has the patient received recommended diagnostic testing to monitor for these complications?

▶ Medication adherence—Are there barriers to the patient taking medications, or side effects from prescribed medications? Does the patient need refills?

▶ Lifestyle compliance—Are there barriers to recommendations made to control the disease and prevent complications? Does the patient need additional education or support?

  Chronic disease management is also one area where medical students can take an active role in patient care. Part of effective care of a patient with a chronic disease is optimizing self-management.[27] As students get more comfortable with patient education, they can begin to deliver patient education to allow for more effective self-management.[28,29]

Feature	Hypertension	COPD
Disease control	Blood pressure is 143/92 mm Hg He denies headaches, vision changes, chest pain, or dyspnea	PFTs last month showed an FEV1/FVC ratio of 0.67 His breathing is reported as "good"
Development of complications	He denies chest pain, changes in urine production or exercise tolerance, or peripheral edema His heart is regular rate and rhythm without extra sounds	He denies increased sputum production or dyspnea His lungs are clear to auscultation, and there is no clubbing or cyanosis
Medication adherence	He frequently misses his nighttime dose of medications, but takes his morning medications	He is using his rescue inhaler three times a week. He is unable to afford his long-acting anticholinergic
Lifestyle adherence	He has been working to lower the sodium in his diet	He continues to smoke one-half pack cigarettes daily, but wants to quit

Table 4.6 ▸ Mr. Clem's History

PFT, pulmonary function test.

To successfully complete a chronic disease follow-up, review the physician's previous note on the patient and help close the loop on any referrals, labs, or tests that were ordered at the previous visit (Chapter 12).

Brian Clem next steps. You determine the information shown in Table 4.6 from chart review and from his history. You plan to discuss strategies for smoking cessation and ways of improving Mr. Clem's control of hypertension, perhaps by changing to a once-daily medication with Dr. Butler. Mr. Clem's COPD seems stable at present without the long-acting medication but you plan to discuss resources to help him with medication costs.

Wellness Visit

What patients often refer to as a "checkup," physicians often refer to as a health maintenance visit. Wellness visits are an opportunity to ensure that the patient has received recommended screening tests and to counsel on lifestyle changes to improve health. While there is no science to support improved outcomes with wellness visits for adults, these visits make up a considerable part of the work of the primary care clinician. Knowing how to focus these visits can ensure efficiency and effectiveness for the patient. Prenatal care visits for pregnant women and well-child care are specialized types of this visit. Table 4.7 presents information on topics to address at wellness visits.

Part of the Affordable Care Act (ACA) states that preventive services with a Grade A or B recommendation by the United States Preventive Services Task Force (USPSTF) should be covered without out-of-pocket expenses for the patient.[30] Therefore, these visits are an opportunity to ensure all patients have received recommended vaccinations, cancer screening, identification of cardiovascular risk factors, and lifestyle counseling. While many organizations make recommendations for screening tests, the ACA and most family physicians rely on recommendations from the USPSTF (www.uspreventiveservicestaskforce.org).

The Agency for Healthcare Research and Quality (AHRQ) Electronic Preventive Services Selector (ePSS) is available on the web at https://epss.ahrq.gov/PDA/index.jsp or as an app for

Table 4.7 ▶ What to Address in Wellness Visits—RISE Mnemonic	
Activity	**Examples**
Risk factor identification	Obesity screening Blood pressure screening
Immunization need/review	Influenza and pneumococcal vaccination
Screening tests to consider	Cancer screening Lipid screening Sexually transmitted infection screening
Education	Exercise counseling Recommendations to pursue a living will and power of attorney

smart phones, and can help you track recommendations based on a patient's age and gender (Fig. 4.1).

In preparation for Octavia Johnson's wellness visit, you identify Grade A and B recommendations from USPSTF. You review her chart to determine the items she has already received, and then make a list of items to address during her visit. These would include vital signs, lifestyle factors, sexually transmitted infection risk, and intimate partner violence.

Procedure Visit

The types of procedures performed will vary based on the patient population being served and the training of the physician. Procedure visits may be scheduled in advance or may be needed if the patient's problem dictates an office procedure.

Prior to observing or assisting with a procedure, it may be helpful to review a video online of the procedure. YouTube is often a good source for these videos, such as this one demonstrating a shave biopsy often performed with patients with suspected basal cell carcinoma, like Mr. Newton (https://www.youtube.com/watch?v=nbdmmukko4s).

Procedure visits generally require written informed consent: a discussion with the patient about the risks, benefits, and alternatives to the recommended procedure and documentation by the patient, the person obtaining consent, and the performing physician. For patients with lower health literacy or non-native English speakers, incorporating written documents or online decision tools may help to achieve truly informed consent.[31]

Students can assist their preceptor by working with office staff to ensure all tools are available and the patient understands the procedure, as well as the plan for follow-up. Depending on the level of training of the student, the complexity of the procedure, and the wishes of the patient and the preceptor, students may also assist with procedures. If assisting an ambulatory procedure, a review of sterile procedures should be performed ahead of time (example at https://www.youtube.com/watch?v=AL0EE8zhNVM).

You review the previous note from your preceptor in the EHR and note that Mr. Newton has a changing lesion on his neck. You ensure that Dr. Butler has all the necessary tools, then talk with Mr. Newton about the procedure and share the video you found on YouTube. Together, you and Dr. Butler perform a successful shave biopsy. The pathology report returns 1 week later and confirms a basal cell carcinoma that was completely excised.

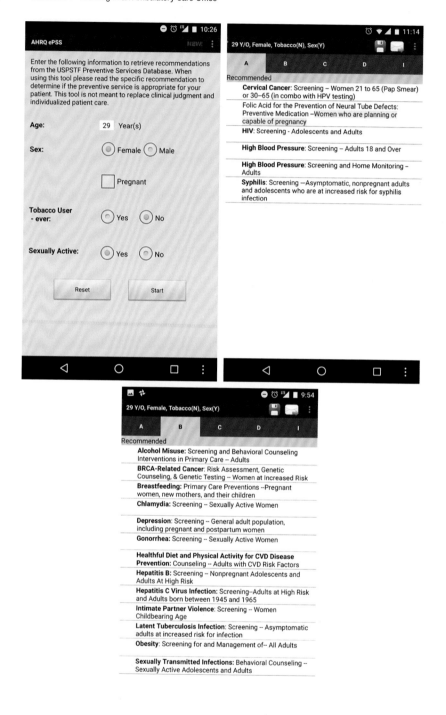

Figure 4.1 ▶ Snapshots from the AHRQ app for iOS platform.

QUESTIONS

1. The best example of the power of the biopsychosocial model in working with patients is:
   A. It commonly uses social workers to ascertain the social context of disease.
   B. It contextualizes care and allows us to recognize that our role is to consider the whole person, medical and psychological, and not just the diagnosis.
   C. It frames healthcare delivery as needing a team to deliver outstanding care.
   D. It addresses common biases in our thinking.

2. Patient presentations as delivered by students and residents to attending physicians often follow a traditional form. SNAPPS encourages a different style of case presentation. Which SNAPPS element is correct:
   A. State the name of the patient you will be presenting.
   B. Note the style that other students use to make their presentations.
   C. Attend to the Affect of the patient while gathering the history.
   D. Preface your presentation with a series of questions you are trying to get answered.
   E. Plan management for the patient's medical issues.

3. All medical students should strive to find ways to make themselves indispensable to those with whom they work. Common categories in which students can often assume greater responsibility in patient care as their skills develop include:
   A. Patient referrals.
   B. Home visits.
   C. Therapy.
   D. Disease management.
   E. Organizing follow-up visits.

4. There are many issues to address during wellness visits. While rapport building and the psychosocial model are very important elements that contribute to a successful visit, RISE is a mnemonic tool that:
   A. Organizes these visits by helping us focus on what to address.
   B. Helps assist our patients in improving their energy levels.
   C. Breaks down each step in the biopsychosocial model.
   D. Gives us detailed information on a patient's immunization needs.
   E. Reliably reduces cost and improves outcomes.

5. Renleigh Mu is 45 years old and has hypertension. She has a 15-minute appointment with you today to assess a lesion on her abdomen that has changed recently. She would also like a mammogram. She has no time for a longer visit today and only wants you to offer an opinion regarding the skin lesion. How would you best characterize this visit?
   A. Chronic disease follow-up.
   B. Procedure.
   C. Wellness visit.
   D. Acute/sick visit.
   E. Not necessary.

ANSWERS

Question 1: The correct answer is B.

The biopsychosocial model recognizes that making a correct diagnosis and prescribing an effective treatment are only part of a physician's role. Physicians must also address the psychological effect of symptoms and diseases on the patient and their social network.

Question 2: The correct answer is E.

The SNAPPS is learner-centered model for case presentations. S stands for Summarize briefly the history and findings; N stands for Narrow the differential to two or three relevant possibilities; A stands for Analyze the differential by comparing and contrasting the possibilities; P for Probe the preceptor by asking questions about uncertainties, difficulties, or alternative approaches; P for Plan management for the patient's medical issues; and S for Select a case-related issue for self-directed learning.

Question 3: The correct answer is D.

Table 4.4 indicates that patient education, patient follow-up, teaching, and disease management are common areas in which students can assume greater responsibility as their skills develop. As students work to make themselves indispensable in whatever environment they find themselves working and learning in, it is useful to keep these categories in mind.

Question 4: The correct answer is A.

The RISE mnemonic, shown in Table 4.7, is introduced to help you organize your thinking about the major themes that need attention during wellness visits. These include risk factor identification (weight, alcohol, multiple sexual partners, food insecurity...), immunization needs, screening tests to consider (based on age, gender, smoking, etc.), and education needs such as exercise counseling.

Question 5: The correct answer is D.

Acute or sick visits are the types of visits students may be most comfortable with from previous education on history-taking. Patients have generally scheduled the appointment recently and want to focus on a couple of key concerns. For Ms. Mu this visit would be best characterized as an acute/sick visit. She is not making herself available for a procedure, this is not a chronic disease follow-up visit, and while the mammogram may traditionally be thought of as part of wellness visit, the primary driver of this visit is a desire to assess a skin lesion; thus it is an acute/sick visit.

REFERENCES

1. Bowen JL, Salerno SM, Chamberlain JK, et al. Changing habits of practice: transforming internal medicine residency education in ambulatory settings. *J Gen Intern Med.* 2005;20(12):1181–1187.
2. Irby DM. Teaching and learning in ambulatory care settings: a thematic review of the literature. *Acad Med J Assoc Am Med Coll.* 1995;70:898–931.
3. Williams CK, Hui Y, Borschel D, et al. A scoping review of undergraduate ambulatory care education. *Med Teach.* 2013;35:444–453.
4. Lawrence SL, Lindemann JC, Gottlieb M. What students value: learning outcomes in a required third-year ambulatory primary care clerkship. *Acad Med.* 1999;74:715–717.
5. Helman CG. Disease versus illness in general practice. *J R Coll Gen Pract.* 1981;31:548–552.
6. Cassell EJ. *The Healer's Art: A New Approach To The Doctor-Patient Relationship.* London: Penguin Books; 1978.
7. Borrell-Carrió F, Suchman AL, Epstein RM. The biopsychosocial model 25 years later: principles, practice, and scientific inquiry. *Ann Fam Med.* 2004;2:576–582.

8. Burkett GL. Culture, illness, and the biopsychosocial model. *Fam Med.* 1991;23:287–291.

9. Egnew TR. The art of medicine: seven skills that promote mastery. *Fam Pract Manag.* 2014;21:25–30.

10. Stewart EE, Fox CH. Encouraging patients to change unhealthy behaviors with motivational interviewing. *Fam Pract Manag.* 2011;18:21–25.

11. Boxer H, Snyder S. Five communication strategies to promote self-management of chronic illness—family practice management. *Fam Pract Manag.* 2009;16:12–16.

12. Funnell MM. Helping patients take charge of their chronic illnesses—family practice management. *Fam Pract Manag.* 2000;7:47–51.

13. Lubarsky S, Dory V, Audétat MC, et al. Using script theory to cultivate illness script formation and clinical reasoning in health professions education. *Can Med Educ J.* 2015;6:e61–e70.

14. Stern SDC, Cifu AS, Altkorn D. *Symptom to Diagnosis: An Evidence-Based Guide.* New York: McGraw-Hill Medical; 2010.

15. Helman CG. The role of context in primary care. *J R Coll Gen Pract.* 1984;34:547–550.

16. Adams J, Murray III R. The general approach to the difficult patient. *Emerg Med Clin North Am.* 1998; 16:689–700.

17. Hull S, Broquet K. How to manage difficult patient encounters—family practice management. *Fam Pract Manag.* 2007;14:30–34.

18. 10 Unwritten rules about surviving the third year. *Medscape.* Available from: http://www.medscape.com/viewarticle/742090. Accessed December 8, 2016.

19. Tips on making the most of each rotation. Available from: http://www.aafp.org/dam/AAFP/documents/medical_education_residency/fmig/tips_rotations.pdf. Accessed December 8, 2016.

20. Wolpaw T, Wolpaw D, Papp K. SNAPPS: a learner-centered model for outpatient education. *Acad Med.* 2003;78(9):893–898.

21. Hammoud MM, Dalymple JL, Christner JG, et al. Medical student documentation in electronic health records: a collaborative statement from the alliance for clinical education. *Teach Learn Med.* 2012;24(3): 257–266.

22. AAMC Compliance Advisory: Electronic Health Records (EHRs) in Academic Health Centers (2014). Available from: https://www.aamc.org/download/316610/data/advisory3achallengefortheelectronichealthrecordsofacademicinsti.pdf. Accessed December 8, 2016.

23. CMS Manual, Transmittal 2303. Teaching physician service (2011). Available from: https://www.cms.gov/Regulations-and-Guidance/Guidance/Transmittals/downloads/R2303CP.pdf. Accessed December 8, 2016.

24. Ventres W, Kooienga S, Marlin R. EHRs in the exam room: tips on patient-centered care—family practice management. *Fam Pract Manag.* 2006;13:45–47.

25. White B. Improving chronic disease care in the real world: a step-by-step approach—family practice management. *Fam Pract Manag.* 1999;6:38–43.

26. Kibbe DC, Johnson K. Do-it-yourself disease management—family practice management. *Fam Pract Manag.* 1998;5:34–42.

27. Von Korff M, Glasgow RE, Sharpe M. Organising care for chronic illness. *BMJ.* 2002;325:92–94.

28. Gorrindo P, Peltz A, Ladner TR, et al. Medical students as health educators at a student-run free clinic: improving the clinical outcomes of diabetic patients. *Acad Med.* 2014;89:625–631.

29. Bell K, Cole BA. Improving medical students' success in promoting health behavior change: a curriculum evaluation. *J Gen Intern Med.* 2008;23:1503–1506.

30. HHS.gov. About the ACA, Preventive Care. Available from: https://www.hhs.gov/healthcare/about-the-aca/preventive-care/index.html

31. Cordasco KM. *Obtaining Informed Consent from Patients: Brief Update Review. Making Health Care Safer II: An Updated Critical Analysis of the Evidence for Patient Safety Practices.* Rockville (MD): Agency for Healthcare Research and Quality; 2013.

Behavior Change

KEY POINTS

1 ▸ Physician communication skills predict adherence, and clinical outcomes improve among patients with chronic illnesses such as diabetes and hypertension with good physician communication.

2 ▸ While biomedicine has traditionally focused on disease, patient-centered care expands upon pathophysiology to include illness—the patient's experience of their disease process and symptoms.

3 ▸ The historical shift from the morbidity and mortality associated with infectious disease to chronic illnesses, which are very much influenced by behavior, adherence, and modifiable risk factors, has changed the physician–patient relationship.

4 ▸ Effective chronic disease prevention and management requires doctor–patient collaboration. The development of effective counseling skills has become a core competency for primary care clinicians.

Patient centered care is one of the six main elements of the Institute of Medicine's quality criteria.[1] This chapter presents three models of patient-centered counseling for primary care clinicians. The first, the **BATHE technique** is useful with both mental health problems as well as psychosocial aspects of both acute and chronic illness. **Stages of Change** counseling and **Motivational Interviewing**, models two and three, are strategies typically used when health-related behaviors such as adherence, smoking, alcohol use, improved diet, and or exercise are the focus of the intervention.

> 30–60% of ambulatory care patients have a psychosocial component to their symptoms

BATHE

One of the distinctive features of family medicine as a specialty is the emphasis on viewing patients within a biopsychosocial context in which biologic, psychological, and social factors interact.[2,3] In addition, patient-centered care expands upon pathophysiology to include illness—the patient's experience of their disease process and symptoms.[4]

Developed by a psychologist and family physician, the BATHE technique typically requires only 5 to 10 minutes.[5] BATHE is an acronym in which each letter is associated with a successive question or statement from the physician, as shown below. Patients receiving BATHE report higher levels of satisfaction with their medical care and are more likely to recommend their physician to others.[6,7]

BATHE questions are typically asked immediately after obtaining a clear picture of the patient's presenting problem and before conducting a physical examination.

Ms. Johnston is a 44-year-old African-American woman who comes to see Dr. Reddy with a concern about headache and fatigue. For the past 2 months, she has felt tired and run down throughout the day. She has had nearly daily headaches, experienced as a tight band around her forehead without nausea, vomiting, or photophobia. She also indicates that she has had trouble staying asleep throughout the night, frequently waking up for about 1 hour at least twice. For the past 3 years, she has been treated for hypertension with losartan and hydrochlorothiazide, with good control. Today, Ms. Johnston's blood pressure is 165/90 mm Hg.

The elements of the **BATHE** interview technique are as follows:

▶ **B**ackground: This begins with an open-ended question that allows the patient to raise relevant physical, psychological, and social concerns. Physicians sometimes fear that open-ended queries will require prolonged, time-consuming patient responses, but most research suggests that this fear is unfounded—most patients verbalize their primary concern within 60 seconds and up to 90% will be finished within 2 minutes.[8]

Dr. Reddy states, "This sounds very difficult. Talk to me more about what has been going on..." Ms. Johnston reports that approximately 4 months ago her mother died. Since then, she has overseen managing her mother's estate. Ms. Johnston indicates that she is the oldest of six adult children and that her siblings "all have an opinion about what I should be doing."

▶ **A**ffect: A patient's affect provides information about the subjective significance of life events as well as influencing the development of rapport. Clinicians should not assume they know how a patient feels, they should ask. For example, for a patient undergoing divorce, one might expect them to be sad because of relationship loss. However, if the relationship has been abusive, the most salient emotion may be relief. Physician attention to the patient's emotional state is positively associated with self-management of chronic disease and reduced anxiety.[9]

Dr. Reddy asks: "Tell me about how you have been feeling about this?" Ms. Johnston reports feeling both sad and irritable. "I'm snapping at my husband, my kids—they really haven't done anything wrong, they don't deserve it."

▶ **T**roubles: A physician should now ask: "What troubles you **most** about this?" This question elicits a specific dimension of the problem that is of greatest concern to the patient. It is particularly helpful in situations where the patient seems to be globally overwhelmed—"I don't know where to start; everything is a mess."

You should not assume that you necessarily know what most troubles the patient. For example, if one just found out about a spouse having an extramarital affair, you might think that being able to trust the partner and feelings of betrayal would be likely responses. However, the patient may already have decided to terminate the relationship and is currently more worried about finances and raising a child as a single parent.

> Dr. Reddy asks: "What troubles you most about this?" Ms. Johnston indicates what bothers her the most about the situation is that her younger siblings are now looking to her for advice and financial support. Her mother had previously filled this role and as the oldest, her siblings are now looking to her to fill this parental role.

▶ **H**andling: This question assesses patients' coping skills. Often, patients are handling the situation as best as could be expected but certainly appreciate the physician's validation of their efforts.

Coping can be divided into two general categories—emotion focused and problem focused.[10] When a situation is uncontrollable, emotion-focused coping leads to better patient outcomes. In uncontrollable situations, such as death of a parent, effort should initially be focused on asking patients how they have handled similar situations in the past. Emotion management can take many forms including scheduled time for exercise, talking with friends, or engaging in recreational activities such as watching movies.

Patients should also be asked to generate **their own solutions to the problem**. The physician should encourage problem solving when patients can directly act to change a difficult situation. For example, for victims of domestic violence, obtaining information about affordable apartments or, if necessary, how to obtain a restraining order, are active coping strategies.

> Dr. Reddy states: "That sounds very difficult. How do you feel you are handling these challenges?" Ms. Johnston reports that she has friends and a supportive social network at her church. She feels she needs to convey to her siblings that she is grieving too and while interested in their well-being, cannot replace their mother's role.

▶ **E**mpathy: By acknowledging the situation and accompanying feelings, the physician validates the patient's experience and confirms that they have genuinely been listening. Empathy can take the form of simple to complex statements. In BATHE, an empathic statement is used to close the brief counseling part of the encounter. In a typical outpatient visit, the clinician would then go to symptom-focused questioning and the physical examination.

> Dr, Reddy states: "Given the circumstances I can completely understand why you would feel that way." Ms. Johnston says that she was not entirely aware how upset she was about the situation until talking about it with the physician. She acknowledges that since her mother's death she may not have been consistent in taking her blood pressure medication. She also wonders if her headaches may be related to stress.

STAGES OF CHANGE (TRANS-THEORETICAL MODEL)

Stages of change emerged from an in-depth study of 18 models of psychotherapy. While specific interventions associated with patient change were fairly well understood, Prochaska and colleagues[11] found that relatively little was known about the process by which patients actually change. As part of their research, they obtained narrative accounts from smokers who had successfully quit and those who had not. While we often think of quitting smoking as an all or nothing event ("going cold turkey"), successful quitters described a series of stages leading to successful smoking cessation. These changes include precontemplation, contemplation, preparation, action, and maintenance (Table 5.1).

Mr. Martindale is a 47-year-old white man seeing you today for frequent coughing of approximately 6-weeks duration, productive of clear mucus. You note in his record that he has been seen for a similar concern several times in the past 2 years. His symptoms are becoming more frequent. He has a 44-pack/year history of smoking and is currently smoking two packs of cigarettes daily. He has been advised to quit smoking multiple times previously. He takes no medication. His blood pressure today is 145/90 mm Hg and his temperature is 99.4°F. Examination reveals coarse rhonchi with wheezing.

Mr. Martindale's increasing cough and bronchitis are likely related to his smoking which provides an opportunity to move his interest in quitting along the stages of change. On questioning, he believes that these coughing episodes are related to smoking and he can now see a benefit to quitting. He has been thinking about quitting but failed in the past, so is reluctant.

Some patients are not able to maintain abstinence from the behavior but return to their previous behavior pattern. In quitting smoking (or abstaining from alcohol), a common cognitive pattern is "abstinence violation effect"[12]: a patient views lapse as evidence of helplessness and inability to change. It is particularly important in this case for the clinician to avoid conveying disappointment or implying that the patient has failed; rather point to the patient's prior successes. For example, the clinician could state "I don't see the situation as hopeless—you didn't smoke for 10 months—that is quite an achievement. You obviously did many things right." Alternatively, the clinician should explore reasons for restarting the behavior. "Tell me about the period in which you were doing well and the situation that triggered drinking—it sounds like something must have caught you off guard—probably something you didn't expect."

Relapse is part of the change process: ex-smokers report an average of 4–5 attempts at quitting[13]

Because of the duration and number of cigarettes Mr. Martindale has been smoking per day, it is likely that he will experience pronounced nicotine withdrawal with quitting. Therefore, nicotine replacement in the form of gum or patches or medication such as bupropion or varenicline would increase the likelihood of success (Chapter 23). After discussion about his prior success with quitting and pitfalls, you provide a prescription for bupropion to begin several weeks before his quit date. You suggest that Mr. Martindale remove smoking-related stimuli from his environment; this may include thoroughly cleaning the carpets and drapes in his home and having his car detailed.

At a 3-month follow-up visit, Mr. Martindale described how he had been at a party where he found several of his friends smoking. One of his friends offered him a cigarette. Mr. Martindale said it was difficult for him because he felt like he was being rude to his friends by not joining them. Smoking on the porch with his friends was a habit for Mr. Martindale and his initial impulse was to accept the cigarette. However, he stated that he thanked his friend, told him he had recently quit smoking and went back inside.

Table 5.1 ▶ The Stages of Change and Questions for the Patient

Stage	Readiness to Change	Questions to Ask the Patient
Precontemplation	No interest in changing; has not considered making changes Clinicians should limit time spent, but provide an opening to discuss in the future	• Do you mind if I ask about your smoking[a]? • Have you thought at all about cutting down on your smoking? • Has your smoking created any problems for you? • What would tell you that it might be time to think about cutting down or stopping smoking?
Contemplation	Considering change in the next 6 months Clinicians should acknowledge intent, and support and provide preparatory information	It sounds like you are seriously thinking about stopping smoking. • What do you see as the benefits from quitting? • What might you miss or have to give up if you quit smoking? • What would be the hardest part of quitting? • How would others in your life respond if you stopped smoking?
Preparation	Patient plans to initiate change within the next 30 days Clinician can help the patient set a quit date, provide support and information to increase success, medication if needed, and follow-up	It sounds like you made up your mind to stop smoking. Tell me more about that. • How can I be of help? • What made you decide it was time? • What specific plan do you have to keep from smoking/drinking?
Action	Patient has made the behavior change but it has been in place for less than 6 months Clinicians should listen, support, help problem solve as needed, and follow up	You are doing great without smoking! You made it through 2 months. That is quite impressive. • Are you experiencing any craving at all? • How have you been managing those episodes of craving? • Did any obstacles come up that you did not expect? • How are others in your life supporting your change? • What has been the most challenging situation so far? How did you handle it?
Maintenance	Behavior change has been present for more than 6 months Clinicians should help patients anticipate slips and provide support and follow-up as needed	• Have you had any periods where you slipped up? • How long did the slip-up last? • What was the trigger? • How did you get yourself back on track? • What did you learn from the experience? • It is hard to predict all the challenges that someone will face; are there other situations that seem to be particularly challenging?

[a]The questions can apply to any type of behavior such as drinking or drug use.

MOTIVATIONAL INTERVIEWING

> "Motivational interviewing is a collaborative conversation style for strengthening a person's own motivation and commitment to change"[14]

Motivational interviewing, originally developed for substance abuse treatment, was a major departure from long-standing counseling practices. In contrast to the confrontational, shame-based treatment approach that was popular through the 1990s, William Miller found that patients were more successful at reducing drug and alcohol use when therapists were empathic and supportive.[15,16] Since Miller's original work, motivational interviewing has been applied in a wide range of medical settings including emergency departments, nephrology clinics, and outpatient primary care.[14] Motivational interviewing has proved useful for increasing adherence with diabetic and asthma treatment regimens as well as diet, exercise, and smoking cessation.

Basic Assumptions

Similar to the stages of change, motivational interviewing recognizes that people experience considerable ambivalence about making major lifestyle changes. However, rather than direct education about the benefits of stopping smoking or reducing drinking, motivational interviewing uses focused, Socratic questioning to elicit the patient's own "change talk." Motivational interviewing also recognizes that because of ambivalence, patients may resist change. Rather than viewing resistance as the patient's problem, motivational interviewing characterizes resistance as a way that the patient maintains autonomy as well as being a signal to the physician about the patient's movement between the poles of ambivalence.

The Spirit of Motivational Interviewing

Practicing motivational interviewing effectively involves more than learning a set of interview techniques. Instead, the physician' worldview must expand beyond rational, directive patient education to **becoming an empathic listener and questioner**. Maintaining a stance of respectful inquisitiveness is often challenging especially when patients do not themselves recognize the risks of their behavior.

There are four basic motivational interviewing dimensions that need to be incorporated to maintain the spirit of motivational interviewing:

▶ **Resist the righting reflex:** When patients are practicing behaviors that are clearly harmful to their health or verbalizing misconceptions about the impact of alcohol use, high fat diets, smoking, or sedentary lifestyle, a normal reaction is to highlight the problem and make recommendations, to try to "fix it." In many cases, however, patients are well aware that they are drinking too much and that smoking is harmful to their health. Paradoxically, additional health education is likely to elicit reactance— exerting autonomy in the face of efforts to persuade. **For motivational interviewing to be effective, patients must generate the reasons for changing themselves. The clinician's job is to keep the patient in conversation and to avoid the righting reflex.**

Signs of the righting reflex

1. "You should…."
2. "I want you to…."
3. "You really need to…."

▸ **Understand patient values:** While reducing the patient's alcohol use may be helpful in maintaining health and reducing the risk of liver disease, the patient may have a different motivation for change, and often does. Often, a key value that motivates health behavior change is to maintain or strengthen relationships with family, coworkers, or friends. **The logical medical reasons for change may not be the patient's priority.**

▸ **Listen carefully: Being carefully and genuinely listened to by someone with a desire to understand is a powerful experience and quickly builds a relationship of trust.** In a busy practice, when a patient is speaking, it is common to be considering a protocol for differential diagnosis or the next symptom-focused question. When your clinical problem solving distracts you from hearing the patient, remind yourself to listen carefully—it will save time in the long run.

▸ **Encourage and highlight patient choice:** When considering smoking cessation, weight loss, dietary change for type 2 diabetes or the optimal time of day for dialysis, patients typically know what will work best for them. However, to enhance patient commitment it is often helpful to ask patients directly how they could best implement lifestyle changes. This creates a collaborative relationship, which will likely enhance patient adherence.

Key Motivational Interview Counseling Principles

Express Empathy

Motivational interviewing is not a form of manipulative counseling designed to get patients to adhere to medical advice, nor is it cheerleading. Instead, the patient's own values and priorities become a driving force for change. Framing effective Socratic questions requires an understanding of what is important to the patient. In addition, patients are less likely to be open to new input if they do not feel understood. While smoking cessation and dietary intervention for the patient with metabolic syndrome may seem logical and straightforward, patients may experience these as major life challenges and doubt their ability to be successful.

Develop Discrepancy

Cognitive dissonance is a major force for propelling the patient to change health behavior. In response to the physician's skillful Socratic questions, the patient verbalizes personal values or goals while coming to recognize that these aspirations are inconsistent with their health behavior. This cognitive dissonance creates discomfort and is associated with a drive toward resolution. The resolution can only occur with a change in core values (which is unlikely) *or* change in the current behavior that is inconsistent with the patient's goals. Again, through the physician's questioning, patients verbalize this discrepancy, themselves.

Roll with Resistance

When patients feel that their autonomy is threatened by an external influence, it is natural to try to preserve independence. When faced with the righting reflex, many patients automatically move toward the "no" end of the ambivalence continuum. Statements of resistance ("I can't stop drinking now—not with this overbearing supervisor I have to deal with every day") often indicate that the patient feels that the physician has not really heard them or appreciates the depth of their struggle. Put differently, the physician has not yet learned how to cooperate with the patient.

Enhance Self-Efficacy

Physicians cannot make the changes that patients need to undertake to move their lives forward. Encourage your patients to explore and recognize that they can achieve their own goals by helping them recognize their own strengths and self-determination. As Miller notes, patients have a "deep well of wisdom and experience" for the physician to activate. Patients know that heavy smoking or drinking is not beneficial but may not experience a level of self-confidence to change.

> Not-so-good motivational interviewing
> https://www.youtube.com/watch?v=80XyNE89eCs
> Good example of motivational interviewing
> https://www.youtube.com/watch?v=URiKA7CKtfc

It can be helpful to ask the patient about challenges that they have overcome in their lives. Patients who have, for a period of time, successfully stopped drinking, smoking, increased their physical activity, maintained a healthy diet, or adhered to a chronic disease medication regimen, have a foundation of success. However, patients may not recognize these strengths unless the physician is deliberate in asking about them. For example, the patient who maintained smoking cessation for 3 months before relapsing has successfully navigated the period in which physical distress and craving is at its peak. A discussion of this success will likely enhance the next smoking cessation attempt.

OARS: Specific Interviewing Techniques for Motivational Interviewing[17]

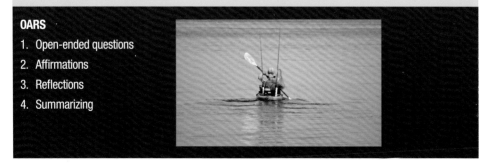

OARS
1. Open-ended questions
2. Affirmations
3. Reflections
4. Summarizing

▶ **Open-Ended Questions:** Begin encounters with an open-ended question. In contrast to symptom specific questions ("How long have you had pain?" or "Where does it hurt the most?"), open-ended queries ("What brings you in today" or "Tell me more about how you are handling this?") encourage the patient to be an active collaborator in their care. While responses to open-ended queries reveal the patient's agenda for the clinical encounter, they often reveal the patient's perspective on the significance of symptoms as well as underlying values.

▶ **Affirmations:** Motivational interviewing uses affirmations to activate patients' strengths. By pointing out how the patient has overcome adversity in the past or their desire to make a genuine lifestyle change, the physician is highlighting patient strengths and competencies that can be built upon. ("I am impressed with your determination to make regular exercise a part of your life.") It is important that the physician's statements are sincere rather than contrived compliments. However, even small steps can be responded to genuine positive recognition. For example, a patient's willingness to tolerate the discomfort of a conversation about the pros and cons of alcohol use is an achievement to be acknowledged.

▶ **Reflections:** Simply re-stating what the patient has told you conveys that you are listening. Reflecting understanding of the patient's concerns is also a useful way to "track" the conversation as well as to be sure that you are accurately understanding the information provided. More sophisticated reflections can highlight both sides of patient ambivalence.

▶ **Summarizing:** A good summary ties together patients' reasons for seeking care, the meaning of their symptoms, an explanation of their condition/symptoms, and serves as the foundation for moving to the next step. Summarizing what the patient has said also conveys that the physician has been listening carefully. In addition, a useful summary conveys the patient's perspective in an integrated way that hopefully leads them to take the next action step. ("Until we discussed it today, you did not really appreciate the effect of using marijuana every day on your ability to concentrate on your schoolwork. Doing well in college is also obviously clearly important to you. What do you think would be the best strategy for cutting down?".)

How to Provide Information within Motivational Interviewing

Up to this point, the focus has been on appreciating the patient's perspective. Physicians, however, also have responsibility for providing relevant information. While motivational interviewing's focus is for the patient to generate their own reasons and motivation for change, patients may be unaware of or operating on misinformation about health risks.

Asking permission before presenting information ("Would it be ok if I shared some information about drinking alcohol during pregnancy?") provides the patient with a sense of control. The patient will also have greater personal investment in the discussion since they are consciously choosing to receive the information. After receiving permission, the physician can relate the information in a neutral, factual manner. After this description, if the patient does not respond, the physician should probe: "What is your reaction to that information?"

Ms. Richardson is a 28-year-old woman seeing you today for a health maintenance visit. The nurse's note indicates she would like to talk about discontinuing her birth control because she has decided she would like to become pregnant. Ms. Richardson and her husband own a restaurant. They routinely have three or four drinks with several of the staff immediately after the restaurant closes.

In the past, you have pointed out to her that consumption of more than three drinks at a time for women is considered excessive drinking. Ms. Richardson's response was: "I'm not an alcoholic, it's just the way that we all wind down after work. If I didn't have a few drinks, I don't think I'd ever get to sleep after getting wound up running that restaurant all night." To eliminate alcohol while pregnant, you will need to address two currently conflicting values—the need to temporarily "de-stress" at work and a desire to have a healthy infant.

You say the following using your best motivational interviewing technique: "Ms. Richardson, before we discuss discontinuing your birth control, I would like to summarize what I'm hearing. Drinking after work is a habit that dates back 7 to 8 years and has been the most consistent strategy that you have used to deal with the stress of a hectic work day. While it relaxes you, you've begun to notice that you feel "foggy" during the early part of the next day and wonder if the alcohol is doing this. You are also interested in getting pregnant within the next year."

After asking for permission to discuss alcohol and pregnancy you proceed: "It is recommended that women not drink alcohol when they are pregnant or actively trying to get pregnant. Drinking during pregnancy is associated with having a baby with both physical problems and developmental delays which they do not outgrow. What are your thoughts about that information?"

Note that phrases such as "your baby" or "You should not…" are deliberately avoided to reduce defensiveness.

Responding to or "Rolling With" Resistance

There are times when patients indicate overtly or covertly that they do not agree with the clinician that their health behavior is a problem. This may be expressed through nonverbal signals such as looking at the floor, sighing, rolling their eyes, or checking their watch. If the patient becomes disengaged during the discussion, it is important to verbally address the behavior in a noncritical manner. If the patient's response is not addressed, the likelihood of adherence or further consideration of behavior change is greatly diminished.

Behavior suggesting a "missed connection"
▶ Nonverbally ignoring the physician
▶ Interrupting
▶ Arguing
▶ Minimizing
▶ Silence

Physicians and patients often have a "missed connection" because the patient does not say anything overt indicating their disagreement with the treatment plan. They may appear inattentive, simply become quiet or change the subject. (*"OK Doctor—I get what you're saying about my drinking but could you look at these calluses on my feet—they really hurt."*) When these behaviors occur, there are several responses that are helpful. Simply saying

"I noticed that you got quiet. Was there something I said that bothered you or made you uncomfortable?" or "When we were talking about your smoking, I sense I may have missed something important to you; could you tell me what that was?" or finally, "I felt like we somehow got disconnected a few minutes ago. Where did we get off track?"

These interactions suggest that the physician has missed something important. You may have misjudged the patient's stage in the trans-theoretical continuum, overestimated the patient's experience of self-efficacy, or simply lapsed into educator mode without asking the patient's permission first. As in these examples, raising your observation will usually get the encounter back on track.

CONCLUSION

Physician communication skills predict adherence and good physician communication leads to improved clinical outcomes for patients with chronic illnesses such as diabetes and hypertension.[18] Several focused counseling strategies have been provided for your work with patients in the ambulatory setting. While BATHE, Stages of Change, and motivational interviewing have been presented as distinct approaches, these techniques often overlap. Primary care patients often do not fit into specific categories. For example, smoking cessation may be a presenting problem, but at the same time the patient may be struggling with symptoms of depression and/or anxiety related to family or work dynamics. In actual practice, you may want to consider using these strategies at the beginning and end of an office visit. For the purposes of differential diagnosis and fact gathering, you will need to ask closed-ended questions and conduct an appropriate physical examination. Open-ended questions, however, often yield richer information and engage patients and physicians more deeply in caring work.

ACTIVITY

▶ **Practice Motivational Interviewing:** Most of us have habits that we would like to change. We might like to improve our diet, increase our exercise level or even our daily intake of fluids. This exercise works best if there are three participants. Have one of the participants present a problem—it can be real or fictional—while the other uses motivational interviewing principles to address the concern. The third person should be an observer who pays attention to the extent to which both the spirit and the specific techniques of motivational interviewing are accurately implemented. Give yourself 5–10 minutes per scenario with subsequent feedback. Both the interviewer and the "patient" should remember that ambivalence is a significant factor in any lifestyle change.

QUESTIONS

1. Motivational Interviewing is best considered as:
   A. Convincing patients to change their lifestyles.
   B. Cheerleading.
   C. Trying to get patients to see the doctor's point of view.
   D. Preventing relapse in patients who have changed their lifestyle.
   E. Facilitated change talk discussion to strengthen a person's motivation to change.

2. During a discussion of a patient's weight, a physician states: "I really think you should set a goal of losing 15 pounds within the next 3 months." This is an example of:
   A. The righting reflex.
   B. Stage of change "action" talk.
   C. Motivational interviewing.
   D. Understanding the patient's values.
   E. Developing discrepancy.

3. You are working with a patient who is trying to reduce or discontinue her problematic alcohol consumption. Choose the best question that will allow a patient who is in the contemplation stage of change to further their thinking.
   A. "Have you thought at all about cutting down on your drinking?"
   B. "What plan have you considered in reducing your alcohol use?"
   C. "It sounds like you are serious about cutting down or quitting…."
   D. "What did you learn about the last experience of trying to quit?"

4. Which one is correct when recalling the BATHE technique?
   A. B = Behavior
   B. A = Affect
   C. T = Thoughts
   D. H = Help
   E. E = Examples

5. In working with a patient who is considering making a change in their illicit drug use, a physician skilled in facilitating behavior change might try to help the patient verbalize personal values or goals while coming to recognize that these aspirations are inconsistent with their health behavior. This process is called which of the following?
   A. Rolling with resistance.
   B. Righting reflex.
   C. Enhancing self-efficacy.
   D. Developing discrepancy or cognitive dissonance.

ANSWERS

Question 1: The correct answer is E.
Motivational interviewing is a collaborative conversation style for strengthening a person's own motivation and commitment to change. Motivational interviewing uses focused, Socratic questioning to elicit the patient's own "change talk."

Question 2: The correct answer is A.
When patients are practicing behaviors that are clearly harmful to their health or verbalizing misconceptions about the impact of alcohol use, high fat diets, smoking, or sedentary lifestyle, a normal reaction is to highlight the problem and make recommendations, to try to "fix it" (the Righting Reflex). Signs of the Righting Reflex are statements beginning with "You should," "I want you," or "You really need to."

Question 3: The correct answer is C.
As shown in Table 5.1, for patients in the contemplative stage of change, clinicians should acknowledge intent, and support and provide preparatory information. Examples of questions to ask patients in this stage include: "It sounds like you are seriously thinking about stopping smoking. What do you see as the benefits from quitting?"

Question 4: The correct answer is B.

BATHE is an interview technique. The acronym BATHE stands for Background, Affect, Troubles (you most), Handling, and Empathy.

Question 5: The correct answer is D.

Cognitive dissonance is a major force for propelling the patient to change health behavior. In response to the physician's skillful Socratic questions, the patient verbalizes personal values or goals while coming to recognize that these aspirations are inconsistent with their health behavior.

REFERENCES

1. Institute of Medicine (IOM). *Crossing the Quality Chasm: A New Health System for the 21st Century.* Washington, DC: National Academy Press; 2001.
2. Friedman CP, Slatt LM, Baker RM, et al. Identifying the content of family medicine for educational purposes: an empirical approach. *Acad Med.* 1983;58(1):51–57.
3. Engel G. The need for a new medical model: A challenge for biomedicine. *Science.* 1977;196:129–136.
4. Kleinman A. *The Illness Narratives: Suffering, Healing, and the Human Condition.* New York, NY: Basic Books; 1988.
5. Stuart M, Lieberman. *The Fifteen Minute Hour: Therapeutic Talk in Primary Care* 5th ed. Abdington, UK: Radcliffe Publishers; 2015.
6. Leiblum SR, Schnall E, Seehuus M, et al. To BATHE or not to BATHE: Patient satisfaction with visits to their family physician. *Fam Med.* 2008;40(6):407–411.
7. Kim JH, Park YN, Park EW, et al. Effects of BATHE interview protocol on patient satisfaction. *Korean J Fam Med.* 2012;33(6):366–371.
8. Roter DL, Stewart M, Putnam SM, et al. Communication patterns of primary care physicians. *JAMA.* 1997; 277(4):350–356.
9. Kalavana TV. Responding to emotions. In: Brown J, Noble LM, Papageorgiou A, Kidd J, eds. *Clinical Communication in Medicine.* Chichester, UK: John Wiley & Sons, Ltd; 2015.
10. Bond FW, Bunce D. Mediators of change in emotion-focused and problem-focused worksite stress management interventions. *J Occup Health Psychol.* 2000;5(1):156–163.
11. Prochaska JO, DiClemente CC, Carlo C. Transtheoretical therapy: Toward a more integrative model of change. *Psychother Res.* 1982;19(3):276–288.
12. Curry S, Marlatt GA, Gordon JR. Abstinence violation effect: Validation of an attributional construct with smoking cessation. *J Consult Clin Psychol.* 1987;55(2):145–149.
13. Borland R, Partos TR, Yong HH, et al. How much unsuccessful quitting activity is going on among adult smokers? Data from the International Tobacco Control Four Country cohort survey. *Addiction.* 2012;107(3):673–682.
14. Miller WR, Rollnick S. *Motivational interviewing: Helping people change.* 3rd ed. New York, NY: Guilford; 2013.
15. Miller WR, Rose GS. Toward a theory of motivational interviewing. *Am Psychol.* 2009;64(6):527–537.
16. Smith J, Carpenter K, Wain R, et al. Motivational interviewing. In: A. Mack, et al. *Clinical Handbook of Addictive Disorders.* New York, NY: Guilford; 2016.
17. Rollnick S, Miller W, Butler C. *Motivational Interviewing in Health Care Settings.* New York, NY: Guilford; 2008.
18. Haskard Zolnierek KB, DiMatteo MR. Physician communication and patient adherence to treatment: A meta-analysis. *Medical Care.* 2009;47(8):826–834.

Patient Safety in Primary Care

KEY POINTS

1 ▶ Medical errors are the mistakes made during the care of patients. They can occur when a correct decision or action is made but does not get carried out appropriately or when the original decision or action is incorrect.

2 ▶ Adverse events are harmful outcomes to patients that occur from medical care. When they are due to error they are called preventable adverse events.

3 ▶ The most common types of errors in family medicine are medication errors, testing process errors, and diagnostic errors. Contributing factors to these errors include communication, systems, and thinking problems.

4 ▶ Family medicine offices are clinical microsystems where physicians, staff, patients, and processes come together for the purpose of quality care for patients. High-quality microsystems are more likely to find errors earlier and have fewer errors and preventable adverse events.

5 ▶ When errors and preventable adverse events occur, physicians should disclose the error to the patient and also care for themselves and their teams.

It's morning huddle time at your family medicine clerkship office. Dr. Jones, her MA, Mark, the front desk clerk, Linda, and you are quickly reviewing today's appointments prior to starting the office session. Helga Johnson is scheduled at 10 AM, to follow up on her diabetes. She hasn't been in the office in 6 months, but was doing pretty well at the last visit. Mark looks up from reviewing the EMR and says, "Dr. Jones, you did a punch biopsy on a skin lesion 6 months ago, and the results showed a skin cancer. I don't see that we ever notified the patient." A scan through the patient's electronic chart by everyone in the huddle confirms that this result was never conveyed to the patient.

Experiences like this are scary for doctors, students, office staff, and patients. Something goes wrong, a mistake is made, and a patient potentially is harmed. While more attention has been paid to errors that occur in the hospital versus the doctor's office, the importance of errors in the office setting has become increasingly studied in recent years. The goal of this chapter is to discuss the most common errors in outpatient settings, how to prevent them, and how to deal with victims of errors (including "second victims"—healthcare workers involved in error). But first, we need to understand exactly what is meant by medical error, and how error, safety, and adverse events relate to each other, and to our care of patients in the office.

Sometimes, patients experience adverse outcomes. If the adverse outcome is due to medical care, rather than the disease or illness, it is called an adverse event (Fig. 6.1A). An unpreventable adverse event happens predictably, like hair loss after chemotherapy for cancer or possibly candida vaginitis after a course of antibiotics. A preventable adverse event occurs when an error occurs, like a rash from amoxicillin prescribed to patient who is allergic to penicillin.

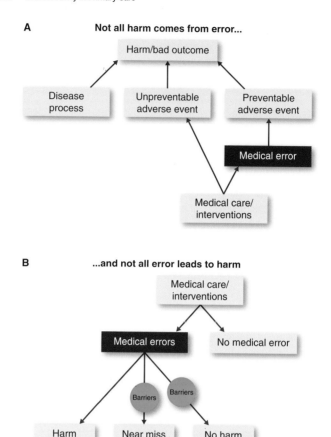

Figure 6.1 ▶ **A.** Causes of adverse outcomes. **B.** Consequences of interventions.

Medical errors are mistakes made while providing care—they occur during the process of care. We can make a wrong decision, like ordering the wrong drug, making the wrong diagnosis, or forgetting to order a treatment. We can also make the correct decision, but something goes wrong in the system of care, like ordering the correct drug, but the wrong dose is dispensed at the pharmacy.

Luckily, many medical errors never reach patients, because they are discovered and corrected (Fig. 6.1B). Patients, or other healthcare providers like pharmacists or nurses, may ask a question or make an observation about a decision, and the error is discovered and changed (Fig. 6.1B, Barrier). These are called near misses. Sometimes an error does reach a patient, but there is no harm done (Fig. 6.1B, Barrier). For example, a test result never returns on a patient, but the result is normal and does not change care decisions. An error happened, but due to good luck, there was no harm done.

Patient safety includes everything we do in medicine to decrease errors and adverse events and keep patients safe. While these definitions seem pretty straightforward, in reality medical error, mistake, adverse event, and adverse incident are often used inter-changeably. It can be confusing, so when talking or reading about medical error, you should pay attention to whether the discussion is about the processes of care or the outcomes of care. Our goal is to improve outcomes, but we need to address processes to get there.

MOST COMMON ERRORS IN OUTPATIENT PRIMARY CARE SETTINGS

Identifying the most common errors in outpatient ambulatory settings is difficult. Studies have examined reports from physicians, nurses, and office staff, analyzed "incident reports," malpractice claims, medical records, billing and quality databases, and required reports to health systems and governments. Some only included errors that caused significant harm to patients, while others included anything that "should not have happened in my office and I do not want to happen again." This has led to a frequency of errors as low as 5/100,000 visits to as high as 24/100.[1-5] The most common and best studied errors in primary care are:

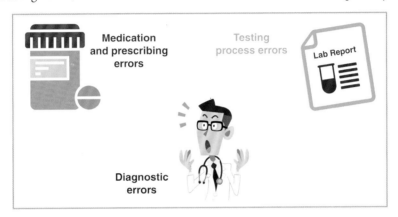

Three big factors contribute to errors:

▶ **Communication:** Doctor–patient, office staff–patient, doctor–office staff, and doctor–doctor are areas where communication occurs every day. In some studies, communication is the number one contributing factor to errors and preventable adverse events.[6]

▶ **Systems:** Our electronic medical records are the most obvious system we use in medicine, but protocols and procedures for everything we do in our offices are also important systems.

▶ **Thinking errors and bias:** Doctors use patterns to help recognize and diagnose illnesses, but sometimes doctors may jump to a wrong diagnosis because of a number of biases that we all have. Many of our patients present with undifferentiated complaints, and we try to be both efficient and cost-effective in our care, making thinking errors a common risk in primary care.

Medication Errors

Ms. Smith came to see Dr. Jones today. She is complaining of nausea, vomiting, diarrhea and weakness for the last week. Two weeks ago, she was started on hydrochlorothiazide (HCTZ) for hypertension. You begin by reviewing all of Ms. Smith's medications in her chart, which include omeprazole from Dr. Jones and citalopram from a psychiatrist at a community mental health clinic. However, Ms. Smith states that her psychiatrist stopped the citalopram and started her on lithium a couple of months ago, because he thinks she has bipolar disorder. The student looks through the chart, but doesn't see that this medication change was noted in her medication list. Dr. Jones and you realize the patient likely has lithium toxicity from the interaction of HCTZ with lithium.

Common medication errors include errors of commission (prescribing the wrong medicine or the wrong dose or medication interactions) and errors of omission (NOT prescribing needed medications). In this case, an incorrect medication list led to a serious medication interaction and the patient suffered a preventable adverse event. It is easy to see that issues with communication and systems contributed to the medical error. One way clinicians systematically evaluate what happened when an adverse event (or even a near miss) occurs is to perform a Root Cause Analysis (RCA). RCAs can involve many people for major events, especially in the hospital setting, but an RCA can also be performed simply in the office setting using the "5 Whys" technique. Start with what you know went wrong and ask "why" and then keep asking "why" for each answer. Usually by the time you get to 4 to 6 whys, you are close to knowing more about the cause of the medical error. An example of a 5 Whys analysis for this problem is shown in Figure 6.2. What other scenarios could you imagine leading to this medication interaction? You can find more information about RCAs on Patient Safety Net (PSNet) (https://psnet.ahrq.gov/primers/primer/10/root-cause-analysis).

Preventing medication errors means improving our systems and our communication, as well as our documentation. Our EMRs are only as good as the information we put into them! Digital prescribing means that we are unlikely to have errors from messy

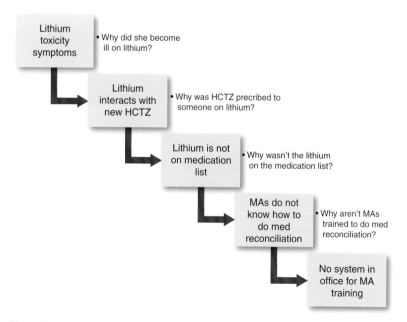

Figure 6.2 ▶ Possible 5 Whys analysis for a medication error in the office.

handwriting, but we can miss potential interactions not only from missing drugs in the medication list but from "alert overload," when we start ignoring EMR alerts for things like drug interactions because they pop-up frequently, often for minor issues. With literally hundreds of EMR systems used by physicians in the United States, there are steep learning curves for physicians as they use these complex systems.

One good tool for preventing errors is "double-checking." This happens all the time when pharmacists review prescriptions before filling them, but we can also ask our patients to serve as double-checkers by bringing their medicines with them to office visits, encouraging them to review their medicines when they get them at the pharmacy, and always asking patients about new medicines or changes they may have made in their medicines (including nonprescription and herbal medications) at every visit. What other ways can you imagine using double-checking to help decrease medication errors? https://www.ismp.org/pressroom/Patient_Broc.pdf is a great pamphlet for patients from the Institute for Safe Medication Practices.

Testing Process Errors

In the example case, we read about a pathology report on a skin biopsy that was never shared with the patient. Laboratory tests are commonly performed in family medicine, with some testing done at the "point of care" (e.g., urinalyses, blood sugars, strep screens) and other testing completed at reference laboratories. The model in Figure 6.3 shows the many steps that commonly occur from the decision to order a test through patient follow through. Some health systems may make results available to the patient at the same time as the physician. This may increase patients' abilities to see their test results quickly, but you can imagine other problems that may occur when patients get their test results before their physicians have had a chance to review and interpret them.

Errors can occur anywhere along the process. Early research reported that most errors in the testing process occurred with ordering and implementing test orders,[7,8] but recently errors in notifying patients and following through with abnormal results have been reported to be more common than previously thought (7.1% failures to inform in a 2009 study and 34% failures to follow up appropriate treatment after an abnormal

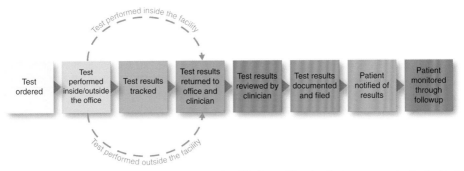

Figure 6.3 ▶ Example of an office testing process. (Modified from: Planning for Improvements. Content last reviewed August 2013. Agency for Healthcare Research and Quality, Rockville, MD. http://www.ahrq.gov/professionals/quality-patient-safety/quality-resources/tools/office-testing-toolkit/officetesting-toolkit5.html.)

result in a 2010 study).[9,10] There can also be delays in notification that can affect both patient anxiety and clinical outcomes. The part of the testing process with the fewest errors is the actual performance of the laboratory test, especially when done in reference laboratories.

The testing process is a great example of how "work systems" create both safe and risky environments for patient care. A work system includes not just the people but also the technology (EMRs, patient portals, glucose meters, etc.) and physical and organizational environment where we perform our clinical tasks. Within this work system, we provide clinical care and achieve clinical outcomes (and other outcomes, too, like creating a good place to work and learn).[11]

To have a safe, error-free testing process, we not only need a good testing process, but also a good work system. Family medicine offices are "clinical microsystems" within larger healthcare systems. A clinical microsystem is a type of work system that includes a small group of people who work together on a regular basis to provide care to discrete subpopulations of patients.[12] Details about clinical microsystems are available at http://clinicalmicrosystem.org. Successful components of a high performing microsystem guide us on how to prevent system-based errors, like those in the testing process.

Why did Dr. Jones not notify Helga Johnson about her abnormal biopsy results? The office might do a 5 Whys RCA to find out the problem, and then look at their testing process within their work system for ways to improve it. Maybe the result came back to the wrong doctor's EMR "inbox" and was ignored by that doctor, who thought Dr. Jones would take care of it. Information technology, education and training, interdependence, and patient focus areas may need attention. Or maybe the result was formatted in such a way in the computer that the abnormality was missed when Dr. Jones reviewed it—information technology, patient focus, and process improvement might be next steps.

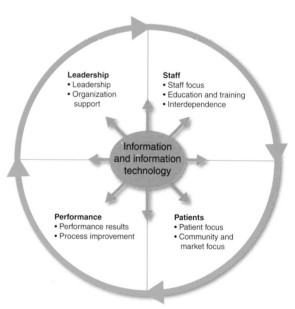

Modified from: Nelson E, Batalden PB, Huber TP, et al. Microsystems in health care: Part 1. Learning from high-performing front-line clinical units. *Jt Comm J Qual Improv.* 2002;28(9):472–493.

Diagnostic Errors

Because of the testing process error, Helga Johnson's cancer diagnosis has been delayed. System errors, especially those in the testing process (for both laboratory and imaging tests) are one of the most common causes of diagnostic delays and misdiagnoses. In one study of ambulatory care, they accounted for 44% of diagnostic errors.[13] The society to improve diagnosis in medicine (http://www.improvediagnosis.org) estimates that 1 in 10 diagnoses are incorrect and that common diagnoses (e.g., heart attack, cancer, and stroke) are among the most common diagnostic errors. In addition to system errors, cognitive or thinking errors are the other main cause of incorrect and delayed diagnoses. Cognitive errors are rarely due to lack of knowledge, but are best understood in the context of how our brains manage and process information.

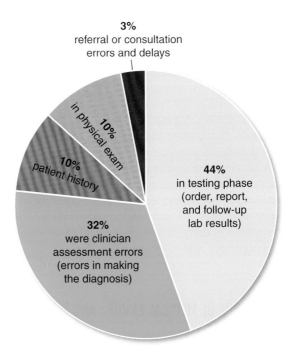

3%
referral or consultation errors and delays

10% in physical exam

10% Patient history

32% were clinician assessment errors (errors in making the diagnosis)

44% in testing phase (order, report, and follow-up lab results)

Eder M, Smith SG, Cappelman J, et al. Improving Your Office Testing Process. A Toolkit for Rapid-Cycle Patient Safety and Quality Improvement. AHRQ Publication No. 13–0035. Rockville, MD: Agency for Healthcare Research and Quality; August 2013.

Our minds make decisions using two different systems of thinking. One system (analytical reasoning or type 2) is conscious, deliberate, explicit, rational, and controlled. The other (nonanalytical reasoning or type 1) is unconscious, associative, implicit, intuitive, and automatic.[14,15] These were popularized recently as "Thinking, Fast and Slow."[16] To be successful physicians, we need both systems of thinking. Pattern recognition—quickly identifying key diagnostic criteria for everything from an upper respiratory infection to appendicitis—is a hallmark of expert decision making and allows experienced physicians to quickly see, diagnose, and manage a large number of patients in a relatively short amount of time. This type of thinking, however, can lead to cognitive errors, which can lead to diagnostic errors. Almost one hundred cognitive errors or biases have been described in medicine, but three of the most common are:

▶ **Context errors:** The physician inappropriately limits consideration to only one set of diagnostic possibilities, in lieu of others. For example, gastrointestinal causes are not considered for a patient presenting with chest pain.

▶ **Availability errors:** The physician chooses the most likely diagnosis over conditions that are rarer, or they choose conditions they are most familiar with or have seen recently. An example would be the patient with a dissecting aortic aneurysm whose chest pain is attributed to a musculoskeletal strain.

▶ **Premature closure:** Once a plausible condition is identified, other possibilities are not fully considered; we just stop thinking. This is similar to anchoring.

Probably you can think of times when you experienced one of these thinking errors. Rather than suggest that all physicians approach every patient concern in a slow, deliberate, and analytic style, recent studies suggest that medical education and work systems need to be designed to train and assist physicians to use the most appropriate thinking, what has been called "metacognition" or thinking about your thinking. This requires that medical students learn about thinking biases and receive feedback when they occur. We need to be aware of emotions and situations that make us more likely to succumb to a cognitive error, such as not liking a patient (or liking a patient too much). In clinical practice, learning a guided structured reflective process for diagnosis and using cognitive forcing strategies (requiring consideration of alternative diagnoses, for example) show promise in improving diagnostic decision making. However, the field of how to improve physicians' thinking is still relatively young.[14]

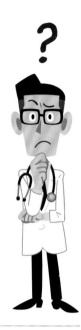

DISCLOSURE OF MEDICAL ERRORS AND THE SECOND VICTIM

Dr. Jones is not having a good week! She now has to tell Ms. Smith that she prescribed HCTZ without appropriate monitoring because her team failed to properly reconcile the medication list AND she has to tell Helga Johnson that she has skin cancer and that she missed the test result 6 months ago. Luckily, Dr. Jones received excellent training about how to disclose medical errors, and while the conversations are still difficult, she knows that her relationships with her patients are more likely to be positive if she is transparent and honest.

Thirty years ago, medicine practiced a "deny and defend" way of dealing with medical errors; physicians and other healthcare providers avoided talking about, and denied ever making, mistakes. Today, in a patient safety culture, errors are sought out so they can be mitigated and prevented, and disclosure to patients is de rigueur. Not only is disclosing errors to patients the ethically correct thing to do, studies overwhelmingly show a positive or neutral effect on the doctor–patient relationship, trust in the physician, and willingness to stay with the physician when disclosure occurs. PSNet has a primer on error disclosure at https://psnet.ahrq.gov/primers/primer/2/error-disclosure. The basic guidelines for how to disclose an error have emerged over the last 20 years and generally include the following components:

▶ Involve insurers, risk management, and the medical team when serious harm has occurred to patient.

- Do not overly delay disclosure waiting for unity, guidance, or decisions.
- Use immediate apology with delayed disclosure, if necessary:
  - Say you are sorry about harm, you believe an error was made, but you do not know all the details yet.
  - Set an appointment with the patient, family in near future for full disclosure to occur.

▶ Take the initiative; do not wait for patients to call and ask.

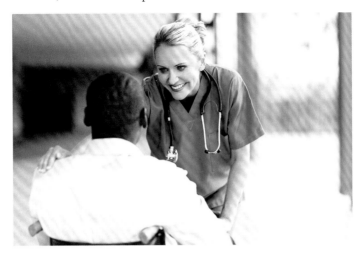

▶ Explain only what you know.
  - Accept personal responsibility, when appropriate.
  - Do not blame others, but do not hide errors of others.
  - Use nontechnical language.
  - Offer to investigate and find out information, when possible.
▶ Apologize.
  - Express sorrow, sympathy.
▶ State the actions being taken to prevent recurrences.
  - What is being done to make sure it does not happen again.
▶ Consider: Offer appropriate financial compensation.
  - Do not charge for your time or office visit.
  - Work with insurers, risk management, and/or legal staff about offering compensation.

Medical students and other learners should never take it upon themselves to disclose an error to a patient—they should be involved with the attending physician or preceptor, but the responsibility lies with the patient's physician. What is a student to do when they observe an error, but the attending does not acknowledge it or disclose it to the patient? This is a very difficult situation to be in, as students are naturally worried about their evaluations and will often think that the attending probably knows best. In such a situation, students should try to speak with the attending in an honest, but not combative manner. If this fails, or cannot be accomplished, the student should go to the course director or college leadership. When students make errors, they should disclose to the attending physician and, along with the physician, make a disclosure to the patient.

While patients should always be the first priority when dealing with a medical error, attention must also be given to healthcare providers, including physicians, staff, and students, who are involved in a medical error.[17] These people have been called the "second victims." One of the first descriptions still resonates with physicians and students today:

"Virtually every practitioner knows the sickening feeling of making a bad mistake. You feel singled out and exposed—seized by the instinct to see if anyone has noticed. You agonize about what to do, whether to tell anyone, what to say. Later, the event replays itself over and over in your mind. You question your competence but fear being discovered. You know you should confess, but dread the prospect of potential punishment and of the patient's anger. You may become overly attentive to the patient or family, lamenting the failure to do so earlier and, if you have not told them, wondering if they know."[18]

Unfortunately, while didactic teaching about medical errors has increased in the last 10 years, students rarely get important role modeling about self-care after involvement in a medical error. Positive coping mechanisms include seeking social support, receiving validation of the decision-making process, getting reaffirmation of professional competency, and reassurance of personal self-worth. This means taking time to talk about the event, and your feelings about it with a peer, a counselor, and/or a friend or loved one. Unfortunately, negative coping mechanisms also happen, including distancing one's self from others, practicing escape-avoidance, loss of confidence, and even leaving

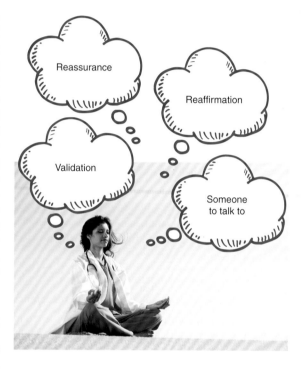

medicine. It is important to remember that medical errors will happen, but improving communication and systems, with time for "thinking about your thinking," may prevent some errors. Always put your patient first, but allow time and resources for the "second victim," as well.

For more information, the PSNet link about second victims is at https://psnet.ahrq.gov/primers/primer/30/support-for-clinicians-involved-in-errors-and-adverse-events-second-victims. Here you can read about ways second victims can not only survive medical errors, but also thrive by making something good come out of the event by getting needed support and working on making clinical changes.

Dr. Jones knows she and her team need to deal with the effect of these recent errors. They spend a staff meeting discussing the causes of the errors and how they can use the quality improvement process to prevent these errors in the future. But they also spend some time acknowledging how they feel, and validating each other as individuals and as a team. As the practice leader, Dr. Jones acknowledges the inevitability of mistakes, while committing the practice to doing all they can to prevent them.

QUESTIONS

1. Which of the following is an example of an error of omission?
   A. Prescribing an antibiotic to a patient with a known allergy to that medication.
   B. Percussing an abdomen using the incorrect technique.
   C. Testing a lipid panel in a patient with normal lipids who had one done a year ago.
   D. Doing a pelvic examination in a patient with chest pain.
   E. Not prescribing aspirin in a middle-aged smoking patient with chest pain and EKG changes.

2. You admit Mrs. Jamison to the hospital with rectal bleeding and an INR of 10.6 while taking Coumadin. You wonder if this could have happened due to something you either did or did not do and you decide to do a 5 Whys Root Cause Analysis. Which "Why" is the best place to begin in this circumstance?
   A. Why did Mrs. Jamison have an INR of 10.6?
   B. Why was she not tested more recently than 3 months ago?
   C. Why did my office not contact her to come in to have her blood tested every month?
   D. Why do not we consider the use of other oral anticoagulants for patients who have difficulty with blood test follow-up?
   E. Why is dosing with Coumadin so difficult?

3. Primary care physicians (like all physicians) are subject to thinking errors and bias. The most important reason for thinking biases in primary care physicians is:
   A. We are not as smart as other specialists.
   B. We have many patients with undifferentiated complaints and we must make decisions using pattern recognition.
   C. We do not have good electronic medical records.
   D. We are not efficient in our thinking.
   E. We have too many competing problems to address.

4. You have made a mistake of considerable significance in the care of an elderly woman with advanced dementia that may have led to her premature death. Which one of the following strategies would be useful in moving forward?
   A. Wait for the patient's family to ask about what happened.
   B. Explain but do not apologize.
   C. Involve insurers, risk management, and the medical team.
   D. Deny any significant event occurred. Her advanced dementia portended a premature death.

ANSWERS

Question 1: The correct answer is E.
Common medication errors include errors of commission (prescribing the wrong medicine or the wrong dose or medication interactions) and errors of omission (NOT prescribing needed medications).

Question 2: The correct answer is A.
A Root Cause Analysis can also be performed simply in the office setting using the "5 Whys" technique. Start with what you know went wrong and ask "why" and then keep asking "why"

for each answer. Usually by the time you get to 4 to 6 whys, you are close to knowing more about the cause of the medical error.

Question 3: The correct answer is B.

Doctors use patterns to help recognize and diagnose illnesses, but sometimes doctors may jump to a wrong diagnosis because of a number of biases that we all have. Many of our patients present with undifferentiated complaints, and we try to be both efficient and cost-effective in our care, making thinking errors a common risk in primary care.

Question 4: The correct answer is C.

The basic guidelines for how to disclose an error have emerged over the last 20 years and generally include the following components: involve insurers, risk management, and the medical team when serious harm has occurred to the patient, take the initiative—don't wait for patients to call and ask, explain only what you know, apologize, state actions to be taken to prevent recurrence, and consider offering appropriate financial compensation.

REFERENCES

1. Elder N, Dovey S. A Classification of medical errors and preventable adverse events in primary care: A synthesis of the literature. *J Fam Pract.* 2002;51:927 932.
2. Elder N, VonderMeulen M, Cassedy A. The identification of medical errors by family physicians during outpatient visits. *Ann Fam Med.* 2004;2(2):125–129.
3. Phillips R, Dovey S, Graham D, et al. Learning from different lenses: Reports of medical errors in primary care by clinicians, staff and patients. *J Patient Safety.* 2006;2(3):140–146.
4. Phillips RL, Jr., Bartholomew LA, Dovey SM, et al. Learning from malpractice claims about negligent, adverse events in primary care in the United States. *Qual Saf Health Care.* 2004;13(2):121–126.
5. Sandars J, Esmail A. The frequency and nature of medical error in primary care: understanding the diversity across studies. *Fam Pract.* 2003;20(3):231–236.
6. Fernald D, Pace W, Harris D, et al. Event reporting to a primary care patient safety reporting system: A report from the ASIPS Collaborative. *Ann Fam Med.* 2004;2:327–232.
7. Hickner J, Graham D, Elder N, et al. Testing process errors and their harms and consequences reported from family medicine practices: A study of the AAFP National Research Network. *Qual Saf Health Care.* 2008;17(3):194–200.
8. Nutting PA, Main DS, Fischer PM, et al. Toward optimal laboratory use. Problems in laboratory testing in primary care. *JAMA.* 1996;275(8):635–639.
9. Casalino LP, Dunham D, Chin MH, et al. Frequency of failure to inform patients of clinically significant outpatient test results. *Arch Intern Med.* 2009;169(12):1123–1129.
10. Chen E, Eder M, Elder N, et al. Crossing the finish line: Follow up of abnormal test results in a multi-site community health center. *J Natl Med Assoc.* 2010;102:720–725.
11. Holden RJ, Carayon P, Gurses AP, et al. SEIPS 2.0: a human factors framework for studying and improving the work of healthcare professionals and patients. *Ergonomics.* 2013;56(11):1669–1686.
12. Mohr JJ, Batalden PB. Improving safety on the front lines: the role of clinical microsystems. *Qual Saf Health Care.* 2002;11(1):45–50.
13. Schiff GD, Hasan O, Kim S, et al. Diagnostic error in medicine: Analysis of 583 physician-reported errors. *Arch Intern Med.* 2009;169(20):1881–1887.
14. Lambe KA, O'Reilly G, Kelly BD, et al. Dual-process cognitive interventions to enhance diagnostic reasoning: a systematic review. *BMJ Qual Saf.* 2016;25(10):808–820.
15. Croskerry P. From mindless to mindful practice—cognitive bias and clinical decision making. *N Engl J Med.* 2013;368(26):2445–2448.
16. Kahneman D. *Thinking, Fast and Slow.* New York: Farrar, Straus and Giroux; 2011.
17. Seys D, Wu AW, Van Gerven E, et al. Health care professionals as second victims after adverse events: a systematic review. *Eval Health Prof.* 2013;36(2):135–162.
18. Wu AW. Medical error: the second victim. *BMJ.* 2000;320:726–727.

Overview of Prevention and Screening

KEY POINTS

1 ▶ Clinical preventive services include immunizations, counseling (e.g., smoking cessation), screening, and chemoprophylaxis (i.e., taking meds to prevent adverse health outcomes).

2 ▶ Immunizations are one of the most effective prevention strategies; family physicians should address patient and parental concerns regarding vaccine safety and reasons for immunizing.

3 ▶ The goal of screening is not merely to find problems but to identify asymptomatic persons for whom an intervention will reduce early disease progression or prevent adverse events.

4 ▶ When considering chemoprophylaxis (e.g., aspirin to prevent myocardial infarction), it is important to balance the potential risk reduction against the potential for harm.

5 ▶ Effectiveness of a prevention activity should be demonstrated before implementation in clinical practice. Most prevention interventions also have the potential for causing harm.

Mrs. Smith is a 56-year-old woman coming to her new primary care provider to establish care and for a routine physical examination. Mrs. Smith is a nursing assistant who recently received health insurance after experiencing a 7-year gap during which time her medical care was scant and only included care for acute indications at the emergency department. She notes on her intake form a family history of breast cancer in a maternal aunt in her 60s and a paternal grandfather who died of rectal cancer at age 72 years. Mrs. Smith is a light smoker with a pack of cigarettes lasting her 2 weeks and has a BMI of 34. She is postmenopausal and has no other past medical or surgical history and takes no medications. She is unmarried and is sexually active with a new partner whom she met 3 months ago.

Using the information and resources in this chapter, devise your own personalized preventive care plan and counseling strategy to help this patient achieve a more optimal state of health and well-being while reducing the acute and chronic illnesses. To guide your thinking, consider the following:

▶ List the grade A and B recommendations from the United States Preventive Services Task Force (USPSTF) with regard to disease prevention and screening. For Mrs. Smith, immediate concerns might be smoking cessation (SOR A), hypertension screening (SOR A), and screening mammography (SOR B). Other options might be depression screening (SOR B), screening for hyperlipidemia (SOR A), attention to cardiovascular risk factors and, if present, offering behavioral counseling for obesity (SOR B), and needed immunizations.

▶ With regard to grades C, D, and I recommendations, consider how you would approach these topics using a shared decision-making model. Screening for and prevention of sexually transmitted infections, given her new partner, could be important.

▶ Identify likely short- and long-term goals that you may wish to assist this patient in setting and consider an appropriate follow-up interval to help sustain behavior change while monitoring her progress. Of the above concerns, the largest benefit for Mrs. Smith might be smoking cessation, but this might not be a priority for her (see Chapter 5).

▶ Identify colleagues and support staff who could provide important services and expertise in helping your patient become empowered in achieving her goals. Your practice might include a health coach for smoking cessation for Mrs. Smith or a nutritionist for assistance with diet.

WHAT IS PREVENTION?

The goal of preventive medicine is to protect, promote, and maintain health and well-being while preventing disease, disability, and premature death. Prevention has traditionally been divided into three different categories—primary, secondary, and tertiary prevention. For primary prevention, the goal is to prevent disease or injury prior to their onset. In secondary prevention, we aim to reduce the morbidity and mortality of a disease, disability, or injury after an event has occurred. At the tertiary level, interventions aim to reduce the impact or disability of an ongoing disease process or injury. Examples are shown in Table 7.1.

Table 7.1 ▶ Levels of Preventive Healthcare

Prevention Measure	Disease	Intervention Level	Examples
Primary prevention	Pneumonia	Individual/clinical	Providing routine immunizations to children during well-child checks
		Population	State-wide regulations requiring school children to be fully immunized prior to enrollment
Secondary prevention	Breast cancer	Individual/clinical	Offering periodic mammograms to women at risk of breast cancer
		Population	Organizing a mass communication campaign to heighten breast cancer awareness and available screening
Tertiary prevention	Cardiovascular disease	Individual/clinical	Refer patients who are recovering from MI to a cardiac rehabilitation program
		Population	Work with local community leaders and policy makers to increase access to and availability of fresh produce in food deserts where CVD prevalence is highest and work on enhancing the built environment to facilitate more people with CVD to exercise

CVD, cardiovascular disease; MI, myocardial infarction.

With the focus being on care throughout the lifespan, much of the work of family physicians falls into one of these categories of prevention. Every patient encounter is an opportunity to individualize preventive approaches to reduce health risks, maintain current state of health, promote healthy behaviors, and consider how to minimize adverse outcomes of established disease.

WHEN SHOULD PREVENTION BE CONSIDERED?

As a clinician, it is important to approach prevention with a clear understanding of what health problem or adverse event you are trying to avoid. Keep in mind that the goal of prevention is to help people live longer or have better quality of life, not merely to detect disease early. We must also recognize that not every health problem can be prevented.

Criteria for assessing benefits for routine preventive care are:

▶ **Measuring the burden of suffering caused by a health problem.** This is determined by the prevalence as well as seriousness of a given health problem in the population. Seriousness of the health problem can be thought of in terms of the "6 Ds."

> Death, Disease, Disability, Discomfort, Dissatisfaction, and Destitution

The more of these associated factors, the more serious the health problem. Another useful way to think about the seriousness of a health problem is in terms of disability adjusted life years (DALYs). DALYs for a health problem are calculated as the sum of the years of life lost due to premature mortality from that problem and the years lost due to disability for incident cases of that health problem. The sum of DALYs across a population can be thought of as a measurement of the gap between current health status and an ideal health situation where the entire population lives to an advanced age, free of disease and disability. For more information on understanding DALYs, visit https://www.youtube.com/watch?v=Exce4gy7aOk.

▶ **Are safe and effective interventions available to improve outcomes?** In primary prevention, the intervention must work to delay or prevent the health problem. For Mrs. Smith, smoking cessation would fall into primary prevention. In secondary prevention (i.e., screening), there must be an effective treatment that prevents disease from advancing and it must be *more* effective when applied at the time asymptomatic disease is found than if applied at the time the patient would have presented with symptoms. This is likely true of early detection of breast cancer for Mrs. Smith or identifying hypertension or a sexually transmitted infection. Because most prevention interventions must be offered to many people for only a few to benefit, we must ensure that benefits clearly outweigh any potential risks.

▶ **Cost-effectiveness.** While preventive efforts tend to reduce long-term health system costs, most prevention interventions initially add cost. The question that must be asked is whether the intervention is worth the cost in terms of lives saved, disability prevented, or quality of life gained. Cost-effectiveness is a particular consideration when there is more than one intervention that could be used to prevent a given health problem.

▶ **Prevention as a population-level activity.** Many patients must participate to reduce disease incidence and prevalence. Typically, a preventive intervention yields large benefits only for a very small number of participants. A large number of participants will be caused minor harms, inconveniences, and expenses; and more substantial harms and costs will accrue to a variable number. For example, a meta-analysis of mammography screening trials found that out of 1,904 women of ages 40 to 49 years who were screened for 10 years by mammography, breast cancer death was prevented in one woman.[1] She is the one who benefits. All 1,904 women undergo the minor harm of an uncomfortable test as well as some radiation exposure while many undergo the more substantial harms of biopsy, worry about a false-positive test, and even unnecessary treatment of overdiagnosed breast cancers. All 1,904 women also have the cost (or cost-sharing) of mammography, and some have the costs of further evaluation and treatment including diagnostic procedures such as biopsy.

WHAT IS SCREENING?

Screening involves testing for a health problem or risk factor when there are no recognized signs or symptoms of that problem or risk factor. The goal of screening is not merely to *find* problems. **The goal of screening is to identify an asymptomatic person for whom an intervention will help reduce the progression of early disease or prevent an adverse health event.** Performing tests in patients who already have symptoms is not screening. Table 7.2 displays characteristics of screening programs that must be considered when evaluating its effectiveness.

Not all screening tests are laboratory tests. A question that you ask an asymptomatic patient on a review of systems can be considered a screening "test." Physical examination maneuvers performed on asymptomatic patients are screening interventions. Questionnaires, radiology studies, and various procedures are all used in certain instances as screening tests. Screening can be the initial intervention that results in a cascade of subsequent events that can ultimately help a person by preventing disease progression or adverse health outcomes. Take, for example, blood pressure (BP) measurement in Mrs. Smith. About two-thirds of people with obesity have hypertension and people with hypertension have an increased risk of heart disease and stroke (see Chapter 12). Repeated BP measurement has adequate specificity and predictive value and is acceptable to patients and the intervention, medication, is effective in preventing disease.

 Table 7.2 ▶ Criteria to Guide Evaluation of a Screening Program

- Significant burden of suffering of the target health problem
- Detectable preclinical phase exists
- Adequate sensitivity, specificity, and predictive value of available screening test
- Intervention that when administered in the detectable preclinical phase is more effective than if given when symptoms develop
- Screening procedure is acceptable to patients
- Program is cost-effective and benefit exceeds harm for the population screened

Alternatively, the cascade of events started by screening could yield no benefit (e.g., pelvic examinations on asymptomatic women) or, in some cases, can lead to harm. For example, Mrs. Smith might have an abnormal mammogram leading to additional testing that proves her mammogram to be a false positive—an extremely stressful event. The net benefits versus harms of a screening test is an important but often difficult concept to articulate during clinical counseling. Clinicians can utilize resources such as the USPSTF to formulate clear recommendations based on available evidence from the peer-reviewed literature. These recommendations are graded according to standardized criteria for a broad list of health conditions. See https://www.uspreventiveservicestaskforce.org/BrowseRec/Index/browse-recommendations for recommendations and https://www.uspreventiveservicestaskforce.org/Page/Name/grade-definitions for an explanation of the grading system. Offer Grade A and B services as these are ones with high certainty that the net benefit is substantial.

As a case study, consider prostate cancer screening as presented by the National Cancer Institute (https://www.cancer.gov/types/prostate/psa-fact-sheet) to understand how a growing evidence base on the risks and benefits of a screening intervention can produce dramatic shifts in national guidelines and clinical practices.

To learn more about screening and individualizing approaches to preventive health services, look at the Centers for Disease Control (CDC) Prevention Checklist: http://www.cdc.gov/prevention/. To assist primary care clinicians in point of care utilization of current guidelines, mobile apps such as the electronic preventive services selector have been developed and are available on multiple platforms. For more details, visit http://epss.ahrq.gov/PDA/index.jsp.

Detectable Preclinical Phase

The condition that screening is to identify must have a preclinical (asymptomatic or latent) phase that can be detected by the screening test. A health problem that causes symptoms immediately or relatively soon after its onset would not be a candidate for a screening program. Influenza, for example, is a common illness for which prevention is available to reduce morbidity and mortality. However, there is no preclinical phase during which "pre-influenza" is detectable. Prevention efforts for influenza must therefore use alternative primary prevention strategies such as immunization, hand-washing, and masks.

A screening program's effectiveness ultimately hinges on whether an intervention given during the detectable preclinical phase works better than an intervention given once the patient becomes symptomatic and is diagnosed clinically. As noted above and in Figure 7.1 (see Tumor B), prostate cancer is a good example of a disease that often has a long preclinical phase, but where treatment during that phase has not been shown to necessarily improve outcomes.

Performance of Test

The screening test itself must perform well according to defined criteria. Screening tests should have high sensitivity as well as adequate specificity (see Chapter 3). Recall that the predictive value of a test is intimately tied to the prevalence of the disease or condition being considered. With screening tests, the prevalence of the condition being sought is usually very low, often even among the so-called "high-risk" groups. Therefore, a highly sensitive test is needed to avoid missing the few cases of disease that are actually present (i.e., minimize false negatives). A screening test also needs to have high specificity to avoid

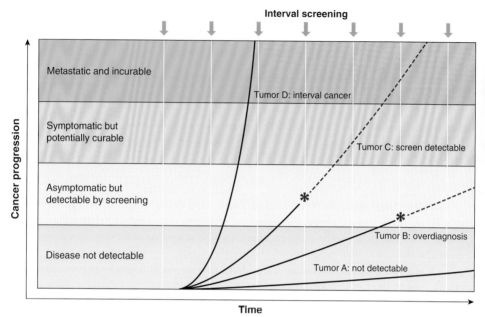

Figure 7.1 ▶ Understanding length-time bias. In this hypothetical example, the probability of detecting disease is related to the growth rate of each tumor. *Tumor A* remains microscopic and undetectable with the current screening test. *Tumor B* eventually becomes detectable by screening (*), but its growth rate is so slow that it will not cause symptoms during the life of the individual; its detection will result in overdiagnosis. *Tumor C* (the only cancer with potential to benefit from screening in this example) is capable of metastasizing, but it grows slowly enough so that it can be detected by screening (*); for some, this early detection will result in survival. *Tumor D* grows very quickly and therefore is usually not detected by screening. This will present in the interval between screening examinations and has a poor prognosis. *Red dashed lines* represent the natural history of these tumors in the absence of detection by screening. (From Gates TJ. Screening for cancer: Concepts and controversies. *Am Fam Physician.* 2014;90(9):625–631; http://www.aafp.org/afp/2014/1101/p625.html.)

additional testing ("work-ups") or treatments for people who do not have the disease (i.e., minimize false positives). Even with a highly sensitive and highly specific screening test, one may expect a significant number of false positives (requiring further testing) when applied to a population.

For a more detailed review on the concepts of sensitivity, specificity, and positive/negative predictive values, check out this video tutorial: https://www.youtube.com/watch?v=QajIM17MZYQ. To quickly calculate the above statistical parameters for any given clinical test, visit https://www.medcalc.org/calc/diagnostic_test.php.

Acceptability to Patients

Successful screening tests are well tolerated by the patient and thereby have higher utilization rates. Blood tests and short questionnaires are generally quite acceptable to patients. Colonoscopy is a good example of an effective screening test that is not acceptable to some patients. Technologic developments including the fecal immunochemical test (FIT) can help increase colorectal cancer screening rates by providing a less invasive and more affordable alternative.[2]

APPROACHES TO PREVENT DISEASE

In addition to screening, four other approaches are used by clinicians to address preventive health. Ideally, these interventions are carried out in well-coordinated interdisciplinary teams and include immunizations, chemoprophylaxis, counseling, and community health programs.

Immunizations

Immunizations are one of the most effective prevention strategies ever introduced. Diseases such as smallpox, measles, and polio—not long ago responsible for significant morbidity and mortality—have either been eradicated or are under much improved control as a result of widespread vaccination (Table 7.3). In addition to being extremely effective, immunizations are also one of the most cost-effective of all primary prevention activities.

Despite the fact that many vaccine-preventable diseases of childhood have been virtually eliminated in the United States, it remains important to continue to strongly promote vaccines. As international travel and migration become more common, the risk of

Table 7.3 ▶ Comparisons of Prevaccine era and Current Estimated Morbidity and Mortality for Vaccine-Preventable Diseases

Disease	Vaccine Dates	Prevaccine Estimated Annual Average		Postvaccine Reported		Reduction (%)	
		Cases	Deaths	Cases (2010)	Deaths (2004)	Cases	Deaths
Diphtheria	1928–1943	21,053 (1936–1945)	1822 (1936–1945)	0	0	100	100
Measles	1963, 1967, and 1968	530,217 (1953–1962)	440 (1953–1962)	63	0	>99	100
Mumps	1940s, 1967	162,344 (1963–1968)	39 (1963–1968)	2,612	0	98	100
Pertussis	1914–1941	200,752 (1934–1943)	4034 (1934–1943)	27,538	27	86	>99
Poliomyelitis (paralytic)	1955, 1961–1963, 1987	16,316 (1941–1950)	1879 (1941–1950)	0	0	100	100
Rubella	1969	47,745 (1966–1968)	17 (1966–1968)	5	0	>99	100
Congenital Rubella Syndrome	1969	152 (1966–1969)	Not available	0	0	100	N/A
Smallpox	1798	29,005 (1900–1949)	337 (1900–1949)	0	0	100	100
Tetanus	1933–1949	580 (1947–1949)	472 (1947–1949)	26	4	96	>99

Data from Hinman AR, Orenstein WA, Schuchat A; Centers for Disease Control and Prevention (CDC). Vaccine-preventable diseases, immunizations, and MMWR—1961–2011. *MMWR Suppl.* 2011;60(4):49–57; Roush SW, Murphy T V. Historical comparisons of morbidity and mortality for vaccine-preventable diseases in the United States. *JAMA.* 2007;298(18):2155–2163.

Table 7.4 ▶ Common Misconceptions About Vaccines

Misconception	Context and Possible Physician Response
Children can get autism from vaccines	A case-series published in the Lancet in 1998 implied a link between MMR vaccine and autism.[a] Several studies subsequently consistently demonstrated that there is no such. In 2010, the Lancet formally fully retracted the 1998 study due to dishonesty in reporting and other ethical violations.[b]
Vaccines can cause the disease they are supposed to prevent	A common example is the myth that influenza vaccine causes the flu. Confusion likely arises from coincidental viral symptoms and vaccine side effects (e.g., mild aches, low-grade fever) perceived as "the flu." Most vaccines manufactured today are made from killed virus which cannot reproduce and cause infection. Even vaccines made from live viruses or bacteria are made with only part of the virus or bacteria. You cannot get the flu from the flu vaccine, because the vaccine is made from a killed virus
Vaccines can cause mercury poisoning	Thimerosal, which is used in development of some vaccines, contains mercury. The amount of mercury present in thimerosal is minute, does not accumulate in the body, and is much less toxic than other forms of mercury. Today, influenza vaccine is the only immunization that contains thimerosal, and preservative-free (thimerosal-free) influenza vaccine is available for young children
Vaccines are dangerous and not tested	Vaccine development and manufacturing follows standard safety protocols. Before being released, vaccines are carefully tested. Following release, vaccine safety is carefully monitored

[a]Wakefield AJ, Murch SH, Anthony A, et al. Ileal-lymphoid-nodular hyperplasia, non-specific colitis, and pervasive developmental disorder in children. *Lancet.* 1998;351(9103):637–41.
[b]Retraction–Ileal-lymphoid-nodular hyperplasia, non-specific colitis, and pervasive developmental disorder in children. *Lancet.* 2010;375(9713):445.

infectious diseases, particularly airborne pathogens, spreading among people across borders is more significant than ever before. For example, China reported 131,441 measles cases (98.4 per million) in 2008 and a large outbreak in Japan resulted in over 18,000 (140.7 per million) reported cases in 2007.[3]

Immunization confers protection in the case of individual exposures. Furthermore, the concept of *herd immunity* applies, whereby high levels of immunization in a population protect the few unimmunized persons from infection. When individuals decline to vaccinate themselves or their family, herd immunity weakens so that unimmunized persons are more likely to become infected and the risk of an epidemic of infection increases, particularly for the very young, elderly, and immunocompromised. You should be prepared to respond to patients' and parents' common misconceptions about vaccines (Table 7.4). For information on talking with those who prefer not to immunize, see http://www.immunize.org/talking-about-vaccines/.

For additional information on immunizations and resources to enhance your patient counseling skills, visit the CDC website http://www.cdc.gov/vaccines/ and the World Health Organization's "Myths and Facts about vaccinations" (http://www.who.int/features/qa/84/en/) and watch the following video: https://www.youtube.com/watch?v=3uVvq7dbf4s. For Mrs. Smith, assuming adequate childhood vaccinations, the CDC website indicates that for adults in her age group, vaccinations that may be needed include influenza and tetanus/diphtheria/pertussis and possibly others based on health status and risk.

Table 7.5 ▶ Examples of Chemoprevention		
Medication	**Preventive Use(s)**	**Potential Harms**
Aspirin	Reduce risk of myocardial infarction in men 45–79 years; reduce risk of ischemic stroke in women 55–79 years	Gastrointestinal bleeding, hemorrhagic stroke
Folic acid	Reduce risk of neural tube defects in women of childbearing age	None
Tamoxifen	Reduce risk of breast cancer in women at high risk	Pulmonary embolism, deep venous thrombosis, hot flashes, endometrial cancer

Chemoprophylaxis

Chemoprophylaxis, also called chemoprevention, is the use of a medication to prevent disease or an adverse health outcome. Examples are shown in Table 7.5.[4,5] Many forms of treatment are actually chemoprevention. Statins, for example, offered to people with elevated cholesterol or diabetes are given to reduce the risk of cardiovascular events and stroke. For Mrs. Smith who has one known cardiovascular risk factor (smoking), if her 10-year cardiovascular disease event risk is 10% or greater (see Chapter 12), she would benefit from a statin. Bisphosphonates, offered to patients with osteoporosis, are really given in hopes of preventing fragility fractures. When considering any chemoprevention, it is important to balance the potential risk reduction against the potential for harm due to adverse effects.

Counseling

Clinicians' efforts to counsel people to exercise, eat healthier, lose weight, quit smoking, and limit alcohol intake are examples of preventive interventions to encourage individuals to change behavior. The effectiveness of such counseling should be subjected to the same scrutiny as other prevention interventions. A successful intervention supported by evidence is tobacco cessation counseling.[6] Even brief advice given by a clinician to a smoker to quit smoking leads to greater cessation attempts and greater cessation rates. Use of the "Five As" (see Chapter 23) and motivational interviewing (see Chapter 5) are among the techniques shown to encourage people to adapt healthier behaviors. Intensive counseling may be effective for some patients with other conditions (e.g., weight loss for obese patients).

For "Five As" approach https://www.youtube.com/watch?v=Ky5P9n40eh0 and for a demonstration, see https://www.youtube.com/watch?v=yzWfgjXsgr4.

Integrating Community Health

Clinical approaches to disease prevention and health promotion should ideally be integrated into comprehensive and multidisciplinary programs utilizing public health, health policy, and community developing and planning activities. By enabling positive health behaviors (e.g., increasing access to green spaces) and disincentivizing negative health behaviors (e.g., restricting smoking in public places), health outcomes stand a significantly greater chance of making sustainable improvements.

The following case studies from the CDC demonstrate the importance of investing in community interventions outside of the clinical space:

▶ Making the Business Case: Community Health Investments Yield Results https://www.youtube.com/watch?v=CI-3FGAqoa4&list=PLvrp9iOILTQakIFMK28M7_0mju-qXnjjV&index=2

▶ Making the Case for Prevention: Community Partnerships Benefit Students, Schools & Health https://www.youtube.com/watch?v=baJxYum63I4&index=7&list=PLvrp9iOILTQakIFMK28M7_0mju-qXnjjV

▶ Making the Business Case for Prevention: Healthy Options Sell in a Food Desert https://www.youtube.com/watch?v=mU5IJQpJFMc&list=PLvrp9iOILTQakIFMK28M7_0mju-qXnjjV&index=10

EVIDENCE FOR SCREENING AND PREVENTION

Clinicians need to be certain that a preventive service will not do more harm than good. Overdiagnosis, labeling as diseased, unnecessary confirmatory tests, side effects of treatment, and even death can be the direct or indirect effects of a preventive intervention. Once a preventive intervention is introduced and undergoes widespread adoption, it is difficult to reverse clinician and patient behavior related to the service. For example, changing patient and physician behavior pertaining to prostate cancer screening is difficult. Such screening was adopted and promoted based on observational studies before better quality evidence existed. Unfortunately, observational designs are problematic when it comes to studying screening.

Sources of Bias in Studies of Screening

Observational studies of the effects of screening generally suffer from two major biases: lead-time bias and length-time bias. *Lead-time bias* occurs when people whose disease was diagnosed by screening *appear* to have longer survival than those whose disease was diagnosed because of symptoms or signs, even if actual years of life were not prolonged (Fig. 7.2). This apparent discrepancy occurs because "survival" is measured from the time

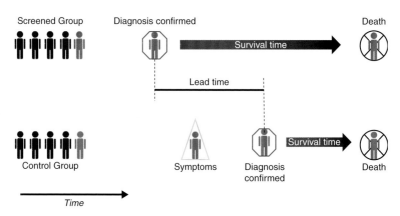

Figure 7.2 ▶ Understanding lead-time bias.

of diagnosis. Hence, a person who is screened may be diagnosed earlier than a person who is not screened but will not live any longer in absolute lifespan.

Consider, as an example, the genetic disease, Huntington disease. The disease is considered progressive and incurable. Although genetic testing allows for the detection of the known DNA mutation, the detection of this disease in its preclinical phase will not alter its course.

Overdiagnosis can be thought of as an extreme form of *length-time bias*. Overdiagnosis is not the same as false-positive tests. In overdiagnosis, histologic cancer is actually detected, but the cancer is one that would never have become clinically relevant (tumor B in Fig. 7.1). Overdiagnosis is one likely explanation why current screening programs for breast and prostate cancer have failed to reduce mortality.[7] Only by finding and adequately reducing the mortality from the aggressive cancers will screening make a difference. At the same time, it is important to develop strategies to reduce the unnecessary treatments for people whose screen-detected disease has little or no true malignant potential.

The way to mitigate these two important biases is to perform randomized controlled trials of screening. Adequate randomization will ensure that there is a balance of people with indolent and aggressive disease in both groups (screened and unscreened). In addition, the point at which people are randomized marks an equivalent starting time in both groups, so that lead-time is avoided. However, these studies are difficult to perform given the ethical concerns of withholding screening tests and the time, financial, and other technical challenges inherent in the design of randomized controlled studies.

GUIDELINES AND RESOURCES

The USPSTF is an independent panel of prevention experts, including family physicians, who conduct rigorous, impartial assessments of the scientific evidence for the effectiveness of a broad range of clinical preventive services including screening, counseling, and chemoprevention. Because of their rigor, explicit methods, and impartiality, the USPSTF recommendations are considered by many to be the "gold standard" for clinical preventive services. The USPSTF regularly updates their recommendations as new evidence accumulates. The USPSTF also provides several patient-friendly options to guide preventive decision making. Their recommendations, systematic reviews, and evidence summaries (also published in peer-reviewed journals) are available at http://www.ahrq.gov/CLINIC/uspstfix.htm.[8]

In guideline development, it is important that conflicts of interest do not influence recommendations. Organizations that advocate for patients with certain diseases may be overly enthusiastic about recommending a prevention strategy, even before the evidence is sufficient. Similarly, the potential for financial gain due to a test or medication may influence guideline development and needs to be guarded against. For example, the current guidelines on whether to screen adults for glaucoma are notably different between the USPSTF and the recommendations of the American Academy of Ophthalmology (AAO).[9,10] The USPSTF concluded that the evidence is insufficient while the AAO recommends that adults be screened as part of comprehensive eye care. Whether these differences are due to vested interest or different interpretations of the evidence is difficult to know.

When Guidelines Conflict

Unfortunately, guidelines about preventive services will sometimes conflict, leaving the clinician and patient in somewhat of a quandary. In most cases, such conflicts will arise when the evidence is simply insufficient. The USPSTF often will classify services lacking good quality evidence in this way. As a clinician, you should become familiar with the issues about the service that are controversial, and where the evidence is weak, it is recommended that you consider using a strategy of shared decision making with patients. That is, you discuss the preventive service and its potential for helping the patient as well as its potential risks. The goal is to reach a mutually agreeable decision that reflects the health preferences of the patient as well as their individual risk factors.

Applying Preventive Care in Clinical Practice

The **RISE** mnemonic (risks, immunizations, screening, education), discussed in Chapter 4, is one approach to help clinicians remember to apply the principles of preventive medicine in daily practice.

SYSTEMS OF CARE

Preventive care is improved by its incorporation into systems of health delivery. Many elements of prevention do not necessarily need to be provided directly by the family physician. For example, reminders for screening tests can be automatically mailed or texted to patients. Office staff can be trained to identify patients in need of recommended preventive care and these patients' charts can be flagged for physician review. Nearly all workers in a health system can help implement screening programs, like the Five As for all patients who use tobacco or to encourage immunizations. Electronic record systems particularly allow for greater ease of tracking preventive care than previous paper charts. However, any system requires frequent updates as changes in recommendations occur, new evidence of effectiveness emerges, or new technologies become available to enhance earlier detection.

QUESTIONS

1. Which of the following is included in clinical preventive services?
   A. Immunizations
   B. Family history
   C. Cognitive behavioral therapy
   D. Medications for treatment

2. An effective screening test will do which one of the following?
   A. Find a disease before it is clinically apparent
   B. Test for a disease that has no cure
   C. Find half of all cases
   D. Find diseases that have little morbidity

3. Which one of the following is an example of chemoprevention?
   A. Antibiotics for pneumonia
   B. Antihypertensive medications to treat high blood pressure
   C. Insulin to treat diabetes
   D. Aspirin to prevent myocardial infarction and stroke

ANSWERS

Question 1: The correct answer is A.

Key point 1. Clinical preventive services include immunizations, counseling (e.g., smoking cessation), screening, and chemoprophylaxis (i.e., taking meds to prevent adverse health outcomes.

Question 2: The correct answer is A.

The goal of screening is to identify an asymptomatic person for whom an intervention will help reduce the progression of early disease or prevent an adverse health event.

Question 3: The correct answer is D.

Chemoprophylaxis, also called chemoprevention, is the use of a medication to prevent disease or an adverse health outcome. Examples, shown in Table 7.5, include aspirin to reduce risk of myocardial infarction in men 45 to 79 years and reduce risk of ischemic stroke in women 55 to 79 years.

REFERENCES

1. Nelson HD, Tyne K, Naik A, et al. Screening for breast cancer: systematic evidence review update for the U. S. Preventive services task force. Ann Intern Med. 2009;(74):95. http://www.ncbi.nlm.nih.gov/books/PMH0005880/
2. Allison JE, Fraser CG, Halloran SP, et al. Population screening for colorectal cancer means getting FIT: the past, present, and future of colorectal cancer screening using the fecal immunochemical test for hemoglobin (FIT). Gut Liver. 2014;8(2):117–130.
3. Centers for Disease Control and Prevention (CDC). Progress toward measles elimination–Japan, 1999–2008. MMWR Morb Mortal Wkly Rep. 2008;57(38):1049–1052.
4. Wolff T, Witkop CT, Miller T, et al. Folic acid supplementation for the prevention of neural tube defects: An update of the evidence for the U.S. preventive services task force. Ann Intern Med. 2009;150(9):632–639.
5. Wolff T, Miller T, Ko S. Aspirin for the primary prevention of cardiovascular events: an update of the evidence for the U.S. Preventive services task force. Ann Intern Med. 2009;150(6):405–410.
6. Patnode CD, Henderson JT, Thompson JH, et al. Behavioral counseling and pharmacotherapy interventions for tobacco cessation in adults, including pregnant women. Agency *for Healthcare Research and Quality (US).* 2015. http://www.ncbi.nlm.nih.gov/pubmed/26491759. Accessed October 26, 2016.
7. Esserman L, Shieh Y, Thompson I. Rethinking screening for breast cancer and prostate cancer. *JAMA.* 2009;302(15):1685–1692.
8. Clinical guidelines and recommendations | agency for healthcare research & quality. http://www.ahrq.gov/professionals/clinicians-providers/guidelines-recommendations/index.html. Accessed October 23, 2016.
9. Get Screened at 40 - American academy of ophthalmology. http://www.aao.org/eye-health/tips-prevention/screening. Accessed October 23, 2016
10. Final recommendation statement: Glaucoma: Screening - US Preventive Services Task Force. https://www.uspreventiveservicestaskforce.org/Page/Document/RecommendationStatementFinal/glaucoma-screening. Accessed October 23, 2016.

Prenatal Care

Family physicians' knowledge, scope of practice, and comprehensive training makes them uniquely suited to provide prenatal care for women and their families. Bonds formed during maternity care can translate into lifelong relationships with families. Prenatal care is a highly rewarding part of family medicine because of this special type of continuity. While only 9.7% of recertifying family physicians reported providing maternity care,[1] a substantial proportion of women (34.4%) receive some form of care from a family physician during pregnancy.[2]

FAMILY PHYSICIANS' APPROACH TO MATERNITY CARE

While family physicians and obstetrician-gynecologists both deliver high-quality maternity care, family physicians who practice obstetrics traditionally use fewer interventions; in a recent hospital database study, family physicians had lower cesarean rates, higher rates of vaginal birth after cesarean section (VBAC), higher rates of vacuum-assisted delivery, and similar rates of labor induction.[3]

Ann is a 25-year-old teacher who presents to the clinic to establish care. She has no significant medical problems and denies tobacco, alcohol, or drug use. She is engaged and plans on getting married next year. She is currently sexually active with her partner and uses condoms for contraception. She has plans for pregnancy in the next few years. She also tells you her sister had a baby with anencephaly, and that this was really hard on their family.

PRECONCEPTION VISIT

A preconception visit addresses expectant parents' health and well-being and is ideally done 3 to 6 months prior to conception. However, with Ann's mention of her sister's baby with anencephaly and her use of a less effective form of contraception, some aspects of a preconception visit are appropriate now. Opportunities for informal preconception guidance include well-woman examinations, visits for contraception or a negative pregnancy test, and follow-up visits after an adverse birth outcome. A summary of recommendations for preconception visits is at the end of this chapter.

BOX 8.1 UNITED STATES RECOMMENDATIONS FOR FOLIC ACID SUPPLEMENTATION

▶ Women of childbearing age: consume 0.4 mg (400 µg) of folate in vitamin form or fortified foods daily, in addition to a diet high in folate-rich foods.

▶ Amount should increase to 0.6 mg/d in pregnancy and 0.5 mg/d during lactation

▶ Women with a history of pregnancy affected by a NTD (e.g., spina bifida) should consume 4–5 mg/d of folic acid (requires a prescription), start at least 1-month preconception.

Occupational Risks

Occupational exposures affect pregnancy in the preconception period and/or during gestation. Untoward effects relate to the fetal gestational age at the time of exposure. Environmental exposures that adversely affect the fetus include solvents (e.g., pesticides, paint thinner/strippers, fertilizers) and heavy metals such as lead, mercury, or arsenic. Women who work in a hospital setting should avoid exposure to ionizing radiation, chemotherapeutic agents, and misoprostol. While Ann's work as a teacher does not pose an occupational risk, a review of her hobbies may expose other risks.

Folic Acid

Folic acid consumption reduces the risk of neural tube defects (NTDs). Box 8.1 lists indications for folic acid supplementation. Ann could benefit from initiating folic acid, with consideration of using a higher dose given her sister's history. Women with certain medical conditions (e.g., diabetes, malabsorption, seizure disorder), genotypes associated with NTDs, and members of high-risk ethnic groups (e.g., Celtic, Sikh, or Northern Chinese ancestry) may also benefit from high-dose folic acid.[4]

Genetic Screening and Counseling

Goals of preconception genetic counseling include counseling women who are at risk for a fetal anomaly or genetic disorder and informing couples about available screening tests (Table 8.1). Carrier testing can be performed before pregnancy in patients with known familial disorders. Women at risk for having a child with sickle cell disease, thalassemia, or cystic fibrosis (CF) should also be screened in the preconception period.

Medical Conditions

Preconception care provides an opportunity for women with medical conditions to optimize their treatment and improve the likelihood of a healthy pregnancy.

Diabetes Mellitus

Infants of mothers with diabetes mellitus are at a fourfold increased risk for congenital malformations like cardiac anomalies and NTDs. Elevated blood glucose levels increase the likelihood of anomalies. Since many pregnancies are unplanned, optimizing glycemic control before conception is essential. The recommended range for fasting blood glucose is 4 to 7 mmol/L; hemoglobin A1C (HgA1C) ideally should be less than 6.

Table 8.1 ▶ Preconception Screening Recommendations for Specific Diseases

Disease	Cause	Heritability	Epidemiology	Screening Available	Recommendations for Screening
Tay–Sachs	Deficiency of the enzyme hexosamini-dase-A	Recessively inherited lysosomal storage disease	1:30 carrier risk in people of Ashkenazi Jewish heritage and French Cana-dians	Enzyme assay for hexosamini-dase-A	Routine preconcep-tion screening for those at risk[a]
Sickle cell anemia	Amino acid substitution of valine for glu-tamic acid on the *HBB* gene of chromosome 11	Autosomal recessive	10% African-Americans are carriers; Indo-Pakistani and Arab ethnic groups	Hemoglobin electrophoresis	Preconception screening for women at risk; for women with sickle cell trait, partner screening recom-mended[a]
Thalassemia alpha and beta type	Abnormality in hemoglobin production with inadequate oxygen carry-ing capability and anemia	Autosomal recessive	1:12 carrier rate in people of Asian or Mediterranean descent	DNA testing for abnormal thalassemia hemoglobin in women with low MCV, nor-mal hemoglobin electrophoresis	Preconception screening for women at risk and partners of women with abnormal hemoglobin genes
Cystic fibro-sis (CF)	Mutations in the CF trans-membrane conductance regulator (CFTR)	Autosomal recessive	1:25 carrier risk in whites of northern European heritage	DNA testing	Offer preconception screening to all patients; screening is most efficacious in non-Hispanic white and Ashkenazi Jew-ish populations[a–c]
Spinal muscular atrophy (SMA)	Mutations in survival motor neuron (SMN1) gene at chromosome 5q11.2–13.3	Most common autosomal recessive neurode-generative disease	1:25–1:50 carrier rate; no specific race or ethnicity iden-tified as high-risk; carrier status lowest in blacks	DNA testing	Offer carrier screen-ing to all couples in the preconception/ prenatal period regardless of race, ethnicity, or history[a,b]

[a]Recommended by ACOG.
[b]Recommended by American College of Medical Genetics.
[c]Recommended by the National Institutes of Health (NIH).

Epilepsy

Infants of women with epilepsy have an increased risk of anomalies (6% vs. 2% to 3% in the general population),[5] especially cardiac and NTDs. It is not clear whether these abnormal-ities are caused by epilepsy or by antiepileptic drugs. Older medications like valproic acid, carbamazepine, and phenytoin are more strongly associated with congenital anomalies; polytherapy further increases risk.

Tobacco and Alcohol

Smoking is associated with placenta previa, placental abruption, preterm premature rupture of membranes (PPROM), intrauterine growth restriction, stillbirth, and ectopic pregnancy (Chapter 23). Women who use tobacco and wish to conceive are strongly encouraged to quit prior to conception.

Fetal effects depend on the amount of alcohol consumed, duration of use, and timing in gestation. Binge drinking (consuming less than five drinks in one sitting) is more dangerous to fetal neurologic development than nonbinge usage. While there is a general consensus that women should not drink excessively during pregnancy, it remains unclear what level of alcohol is harmful. Many US authorities recommend against the consumption of any alcohol during pregnancy.

Medication History

Use of all prescription and nonprescription drugs, herbal supplements, and vitamins should be reviewed and documented at the preconception visit. When asked about medications, patients like Ann, who do not take prescription medications, may forget to mention nonprescription drugs and supplements. If a woman requires a drug with teratogenic potential (e.g., misoprostol, isotretinoin, warfarin, or HMG-CoA reductase inhibitors), informed consent and a discussion about safer options is necessary.

As part of a broader effort to further improve the content and format of prescription drug labeling, the US Food and Drug Administration is currently replacing the pregnancy labeling categories (A, B, C, D, or X) using the new Pregnancy and Lactation Labeling Rule (PLLR). Under this system, letter designations will be replaced by a narrative summary of known risks for drugs/biologics during pregnancy and lactation.[6]

Immunizations

The preconception visit is a useful time to update immunization status. Screen for rubella susceptibility by history, prior vaccination, or serology and, if nonimmune, immunize with MMR. Similarly, document immunity to varicella by history or serology (85% to 90% of individuals who deny having varicella are actually immune) and, if titers are negative, immunize with Varivax prior to conception. Although women have historically been counseled not to conceive within 3 months of MMR immunization, the likelihood of the fetus developing congenital rubella syndrome is largely theoretical.[7] Influenza vaccination is recommended for pregnant women by the Centers for Disease Control and Prevention (CDC) and can be administered during any trimester.

After discussing Ann's family's experience with her sister's pregnancy loss, you do a brief preconception visit and advise her to take 4 to 5 mg of folic acid daily (Box 8.1). You review her medications and herbal supplements. She is unsure if she ever had chicken pox, so you check a titer. Her last MMR and flu shot are up to date, and she got a pertussis booster after her sister had her baby.

PRENATAL CARE

The Institutes of Medicine recognized prenatal care as a national policy issue in 1985. Congress later enacted legislation that expanded Medicaid coverage for pregnant women. In 2007, 70.5% of US women received prenatal care considered both early (first trimester) and adequate.[8]

Despite widespread use of prenatal care, evidence of its effectiveness is lacking. Rates of preterm delivery and low birth weight (LBW) have not improved over the past decades. Although the United States has some of the highest per capita healthcare expenditures of industrialized nations, maternal and infant mortality rates lag behind most other industrialized nations (Chapter 1). Major racial disparities continue to exist. The maternal mortality rate for black women is four times higher than for white women (41.1 per 100,000 vs. 11.8 per 100,000 in whites and 15.7 deaths per 100,000 in women of other races) and preterm birth rates among black women in 2015 were 50% higher than for white women (13% vs. 9%).[9,10] Some studies suggest that prenatal care may not be effective for improving aggregate birth outcomes because most pregnancy complications result from prepregnancy behaviors or life circumstances that are difficult to reverse.[11] However, women may be more amenable to healthy lifestyle changes when they are pregnant.

> Denise, a 28-year-old accountant, comes to your office worried that her period is late. She has very regular cycles, and states that her period is almost a month late. She is sexually active but does not use contraception because she worries about the influence of hormones on her body. She has noticed some breast tenderness and felt nauseated for the past week. She also feels "exhausted." She took a home pregnancy test that was positive. She is not unhappy about a pregnancy.

Diagnosing and Dating Pregnancy (Confirmation of Pregnancy)

Amenorrhea, nausea, fatigue, and breast tenderness are the most common symptoms of early pregnancy. While none of these individual symptoms has a high sensitivity for diagnosing pregnancy, nausea gravidarum, also known as morning sickness, has a specificity of 86%.[12] Combinations of symptoms increase predictive value over single symptoms.

The first day of the most recent menstrual cycle is traditionally used to calculate the estimated date of delivery (EDD). In women with reliable menstrual histories and regular cycles, Naegele's rule can be used to estimate the EDD. Many apps exist to calculate EDD as well (https://itunes.apple.com/us/app/acog/id616323665?mt=8).

> Naegele's Rule: EDD = (LMP – 3 months) + 7 days

Pregnancy tests use urine or serum to check for beta human chorionic gonadotropin (β-HCG). β-HCG is detectable in the blood almost immediately after conception. Urine tests are nearly always positive around the time of the first missed period. β-HCG concentrations in the range of 25 to 50 mIU/mL are detectible on qualitative urine samples. Serum pregnancy tests detect β-HCG at levels as low as 10 to 15 mIU/mL. β-HCG levels:

▶ Correspond closely with gestational age during the first trimester

▶ Increase exponentially until 8 to 10 weeks, then plateau

▶ Double every 1.4 to 2 days in healthy pregnancies with a minimum increase of 53% expected every 48 hours

An appropriate rise in β-HCG levels on two quantitative (serum) pregnancy tests drawn 48 hours apart is reassuring for normal pregnancy.

Transvaginal ultrasound is the most accurate test for documenting and dating intrauterine pregnancy. First trimester transvaginal ultrasound confirms gestational age within ±4 days by measuring the gestational sac and fetal crown to rump length.

Ultrasound findings at specific HCG levels (estimated gestational age)

▶ Gestational sac is seen when HCG is >1,000 mIU/mL (4.5–5 weeks EGA)

▶ Yolk sac is seen when HCG is >2,500 mIU/mL (6 weeks EGA)

▶ Fetal pole is seen when HCG is >5,000 mIU/mL (7 weeks EGA)

Early Pregnancy Loss and Ectopic Pregnancy

Ten to fifteen percent of clinically-recognized pregnancies end in fetal loss. Increased maternal age, previous spontaneous abortion, smoking, certain infectious diseases, and immunologic dysfunction are all risk factors.

Vaginal bleeding occurs in approximately one quarter of women during the first trimester. Half of these women have uneventful prenatal courses. Cramping and abdominal pain increase the likelihood of spontaneous abortion (miscarriage). Transvaginal ultrasound and serial β-HCG levels help in the assessment of viability.

Ruling out ectopic pregnancy in cases of first trimester bleeding is critical. Ectopic gestation occurs in 2% of total pregnancies and is the leading cause of maternal mortality during the first trimester. Risk factors include previous pelvic inflammatory disease, history of ectopic pregnancy, tubal surgery, assisted reproductive technology, and current use of an intrauterine device. Patients may have first trimester bleeding and/or pelvic pain or be asymptomatic. Early diagnosis is augmented using quantitative β-HCG and transvaginal ultrasound. Ultrasound may show a fetal pole or heartbeat visible outside the uterine cavity or a thick-walled adnexal mass without a yolk sac or fetal pole.

Risk Assessment

A summary of evidence-based recommendations for prenatal care is at the end of this chapter.

Obstetric History

Documentation of past obstetric history includes all pregnancies, deliveries, and number of children (Table 8.2). The strongest risk factor for preterm delivery in the current pregnancy is a history of preterm delivery.

Table 8.2 ▶ Documentation of Obstetric History

Term	Definition	Examples
Gravida	Number of times a woman has been pregnant, regardless of whether or not it resulted in a live birth	Nulligravida = never been pregnant (G0) Primigravida = pregnant once (G1) Multigravida = pregnant more than once (G number of pregnancies)
Parity (Para)	Number of pregnancies carried past 20 weeks of gestation	Nullipara = never carried pregnancy past 20 weeks Primipara = one pregnancy past 20 weeks Multiple gestation pregnancies count as 1 parity
Term	Number of deliveries after 37 weeks of gestation	
Preterm	Number of deliveries prior to 37 weeks of gestation	
Aborted	Combined number of spontaneous abortions (miscarriage) and elective abortions	
Living	Number of living children (for multiple gestation pregnancies, each living child counts as one)	

Example: You are seeing a 32-year-old woman who had twins delivered at term, a miscarriage, and an elective abortion. What are her Gs and Ps?
Answer: She is a G3 (3 pregnancies) and P1 (1 delivery at term), 0 (no preterm deliveries), 2 (2 aborted), 2 (2 living children)—so G3P1022.

Current Medical and Past Surgical History

Medical, surgical, family, and social history contribute to successful prenatal care. Prenatal care intake forms are often used to guide you through the relevant history including chronic illnesses; medications; prior uterine/other surgery; tobacco, alcohol, and substance use; occupational risks; and immunizations.

> Denise's in-office qualitative urine pregnancy test is positive. As her cycles are regular, you calculate her EDD. A quick look at the transvaginal ultrasound shows a yolk sac inside a normally shaped gestational sac. On further history, you note that she smokes ½ packs of cigarettes daily and occasionally drinks alcohol. She asks what you can do to help her quit smoking and how much alcohol is safe during pregnancy.

Health Habits

Pregnant women should be counseled about behavioral methods to quit smoking. Both bupropion and nicotine patch replacement have been used during pregnancy and appear effective.[13] The nicotine patch is associated with decreased prematurity risk and small-for-gestational-age infants and bupropion is associated with a lower risk of prematurity compared to smoking. Denise decided to try a nicotine patch and to avoid alcohol.

Nutrition

Additional nutrients needed during pregnancy include folic acid, iron (30 g daily), and calcium (1,200 mg daily). Pregnant women taking iron or iron and folic acid are less likely to have anemia or iron deficiency at term.[14] Preterm birth, LBW, perinatal mortality, stillbirth, and neonatal mortality are also positively impacted, especially in developing countries.

Prenatal Visits

Continuity of care during pregnancy by one provider or a small team seems to benefit women. Women receiving prenatal care from a single physician are likely to receive more prenatal care, which has been correlated with increased maternal weight gain and infant birth weight.[15] A Cochrane review concluded that low-risk prenatal care provided by family physicians, obstetricians, and midwives is equally effective, although women seem more satisfied with care provided by family physicians and midwives.[16] Group prenatal visits, where women attend visits with a cohort of similar gestational age pregnancies, are another form of prenatal care.[17]

Schedule of prenatal visits

▶ First visit at 6–8 weeks of gestation

▶ Monthly visits until 28 weeks of gestation

▶ Biweekly visits from 28–36 weeks

▶ Weekly visits after 36 weeks until delivery

First Trimester Prenatal Care

The first 13 weeks of pregnancy are the most critical period in fetal development because the majority of organogenesis occurs during this time. This is when the embryo/fetus is most susceptible to environmental and teratogenic insults.

Physical Examination

Most clinical guidelines for routine prenatal care recommend measuring blood pressure (BP) at the initial and subsequent prenatal visits. Levels over 140 mm Hg systolic or 90 mm Hg diastolic recorded on two occasions more than 6 hours apart indicate hypertension. At a gestational age of <20 weeks, BP elevation is usually attributed to chronic hypertension unless trophoblastic (molar) disease or multiple gestation is present. **Gestational hypertension** is defined as hypertension after 20 weeks of pregnancy that is not associated with proteinuria.

Height and weight are measured at the initial physical examination to calculate the patient's body mass index (BMI). Significantly under- or overweight status should be noted. Recommended weight gain during pregnancy is based on prepregnancy BMI as shown in Table 8.3.

A physical examination should be performed at the initial visit, unless the woman had one during preconception care. Poor dentition, specifically gingival disease, increases the risk of preterm delivery. Patellar and ankle reflexes are checked and documented because pre-eclampsia often manifests with hyperreflexia. The clinical breast examination is used to detect abnormalities such as cancer or fibrocystic disease. Randomized clinical trials (RCTs) do not show that either nipple shields or Hoffman's exercises influence success with breastfeeding and suggest discontinuing routine examination of the nipples for inversion.

Table 8.3 ▶ Institute of Medicine Recommendations for Pregnancy Weight Gain

Prepregnancy BMI	Suggested Weight Gain (lb)
<19.8 (Low)	28–40
19.8–26.0 (Normal)	25–35
26.1–29.0 (Overweight)	15–25
>29.0 (Obese)	11–20

Data from: http://nationalacademies.org/hmd/~/media/Files/Report%20Files/2009/Weight-Gain-During-Pregnancy-Reexamining-the-Guidelines/Report%20Brief%20-%20Weight%20Gain%20During%20Pregnancy.pdf

An initial pelvic examination is used to detect anatomic defects of the reproductive tract and screen for sexually transmitted infections (STIs), including genital abnormalities such as herpetic lesions or condyloma.

While cervical length, dilation, effacement, and position should be documented at the initial examination, routine cervical checks at every prenatal visit are ineffective for predicting preterm birth and not recommended. The bimanual examination is useful for evaluating the adnexa and estimating uterine size. Clinical pelvimetry is no longer recommended.

Laboratory Testing

Table 8.4 displays the recommended laboratory testing at the first prenatal visit. Situations that result in maternal–fetal blood exchange (i.e., amniocentesis, abruptio placentae, trauma, threatened pregnancy loss, and elective termination) necessitate RhoGAM administration in Rh(D)-negative women.

Bacterial vaginosis (BV) is present in 15% to 45% of women and confers a 2- to 4-fold increased risk for preterm delivery and PPROM.[18] The U.S. Preventive Services Task Force (USPSTF) and the American Congress of Obstetricians and Gynecologists (ACOG) currently recommend against screening women at average risk for preterm delivery for BV because screening and treating all pregnant women with BV does not appear to prevent preterm delivery. Women with a history of preterm delivery may benefit from BV screening/treatment.

Human immunodeficiency virus (HIV) testing is recommended for all pregnant women in the first trimester with repeat testing in the third trimester for women at increased risk. Combinations of medications (lamivudine [Epivir], zidovudine [Retrovir], and nevirapine [Viramune]) reduce fetal transmission. While elective cesarean may decrease risk of HIV transmission, recent US studies show no benefit beyond that of use of highly active antiretroviral therapy in women who have a viral load <1,000 copies/mL.[19]

Immunization

Vaccination against hepatitis B is safe in pregnancy and can be offered to women at increased risk. Repeat screening of women at risk is also recommended in some guidelines. Newborns of mothers who are hepatitis B surface antigen positive should receive hepatitis B vaccination and hepatitis B immunoglobulin immediately after delivery.

Ultrasound

Ultrasound at 18 to 20 weeks of gestation is commonly performed, even though evidence does not correlate routine ultrasound screening with improved pregnancy outcomes. Authors of a Cochrane review concluded that routine ultrasound prior to 24 weeks improved pregnancy dating and decreased need for postdate induction. The National Institutes of Health and ACOG recommend ultrasound for specific indications (Table 8.5) rather than routinely in low-risk pregnancies. Denise has had an uneventful pregnancy at 20 weeks and understands that your practice does not routinely order ultrasounds.

Genetic Screening

Available options to detect fetal structural and chromosomal anomalies include ultrasound, maternal serum screening, and noninvasive prenatal testing using fetal cell free DNA. The goal of screening is to identify fetal anomalies that are either not compatible with life or are associated with long-term disability and morbidity.

Table 8.4 ▶ Laboratory Tests Performed During Routine Prenatal Care

Test	Maternal Effects	Risks to Fetus	SOR
ABO type, Rh, and antibody screen	If RhoGAM is not given to an Rh– mother, 0.7–1.8% of women develop antenatal isoimmunization; 8–17% during delivery	Without treatment, one-third of fetuses develop hemolytic anemia and hyperbilirubinemia, and another quarter develop hydrops resulting in death	A
Hemoglobin/ hematocrit	Most common cause of anemia in pregnancy is iron deficiency[a]		B: First visit C: Repeat testing in asymptomatic low-risk women
RPR/VDRL for syphilis	Premature delivery occurs in 20% of cases of maternal syphilis; vertical transmission is estimated at 60–80%	Congenital syphilis causes fetal anemia, pneumonia, hepato-splenomegaly, and nonimmune hydrops.	A: Rescreen in third trimester if high risk
Rubella titer		Congenital rubella causes senso-rineural deafness, micro-ophthal-mia, encephalopathy, cataracts, and cardiac abnormalities	B: Screen child-bearing-aged women by vacci-nation history or serology
Hepatitis B surface antigen (HBsAg)		When a pregnant woman is pos-itive for HBsAg or e-antigen, the fetus has a 70–90% chance of acquiring hepatitis B; 85–90% of infected infants become chronic carriers	A: Rescreen in third trimester if high risk
Gonorrhea	Infection strongly linked with preterm delivery	Fetal infection can result in spon-taneous abortion and stillbirth; neonatal infection causes gonococcal ophthalmia, arthritis, and sepsis	B: High risk C: Universal screening
Chlamydia	Infection associated with higher rates of preterm deliv-ery and intrauterine growth restriction	Pneumonia and ophthalmia neo-natorum in 30–50% of cases	B: High risk C: Universal screening
Papanicolaou test		If due	A
Urine culture	ASB in pregnancy is a risk factor for pyelonephritis and preterm delivery	Prematurity and low birth weight.	A
Human immu-nodeficiency virus (HIV)	Maternal treatment with zidovudine reduces vertical transmission of HIV from 25–8.3%	HIV infection	A: High risk C: Universal screening

[a]Treat anemia with iron supplements if hemoglobin <11 g/dL in first and third trimesters or <10 g/dL in second trimester
ASB, asymptomatic bacteriuria; hx, history.

Table 8.5 ▶ Indications for Ultrasound During Pregnancy

Indications

- Estimation of gestational age
- Vaginal bleeding
- Evaluation of fetal growth
- Evaluation for placentation/multiple gestation pregnancy
- Suspected hydatidiform mole
- Suspected ectopic pregnancy
- Size/dates discrepancy
- Suspected polyhydramnios or oligohydramnios
- Evaluation of abnormal genetic screening tests
- Fetal anomaly assessment
- History of previous fetal anomaly/congenital defects

Data from: American College of Radiology. ACR practice guidelines for the performance of antepartum obstetrical ultrasound. In: *ACR Practice Guidelines and Technical Standards,* 2003. Philadelphia, PA: ACR; 2003;625–631.

The risk of Down syndrome increases with maternal age. The odds of having an infant with Down syndrome at age 20 years are approximately 1:1,440, increasing to 1:338 at age 35 years and 1:32 at 45 years of age.[20] All pregnant women 35 years or older at the time of delivery should be offered genetic counseling and chorionic villus sampling (CVS) or amniocentesis for the diagnosis of genetic abnormalities. Thirty-five years is the threshold for offering amniocentesis because this is the age when the risk of having a fetus with a chromosomal defect equals the rate of fetal loss from amniocentesis.

Nuchal translucency of the fetal neck on ultrasound is often combined with β-HCG and Pappalysin-1 in first trimester screening. Increased fetal nuchal thickness is a marker for Down syndrome. Noninvasive prenatal testing (NIPT) analyzes cell-free fetal DNA in maternal blood from which the fetal karyotype can be determined. Sensitivity is 99% with 0.1% specificity.[21] NIPT is not recommended for low-risk pregnancies, multiple gestations, or pregnancies with ultrasound-detected anomalies; maternal obesity can also lead to decreased sensitivity.

Women with an abnormal first-trimester genetic screening are offered CVS between 10 and 12 weeks' of gestation or amniocentesis between 15 and 20 weeks of gestation. Placental tissue is obtained using ultrasound-guided needle biopsy of the placental villi. CVS cannot be used to diagnose NTDs.

Second and Third Trimester Prenatal Care

Traditional components of subsequent prenatal visits include measurement of weight, BP, fundal height, and fetal heart tones.

Physical Examination

Inadequate weight gain may be associated with LBW, preterm delivery, and intrauterine growth restriction. Obese women have an increased risk of gestational diabetes (GDM), pre-eclampsia, preterm delivery, vacuum or forceps delivery, and cesarean.[22]

Most guidelines recommend **measuring BP at every prenatal visit**. Early detection of an elevated BP trend persisting over time is the best screening strategy for gestational hypertensive disorders.

In the second and third trimester, **fundal height** is a good estimate of uterine size and gestational age. Fundal height is measured as the distance in centimeters between the superior edge of the pubic symphysis and the top of the uterine fundus (see https://www.youtube.com/watch?v=nyfUh5zlB1U). At 20 weeks of gestation, the fundus should be at the level of the umbilicus. During each week between 20 and 36 weeks of gestation, the fundal height increases by about 1 cm. Measurements deviating by more than 2 cm may indicate problems with fetal growth.

Auscultation of the fetal heart rate is generally done at all follow-up visits. Normal fetal heart rate ranges from 110 to 160 beats per minute.

Laboratory Testing

Routine urine dipstick tests for protein and glucose are no longer recommended during prenatal visits. They are unreliable in detecting the moderate or variable elevations of albumin that occur with pre-eclampsia.

The American College of Obstetricians and Gynecologists recommends that all pregnant women be **screened for GDM**, whether by patient medical history, clinical risk factors, or laboratory screening blood glucose results.[23] In women with risk factors, early screening at prenatal intake may be considered to detect women with preexisting undiagnosed type 2 diabetes. These **risk factors** include previous history of GDM, history of or current impaired glucose metabolism, and BMI >30. If early screening is normal, repeat screening is done at 24 to 28 weeks gestation

Screening for GDM is generally performed at 24 to 28 weeks' gestation. The 1-hour test measures blood glucose 1 hour after oral ingestion of 50 g glucose. The upper limit of normal for the 1-hour test is between 130 and 140 mg/dL.

If the 1-hour test is abnormal, a 3-hour glucose tolerance test (GTT) should be administered. After a fasting blood glucose is measured, a 100-g oral glucose load is given, with blood glucose drawn hourly for three consecutive samples. A diagnosis of GDM is made when elevation occurs with either the fasting glucose alone or with two or more of the 3-hour measurements.

When diet alone is ineffective for controlling blood glucose, medication is generally instituted. Use of oral diabetes medications (sulfonylureas and metformin) is increasingly common, although insulin continues to be the therapy with the best-known safety profile.

An **antibody screen for isoimmunization** in women who are Rh negative is done at 28 weeks' gestation. Rho(D) immune globulin is given to Rh-negative women with a negative screen. Women with a positive antibody screen do not benefit from Rho(D) injection and should be evaluated for Rh hemolytic disease.

Retesting for anemia with a hematocrit or hemoglobin at 28 weeks' gestation is appropriate because maternal blood volume expands during the second trimester.

In the third trimester, both ACOG and USPSTF recommend **repeat screening for hepatitis B, syphilis, gonorrhea, and chlamydia in high-risk populations**. High-risk populations include women younger than age 25 with two or more sexual contacts, women who work in the sex trade, and women with prior history of syphilis or gonorrhea.

Patients and their partners should be asked about a history of genital and oro-labial **herpes simplex infection (HSV)**. Rates of vertical transmission at delivery are 57% in primary HSV infection, 25% in nonprimary first episodes, and 2% for recurrent infection.[24]

The infection is transmitted to the fetus as it passes through the birth canal, with localized disease-causing lesions on the neonate's face, eyes and mouth. More severe infection involving the central nervous system carries a 4% mortality rate, while disseminated HSV infection causes 30% mortality in neonates.[25] **ACOG recommends antiviral therapy for women with primary HSV infections and those at risk for recurrent infections after 36 weeks' gestation** (strength of recommendation [SOR] C). Delivery by cesarean is recommended for women who have active genital herpes lesions present at the time of labor.

Group B streptococcus (GBS) is a leading cause of neonatal morbidity and mortality. GBS in the genital and gastrointestinal tract affects 6.6% to 20% of pregnant women in the United States. The CDC, ACOG, and the American Academy of Pediatricians (AAP) all recommend that women be offered screening for GBS at 35 to 37 weeks of gestation. Women who are culture positive for GBS should receive antibiotic prophylaxis (intravenous penicillin G) during labor. A free online app from the Center for Disease Control is available at http://www.cdc.gov/groupbstrep/guidelines/prevention-app.html.

PATIENT EDUCATION AND PSYCHOSOCIAL SUPPORT

Denise continues to come for her routine prenatal care and confides in you that the father of the baby is no longer involved. Her family has been very supportive and she plans to move in with her sister for a while. She has questions about her diet, but is gaining weight normally. She also wants to know if it is safe to wear her seat belt now that her belly is so big and what she can do for constipation.

Diet and Dietary Supplements

Pregnant women are encouraged to eat a varied diet. Most pregnant women require an additional 150 calories daily during the first trimester and 300 to 500 extra calories daily in the second and third trimesters.

Pregnant women are at risk from certain foods during pregnancy. Consumption of monkfish, swordfish, shark, king mackerel, tilefish, and tuna is linked to mercury exposure. Mercury can adversely affect fetal neurologic development, and the Food and Drug Administration (FDA) advises pregnant women to consume no more than 12 ounces of tuna weekly.[26] Oysters, certain types of sushi, and raw shellfish may harbor *Vibrio cholera*, *Vibrio parahaemolyticus*, hepatitis A, or parasites and are best avoided during pregnancy. *Escherichia coli* (*E. coli*) food poisoning can result from eating beef that is not thoroughly cooked. Listeriosis is a bacterial infection associated with milk, fruit juice, cheese, or dairy products that are not pasteurized. Listeriosis is associated with chorioamnionitis, preterm delivery, and fetal demise. Pregnant women should avoid soft, unpasteurized cheeses such as brie and camembert, and all varieties of pâté.

Artificial sweeteners such as Aspartame and Splenda are unlikely to cause fetal toxicity. Insufficient evidence is available as to whether caffeine affects infant birth weight or other pregnancy outcomes.[27]

Lifestyle Topics

Most couples can safely continue normal sexual relations. Sexual intercourse is contraindicated with placenta previa, preterm labor, and cervical insufficiency. Condoms are advised if exposure to STI is a possibility.

Commercial air travel is generally safe and women with uncomplicated singleton gestations can fly until 36 weeks of gestation. Recommendations include sitting in an aisle seat, performing isometric calf exercises to reduce venous thrombus formation, walking in the cabin when possible, and drinking water to prevent dehydration (SOR C).

Pregnant women should wear seat belts in cars. Motor vehicle accidents are a leading cause of death and disability in pregnant women. The lap belt should be worn under the uterus and across the hips, and the shoulder belt worn above the fundus and between the breasts. The fit should be snug and belts should never be worn over the fundus.

Strong evidence suggests that exercise in pregnancy is safe and beneficial. Regular exercise improves maternal fitness and wellbeing, reduces musculoskeletal complaints, and moderates maternal weight gain. In the absence of medical or obstetric contraindications, most women who are active prior to pregnancy can continue their usual activities. Recommend at least 20 to 30 minutes of moderate-intensity exercise (e.g., walking, swimming, and water aerobics) daily or on most days per week.

Medication Use

Prescribing medications during pregnancy involves balancing maternal benefit with potential risks to the fetus. Women who require drugs with known risk should be transitioned to medication with less risk when possible, especially during organogenesis.

Nearly half of all women use complementary and alternative therapies. The safety and efficacy of the majority of complementary therapies used during pregnancy have not been established. Ginger reduces nausea and vomiting in early pregnancy by blocking 5-HT3 receptors and suppressing the neural pathway between the emetic center in the medulla and the stomach. Red raspberry leaf in tea or capsule form is purported to stimulate labor. Neither ginger nor raspberry leaf is associated with adverse pregnancy outcomes.[28]

Intimate Partner Violence

Intimate partner violence (IPV) affects up to 20% of pregnant women (Chapter 21). Abuse often intensifies during pregnancy, and women who are abused may be less likely to obtain prenatal care. IPV screening during pregnancy is done at the initial prenatal visit using a brief interview question. Placental abruption, LBW, fetal loss, and postpartum depression are associated with IPV.

Denise had a normal 1-hour glucose tolerance test at 26 weeks and comes back in for her group B streptococcus (GBS) screen at 36 weeks. She has been having heartburn over the past 2 weeks, and also says that her back hurts after she has been at work all day. Her fundal height is 36 cm and is consistent with her dates. She wants to discuss breast feeding. Her mother did not breastfeed her but she wants to do what is best for the baby.

Common Problems

Subsequent visits are an appropriate time for anticipatory guidance about normal pregnancy-related issues (Table 8.6). Reassuring women that these changes are normal, common, and transient is important.

Large amounts of information are available about pregnancy through books, videos, and the internet and many women have specific ideas about what they want during labor. Use of epidural, breastfeeding, infant rooming-in versus nursery care, pacifier use, and

Table 8.6 ▶ Common Problems in Pregnancy

Problem	Cause	Counseling Tips
Heartburn	Relaxation of the lower esophageal sphincter and increased bowel transit due to increased progesterone	Eating smaller meals and avoiding greasy foods often improves symptoms. Antacids containing calcium carbonate can be helpful as can H2 blockers
Urinary frequency/stress urinary incontinence	Common in first and third trimesters	Symptoms usually resolve post pregnancy. Kegel exercises to strengthen pelvic floor
Hemorrhoids	Worsen in pregnancy due to increased venous congestion in the rectal vascular plexus	Topical treatments (witch hazel pads, external hemorrhoid cream and sitz baths). Several prenatal vitamins contain prophylactic stool softeners like docusate sodium (Colace)
Backache	Common in later pregnancy due to compensatory lordosis from enlarging uterus; relaxin loosens ligaments in the pubic symphysis, back, and pelvis	Wear flat-heeled shoes and maintain good posture to counter changes in center of gravity
Round ligament pain	Spasm of round ligaments Sharp, stabbing, sporadic pain located in the inguinal area. Worse in multiparas; not harmful to the fetus.	Exercise, warm baths, a pregnancy girdle, and acetaminophen sometimes help
Leukorrhea	Heavy, whitish vaginal discharge seen in pregnancy Results from increased vaginal blood flow and increased estrogen levels	Reassurance that discharge is physiologic and not due to infection

circumcision can all be addressed as part of the birth plan. Discussing the planned course early allows the physician flexibility in accommodating the patient's wishes. Developing a birth plan can facilitate a discussion of labor options between a pregnant woman and her family physician. Many hospital websites have sample birth plans.

Breastfeeding support/education provided by professionals and peers to individual women, regardless of maternal age, is associated with an increase in the duration of any and exclusive breastfeeding.[29] Babies who are breastfed are less likely to develop otitis media, gastroenteritis, upper respiratory infections, and urinary tract infections.

Physicians often recommend structured educational programs for childbirth and parenting. Several observational studies demonstrate improved performance in labor in expectant women who attend childbirth classes. Knowing what to expect during labor helps parents play a more active and informed role.

Trial of Labor after Cesarean/Vaginal Birth after Cesarean

Discussing delivery plans with women who have had a previous cesarean delivery is usually done prior to the late second trimester. For many women, trial of labor after cesarean (TOLAC) is preferred over elective repeat cesarean.

Both ACOG and the American Academy of Family Physicians (AAFP) have issued guidelines for women considering TOLAC/VBAC (http://www.aafp.org/afp/2005/1115/p2126.html and http://www.seminperinat.com/article/S0146-0005(10)00056-X/abstract). Women with one previous cesarean delivery with a low transverse uterine incision should be offered a trial of labor.

About three quarters of women who attempt TOLAC are successful. A calculator to estimate the chances for successful TOLAC can be found at https://mfmu.bsc.gwu.edu/PublicBSC/MFMU/VGBirthCalc/vagbirth.html. No evidence-based recommendations are available regarding the best method for presenting risks and benefits of TOLAC to patients.

Denise is now 41 weeks of estimated gestation age and she comes in to discuss plans. She elects to proceed with a medical induction and receives intravaginal misoprostol (cytotec) followed by Pitocin. She delivers a 7-lb 5-oz female with Apgars of 9 and 9.

Postdate Pregnancy

In the absence of medical or obstetric indications, induction of labor should not be performed earlier than 39 weeks of gestation. One-tenth of pregnancies continue to at least 42 weeks of gestation and are considered postdates. Maternal risks associated with postdate pregnancy include dystocia, postpartum hemorrhage, and emergent surgical delivery. Fetal risks include asphyxia, meconium aspiration, septicemia, and death.

The most common cause of postdate pregnancy is inaccurate dating. A Cochrane review of 22 RCTs found that routine labor induction at 41 weeks is associated with fewer perinatal deaths and fewer cesareans.[30]

The ACOG recommends fetal assessment beginning at 41 weeks of gestation.[31] When a physician and patient elect to manage a postdate pregnancy expectantly, fetal monitoring is indicated. A combination of twice-weekly nonstress testing (NST), amniotic fluid index, or biophysical profile (BPP) is used, although evidence of benefit is unclear and no single test is better than another.

The interpretation of NST uses three categories to assess risk (Table 8.7).[32] A category 1 NST has a negative predictive value (NPV) for stillbirth of 99.8% and a positive predictive value (PPV) of 10%. The BPP (http://perinatology.com/Reference/glossary/B/Biophysical%20profile.htm) has an NPV of 99.9% and a PPV of 40% (Chapter 3).[33]

Table 8.7 ▶ Postdate Pregnancy Surveillance Using Nonstress Testing

Nonstress Test Result	Criteria
Category 1 (normal)	Two or more fetal heart rate accelerations over a 20-minute period; each acceleration must be at least 15 beats above the baseline heart rate and last at least 15 seconds; testing may be extended to 40 minutes to account for fetal sleep–wake cycles
Category 2 (equivocal)	Further testing required
Category 3 (abnormal)	No accelerations seen over a 40-minute period; if strip does not normalize, consider delivery

Data from: ACOG practice bulletin. Antepartum fetal surveillance. Number 9, October 1999. Clinical management guidelines for obstetrician-gynecologists. *Int J Gynaecol Obstet.* 2000;68:175–185; ACOG Practice Bulletin No. 106. Intrapartum fetal heart rate monitoring: nomenclature, interpretation, and general management principles. *Obstet Gyncol.* 2009;114(1):192–202.

FAMILY PHYSICIANS AND OBSTETRIC CONSULTANTS

Family physicians work closely with their obstetric consultants in caring for pregnant women who require higher acuity care. When the consultation process works effectively, the patient benefits from a specialty opinion while maintaining the continuity relationship with the primary physician. The AAFP–ACOG liaison committee has published guidelines for consultations between family physicians and obstetrician gynecologists.[34] Family physicians are encouraged to request consults in a timely fashion, clearly discuss the reasons for consultation, and maintain collegial relationships with physicians who provide back-up.

Summary of Evidence-Based Recommendations

Preconception Care

Recommendation	Strength of Recommendation[a]
Women considering becoming pregnant and pregnant women should be counseled that dietary supplementation with folic acid (400 μg) before conception and during the first trimester decreases the risk of NTDs in the fetus[35]	A
Intensive preconception glycemic control in women with diabetes prevents major congenital anomalies in offspring[36]	A
Women with epilepsy planning to conceive should be changed to monotherapy or less teratogenic medications when possible, and advised to take at least 1 mg of folic acid daily prior to conception[37]	B
Smoking cessation should be advised for all women who anticipate becoming pregnant[38]	A

Pregnancy Care

Recommendation	SOR[a]
The traditional visit schedule can be abbreviated without an increase in adverse maternal or neonatal outcomes[16]	A
Women with a continuity provider are more likely to attend prenatal education, discuss concerns, require less analgesia in labor, and feel prepared for delivery and infant care[15]	A
Maternal weight and height should be measured at the first antenatal appointment in order to calculate the body mass index (BMI)[20,39]	B
Blood pressure measurement is recommended at each prenatal visit[20,39]	C
Routine breast examination during antenatal care is not recommended for the promotion of postpartum breast feeding[20]	A
Routine cervical examination is not effective for predicting preterm birth[20]	A
Pregnant women should be offered fundal height measurements at each prenatal visit to detect small or large for gestation fetuses[20]	B
Routine ultrasound prior to 24 weeks allows for better estimation of gestational age and decreased need for labor induction for postdate pregnancy. No significant difference in clinical outcomes is apparent[40]	A

Pregnancy Care Recommendation	SOR[a]
Pregnant women over age 35 years or with an abnormal screening test (triple screen, quadruple screen) should be offered screening for Down syndrome[20]	B
Healthy, pregnant women are encouraged to participate in mild to moderate exercise three or more times weekly[41]	A
Individualized exercise programs should consider each pregnant woman's prepregnancy activity and fitness levels[41]	B
Pregnant women should be counseled as to the proper use and positioning of seat belts (three-point restraints located across the hips and above the fundus)[42]	B
Sexual intercourse during pregnancy is not associated with harmful effects in the absence of obstetric contraindications[20]	B

[a]A, consistent, good-quality patient-oriented evidence; B, inconsistent or limited-quality patient-oriented evidence; C, consensus, disease-oriented evidence, usual practice, expert opinion, or case series.
For information about the SORT evidence rating system, see http://www.aafp.org/afpsort.xml.

QUESTIONS

1. Which of the following should be done at a preconception visit?
   A. Ultrasound
   B. Pap smear
   C. Iron supplementation
   D. Genetic risk assessment

2. Folic acid reduces the risk of which one of the following conditions?
   A. Gestational hypertension
   B. Preterm labor
   C. Neural tube defects
   D. Pre-eclampsia
   E. Fetal anemia

3. Family physicians have worse obstetric outcomes than obstetricians for similar risk patients.
   A. True
   B. False

4. Which one of the following is a risk factor for gestational diabetes?
   A. Age greater than 25 years
   B. BMI > 30
   C. African-American race
   D. Poor gestational weight gain

5. Which one of the following is part of management for pregnant women with a history of genital herpes?
   A. Start antiviral prophylaxis at 28 weeks
   B. Have a cesarean section delivery
   C. Start antiviral prophylaxis after 36 weeks
   D. Not worry since neonatal herpes is very rare
   E. Not take antiviral medications since they are contraindicated in pregnancy

ANSWERS

Question 1: The correct answer is D.
Goals of preconception genetic counseling include counseling women who are at risk for a fetal anomaly or genetic disorder and informing couples about available screening tests. Carrier testing can be performed before pregnancy in patients with known familial disorders. Women at risk for having a child with sickle cell disease, thalassemia, or cystic fibrosis should also be screened in the preconception period.

Question 2: The correct answer is C.
Folic acid consumption reduces the risk of neural tube defects (NTDs).

Question 3: The correct answer is B.
A Cochrane review concluded that low-risk prenatal care provided by family physicians, obstetricians, and midwives is equally effective, although women seem more satisfied with care provided by family physicians and midwives.

Question 4: The correct answer is B.
Obese women have an increased risk of gestational diabetes, pre-eclampsia, preterm delivery, vacuum or forceps delivery, and cesarean.

Question 5: The correct answer is C.
American Congress of Obstetricians and Gynecologists recommends antiviral therapy for women with primary herpes simplex virus infections and those at risk for recurrent infections after 36 weeks of gestation.

REFERENCES

1. Tong STC, Makaroff LA, Xierali IM, et al. Proportion of family physicians providing maternity care continues to decline. *J Am Board Fam Med.* 2012;25(3):270–271.
2. Kozhimannil KB, Fontaine P. Care from family physicians reported by pregnancy women in the United States. *Ann Fam Med.* 2013;11(4):350–354.
3. Avery DM, Graettinger KR, Waits S, et al. Comparison of delivery procedure rates among obstetrician-gynecologists and family physicians practicing obstetrics. *Am J Clin Med.* 2014;10(1):16–20.
4. Kennedy D, Koren G. Identifying women who might benefit from higher doses of folic acid in pregnancy. *Can Fam Physician.* 2012;58(4):394–397.
5. Lagana AS, Triolo O, D'Amico V, et al. Management of women with epilepsy: From preconception to postpartum. *Arch Gynecol Obstet.* 2016;293:493–503.
6. Gruber R. The US FDA pregnancy lactation and labeling rule- implications for maternal immunization. *Vaccine.* 2015;33:6499–6500.
7. Castillo-Solorzano C, Reef SE, Morice A, et al. Rubella vaccination of unknowingly pregnant women during mass campaigns for rubella and congenital rubella syndrome elimination, the Americas 2001–2008. *J Infect Dis.* 2011;204(Suppl 2):S713–S717.
8. DATA 2020. Healthy people 2020 database. MICH 10.2 Percent of US women receiving early and adequate prenatal care. *Available from:* https://www.healthypeople.gov/2020/topics-objectives/objective/mich-102. Accessed November 2016.
9. Centers for Disease Control and Prevention. Pregnancy mortality surveillance system. Available from: http://www.cdc.gov/reproductivehealth/maternalinfanthealth/pmss.html. Accessed November 2016.
10. Centers for Disease Control and Prevention. Preterm birth. Available from: http://www.cdc.gov/reproductivehealth/MaternalInfantHealth/PretermBirth.htm. Accessed November 2016.
11. Reichman NE, Teitler JO. Timing of enhanced prenatal care and birth outcomes in New Jersey's Health Start Program. *Mat Child Health J.* 2005;9(2):151–158.

12. Paul M, Schaff E, Nichols M. The roles of clinical assessment, human chorionic gonadotrophin assays, and ultrasonography in medical abortion practice. *Am J Obstet Gynecol.* 2000;183(2 Supplement):S34–S43.
13. Berard A, Zhao J, Sheehy O. Success of smoking cessation interventions during pregnancy. *Am J Obstet Gynecol.* 2016;215(5):611.e1–611.e8.
14. Haider BA, Bhutta ZA. Multiple-micronutrient supplementation for women during pregnancy. *Cochrane Database Syst Rev.* 2015;(11):CD004905.
15. Boss DJ, Timbrook RE. Clinical obstetric outcomes related to continuity in prenatal care. *J Am Board Fam Pract.* 2001;14:418–423.
16. Villar J, Carroli G, Khan-Neelofur D, et al. Patterns of routine antenatal care for low-risk pregnancy. *Cochrane Database Syst Rev.* 2001;(4):CD000934.
17. Craswell A, Kearney L, Reed R. Expecting and connecting group pregnancy care: Evaluation of a collaborative clinic. *Women Birth.* 2016;29(5):416–422.
18. Hendler I, Andrews WW, Carey CJ, et al. The relationship between resolution of asymptomatic bacterial vaginosis and spontaneous preterm birth in fetal-fibronectin positive women. *Am J Obstet Gynecol.* 2007;197:488.e1–488.e5.
19. Briand N, Jasseron C, Sibiude J, et al. Cesarean section for HIV-infected women in the combination antiretroviral therapies era, 2000–2010. *Am J Obstet Gynecol.* 2013;209(4):335.e1–335.e12.
20. National Collaborating Centre for Women's and Children's Health. Antenatal care: routine care for the healthy prenatal woman. Clinical Guideline October 2012; Royal College of Obstetricians and Gynecologists. Available from: http://www.vcog.org.uk/resources/Public/Antenatal_care.pdf. Accessed January 2017.
21. Connor P, Gustafsson S, Kublickas M. First trimester contingent testing with either nuchal translucency of cell-free DNA. Cost efficiency and the role of ultrasound dating. *Acta Obstret Gynecol Scand.* 2015;94:368–375.
22. Ma RC, Schmidt MI, Tam WH, et al. Clinical management of pregnancy in the obese mother: before conception, during pregnancy, and postpartum. *Lancet Diabetes Endocrinol.* 2016;4(12)1037–1049.
23. American College of Obstetricians and Gynecologists. Gestational diabetes mellitus. *Obstet Gynecol.* 2013;122(2):406–416.
24. Brown ZA, Wald A, Morrow RA, et al. Effect of serologic status and cesarean delivery on transmission rates of herpes simplex virus from mother to infant. *JAMA.* 2003;289:203–209.
25. ACOG Practice Bulletin. No. 82. Management of herpes in pregnancy. *Obstet Gynecol.* 2007;109(6):1489–1498.
26. U.S. Food and Drug Administration. What you need to know about mercury in fish and shellfish. Available from: http://www.fda.gov/ResourcesForYou/consumers/ucm110591.htm. Accessed November 2016.
27. Jahanfar S, Jaafar SH. Effects of restricted caffeine intake by mother on fetal, neonatal and pregnancy outcomes. *Cochrane Database Syst Rev.* 2015;(6):CD006965.
28. Dante G, Bellei G, Neri I, et al. Herbal therapies in pregnancy: What works? *Curr Opin Obstet Gynecol.* 2014;26(2):83–91.
29. Patnode CD, Henninger ML, Senger CA, et al. Primary care interventions to support breastfeeding: Updated systematic review for the U.S. Preventive Services Task Force; Rockville (MD): Agency for Healthcare Research and Quality (US); 2016 Oct. Report No.: 15-05218-EF-1.
30. Gulmezoglu AM, Crowther CA, Middleton P, et al. Induction of labour for improving birth outcomes for women at or beyond term. *Cochrane Database Syst Rev.* 2012;(6):CD004945.
31. ACOG Practice Bulletin No. 146. Management of late-term and postterm pregnancies. *Obstet Gynecol.* 2014;124(2 Pt 1):390–396.
32. ACOG Practice Bulletin No. 106. Intrapartum fetal heart rate monitoring: nomenclature, interpretation, and general management principles. *Obstet Gyncol.* 2009;114(1):192–202.
33. ACOG Practice Bulletin. No. 145. Anterpartum fetal surveillance. *Obstet Gynecol.* 2014;124(1):182–192.
34. The American Academy of Family Physicians and the American College of Obstetricians and Gynecologists. AAFP-ACOG joint statement on cooperative practice and hospital privileges. AAFP-ACOG Liaison Committee position statement. Available from: http://www.aafp.org/online/en/home/policy/policies/o/obstetric.html. Accessed January 2017.
35. De-Regil LM, Pena-Rosas JP, Fernandez-Gaxiola AC, et al. Effects and safety of periconceptional oral folate supplementation for preventing birth defects. *Cochrane Database Syst Rev.* 2015;(12):CD007950.
36. Tennant PW, Gliniania SV, Bilous RW, et al. Pre-existing diabetes, maternal glycated haemoglobin, and the risks of fetal and infant death: a population-based study. *Diabetologia.* 2014;57(2):285–294.

37. Borgelt LM, Hart FM, Bainbridge JL. Epilepsy during pregnancy: Focus on management strategies. *Int J Women's Health.* 2016;8:505–517.
38. Lindson-Hawley N, Hartmann-Boyce J, Fanshawe TR, et al. Interventions to reduce harm from continued tobacco use. *Cochrane Database Syst Rev.* 2016;(10):CD005231.
39. Akkerman D, Cleland L, Croft G, et al. Institute for Clinical Systems Improvement. Routine prenatal care. Updated July 2012. Institute for Clinical Systems Improvement (ICSI). Available from: https://www.icsi.org/_asset/13n9y4/Prenatal.pdf. Accessed November 2016.
40. Whitworth M, Bricker K, Mullan C. Ultrasound for fetal assessment in early pregnancy. *Cochrane Database Syst Rev.* 2015;14(7):CD007058.
41. American College of Obstetricians and Gynecologists. ACOG Committee Opinion No. 650: Physical activity and exercise during pregnancy and the postpartum period. *Obstet Gynecol.* 2015;126(6):e135–e142.
42. Klinich KD, Flannagan CA, Rupp JD, et al. Fetal outcome in motor-vehicle crashes: Effects of crash characteristics and maternal restraint. *Am J Obstet Gynecol.* 2008;198(4):450.e1–450.e9.

The Pediatric Well-Child Check

KEY POINTS

1 ▶ The pediatric well-child visit allows the provider to monitor growth and development and provide anticipatory guidance to children and their families.

2 ▶ Screen for potential causes of poor health including health habits, exposures, and risk factors at these visits.

3 ▶ Assure that children receive all of their immunizations in a timely manner.

4 ▶ Use these opportunities to develop strong relationships with the child and their family over time; this is a source of great satisfaction for families and providers alike.

The pediatric well-child check is the cornerstone of care for the pediatric patient. This chapter is organized by age group to tailor discussion of important health concerns, screening protocols, risk assessment and harm reduction, and appropriate education.

AGES 0 TO 2 YEARS

You are seeing a 3-day-old newborn, Jay, born at term via uneventful vaginal delivery. You don't know the family well, but met the mother during one of her prenatal visits during which she expressed an interest in "trying to breastfeed this time." You learn that she lives with her partner and their 6-year-old daughter in a two-bedroom apartment. Her partner's mother is currently staying with them.

The frequency and content of the newborn visits provide an opportunity to build a collaborative and trusting relationship with parents. In the course of routine well-child care, we can empower the parents as experts in the care of their child while also monitoring the growth and development of the child and supporting the parents as their life as a family unfolds.

Newborn Issues

Newborns should be seen for an outpatient visit by day 3 to 5 of life to assess hyperbilirubinemia.[1] If they are discharged before 48 hours of age, it is recommended that they been seen as an outpatient within 48 hours of hospital discharge.[2] Two issues to address are jaundice and weight.

▶ Assess jaundice at each outpatient visit in the newborn period. Its presence may be an additional reason to supplement breastfeeding (http://pediatrics.aappublications.org/content/pediatrics/124/4/1193.full.pdf). Jay does not appear jaundiced, but you plan to discuss breastfeeding with his mother and note that optimal breastfeeding of 8 to 12 feedings per day can help decrease the incidence of hyperbilirubinemia.

▶ The nadir of infant weight occurs around 72 hours of life following vaginal deliveries, but can be a bit later for operative births.[3] Jay has lost 5% of his birthweight. Average daily weight gain in the newborn period is 5 to 7 oz/week, or approximately 1 oz/day, once the baby starts gaining weight. If weight loss is noted, consider supplementation or increased feeding of the breastfed baby if[4]:

- Weight loss is 8% to 10% from birth
- There are signs of dehydration
- There is delayed lactogenesis or problems with milk transfer
- There is continued meconium on day 5 of life

> Clinicians providing care for newborns may benefit from training in breastfeeding medicine so that they can provide adequate education and support to breastfeeding patients; physician support of breastfeeding is instrumental in families' success in meeting their breastfeeding goals. (See www.bfmed.org for additional information.)

A summary of the well newborn can be found at: http://pedsinreview.aappublications. org/content/pedsinreview/33/1/4.full.pdf. Parents may need reassurance about typical newborn examination findings. The Stanford University Newborn Nursery Photo Gallery is an excellent resource for reviewing normal and abnormal newborn examination findings: http://med.stanford.edu/newborns/professional-education/photo-gallery.html. Table 9.1 lists items to review at the first outpatient visit.

If there are no concerns about weight, feeding, or jaundice at the first outpatient visit, the next routine visit occurs at 2 weeks of life. However, jaundice or weight gain concerns should prompt much closer follow-up, as often as daily or every 48 hours.

For first-time parents, especially with infants who are breastfeeding, a visit at 1 week of life is useful to assess adequacy of feeding and continue to provide family support. Many clinicians recommend a visit at 1 month of life as well, in order to continue to ensure normal newborn growth and development. As the American Academy of Pediatrics (AAP) recommends clinicians screen mothers for postpartum depression at well-child checks, these visits allow for screening and family support. Otherwise, routine visits occur at 2, 4, 6, 9, 12, 15, 18, and 24 months.

Table 9.1 ▶ First Outpatient Visit: History

Topic	Review
Prenatal and delivery course	Gestational age, known abnormalities, health risks, Apgar scores, initial newborn examination findings
Newborn testing	Newborn screen results, congenital heart defects screen, hearing screen
Examination finding, growth, and development	Birth trauma, hip dysplasia, percent weight loss since birth, feeding patterns and content of feeds, stooling and urination patterns, jaundice, and any treatment needed for these or other health concerns to date
Family habits, safety, and adjustment	Screening for postpartum depression, tobacco exposure, safe sleep for baby, effects of sleep deprivation on parents, child care planning

Newborn Screening

General information about the panel of blood tests obtained via heel stick at 24 hours of life or more, commonly called the "newborn screen," can be found on the CDC website at: http://www.cdc.gov/ncbddd/newbornscreening/. State specific information can be found at: http://www.babysfirsttest.org/newborn-screening/states.

The US Health Resources and Service Administration (HRSA) has issued a report that recommends screening for 32 specific conditions, but states are not required to screen for this uniform panel.[5] Some states screen for additional conditions as well. You let Jay's mother know that these test results will be available in a few weeks and that the office will notify her if any of the tests are positive and what will happen next.

Hearing Screening

CDC recommends that all babies have hearing screening performed before they reach 1 month of age; this is routinely performed before hospital discharge via Brainstem Auditory Evoked Response testing. You note that Jay had a normal test prior to discharge. Newborns who do not pass the hearing screen should have a full audiology evaluation as soon as possible, and no later than 3 months of age.[6]

Growth

Measurement and monitoring of growth is one of the primary reasons for routine well-child checks. From birth to 24 months of age, growth should be plotted on the World Health Organization (WHO) growth curves (http://depts.washington.edu/growth/). These curves are based on using a healthy, breastfed infant as the standard against which growth should be tracked; they should be used regardless of feeding method.

Newborns should regain any initial weight lost so that they are at least back to their birth weight by day 14 of life. Infants gain an average of 1 kg/month from age 0 to 3 months and 0.5 kg/month from age 3 to 6 months. The growth rate continues to slow thereafter with infants and toddlers gaining approximately 0.25 kg/month from age 9 to 24 months.[7]

Specific growth curves are available for children with certain health conditions that affect growth such as Down syndrome or very-low-birth weight (http://depts.washington.edu/growth/).

Failure to thrive should be considered if the infant's weight-for-age falls below the 5th percentile or if the growth rate decelerates such that the trajectory crosses two major percentile lines on the growth chart. In the United States, failure to thrive is seen in 5% to 10% of children in outpatient primary care settings; the majority of cases present before 18 months of age.[8] Inadequate growth can herald endocrine, cardiac, renal, or metabolic disorders but is more commonly a result of inadequate nutrition or social stressors.

Developmental Milestones

In addition to monitoring growth, the well-child visits provide an opportunity to monitor development. The AAP recommends that all children be screened for developmental delays and disabilities in a systematic manner at 9, 18, 24, and 30 months of age.[9] Multiple tools for assessing development exist; a comparison can be found at: http://agesandstages.com/wp-content/uploads/2015/03/Comparison-Chart1.pdf.

Dedicated screening for Autism Spectrum Disorders is recommended at 18 and 24 months.[10] Each state has an early intervention program for children from birth to 3 years of age. Referral to these programs is recommended when concerns arise about development (http://www.parentcenterhub.org/repository/ei-overview/).

Risks Assessment and Harm Reduction

Hazards

As infants and toddlers grow and become more mobile, their exposure to potential environment threats increases. Unintentional injury is the fifth leading cause of death in children age <1 year and the leading cause of death in children of age 1 to 4 years.[11] Unintentional suffocation is the leading type of injury in children <1 year and unintentional drowning is the most prevalent injury type in children of age 1 to 4 years.[11] The following website provides useful guidance for parents on these issues: http://www.webmd.com/parenting/baby/tc/health-and-safety-birth-to-2-years-safety-measures-around-the-home#1.

Abuse

The "Tip Sheets" available from the following site can be useful starting points: https://www.childwelfare.gov/topics/preventing/preventionmonth/resource-guide/tip-sheets/ (Chapter 21).

Parental Education

The AAP recommends exclusive breastfeeding for about 6 months, with continuation for 1 year or longer as mutually desired by mother and infant; a recommendation concurred with by the WHO and the Institute of Medicine. Additional advice for parents is shown in Table 9.2.

Anticipatory Guidance

The rapidity with which infants and toddlers grow and develop is such that they are constantly learning new skills and passing through new developmental stages. The well-child visits provide a forum for monitoring development as well as coaching parents on upcoming developmental stages. You review the well-child visit schedule with Jay's mother and provide her with information on breast feeding support. The ***Bright Futures Pocket Guide*** nicely summarizes anticipatory counseling for each visit. For example, potentially frustrating toddler behavior can be less frustrating when parents know it is part of a normal and expected developmental stage.[15]

> Jay is now 11 months old. He is doing well and is current on his vaccinations. Mom has been successfully breastfeeding him and wonders how long she should do so. She is thinking of weaning soon as she wants to try to conceive again, but ultimately wants to "do what is best" for him. After guiding her through the WHO and AAP recommendations and helping her balance those with her desire to conceive, you provide information and discuss weaning strategies and internet resources.

Common Parental Concerns

Sleep

In addition to clarifying questions about sleep safety (Table 9.2), parents of newborns often benefit from support and education about infant sleep patterns. Newborns sleep the majority of each day (16 to 20 hours, on average), but wake often to feed. The majority of infants

Table 9.2 ▸ Advice for Parents of Newborns and Toddlers

Topic	Advice
Car seat safety[a]	Children should remain rear-facing in the car seat until age 2 years, secured in appropriately adjusted 5-point harness. Car seats should only be placed in the back seat of the car. The harnesses will need to be adjusted as the infant grows
Nutrition: vitamin D[12]	Breastfed infants and formula-fed infants ingesting <1 L of vitamin D fortified formula daily should receive vitamin D supplementation with 400 IU daily or supplementing the breastfeeding mother with 6,400 IU daily; supplementation should begin in the first few days of the infant's life
Nutrition: iron[13]	AAP recommends giving breastfed infants 1 mg/kg/day of a liquid iron supplement until iron-containing solid foods are introduced at about 6 months of age and that all babies be screened at 12 months of age for iron deficiency and iron deficiency anemia. The USPSTF found insufficient evidence for screening for iron deficiency anemia in children ages 6 to 24 months
Nutrition: food choices[b]	Encourage a variety of appropriately textured healthy foods. With the exception of honey due to botulism risk, there are no longer any contraindications to giving infants specific foods. Cow's milk should not be introduced until 12 months of age
Safe sleep[14]	AAP recommends supine positioning on a firm sleep surface; room-sharing without bed-sharing; consideration of pacifier use; and avoidance of soft bedding, overheating, and exposure to tobacco smoke, alcohol, and illicit drugs

[a]See http://www.safercar.gov/parents/CarSeats/Car-Seat-Safety.htm?view=full
[b]The Healthy Children website contains information about readiness for solid foods and age appropriate feeding: https://www.healthychildren.org/English/ages-stages/baby/feeding-nutrition/Pages/Switching-To-Solid-Foods.aspx

do not "sleep through the night" with a 6-hour stretch of sleep until at least 3 months of age, and sometimes much closer to 1 year.

A 2006 systematic review indicates both extinction of crying, often called the "cry it out" method, and parental education about sleep expectations are effective provided the infant is healthy, safe, and not otherwise in danger.[16]

Bowel Movements

Parents of newborns, especially breast fed newborn, often voice concern that their babies have diarrhea. Normal newborn stool has the appearance of a seedy mustard, with a yellowish-green to light brown hue. Normal stooling frequency varies from several stools a day to one stool every several days. It can be normal for infants to become flushed in the face and appear to be straining when they are stooling. In the absence of vomiting, fever, dehydration, abnormal abdominal examination, or other concerning findings, reassurance can be given that this flushing and apparent straining is harmless.

As they enter toddlerhood, some children become constipated once cow's milk is introduced. Reducing the amount of milk ingested or eliminating cow's milk for children with chronic constipation may be helpful.[17] Polyethylene glycol is an effective and safe constipation treatment for use in infants above 6 months of age.[18]

Fussy Baby

It is normal for infants to cry a total of 2 to 3 hr/day. Often this is divided into short intervals and the infant can be calmed with usual caregiving behaviors. Colic is defined as inconsolable crying for 3 or more hours 3 days in any a week, lasting at least 3 weeks. Education and support for parents is important as frustration with the infant's crying is the leading cause of shaken baby syndrome. Though the cause of colic is unknown, studies show that probiotics given to the infant daily can decrease crying time.[19] The 5 Ss for Soothing Babies are discussed at https://happiestbaby.com/using-the-5-ss/.

Tantrums

Tantrums and actions that challenge limits parents set are common and a normal part of toddlers' development as the toddler learns to interact with and negotiate the environment. Many resources exist to help parents navigate these behaviors, including:

▶ Murphy J. The Secret Lives of Toddlers: A Parent's Guide to the Wonderful, Terrible, Fascinating Behavior of Children Ages 1–3. New York: The Berkley Publishing Group; 2004.

▶ The Center for Parenting Education: http://centerforparentingeducation.org/recommended-parenting-books/.

▶ Child Development Institute: https://childdevelopmentinfo.com/ages-stages/toddler-preschooler-development-parenting/.

Immunizations

Vaccination greatly reduces disease, disability, and death worldwide, with only the provision of clean water having a greater influence on these parameters.[20] A 2014 meta-analysis confirms that vaccines are not associated with the development of autism.[21] Vaccines should be provided according to the CDC schedules (https://www.cdc.gov/vaccines/schedules/) unless there is a contraindication for doing so. Information about vaccine contraindications and precautions can be found at http://www.cdc.gov/vaccines/hcp/admin/contraindications-vacc.html. Alternate vaccine schedules have been proposed, but they are not as well studied for safety and efficacy. Common misperceptions about vaccinations are discussed in Chapter 7 (Table 7.4). You offer to provide Jay with an influenza vaccination as it is November and his mother agrees.

> At 18 months, Jay is growing well. He is walking and his fine motor skills are appropriate for his age. His parents note that he does not talk much yet and are wondering what to do about it. After exploring this further with the parents, you recognize that his verbal skills are within the normal range. You elect to reassess in another 3 months.

AGES 2 TO 11 YEARS

> Jay's sister, Justina, is now 8 years old. Her parents bring her for a well-child check and have a few questions. They notice that she has been a bit constipated sometimes and will occasionally complain of a stomach ache that seems to resolve without much intervention. She has been a healthy child so far who is usually around the 65th percentile for BMI. At this visit, you notice her BMI has jumped to the 85th percentile. She used to play soccer but didn't want to play this year because "some of the kids are mean." Her parents tell you she has plenty of friends and does well in school.

Well-child visits typically occur yearly between the ages of 2 and 11 years. Often clinicians will recommend a visit at 30 months (2 1/2 year) as well.

Screening

A summary of the United States Preventive Screening Task Force (USPSTF) screening recommendations can be found at the end of this chapter.

Vision and Hearing

Vision screening should be provided for all children at least once between the ages of 3 and 5 years. Children with abnormal screening results should be referred appropriately. Schools often provide both vision and hearing testing, as well. Audiology or ophthalmology referrals may be needed for children who do not pass the screening tests.

Growth

CDC growth curves should be used to plot growth once a child has reached 2 years of age. Most children will have established their growth trajectories by age 2 years, though there can be some discrepancy in percentiles with the change from the WHO to the CDC curves. Growth curves can be found at http://www.cdc.gov/growthcharts/clinical_charts.htm. Deviations from expected growth patterns should raise concern for inappropriate nutritional practices, hormonal, gastrointestinal, or metabolic derangements, food insecurity, stress in the home environment, or abuse/neglect. You share Justina's growth curve with the child and her parents showing her increased weight percentile. A discussion of heathy eating ensues and you suggest eliminating soda in favor of increasing her water intake, which may help with constipation. Justina notes that her friend has started a dance class and she would be interested in attending to increase exercise.

Development

Clinicians partner with parents to monitor development and act upon concerns that arise. Development encompasses expected changes in physical, intellectual, emotional, and social growth.

A Useful Introduction to Child Development

▶ The Science of Early Childhood Development: https://www.youtube.com/watch?v=tLiP4b-TPCA

▶ Age 2: https://www.youtube.com/watch?v=y9Mm85UAWvM

▶ Age 3: https://www.youtube.com/watch?v=w5DWCwUcOxc

▶ Age 4: https://www.youtube.com/watch?v=o0TGczdbiV4

▶ Developmental milestones for school-aged children: https://www.youtube.com/watch?v=oMliXKTd9sk

The child's behavior can be best understood when it is viewed in the context of the child's developmental stage. For example, toddler behavior often viewed as oppositional is an expected part of development. Sharing this information with parents can equip them to handle the behavior more effectively.

Prepuberty and Puberty

For girls, the average age of pubertal onset is 10.5 years, with average age of menarche at 12.5 years. For boys, average onset is 11.5 years. Breast development and testicular growth are usually the first changes in girls and boys, respectively. Premature puberty is more common in girls than in boys, in obese children, and in children of black or Latino heritage.[22]

Planned Parenthood resources for talking with children about puberty can be found at: https://www.plannedparenthood.org/parents/puberty-101-for-parents.

Risk Assessment and Harm Reduction

As children grow and gain more independence, factors outside of the home environment have a growing influence on their decisions, beliefs, and habits that they build. During the well-child visit, the clinician should assess these factors to identify potential health risks and help the child build healthy habits. A structured tool to do this is the HEEADSSS interview (http://contemporarypediatrics.modernmedicine.com/contemporary-pediatrics/content/tags/adolescent-medicine/heeadsss-30-psychosocial-interview-adolesce?page=full).

For additional information, see https://www.youtube.com/watch?v=DopIg517o00.

HEEADSSS

Home environment	Drugs
Education and employment	Sexuality
Eating	Suicide/depression
peer-related Activities	Safety from injury and violence

Bullying

Bullying and cyber-bullying are prevalent. The following site has useful information on this issue: http://www.stopbullying.gov/index.html. As Justina mentioned some "mean kids," you take the opportunity to talk about bullying, ways to address it, and encourage her to keep her parents and teacher informed.

Car Seats

Children may be turned from rear-facing to forward facing at age 2 years, but should remain in a seat with a five-point harness until they reach at least 4 years of age, 40 pounds, and can sit in a proper seated position for the duration of the car ride. They should then ride in a belt-positioning booster seat until they are at least 4'9" tall and weigh 80 pounds. Children should remain in the back seat of the car until they are at least 13 years.

Internet Safety

Internet safety is also a growing concern. Links to information about keeping children safe online can be found at: http://www.nationalcac.org/internet-safety-tips/.

Other Safety Issues

It can be useful to check in with families about the use of bike helmets, sports, and hobby safety equipment including safe gun storage and use, and age-appropriate discussions about stranger safety and safe touch.

Table 9.3 ▶ Advice for Parents of Children	
Topic	**Advice**
Nutrition	The Academy of Nutrition and Dietetics' position paper on nutritional recommendations for children ages 2–11 years can be found at http://www.eatrightpro.org
Oral health (an oral examination is part of the well-child visit)	To prevent early childhood caries, parents should be counseled to never put their infant to bed with a bottle. The American Dental Association recommends that as soon as teeth appear, they should be brushed at least twice a day for 2 minutes each time, using a soft-bristled brush and fluoridated toothpaste.[23] Parents should use a toothpaste smear the size of a grain of rice for children under age 3 years and a pea size amount for those of ages 3–6 years. Teeth should be flossed daily once the teeth begin to touch. Smiles for Life is a useful oral health resource (http://smilesforlifeoralhealth.org/)
Physical activity[24]	Children and adolescents (age 6–17 years) should have 1 hour or more of physical activity daily. Most of this activity should be either moderate- or vigorous-intensity aerobic physical activity and should include vigorous-intensity physical activity (e.g., running, biking, swimming) at least 3 days per week. Muscle-strengthening physical activity and bone-strengthening activity should occur on at least 3 days per week (using muscles against resistance and weight-bearing activity, respectively). See Youth Physical Activity Guidelines Toolkit at https://www.cdc.gov/healthyschools/physicalactivity/guidelines.htm

Education

Well-child visits during the preschool and elementary school years continue to provide a venue for guiding parents and children in making healthy choices. For preschool and school-aged children, eating and activity habits often mirror those of their parents. Therefore, it can be useful to assess habits, interests, and activities of the whole family. As children grow, the clinician should work to empower the child as an agent in his or her own health. This can start at a young age by addressing questions about daily habits to the child rather than just to the parents.

In addition to discussing nutrition and activity, clinicians should encourage families to limit nonschoolwork-related screen time and encourage reading with their children. Reach Out and Read (http://www.reachoutandread.org/) is an evidence-based program designed to promote early literacy; it can be easily incorporated into the well-child check, with use both as a tool for developmental assessment as well as a way to encourage and support reading. Other educational topics are presented in Table 9.3.

Common Parental Concerns

Sleep

As per the American Academy of Sleep Medicine and the AAP, childhood sleep guidelines to promote optimal health are as follows:[25]

▶ Children 1 to 2 years: sleep 11 to 14 hrs/24 hrs (including naps) on a regular basis.

▶ Children 3 to 5 years: sleep 10 to 13 hrs/24 hrs (including naps) on a regular basis.

▶ Children 6 to 12 years: sleep 9 to 12 hrs/24 hrs on a regular basis.

As per the National Sleep Foundation, watching TV close to bedtime has been associated with bedtime resistance, difficulty falling asleep, anxiety around sleep, and sleeping fewer hours.[26] AAP recommends:

▶ No televisions in children's rooms.

▶ No more than 1 to 2 hours of screen time.

▶ No TV for children under 2 years old.

Discipline

Effective discipline that serves to guide and teach children should be tailored to the age and developmental stage of the child. Physicians should discourage spanking at any age as it has shown not to be an effective technique in correcting the child's behavior and it presents potential immediate and lasting harms.

Challenging behavior in children, beyond what might be expected with the normal developmental stages, can stem from a variety of causes. These include lack of adequate sleep or proper nutrition, stress in the home environment, developmental disorders (including a history of prenatal substance exposure), and uncontrolled mental health or medical issues. These should be explored when behavior problems are reported.

School Readiness

Parents of children whose birthdays are near the cut-off for starting kindergarten may have questions about whether or not holding the child back a year so that he or she is not the youngest in the class will benefit their child.[27] This decision should be made on a case by case basis; however, research suggests that children who are held back do not perform any better academically than children who enter at the usual age and children who are old for their grade may be at higher risk for behavioral issues during adolescence. Parental engagement with fostering school readiness by establishing routines, promoting socialization, and reading regularly with their children can help children succeed in school.

Peer relationships become very important during the elementary school years. The following site contains age-appropriate recommendations on supporting healthy relationships and friendships in school-aged children: http://raisingchildren.net.au/articles/supporting_schoolage_friendships.html/context/288.

Attention Deficit Hyperactivity Disorder

Certain attention deficit or behavior concerns can present or become more prominent during elementary school years. A multidisciplinary approach involving behavioral health support and input from teachers is recommended to gain an accurate assessment of the issues and build a treatment plan.

Immunization

Vaccines should continue to be provided according to the CDC schedule unless there is a contraindication for doing so (https://www.cdc.gov/vaccines/schedules/). This tip sheet provides guidance in talking with parents about the HPV vaccine: https://www.aap.org/en-us/Documents/hpvtoolkit_RI_Success_Resources_2015_Sept.pdf.

AGES 12 TO 18 YEARS

You are seeing a 14-year-old young girl, Jenna, for her sports physical for basketball this fall. Jenna has been healthy throughout her childhood. She is doing well in school and was a star player on her middle school basketball team. Her mother is concerned about Jenna's relationship with her boyfriend and that they may be getting "too serious." After discussing mom's concerns, you conduct the visit with Jenna alone. After discussing confidentiality, Jenna discloses that she has been considering having vaginal intercourse with her boyfriend but doesn't want her parents to know. She denies any substance use as she wants to stay eligible for basketball.

Well-child visit should continue to occur yearly between the ages of 12 and 18 years, and often at least biannual visits are required for organized sports participation in this age group. Risk assessment and harm reduction is of utmost importance during this age range and, as corollary, care of the adolescent hinges on patient confidentiality. As this age range marks the transition from childhood to adult healthcare, providers should request that the adolescent be interviewed alone during the visit as a matter of practice.

Confidentiality

Up to one-third of patients of ages 12 to 18 years report they will not disclose sensitive issues to their provider due to "fear that parents will find out."[28] Laws vary from state to state about what information can and must be shared with parents or guardians, so it is important to know the minor consent laws in your area. In many states, **mature minors**, that is adolescents who are deemed by their provider to have the cognitive maturity to give informed consent and generally over the age of 14 years, are able to receive healthcare without parental notification as are **emancipated minors**, those who are legally responsible for themselves. It should be kept in mind that even if an adolescent's care is kept confidential, billing records may be available to the parent.[29,30]

Suggested Script to Explain Mandatory Reporting

"Your confidentiality is very important to me. I will try to make sure that anything you tell me isn't shared without your permission; however, there are some exceptions. I am required to report child abuse. Also, if I'm very concerned about your safety, I may need to tell another adult or someone who can better help you. Before I tell someone, I will make every effort to talk to you first to let you know that I am going to tell someone. Do you have any questions? And if at any point you have questions, you can always ask me."

From Wisconsin Coalition against Domestic Violence "Teens and Mandatory Reporting: Sample language for mandated reporters when talking to youth" (http://www.endabusewi.org/).

Screening

A summary of the USPSTF screening recommendations can be found at the end of this chapter. As with younger children the CDC growth curves should be used to monitor height, weight, BMI, and blood pressure. The evidence for blood pressure screening in adolescents was determined to be inconclusive by the USPSTF; however, it is recommended by the AAP and should especially be considered in adolescents with risk factors (e.g., obesity, history of low birth weight, or family history of hypertension).

Depression

The USPSTF recommends screening for depression for adolescents aged 12 to 18 years (SOR B), assuring that there are systems in place to ensure diagnosis and appropriate treatment. Up to a third of adolescents on the Youth Risk Behavior Survey reported feeling "sad or hopeless" and 8.3% reported having experienced major depression at some time in the preceding year (https://nccd.cdc.gov/youthonline/App/Default.aspx).[31]

There are two validated screening tools for teenagers: Patient Health Questionnaire for Adolescents: file://uwhfs/shares/TSProfiles/sbs2/Downloads/APA_DSM5_Severity-Measure-For-Depression-Child-Age-11-to-17%20(1).pdf and the Beck Depression Inventory: https://static1.squarespace.com/static/5205b3d1e4b08b89e5d18f2a/t/520ae965e4b0bc-18c970b0f0/1376446821340/Beck-Depression-Inventory-and-Scoring-Key1.pdf. Although you do not employ a depression screening tool in your practice, you routinely ask about depression and Jenna denies feeling depressed.

Sexual Health

Sexually active adolescents should be screened for gonorrhea and chlamydia at least annually and for HIV at least once after the age of 15 years (or younger if at risk).[32] Despite representing a quarter of the sexually active population, adolescents contract over half of the STIs in the United States.[33] This is in part due to higher risk behaviors (e.g., inadequate barrier contraceptives and multiple partners) as well as biologic factors including the immaturity of the cervix.

Sports Preparticipation Screening

The majority of these visits include the components of a regular well visit; however, there is a special emphasis on the cardiac, respiratory, and musculoskeletal systems. A review of the preparticipation physical can be found in the following article: http://www.aafp.org/afp/2015/0901/p371.html. Jenna has no cardiorespiratory symptoms with exercise, her blood pressure is normal, and her examination—focused on heart, lungs, and musculoskeletal examination—is unremarkable. You complete her school sports physical form to allow participation in basketball.

Development

No formal cognitive developmental screening is recommended in the adolescent years. School performance is a good surrogate for this development and asking about school can also help to build rapport and elicit concerns from the adolescent patient.

Puberty

A physical examination for the adolescent includes tanner staging for pubertal development. Though it is outside of the scope of this chapter, it is important to keep in mind that puberty can be an exceptionally challenging time for transgender adolescents as it may increase gender dysphoria as secondary sex characteristics begin to emerge.[34] Tanner stage tables: http://www.childgrowthfoundation.org/CMS/FILES/Puberty_and_the_Tanner_Stages.pdf.

Risk Assessment and Harm Reduction

The bulk of the adolescent well visit should be spent conducting risk assessment and harm reduction. Adolescents engage in a higher proportion of high-risk activities, including reckless driving, substance abuse, unprotected sex, and violent behavior than any other group.[35] Most risk-assessment topics for adolescents are given an insufficient evidence (I) recommendation from the USPSTF. The AAP and AAFP recommend both screening for risk behavior in adolescents and providing appropriate interventions for a positive screen. You commend Jenna for avoiding substance use and for wearing her seatbelt. You discover that Jenna feels safe in her relationship with her boyfriend and is empowered to say no to activities with which she is uncomfortable. You briefly review with her the most protective contraceptive options.

Adolescents report that they prefer when a provider raises these topics and that they would not have raised these concerns without the provider query.[36] Forms that ask adolescents directly about risk behaviors can also be helpful. There is an excellent toolkit available through the University of Michigan: http://www.umhs-adolescenthealth.org/about-us/.

Nutrition and activity counseling continue to be important in this age range.

Personal Safety

Unintentional injury is the leading cause of death in this age group, followed by suicide, and in 15- to 24-year olds, homicide.[36] Developmentally adolescents are more inclined to take risks as they have a heightened feeling of invincibility and have not yet fully developed executive function. Risks and risk behaviors to ask about include abuse, driving, substance use, and sexual behavior (Table 9.4).[36]

Education

Education for the adolescent patient is primary directed at the issues elicited by the risk assessment. Consider use of a tool such as the PASTE mnemonic (**P**roblem, **A**lternatives, **S**elect an alternative, **T**ry it, **E**valuate your choice and modify as needed) to help adolescents identify a plan to decrease their risk behaviors.[37]

Common Parental Concerns

Parents frequently struggle with having difficult conversations about the risk behaviors discussed above. Coaching parents on bringing up these topics in an open and conversational manner can be helpful. The AAP recommends that when tackling these topics, parents should listen without judgment or reaction, avoid catastrophizing and over empathizing, share their values and opinions in a calm manner without condescension or personal attack, and avoid lectures. There is a parental toolkit from the Department of Health & Human Services Office of Adolescent health that can be found: http://www.hhs.gov/ash/oah/resources-and-publications/info/parents/conversation-tools/.

Immunization

Vaccines should continue to be provided according to the CDC schedule unless there is a contraindication for doing so (https://www.cdc.gov/vaccines/schedules/).

> Once back together with Jenna and her mother, you discuss contraception and safety in sexual relationships but keep Jenna's plans for initiating sexual activity confidential. You encourage her to discuss her plans with her mother and discuss with her mother some tools for initiating difficult conversations with her daughter. You also discuss the importance of core strength and cross training in injury prevention during her basketball season.

Table 9.4 ▶ Safety Concerns and Resources for Adolescents[36]

Concern	Resource
IPV	One in ten young people report being hit or physically hurt by a partner at least once in the preceding year, and 6.7% reporting being forced to have intercourse against their will in 2015. An interactive online training for screening for and responding to teen IPV: https://vetoviolence.cdc.gov/apps/datingmatters/
Driving	The bulk of adolescent MVAs are due to inexperience; however, nearly half of teens report texting while driving, 7.8% drove while intoxicated, and 1 in 5 adolescents reported riding with an intoxicated driver on the YRBS. The National Safety Council has information addressing teen driving risks: http://www.nsc.org/learn/NSC-Initiatives/Pages/teen-driving.aspx?var=mnd
Sexual activity	Up to 41% of adolescents report engaging in vaginal intercourse by age 18 years; of those, 43% did not use condoms and 14% did not use any form of contraception. At least one same-sex partner was reported by 2.5% of males and 11% of females of ages 15–19 years in another study. See Chapter 15 for information on obtaining a sexual history. Counseling about delaying sexual activity, use of adequate barrier protection, and methods of contraception is an essential part of the adolescent visit. Online resources include https://bedsider.org/ and http://www.reproductiveaccess.org/
Substance use: alcohol	See Chapter 23. Nearly one-third of adolescents report at least one drink and 17.7% report at least one episode of binge drinking in the previous 30 days. The USPSTF recommends that all adolescents between 12 and 18 years be screened for alcohol misuse (SOR B). Two tools have been validated in adolescents: CRAFFT tool: www.ceasar.org/CRAFFT/pdf/CRAFFT_English.pdf AUDIT tool: https://www.drugabuse.gov/sites/default/files/files/AUDIT.pdf Information on underage drinking: https://www.stopalcoholabuse.gov
Substance use: tobacco	Current cigarette smoking is reported in 10.8% of adolescents, and 24.1% currently using electronic vapor products. Most adult smokers (88%) began smoking before age 18 years. Information including a physician conversation card can be found at the CDC: http://www.cdc.gov/tobacco/data_statistics/sgr/2012/index.htm Patients can download a free app created for teens to help with cessation at: http://www.teen.smokefree.gov/sftapps.aspx#tab_quit_start

CDC, Center for Disease Control; IPV, intimate partner violence; MVA, motor vehicle accident; YRBS, Youth Risk Behavior Survey.

Additional Resources

▶ Bright Futures well visit pocket guide: https://brightfutures.aap.org/materials-and-tools/guidelines-and-pocket-guide/Pages/default.aspx

▶ CDC Resource list with links to useful resources for physicians and families: http://www.cdc.gov/ncbddd/childdevelopment/links.html

▶ HealthyChildren.org Schedule of well-child visits: https://www.healthychildren.org/English/family-life/health-management/Pages/Well-Child-Care-A-Check-Up-for-Success.aspx

▶ American Girl "Advice Library" is a collection of books about self-care, friendship, puberty, and other topics geared toward school aged and preteen girls: http://www.americangirl.com/shop/bookstore/advice-library

USPSTF Screening Recommendations for Children and Adolescents

Level A

Prophylactic ocular topical medication **for prevention of gonococcal ophthalmia neonatorum**	**All newborns** should receive prophylaxis within 24 hours after birth
Human immunodeficiency virus (HIV)	Screen for HIV infection in **all adolescents over age 15 years** and adolescents under age 15 who are at increased risk; one-time screening recommended unless at increased risk

Level B

Dental health: fluoride	For children from birth through age 5 years: • Prescribe oral fluoride supplement **starting at age 6 months for children whose water supply is deficient in fluoride** • Apply fluoride **varnish to primary teeth of all infants and children** starting at the age of primary tooth eruption
Obesity	Screen **children age 6 years and older** for obesity Refer patients to comprehensive moderate- to high-intensity programs that include dietary, physical activity, and behavioral counseling No evidence was found on appropriate screening intervals
Tobacco	Provide education or brief counseling to prevent initiation of tobacco use to **all school-aged children and adolescents**
Visual impairment	Provide vision screening for **all children at least once between the ages of 3–5 years** to detect presence of amblyopia or its risk factors *(Level I for age under 3 years)*
Depression	Screen for major depressive disorder in adolescents **aged 12–18 years**. Screening should be implemented with adequate systems in place to ensure accurate diagnosis, effective treatment, and appropriate follow-up *(Level I for age under 11 years)*
Chlamydia and gonorrhea	Screen for chlamydia in sexually active women **aged 24 years and younger** *(Level I for men)*

Level D (advised against)

Lead	**Do not screen** for elevated blood lead levels in asymptomatic children ages 1–5 years who are at average risk *(level I for screening in asymptomatic children ages 1–5 years who are at increased risk)*
Cervical cancer	**Do not screen** women **younger than age 21 years** for cervical cancer
Genital herpes	**Do not perform** routine serologic screening for HSV in **asymptomatic adolescents**
Idiopathic scoliosis	**Do not screen asymptomatic adolescents** for idiopathic scoliosis

QUESTIONS

1. How often should a child be screened for developmental delays?
   A. Once a year
   B. At 9 months, 18 months, 24 months, and 30 months

C. At age 2 years

D. At every well-child visit

2. Failure to thrive is diagnosed if the child's weight is below the 10th percentile.

A. True

B. False

3. Many physicians use the HEEADSSS questions for pediatric risk assessment. In this pneumonic, the H stands for which one of the following?

A. History

B. Health status

C. Home environment

D. Harm reduction

4. You are seeing a 16-year-old sexually active female. Which of the following is appropriate management?

A. Screen for chlamydia

B. Perform a pelvic examination

C. Do a Pap smear

D. Call her mother to inform her about her daughter's sexual activity

ANSWERS

Question 1: The correct answer is B.

The AAP recommends that all children be screened for developmental delays and disabilities in a systematic manner at 9, 18, 24, and 30 months of age.

Question 2: The correct answer is B.

Failure to thrive should be considered if the infant's weight-for-age falls below the 5th percentile or if the growth rate decelerates such that the trajectory crosses two major percentile lines on the growth chart.

Question 3: The correct answer is C.

HEEADSSS *stands for Home environment, Education and employment, Eating, peer-related Activities, Drugs, Sexuality, Suicide/depression, Safety from injury and violence.*

Question 4: The correct answer is A.

Sexually active adolescents should be screened for gonorrhea and chlamydia at least annually and for HIV at least once after the age of 15 years (or younger if at risk).

REFERENCES

1. Maisels MJ, Bhutani VK, Bogen D, et al. Hyperbilirubinemia in the newborn infant > or = to 35 weeks' gestation: an update with clarifications. *Pediatrics.* 2009;124(4):1193–1198.
2. Benitz WE. Committee on fetus and newborn. American Academy of Pediatrics. Hospital stay for healthy term newborn infants. *Pediatrics.* 2015;135(5):948–953.
3. Flaherman V, Schaefer E, Kuzniewicz M, et al. Early weight loss nomograms for exclusively breastfed newborns. *Pediatrics.* 2015;135(1):e16–e23.
4. ABM Clinical Protocol #3. Hospital guidelines for the use of supplementary feedings in the healthy term breastfed neonate, Revised 2009. *Breastfeeding Med.* 2009;22(3):175–182.

5. U.S. Department of Health and Human Services. Recommended Uniform Screening Panel Core Conditions (as of March 2015). Available from: http://www.hrsa.gov/advisorycommittees/mchbadvisory/heritabledisorders/recommendedpanel/. Accessed December, 2016.

6. Center for Disease Control and Prevention. Hearing Loss in Children. Available from: http://www.cdc.gov/ncbddd/hearingloss/screening.html. Accessed December 2016.

7. Center for Disease Control and Prevention. WHO Growth Standards Are Recommended for Use in the U.S. for Infants and Children 0 to 2 Years of Age. Available from: http://www.cdc.gov/growthcharts/who_charts.htm. Accessed December 2016.

8. Cole SZ, Lanham JS. Failure to thrive: An update. *Am Fam Physician.* 2011;83(7):829–834.

9. Center for Disease Control and Prevention. Developmental monitoring and screening. Available from: http://www.cdc.gov/ncbddd/childdevelopment/screening.html. Accessed December 2016.

10. Armstrong C. AAP releases guidelines on identification of children with Autism Spectrum Disorders. *Am Fam Physician.* 2008;78(11):1301–1305.

11. National Center for Injury Prevention and Control CDC. 10 Leading Causes of Death by Age Group, United States–2014. Available from: http://www.cdc.gov/injury/wisqars/pdf/leading_causes_of_death_by_age_group_2014-a.pdf; http://www.cdc.gov/injury/wisqars/pdf/leading_causes_of_injury_deaths_highlighting_unintentional_injury_2014-a.pdf. Accessed December 2016.

12. Hollis BW, Wagner CL, Howard CR, et al. Maternal Versus Infant Vitamin D supplementation during lactation: A randomized controlled trial. *Pediatrics.* 2015;136(4):625–634.

13. Baker RD, Greer FR. The committee on nutrition. Clinical report—diagnosis and prevention of iron deficiency and iron-deficiency anemia in infants and young children (0–3 years of age). *Pediatrics.* 2010;126(5):1–11.

14. Task force on sudden infant death syndrome. SIDS and other sleep-related infant deaths: Updated 2016 recommendations for a safe infant sleeping environment. *Pediatrics.* 2016;38(5):1–17.

15. Hagan JF, Shaw JS, Duncan P, eds. *Bright Futures: Guidelines for Health Supervision of Infants, Children, and Adolescents. Pocket Guide.* 3rd ed. Elk Grove Village, IL: American Academy of Pediatrics; 2008. Available from: https://brightfutures.aap.org/Bright%20Futures%20Documents/BF3%20pocket%20guide_final.pdf. Accessed December 2016.

16. Mindell JA, Kuhn B, Lewin DS, et al. Behavioral treatment of bedtime problems and night wakings in infants and young children. *Sleep.* 2006;29(10):1263–1276.

17. Irastorza I, Ibañez B, Delgado-Sanzonetti L, et al. Cow's-milk–free diet as a therapeutic option in childhood chronic constipation. *J Pediatr Gastroenterol Nutr.* 2010;51(2):171–176.

18. Hahn TW, Lee J. What is the safest treatment for constipation in children? Evidence-Based Practice. February 2015, p. 6. Available from: https://mospace.umsystem.edu/xmlui/bitstream/handle/10355/45064/EBPediatricsConstipationinChildren.pdf?sequence=1&isAllowed=y. Accessed December 2016.

19. Koonce T, Mounsey A, Rowland K. Colicky baby? Here's a surprising remedy. *J Fam Pract.* 2011;60(1):34–36.

20. Andre FE, Booy R, Bock HL, et al. Vaccination greatly reduces disease, disability, death and inequity worldwide. *Bull World Health Organ.* 2008;86(2):81–160.

21. Taylor L, Swerdfeger A, Eslick G. Vaccines are not associated with autism: An evidence-based meta-analysis of case-control and cohort studies. *Vaccine.* 2014;32:3623–3629.

22. Duke Primary Care. When is puberty too early? October 01, 2013. Available from: https://www.dukehealth.org/blog/when-puberty-too-early. Accessed December 2016.

23. Wright JT, Hanson N, Ristic H, et al. Fluoride toothpaste efficacy and safety in children younger than 6 years: A systematic review. *J Amer Dent Assoc.* 2014;145:182–189.

24. U.S. Department of Health and Human Services. *Physical Activity Guidelines for Americans.* Washington, DC: U.S. Department of Health and Human Services; 2008.

25. American Academy of Pediatrics. *American Academy of Pediatrics Supports Childhood Sleep Guidelines.* Available from: https://www.aap.org/en-us/about-the-aap/aap-press-room/pages/American-Academy-of-Pediatrics-Supports-Childhood-Sleep-Guidelines.aspx. Accessed December 2016.

26. National Sleep Foundation. Children and sleep. Available from: https://sleepfoundation.org/sleep-topics/children-and-sleep/page/0/2. Accessed December 2016.

27. Mayo Clinic. Are there benefits to delaying a child's enrollment in kindergarten? Available from: http://www.mayoclinic.org/healthy-lifestyle/childrens-health/in-depth/kindergarten-readiness/art-20048432?pg=2. Accessed December 2016.

28. Klein J, Wilson KM, McNulty M, et al. Access to medical care for adolescents: Results from the 1997 Commonwealth Fund Survey of the Health of Adolescent Girls. *J Adolesc Health.* 1999;25(2):120–130.

29. English A, Ford CA. The HIPAA privacy rule and adolescents: Legal questions and clinical challenges. *Perspec Sex Reprod Health.* 2004;36(2):80–86.

30. Society for Adolescent Health and Medicine; American Academy of Pediatrics. Confidentiality protections for adolescents and young adults in the health care billing and insurance claims process. *J Adolesc Health.* 2016;58(3):374–377.

31. Current epidemiologic data on adolescent risk behaviors from a local to national level is available in searchable form through the Youth Risk Behavioral Survey (YRBS). Available from: https://nccd.cdc.gov/youthonline/App/Default.aspx. Accessed December 2016.

32. American Academy of Pediatrics. AAP releases policy statement on screening for nonviral sexually transmitted infections in adolescents and young adults. *Am Fam Physician.* 2015;91(9):652–654.

33. Tulloch T, Kaufman M. Adolescent sexuality. *Pediatr Rev.* 2013;34(1):29–37.

34. Vance SR Jr, Ehrensaft D, Rosenthal SM. Psychological and medical care of gender nonconforming youth. *Pediatrics.* 2014;134(6):1184–1192.

35. Committee on Adolescents. Achieving quality health services for adolescents. *Pediatrics.* 2016;128(2):pii: e20161347.

36. Ham P, Allen C. Adolescent health screening and counseling. *Am Fam Physician.* 2012;86(12):1109–1116.

37. Sacks D, Westwood MB. An approach to interviewing adolescents. *Paediatr Child Health.* 2003;8(9):554–556.

10

Care for the Aging Patient

KEY POINTS

1 ▶ Geriatric assessment for common geriatric syndromes and preventative care is very important.

2 ▶ Care for the elderly involves interprofessional teams and sometimes a caregiver.

3 ▶ Altered mental status is the tip of the iceberg for medical illness.

4 ▶ Do not give a pill for every illness.

5 ▶ Social and psychological problems are common, as is atypical presentation of disease.

6 ▶ Palliative care and end-of-life care plan must be discussed early.

As part of a geriatric assessment, you are seeing Doris, a 79-year-old woman with hypertension, hyperlipidemia, coronary artery disease (CAD), and end-stage renal disease on hemodialysis. The patient began having memory problems 5 years ago; these worsened significantly in the last 2 years after she was placed on hemodialysis. She is easily agitated and irritable, as well as exhibiting verbal and physical aggression toward her husband and others. The patient was recently seen by her primary care physician for these issues. He obtained laboratory tests and a magnetic resonance image (MRI) of the brain which were normal.

Doris reports a good appetite and intake. She denies problems with sleeping, depression, or visual/auditory hallucinations. She states that she is worried about her worsening memory. The patient's St. Louis University Mental Status (SLUMS) examination score is 15/30, and her Cornell Scale for Depression in Dementia score is 16. She needs significant help from her husband with some instrumental activities of daily living (IADLs) including shopping, finances, and driving. She is independent in her activities of daily living (ADLs) except for bathing.

ADDRESSING PREVENTIVE CARE IN OLDER ADULTS

There is a demographic shift toward aging populations in many regions of the world. For example, the population of the United States older than age 65 years is expected to double in the next 30 years.[1] Life expectancy is at an all-time high. Care of the aging population has become dominated by management of chronic disease, which now accounts for approximately 80% of healthcare spending in this population.[2]

Despite the growing number and disease burden of older adults, they remain the most heterogeneous age segment of the population in terms of health and functional status. Significant numbers of elderly are free of disease and fully functional while a considerable portion carry high disease burden and disability.

Table 10.1 ▶ Health Status Population Segments

	Healthy	Chronically Ill	Frail	Dying
Types of conditions	Acute illness; early chronic disease	One or more advanced chronic diseases	Multiple chronic diseases; geriatric syndromes	Terminal illness; death expected in days to months
Degree to which conditions significantly impact quality of life	Little	Some, including financial resources	Profound; may include social isolation	Profound
ADL functional status[a]	Independent	Independent	Dependent, fall risk	Dependent
IADL functional status[b]	Independent	Partially dependent	Dependent	Dependent
Approximate frequency of segment in middle-aged population	85–90%	8–12%	2–3%	1%
Approximate frequency of segment in geriatric population	50–65%	25–40%	5–10%	1–2%

[a]ADLs: Bathing, dressing, grooming, toileting, transferring, eating, continence.
[b]IADLs: Food preparation, housekeeping, laundry, shopping, managing finances, medication administration, transportation, telephone use.

Addressing care for the older adult populations warrants classification of this heterogeneity in health status, recognition of the types of conditions that affect them, careful consideration of the overall goals of medical care, incorporation of life expectancy into decision making, and broadening the definition of activities typically included under the umbrella of "prevention."

Heterogeneity of the Older Adult Population

Usual aging is associated with functional change. It might include a decline in muscle strength and aerobic capacity; reduced bone density; decreased cardiac output; vasomotor instability; diminished pulmonary ventilation; decreased drug metabolism; changes in kidney function; altered sensory continence, appetite, and thirst; and a tendency toward constipation and urinary incontinence.

In general, populations of patients can be divided into four categories of health and functional status shown in Table 10.1.

Table 10.2 ▶ Remaining Life Expectancy (Yr), (United States)[a] by Age

Age		65			70			75	
Remaining Life Expectancy in Years	Percentile	25th	50th	75th	25th	50th	75th	25th	50th	75th
	Male	11	17	24	8	14	19	6	11	15
	Female	14	20	27	10	16	22	7	13	17

Age		80			85			90			95		
Remaining Life Expectancy in Years	Percentile	25th	50th	75th	25th	50th	75th	25th	50th	75th	25th	50th	75th
	Male	4	8	12	2	6	8	2	4	6	1	3	4
	Female	5	10	13	3	7	10	2	5	7	1	3	5

[a]In a cohort of 65-year-old men, 25% will be dead in 11 years (by age 76 years), 50% will be dead in 17 years, and 75% in 24 years. Data from: Arias E. United States Life Tables, 2008. *Natl Vital Stat Rep.* 2012;61(3):1–63.

These four health status categories have differing frequencies among middle-aged and older adults, the most significant of which is the dramatic increase of the chronically ill and frail segments observed in the geriatric population. Doris would be in the category of chronically ill.

Life Expectancy

Preventive medicine represents a tradeoff between short-term morbidity (e.g., the discomfort, inconvenience and expense of a colonoscopy) and long-term gain (e.g., reduction of morbidity and mortality from colon cancer) associated with the preventive intervention. A patient engaging in prevention must live long enough to realize its long-term benefit, a consideration that comes into play more often with chronically ill and older patients.

Tools to help clinicians in predicting life expectancy can help assess life expectancy against age benchmarks (referred to as "remaining life expectancy") as shown in Table 10.2. When the length of time needed for a preventive activity to "pay off" reaches or exceeds remaining life expectancy, it becomes unlikely that an individual patient will benefit from the intervention and more likely it will create harm. A related, and perhaps more relevant concept, is that of "active life expectancy" (ALE; i.e., the number of years of disability-free existence).

Care of the elderly should address five domains: (1) patient preferences, (2) interpreting the evidence, (3) prognosis, (4) clinical feasibility, and (5) optimizing therapies and care plans. A stepwise approach to evaluation and management of the elderly, incorporating these domains, is shown in Figure 10.1.

COMMON CONDITIONS CAUSING MORBIDITY AND MORTALITY IN OLDER ADULTS

The common causes of morbidity and mortality in each age group are in Table 10.3, the diseases primarily responsible for killing older adults (mortality) are not congruent with those responsible for making them feel poorly (morbidity). Diseases causing mortality tend to have a shorter period of morbidity before causing death, such as that seen with cancer, stroke, and pneumonia. Diseases causing morbidity often have long periods (from years to decades) of increasing morbidity until a catastrophic or fatal endpoint, such as diabetes leading to limb loss or osteoporosis resulting in hip fracture.

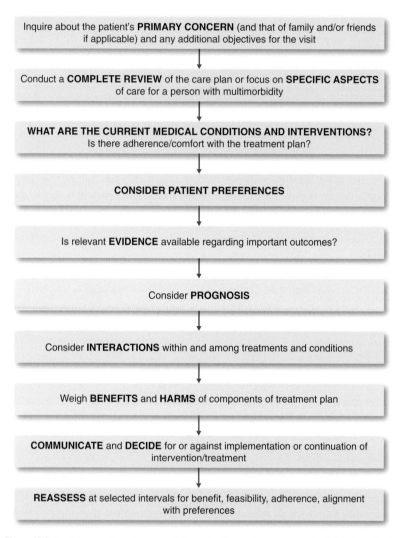

Inquire about the patient's **PRIMARY CONCERN** (and that of family and/or friends if applicable) and any additional objectives for the visit

Conduct a **COMPLETE REVIEW** of the care plan or focus on **SPECIFIC ASPECTS** of care for a person with multimorbidity

WHAT ARE THE CURRENT MEDICAL CONDITIONS AND INTERVENTIONS? Is there adherence/comfort with the treatment plan?

CONSIDER PATIENT PREFERENCES

Is relevant **EVIDENCE** available regarding important outcomes?

Consider **PROGNOSIS**

Consider **INTERACTIONS** within and among treatments and conditions

Weigh **BENEFITS** and **HARMS** of components of treatment plan

COMMUNICATE and **DECIDE** for or against implementation or continuation of intervention/treatment

REASSESS at selected intervals for benefit, feasibility, adherence, alignment with preferences

Figure 10.1 ▶ Evidence-based approach to evaluation and management of elderly patients.

The common geriatric syndromes one will encounter in clinical practice are reviewed in Table 10.4 and the common problems that may require special attention in elderly patients are described in Table 10.5. Although Doris is not presenting with any of the common geriatric syndromes or problems listed in the tables, her memory problems and aggressive behavior are of concern.

The causes for morbidity and mortality for Doris are hypertension, hyperlipidemia, CAD, and end-stage renal disease. Her increasing confusion, suspiciousness, and aggressiveness may be an atypical disease manifestation for disease entities like delirium, sepsis, intra-abdominal pathology, or dementia with behavioral disorder, and requires evaluation.

Table 10.3 ▶ Top 10 Causes of Mortality and Morbidity for People of Age 65 Years and Older in Descending Order

Mortality[a]	Morbidity[b]
• Heart disease	• Arthritis
• Cancer	• Hypertension
• Cerebrovascular disease	• Hearing impairment
• Chronic lung disease	• Heart disease
• Alzheimer disease	• Orthopedic problems
• Diabetes mellitus	• Chronic sinusitis
• Influenza and pneumonia	• Cataracts
• Kidney disease	• Diabetes
• Accidents	• Tinnitus
• Septicemia	• Allergic rhinitis

[a]Centers for Disease Control and Prevention. Deaths, Percent of Total Deaths, and Death Rates for the 15 Leading Causes of Death in Selected Age Groups, by Race and Sex: United States, 1999–2006. http://www.cdc.gov/nchs/nvss/mortality/lcwk3.htm
[b]Centers for Disease Control and Prevention. Prevalence of Selected Chronic Conditions: United States, 1990–1992. http://www.cdc.gov/nchs/data/series/sr_10/sr10_194.pdf

Table 10.4 ▶ Geriatric Syndromes

Syndrome	Background	Screening	Management
Hyperkyphosis	Defined as increased thoracic spine curvature of ≥40 degrees; progression leads to balance problems, slower gait speed, lower grip strength, and falls	The occiput to wall distance should be measured with the patient standing against a wall	Fall prevention; PT for extensor spinal muscle strength is essential. Educate on diaphragmatic breathing to engage core muscles
Weight loss	Involuntary weight loss of 10 lb (4.5 kg) or >5% of body weight over 6 months, or BMI <17 kg/m²	10-item DETERMINE checklist, 18-item mini-nutritional assessment, SNAQ[a]	Consider nutritional therapy under dietician guidance. Use herbs and spices to compensate for age-related changes in smell and taste. Avoid using prescription stimulants to treat
Malnutrition	Diet not adequate to maintain health; with aging, bone mass, lean mass, water content, and basal metabolic rate decrease and fat mass increases. Medications can also cause anorexia	Mini Nutritional Assessment (http://www.mna-elderly.com/). Check oral cavity for oral ulcers, dental caries, periodontal inflammation. Lab: prealbumin and albumin; total cholesterol <160 mg/dL without meds indicates underlying disease	Nutrition guidelines available at: www.choosemyplate.gov. Meals on wheels. Dietary supplements helpful but not superior to regular food intake. Hand to mouth feeding by caregiver most beneficial in patients with dementia. Limited evidence to support appetite stimulant drugs

(continued)

Table 10.4 ▸ Geriatric Syndromes *(Continued)*

Syndrome	Background	Screening	Management
Pressure ulcers	A pressure ulcer is a localized skin injury over a bony prominence, resulting from pressure in combination with shear. Four stages categorize pressure ulcers from redness to loss of full-thickness skin	The Braden Scale for predicting pressure ulcer risk and the Norton Scale for assessing risk of pressure ulcers are used to evaluate ulcers[b]	The National Pressure Ulcer Advisory Panel guidelines (www.npuap.org/) recommend performing skin care, optimizing nutrition, and repositioning at least once every 2 hours plus use of pressure redistribution devices
Frailty	More than three of: exhaustion, unintentional loss >10 lb (4.5 kg) in past year, low physical activity (<270 kcal/week), decreased grip strength, slowness (time to walk 15 feet [4.57 m])	Clinical frailty scale[c]. Walking speed: instruct patient to walk 1–4 m at own speed (<0.6 m/sec: high risk, 0.6 m/sec to 1 m/sec: medium risk, >1 m/sec: low risk)	Comprehensive geriatric assessment and multidisciplinary team-based care. Prevent loss of independence with aerobic and resistance/strengthening exercise and gait training/tai chi for balance; add nutritional support through protein supplementation
Urinary incontinence (UI)	Increases with age. Independent risk factor for NH placement; impairs quality of life. Types: urge, stress, mixed, functional, and overflow. Age-related changes: decreased urethral closing pressure, bladder capacity and contractility, nocturia, vaginal atrophy	Advise bladder diary, check postvoid residual (>200 mL significant). Check for hematuria, urine culture and sensitivity, serum glucose, renal function tests, vitamin B_{12}. Urodynamic testing if diagnosis unclear	Remove offending factors (e.g., caffeine, night-time diuretic) and manage underlying conditions (e.g., constipation). Scheduled voiding, behavioral therapy. Kegel exercises for stress incontinence and antimuscarinic agents or beta 3 agonist. Sacral nerve neuromodulation effective for refractory urge UI. Consider pessaries in stress and urge UI
Falls	Multifactorial causes: Intrinsic (e.g., poor balance, weakness, chronic illness, cognitive or visual impairment), extrinsic (e.g., polypharmacy), and environmental (e.g., poor lighting, no safety equipment, loose carpets)	USPSTF does not advise routine screening. Fall risk assessment: Timed Get up & Go test, Morse Fall scale (helpful in NH), Hendrich II fall risk tool (for hospitalized patients).[d] Assess balance using: Functional reach test, Berg balance scale	Aerobic and resistance exercises, gait and balance training, PT, OT. CBT for fear of falling syndrome. Discontinue or taper medications causing falls (e.g., benzodiazepines, antipsychotics, hypnotics, cardiovascular meds). Modify environmental factors (e.g., improved lighting, assistive devices)

[a]DETERMINE can be found at https://www.dads.state.tx.us/providers/AAA/Forms/standardized/NRA.pdf; SNAQ can be found at: http://www.fightmalnutrition.eu/toolkits/summary-screening-tools
[b]http://www.health.vic.gov.au/__data/assets/file/0010/233668/Norton-scale.pdf and https://secure.in.gov/isdh/files/Braden_Scale.pdf
[c]http://geriatricresearch.medicine.dal.ca/clinical_frailty_scale.htm Timed Get up & Go test: http://www.cdc.gov/steadi/pdf/tug_test-a.pdf
[d]Hendrich fall risk tool: https://consultgeri.org/try-this/general-assessment/issue-8.pdf
BMI, body mass index; CBT, cognitive behavioral therapy; LUTS, lower urinary tract symptoms; NH, nursing home; PT, physical therapy; OT, occupational therapy; SNAQ, simplified nutritional assessment questionnaire; USPSTF, United States Preventive Services Task Force.
Data from: Schneider DL. Hyperkyphosis: a new geriatric syndrome. *Today's Geriatric Med.* 2016;9(3):16. Available at: http://www.todaysgeriatricmedicine.com/archive/MJ16p16.shtml. Accessed September 3, 2016; *Evaluation and Management Tools (Geriatrics E&M Tools) Geriatrics Review Syllabus: A Core Curriculum in Geriatric Medicine.* 9th ed. American Geriatrics Society; 2016. Accessed September 3, 2016.; Vaught S. Gait, balance and fall prevention, *Ochsner J.* 2001;3(2):94–97.

Table 10.5 ▶ Problems Common Among Elderly Patients

Problem	Background	Screening	Management
BPH	Common (more than half by 60 years). New or worsening UI or LUTS are indications for screening	AUA Symptom Index[a] to assess LUTS (score of ≥8 notes severe LUTS); further testing may be warranted (e.g., outlet obstruction, stones)	Avoid caffeine, alcohol, and fluids after 4 PM. Consider use of alpha adrenergic agonists (e.g., clonidine, Catapres) and 5-alpha reductase inhibitors (e.g., finasteride); TURP in severe cases
Insomnia	Difficulty falling or staying asleep, waking too early, or experiencing poor sleep quality. Present in one-third of those aged ≥65 years	Screen annually with a sleep questionnaire[b] designed by the American Academy of Sleep Medicine[b]	Behavioral interventions: stimulus control, daytime sleep restriction, use of bright lights and CBT. Drug therapy: short-acting (to fall asleep) or intermediate-acting (to remain asleep) benzodiazepine
Osteoporosis (Chapter 12)	Per USPSTF: screen includes women aged ≥65 years and women aged <65 years with 10-year high-fracture risk and at-risk men aged ≥50 years	BMD of the proximal femur and lumbar spine is required. Use FRAX (https://www.shef.ac.uk/FRAX/) to assess fracture risk. Take BMD measurements more than once every 2 years.	Reduce risk via lifestyle modification (e.g., weight-bearing exercise at least five times/week for 30 minutes). Take calcium and vitamin D. Drug therapy includes bisphosphonates, denosumab, raloxifene, and teriparatide
Visual impairment	Increases with age (20%–30% >75 years). Cataract and refractive error (causes >20% of IADLs dysfunction) are most common; other common causes are macular degeneration, glaucoma, diabetic retinopathy	Visual acuity and visual field testing annually or as needed (confrontation method), ophthalmoscopy, medication review	Cataract: cataract surgery; Macular degeneration: vitamin supplements, zinc, beta carotene, laser or intravitreal injections of endothelial growth factor inhibitor; Glaucoma: β-blocker drops; Diabetic retinopathy: laser treatment and intravitreal injections, tight glucose control
Hearing impairment	Affects quality of life by family discord, social isolation, depression, anger, loss of self-esteem. Male, white, and low-education increase risk. Most common is presbycusis	Insidious onset; tinnitus an early sign of hearing loss. Screen with Hearing Handicap Inventory for the elderly or whisper test.[c] Handheld audioscope showing loss of 40 db or more.	Communication is key: Pay attention, remove background noise, face-to-face, speak slowly and clearly toward ear, spell words, write down directions, ask patient to repeat the discussion. Options: cerumen removal, hearing aids, assistive listening devices, and cochlear implants.

(continued)

Table 10.5 ▶ Problems Common Among Elderly Patients *(Continued)*

Problem	Background	Screening	Management
Dizziness	Can be vertigo, presyncope, disequilibrium, or mixed. Associated with fear of falling, functional disability, and depression	Orthostatic BP, Dix Hall Pike test, look for nystagmus. Hearing and vision testing, Timed Get up and Go test, Head thrust test, Fukuda stepping test,[d] ECG, BUN, TSH, vitamin B_{12}, folic acid, electrolytes, glucose. Tests NOT done routinely: ENG, rotational chair testing, posturography CT, MRI	Identify and treat cause. Consider adverse effects of meds, treatment of depression, vision, hearing loss. Meclizine for short-term symptomatic management; long-term use causes worsening. Vestibular rehab therapy, Epley maneuver,[e] and exercise. Surgery such as transmastoid labyrinthectomy, partial vestibular neurectomy for Meniere disease
Syncope	Frequency: vasovagal (20%), cardiac (10%), orthostatic (9%), medications (7%), seizure (5%), stroke/TIA (4%), other (8%), unknown (37%)[3]	Obtain history of before, during, and after syncope, perform cardiovascular and neurologic examination, orthostatic BP. Consider ECG, stress test, echocardiogram, carotid Doppler, EEG, Holter, Tilt test & electrophysiology studies	Treat underlying cause. Options: compression stockings, abdominal binders, small meals for postprandial syncope, meds such as midodrine, fludrocortisone, etilefrine, pyridostigmine (vasodepressor syncope), volume expansion, pacemaker (symptomatic bradycardia)
Eating disorders	Taste sensation and olfactory sense decrease with age but not taste discrimination. Edentulousness worsens ability to chew, sarcopenia (loss of muscle tissue) causes difficulty swallowing. Dysphagia (oral, pharyngeal, esophageal) and aspiration are important to identify	Dementia most common cause for oral dysphagia. Pharyngeal dysphagia: ask about choking, coughing, or nasal regurgitation; most common cause is stroke but seen in Parkinson disease, normal aging, MG, CNS tumor. Esophageal dysphagia: ask about food stuck in throat and difficulty swallowing both solids and liquids. Video fluoroscopy and nasopharyngeal laryngoscopy to assess swallowing	Oral and pharyngeal dysphagia: treat underlying cause. Meds: amantadine, angiotensin receptor blockers help in some conditions like Parkinson disease, stroke, and normal aging. Hand to mouth feeding by caregiver. Percutaneous endoscopic gastrostomy tubes will not prevent aspiration and do not improve mortality or morbidity in severely demented patients.

[a]http://www.urologychannel.com/uro/Forms/aua.pdf
[b]http://epworthsleepinessscale.com/
[c]Hearing Handicap Inventory: www.earaudiology.com/hhie.pdf; whisper test: https://www.healthcare.uiowa.edu/igec/tools/sensory/whisperedVoice.pdf and http://www.bmj.com/content/327/7421/967
[d]Dix Hall Pike test https://www.youtube.com/watch?v=kEM9p4EX1jk, Timed Get up and Go test (Timed Get up & Go test: http://www.cdc.gov/steadi/pdf/tug_test-a.pdf), head thrust test (http://www.advancedotology.org/sayilar/56/buyuk/Kaplan1.pdf), Fukuda stepping test (https://www.verywell.com/the-fukuda-stepping-test-2696228)
[e]Epley maneuver: (https://www.activator.com/wp-content/uploads/Home%20Epley%20Handouts.pdf)
AUA, American Urological Association; BMD, bone mineral density; BP, blood pressure; BPH, benign prostatic hyperplasia; BUN, blood urea nitrogen; CBT, cognitive behavioral therapy; CNS, central nervous system; ECG, electrocardiogram; EEG, electroencephalogram; ENG, electronystagmography; FRAX, Fracture Risk Assessment Tool; IADL, instrumental activities of daily living; LUTS, lower urinary tract symptoms; MG, myasthenia gravis; SNAQ, Simplified nutritional assessment questionnaire; TIA, transient ischemic attack; TURP, transurethral resection of the prostate; USPSTF, United States Preventive Services Task Force
Data from: *Evaluation and Management Tools (Geriatrics E&M Tools) Geriatrics Review Syllabus: A Core Curriculum in Geriatric Medicine.* 9th ed. American Geriatrics Society; 2016.

ATYPICAL PRESENTATION

Common conditions like pneumonia and urinary tract infections may present atypically in older adults. An atypical presentation involves vague or nonspecific symptoms, unusual or altered symptoms, or a complete lack of symptoms.[4] For example, a patient presenting with confusion may not have a neurologic problem, but rather an infection. In our case, Doris's limited kidney function requiring dialysis may be a contributing factor to her declining mental status. Several examples are described in Table 10.6. A retrospective study on older adult emergency visits indicated that the prevalence of atypical presentations is 30%.[5]

A possible cause of atypical presentation of illness is age-related physiologic changes with loss of physiologic reserves. In addition, there is interaction of chronic conditions with acute illnesses, polypharmacy, and older age. The most common atypical presentation is absence of fever in disease known to cause fever.

An altered mental state is the tip of the iceberg for medical illnesses in geriatric patients. Patients with geriatric syndromes like dementia and frailty have a significantly increased risk of atypical presentations. Classic disease presentations can also be masked by social and psychological factors. Early awareness of nonspecific presentations and the application of comprehensive geriatric assessments are crucial to preventing the delayed diagnoses and complications associated with delayed treatment; these include longer hospital stays, falls, delirium, morbidity and mortality, and an overall increase in health-care costs.[4]

On further questioning, Doris had gradual decline that worsened after hemodialysis and her confusion worsened after each dialysis treatment. She was seen in the clinic for geriatric assessment and advised to obtain laboratory tests and radiologic investigation. However, for the past week she has been getting very aggressive and before her next appointment, Doris is admitted to the hospital with worsening confusion.

Table 10.6 ▶ Illness Presentations in Older adults

Disorder	"Typical" Presentation	"Atypical" Presentation
Pneumonia	Cough, SOB, sputum production	Absence of usual symptoms, malaise, anorexia, confusion
Myocardial infarction	Severe, substernal chest pain; SOB; nausea	Mild or no chest pain, confusion, weakness, dizziness
Urinary tract infection	Dysuria, frequency, hematuria	Absence of dysuria, confusion, incontinence, anorexia
Thyrotoxicosis (hyperthyroid emergency)	Rapid heart rate, restlessness, agitation, tremor	Lethargy, cardiac arrhythmias, fatigue, weight loss
Acute appendicitis	Right lower quadrant abdominal pain, fever, tachycardia	Diffuse abdominal pain, confusion, urinary urgency, absence of fever or tachycardia
Infection	Fever, tachycardia, elevated white blood cell count	Temperature normal or below normal, absence of tachycardia, slightly elevated white blood cell count
Depression	Sad mood, increased sleep time, fluctuations in weight	Confusion, apathy, absence of subjective feeling of depression

HAZARDS OF HOSPITALIZATION

The age-associated dysregulation of homeostatic processes, multiple chronic illness, and frailty renders older adults more vulnerable to adverse effects relating to medical care. Frequently, in the hospital, treatment prescribed by multiple providers makes a complex situation worse. It is essential for the primary care provider to coordinate care to minimize iatrogenic illness.

Hospitalization hazards include falls, delirium, sleep deprivation, nosocomial infections, complications from hospital procedures, pressure ulcers, and adverse drug events.[6] Hospital beds should be kept as low as possible when patients are unattended, and ambulation and socialization must be facilitated to prevent irreversible functional decline.

Among hazards of hospitalization, delirium is often unrecognized and is present in 10% to 15% on admission and develops in up to 30% on medicine floors. In postoperative patients, rates are 15% to 53% and 70% to 87% in Intensive Care Units. Physicians recognize delirium in 20% and nurses in 50% of admitted patients.[6] The Confusion Assessment Method is the best screening tool (www.medscape.com/viewarticle/481726).

The timeframe of cognitive changes and the patient's baseline status are important in distinguishing between delirium and dementia. In a patient with delirium in the outpatient setting, consider infection (especially of the urinary tract), and look for signs of abuse such as bruising or neglect (does the patient look well cared for and clean).

Prevention is the best management when identifying and treating reversible contributors such as polypharmacy, infection, dehydration, pain, and sensory deprivation. The implementation of shared goals and objectives by an interdisciplinary team is key in preventing delirium. Antipsychotic agents can be used cautiously in cases where the patient's or caregiver's safety is affected.[7]

During both inpatient admissions and outpatient settings, **medication reconciliation** is a quality indicator. An evidence-based approach to reduce unnecessary medication is presented in Figure 10.2.

Doris improves with intravenous fluids and replacement of electrolytes leading the team to believe her delirium was due to electrolyte imbalance and dehydration after dialysis. As Doris has mental health issues (easily agitated and exhibiting verbal and physical aggression toward her husband) a consultation is arranged with a psychiatrist to evaluate her for delirium, dementia, depression, and social domains and quality of life. Doris had delirium due to electrolyte imbalance and dehydration. The psychiatrist dementia evaluation revealed worsening of her scores when compared to our clinic assessment. Also, she has behaviors that may need a different living situation, at least temporarily, to alleviate caregiver burden and stress. After admission to the hospital, the interdisciplinary team discusses the increased demands on the husband in taking care of his wife. The social worker presents a list of sites/facilities so that the husband and family can choose a facility to deliver care transitions.

CARE SITES FOR ELDERLY AND TRANSITIONS OF CARE

"Transitions of care" refer to the movement of patients between healthcare practitioners, settings, and home as their condition and care needs change, most commonly discharge from acute hospital care to another care facility or to home. Care sites in elderly where

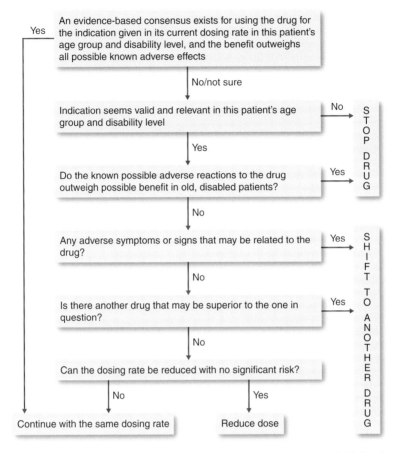

Figure 10.2 ► The good palliative-geriatric practice algorithm. (From Garfinkel D, Zur-Gil S, Ben-Israel J. The war against polypharmacy: a new cost-effective geriatric-palliative approach for improving drug therapy in disabled elderly people. *Isr Med Assoc J.* 2007;9(6):430–434; with permission.)

these transitions occur are listed in Table 10.7. Following her hospitalization, Doris was sent for rehabilitation to a skilled nursing facility for few weeks to improve her strength while arrangements were made to bring in a certified nurse assistant as a caregiver at home.

Unfortunately, transitions do not always go smoothly. Transitions are often marred by a lack of communication between providers at each end of the transition, resulting in errors of overuse, underuse, and inappropriate use of medications and treatments. Ineffective care transition processes not only lead to adverse events but higher hospital readmission rates and increased healthcare expenditure.

Geriatric evaluation and management, when properly targeted to frail older inpatients or outpatients with multidisciplinary needs, has been effective in reducing iatrogenic problems such as adverse drug events or hospital readmission for relapses of chronic illnesses. Problems with care transitions can be ameliorated by timely transfer of information between sites, proactive discharge planning and care coordination, education and preparation of the patient and family about the transition, a self-management plan for after the transfer, and a

Table 10.7 ▶ Care Sites for the Elderly

Site	Patient Needs and Services	Principle Funding Source
Acute care units (ACE) for elders	Specialized "inpatient care" units for geriatric hospital admissions. A patient-centered care plan is developed collaboratively by the interdisciplinary team. These units usually require environmental modifications to promote a homelike atmosphere, safe mobility, and cognitive stimulation, such as transfer-friendly furniture; handrails; the use of color contrast for low vision; family pictures and familiar objects in patients' rooms; and a group activity room for art or music therapy	Medicare Part A
Long-term acute care hospital (LTACH)	Patients with complex medical problems who require long-term care for more than 25 days qualify for LTACH admission. LTACHs are mostly attached to acute care hospitals, but are sometimes a separate unit. LTACHS specialize in taking care of patients, mostly from intensive care units, who require ventilator/respiratory care. They also provide rehabilitation services for stroke patients after their discharge	Medicare Part A, private pay, Medicaid
Inpatient rehabilitation facility (IRF)	If patients can participate in at least 3 hours of PT, they are eligible to be admitted to IRF, which is usually attached to a hospital. Admission generally requires a psychiatric evaluation. These facilities help patients to access short-term rehab focused on improving function. IRFs act as a bridge between acute hospitals and homes. Patients who are not able to perform 3 hours of intensive rehab but can do 1–2 hours are admitted to a subacute (step-down) or postacute care facility, or to a transitional care unit	Medicare Part A
Skilled nursing facility (SNF) Subacute or transitional care for short stay or long-term care	An SNF is a place where patients receive 24-hour care due to their chronic medical problems or problems with ADLs due to impaired memory or physical disabilities. The terms NH, SNF, and long-term care (LTC) facility are interchangeable. An LTC facility that provides short-term rehab (1–2 hours per patient per day) is also considered an SNF. Many SNFs also provide services such as hemodialysis and ventilation	Medicare Part A (short stay/rehabilitation), long-term care (private pay, Medicaid)
Assisted living community (ALC)	An ALC provides care for patients who require minimal help with their ADLs and want to live independently. These communities act as a bridge between independent living and NHs. While 24-hour supervision is provided by most facilities, this is often provided by nonlicensed staff. The types of services vary but may include dementia care services and medication management. Usually, the facility is responsible for some ADL support and other social activities unrelated to physician visits	Private pay, Medicaid (some facilities)

Site	Patient Needs and Services	Principle Funding Source
Continuing care retirement community (CCRC) or life care facility	A CCRC offers services at many levels including independent living, assisted living, long-term care services, and SNF care. Some CCRCs also offer special care units (e.g., for patients with Alzheimer disease). CCRC residents typically move from independent to assisted living, and then to LTC services with age and changes in health status	Private pay
Senior housing	Per the Fair Housing Act, "senior housing" is specifically designed for older adults under a federal, state, or local government program. People aged 62 years or older are eligible, or at least one person of 55 years or older should be in at least 80% of the occupied units. These facilities provide transportation and community activities. They also have safety-equipped (handrails, pull cords) units with security features. Housing options may include rent-assisted/low-income housing, moderate apartment-style living, and luxury retirement living	Private pay
Adult daycare	This essentially mimics child daycare centers. These centers are beneficial for families with obligations preventing care to family members during the day. Adult daycare can offer supervision, social and recreational activities, food, and possibly health-related supervision	Private pay
Home care/home healthcare	Nurse aids offer home care such as medical, nursing, social, and therapeutic treatment or assistance with essential ADLs in the home environment. Other services like PT, OT, ST, and respiratory therapy are delivered at home to recovering, disabled, and chronically or terminally ill patients. Housekeeping, nutrition counseling, social services, emergency response, and case management are included in home care. Face-to-face visits with the physician are essential to enrolling patients in home healthcare services	Private pay for caregiving services. Medicare[a]
Palliative care	Focuses on patient and family-centered care to improve quality of life, proactively prevent symptoms and treat suffering. Addresses physical, intellectual, social, emotional, spiritual needs and promote patient autonomy. Benefits include decreased intensive care unit stays and pharmacy costs in hospital. Reduces unnecessary tests and improves care coordination. Can use life-prolonging medications. Patient may not be terminally ill. No time limit to palliative care stay. Team includes doctors, mid-level providers, nurses, social workers, pharmacists, and chaplains.	Private pay or fee for service with insurance, including Medicare and Medicaid

(continued)

Table 10.7 ▶ Care Sites for the Elderly *(Continued)*

Site	Patient Needs and Services	Principle Funding Source
Hospice care	Focuses on terminal care with life expectancy less than 6 months in some states and 12 months in a few states. Two physicians must certify for eligibility. Active treatments are not pursued and life-prolonging medications not used unless for comfort. Patient or proxy of patient must agree for services. Team consists of nurse/care manager, physician and mid-level providers, social worker, aides, volunteers, physical therapist, occupational therapist, dietician, chaplain. Covers durable medical equipment; tests and treatments are fully covered if they are related to primary hospice diagnosis. Patient can choose the site of care to receive hospice care	Medicare hospice benefit and Medicaid

aPart A for nonphysician home care services (nursing, OT, PT, ST) and part B for outpatient physician services, and outpatient PT, ST, OT services independent of home care agency.
NH, nursing home; OT, occupational therapy; PT, physical therapy; ST, speech therapy.
Data from: Flood F, Allen K. ACE units improving complex care management. *Today's Geriatric Med.* 2013;6(5):28. Available from: http://www.todaysgeriatricmedicine.com/archive/090913p28.shtml. Accessed September 2016; Clark K, Doyle J, Duco S, et al Hot topics in Health Care. Transitions of Care: The need for a more effective approach to continuing patient care. Available from: https://www.jointcommission.org/assets/1/18/Hot_Topics_Transitions_of_Care.pdf. Accessed December 2017.

way for the patient and/or caregiver to be empowered to assert preferences for care. Use of "transition coaches" can help guide patients through care transitions.

> Doris did very well once she came home from the rehabilitation facility, with initial nursing care of 8 hours per day, later increased to 24-hour care when she became dependent on all ADLs. A hospice consultation was requested by the primary care doctor and a hospice worker provided additional care for few hours each day, which was fully covered by Medicare. Doris was in hospice for several months and died peacefully at home.

MENTAL HEALTH

Dementia affects approximately 2.4 to 5.5 million Americans. Prevalence increases with age, to 5% in persons aged 71 to 79 years, 24% in those aged 80 to 89 years, and 37% in those older than 90 years. Mild cognitive impairment (MCI) is different from dementia in that the cognitive impairment is not severe enough to interfere with IADLs. Estimates of MCI prevalence vary widely, from 3% to 42% in adults aged 65 years and older.[8]

Cognitive Screening

Screening for MCI or dementia in asymptomatic adults remains controversial. The United States Preventive Services Task Force (USPSTF) found insufficient evidence to balance the benefits or harms of screening. For those who have symptoms of memory loss, misplacing things, getting lost, or loss of ADLs or IADLS, there are several quick and easy tools to use for assessing patients with cognitive impairment; these are displayed in Table 10.8.

Table 10.8 ▶ Validated Neuropsychiatric Tests to Assess Cognitive Impairment

Study	Tests	Available	About
Mini mental state examination	Orientation, immediate recall, delayed recall, concentration/calculation, language and visual spatial domains	http://www.dementiatoday.com/wp-content/uploads/2012/06/MiniMentalStateExamination.pdf	Widely used, copyrighted, and must be purchased
MOCA	Orientation, recall, attention, naming, repetition, verbal fluency, abstraction, executive function, visuospatial	www.mocatest.org	Higher sensitivity and specificity than MMSE
Mini-cog	Visuospatial, executive function, recall	http://geriatrics.uthscsa.edu/tools/MINICog.pdf	Quick to administer, on two items
SLUMS	Orientation, recall, attention, naming, repetition, verbal fluency, abstraction, executive function, visuospatial	http://aging.slu.edu/index.php?page=saint-louis-university-mental-status-slums-exam	

Memory loss occurs as part of normal aging but can be associated with many conditions, especially if accompanied by dementia. As people live longer, there are more people alive with dementia. Alzheimer disease is the most common cause of dementia, causing 60% to 70% of all cases and affecting over one-third of people over the age of 85 years.[9,10] Alzheimer disease is most common in people over 65 years, and two-thirds of all affected are women.

Cognitive screening should also include ruling out reversible causes like depression, substance abuse, endocrine disorders (relating to vitamin B_{12} and thyroid conditions), and medications (e.g., anticholinergic agents, benzodiazepine, narcotic agents, histamine H2-receptor antagonists, β blockers, and digoxin). A physical examination and laboratory studies (complete blood count, basic metabolic panel, thyroid-stimulating hormone [TSH], vitamin B_{12}, and venereal disease research laboratory [VDRL] test) should be completed along with screening for depression and substance abuse and imaging studies like computed tomography (CT) scan/MRI of the brain.[7] If cognitive impairment is associated with motor abnormalities, consider Parkinson disease, a neurodegenerative disease like progressive supranuclear palsy, or cerebrovascular disease.

Diagnosis of dementia requires that at least two of the core mental functions are impaired enough to impact daily life. They are memory, language skills, ability to focus and pay attention, ability to reason and solve problems, and visual perception.

Patients with dementia should be screened for behavioral and psychological symptoms of dementia (BPSD). These symptoms can increase caregiver stress, patient injury, institutionalization, and morbidity. They also affect the quality of life and cost of care. Several screening methods are available including the Cohen-Mansfield Agitation Inventory, the Neuropsychiatric Inventory, and the Behavioral Pathology in Alzheimer Disease Rating Scale.[7]

Table 10.9 displays the differential diagnosis for patients with memory loss concerns along with key features and prognosis. Many patients and their families are primarily

Table 10.9 ▶ Differential Diagnosis for Patients Presenting with Memory Loss

Dementia Diagnosis	Key Features	Key Findings	Prognosis
Normal aging	Occasionally forgetful, word finding difficulty	Normal neurologic examination. MRI may show mild generalized cortical atrophy and nonspecific changes	Good
Mild cognitive impairment	Impaired short-term memory	Variable medial temporal lobe atrophy on MRI	Increased risk of AD
Delirium	Often toxic, metabolic, or infectious etiology; altered mental status	Impaired attention, fidgety; EEG slowing, evidence of systemic abnormalities	Depends on etiology and severity
Alzheimer disease (AD)	Gradually progressive; short-term memory loss with abnormalities in language, reason, focus, mood, or personality	Normal neurologic examination, medial temporal and parietal lobe atrophy on MRI	Course 4–20 years (average 8 years)
Vascular dementia	History of multiple stroke-like events, vascular risk factors	Evidence of significant cerebrovascular disease on MRI (infarcts, small vessel disease)	Course static or progressive (often coexists with AD)
Frontotemporal dementia	Typically presents with change in behavior, personality (apathy, disinhibition), or language	MRI may show atrophy in frontal and/or temporal lobes	Variable course, progressive speech, and swallowing difficulties
Lewy body dementia	Fluctuating attention, visual hallucinations, parkinsonian motor signs, sleep disorders	Limb rigidity, bradykinesia, may see intention tremor and gait disturbance	Variable course, may see more rapid functional decline versus AD
Parkinson dementia	Parkinson disease with later-onset cognitive dysfunction	Limb rigidity, bradykinesia, resting tremor, gait disturbance	Variable course, may have severe motor disability when dementia occurs

Data from: Emmett KR. Nonspecific and atypical presentation of disease in the older patient. *Geriatrics*. 1998;53(20):50–60; O'Neill PA. *Caring for the Older Adult: A Health Promotion Perspective*. Philadelphia, PA: WB Saunders; 2002.

worried that memory loss represents the onset of Alzheimer disease. Suspect Alzheimer disease in patients with:

▶ Memory loss that disrupts daily life

▶ Difficulty completing familiar tasks or solving problems

▶ Confusion with time and place

▶ Trouble understanding visual images and special relationships

▶ New problems with words in speaking or writing

▶ Misplacing things and losing ability to retrace steps

▶ Decreased or poor judgment

▶ Withdrawal from work or social activities

▶ Changes in mood or personality

For patients with mild dementia, supportive care, adaptive aids, enhanced social activities, and continued learning opportunities are suggested (e.g., source of recommendation C [SOR C]). There are no available medications for non-Alzheimer–type dementia.

Initially, nonpharmacologic interventions should be attempted when managing BPSD. Underlying physiologic and environmental triggers should be identified and controlled, as possible. Pharmacologic treatment (e.g., antipsychotic agents and mood stabilizers) can be used if nonpharmacologic interventions have proved to be ineffective or if there are concerns about patient or caregiver safety.[7]

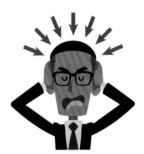

For patients with Alzheimer disease, in addition to behavioral support, a trial of an acetylcholinesterase inhibitor (e.g., donepezil, galantamine, rivastigmine) for those with mild to moderate dementia[11] or the N-methyl-d-aspartate (NMDA) receptor antagonist memantine (Namenda), for those with moderate to severe dementia, is recommended.[12]

Emotional Wellbeing

Satisfaction in one's life, happiness, sadness, and feeling of purpose, are strongly associated with health. Healthcare providers and systems of care should not only focus on morbidity but should also address the patient's emotional wellbeing.

Eight per cent to 40% of older adults in the outpatient setting have minor depression, while major depression has been reported in 6% to 10%. The corresponding figures for nursing home residents are 12% to 20% and 11% to 45% for hospitalized older adults.[13]

Depression and anxiety can decrease adherence to medication functional ability, and hasten disease progression. Medical care givers should be included in the evaluation and screening of depression and anxiety as patients sometimes minimize their symptoms. The first two questions of the patient health questionnaire (PHQ) 9 (www.phqscreeners.com) and the first two questions from the generalized anxiety disorder (GAD) 7 screening tool (http://www.integration.samhsa.gov/clinical-practice/GAD708.19.08Cartwright.pdf) are quick screens for depression and anxiety.[13]

Nonpharmacologic management includes psychotherapy, aerobic exercises, and electroconvulsive therapy. Selective serotonin reuptake inhibitors and serotonin–norepinephrine reuptake inhibitors are the preferred agents (Chapter 22).[7]

ENVIRONMENTAL ASSESSMENT

As part of a comprehensive social assessment, several socioeconomic and environmental elements should be assessed including the patient's ethnic, spiritual, and cultural background; the patient's special needs such as caregivers and their availability; the caregiver burden; safety of the home environment; the possibility of mistreatment of the patient; the patient's economic well-being; and the individual's prior requests. A comprehensive social assessment is time-consuming and may not be feasible in a busy office practice. However, healthcare providers should acknowledge the importance of these social aspects on the patient's quality of life.

Home Safety and Evaluation

The U.S. Census Bureau indicates that 30% of community indwelling older adults live alone, while the remaining 70% live with their spouses or extended families. Establishing a baseline functional status in older people's living environments is an essential aspect of monitoring disease progress and evaluating the effects of the prevention interventions. Home safety and evaluation not only help establish a baseline but also uncovers unmet needs as well as safety and environmental hazards.

An environmental assessment begins with questions about the home situation. A home safety checklist is essential and can be obtained by nonphysician members of the care team. This should cover the patient's socioenvironmental circumstances and special needs, availability of support resources, and the patient's social interaction network. For older adults, particularly those who are frail and lack social support, a home visit is extremely helpful.[14] Tools like the Home Safety Self-Assessment Tool (HSSAT), SAFER-HOME v3, and I-HOPE can guide the visit (http://www.aota.org/practice/productive-aging/home-mods/rebuilding-together/assessments.aspx).

The following should be performed during a formal home assessment:

▶ Observe the patient's daily routine and performance of ADLs such as dressing and transferring.

▶ Assess environmental hazards such as cluttered walking surfaces, improper bed height, poor lighting, and lack of railings that increase risk of fall.

▶ Suggest environmental modifications such as nonslip bath mats, installing support structures (especially in the bathroom), and improved lighting, especially at night.

▶ Discuss the need for assistive devices, such as special utensils, "reachers," and adapted telephones.

Evidence indicates that home safety interventions appear to be more effective when performed by an occupational therapist.[14] Finally, the needs of caregivers, which include training, support, and counseling, need to be recognized and addressed.[15]

PHYSICAL ASSESSMENT

Assess functional status by asking about ADLs and IADLs (Table 10.1). If a patient needs help with these, referrals for physical therapy (PT) and occupational therapy (OT) will help. Emphasis should be on strengthening quadriceps and hamstrings using both isotonic and isometric exercises. At every patient visit, inquire about two or more falls in the past year or fear of falling due to gait and balance problems (Fig. 10.3). Gait and balance assessment must include orthostatic blood pressure (BP) measurement and heart rate, observing the patient getting up and walking, Romberg's and semi-tandem stand test (https://youtu.be/UQ6-7TrmKxU).

Driving is sometimes referred to as "The Ultimate IADL," so it is important to ask about driving as older adults suffer more harmful injuries in motor vehicle accidents (MVAs) than

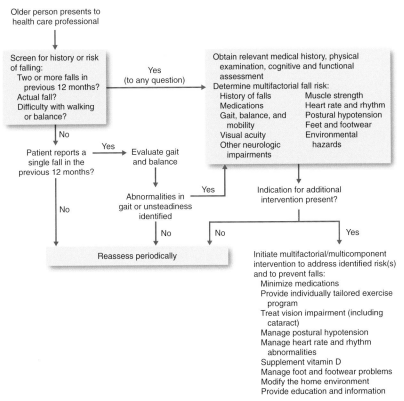

Figure 10.3 ▶ Balance assessment and management. (Adapted from: Kenny RA, Rubenstein LZ, Tinetti ME, et al. Summary of the updated American Geriatrics Society/British Geriatrics Society clinical practice guideline for prevention of falls in older persons. *J Am Geriatr Soc*. 2011;59(1):148–157.)

any other age group. Vision, motor/sensory changes, and cognitive changes that are related to aging, chronic medical conditions, and associated medications can all affect driving skills and safety.

Self-assessment is not an adequate measure of driving ability. No single assessment tool can accurately predict how capable a person is to drive, so a mixture of several assessment tools should be used to determine ability to drive safety. Asking about IADLs provides important clues for assessing functional decline in geriatric patients. The early stages of visual field loss are not noticeable to most older adults; therefore, screening for visual field cuts is important.

The Clinical Assessment of Driving Related Skills (CADReS) is an evidence-based, practical toolbox that can be used in an office-based setting.[16] This toolbox can identify some of the cognitive functional deficits that affect driving performance. Failure to pass the CADReS may warrant referral to a specialist, such as OT, speech therapy (ST), a neuropsychologist, driving rehabilitation specialist (DRS), or another medical specialist, depending on the type of deficit. A DRS is a healthcare professional who can perform a comprehensive driving evaluation to make a fitness-to-drive decision in at-risk older adults who have physical, visual, or cognitive functional impairments.

Healthcare providers should aim to identify, correct, or stabilize functional deficits rather than simply prohibiting older adults from driving. It is recommended that older adults 60 years or above be screened for driving safety annually. Healthcare professionals should always discuss a "driving retirement plan" with people before they receive a "do not drive" prescription. In some states (CA, DE, NJ, NV, OR, PA), it is mandatory to report older adult drivers who are at risk of having MVAs.

SOCIAL ASSESSMENT

Advance Directives

Although extension of life can tacitly be understood to be a goal, the medical management of patients with incapacitating illnesses is based on goals of care agreed upon in shared decision making by the patient, family, and doctor. Healthcare choices are decided in advance directives, which are legal documents prepared by patients before any incapacitating illness. Although the laws vary among states in the United States, there are two basic kinds of directives: **living wills and healthcare proxy** (or durable healthcare power of attorney) (Table 10.10). These directives go into effect only when the patient becomes incapacitated and is unable to make decisions regarding care.

Advance directives can be drafted with the help of a healthcare provider, attorney, local Area Agency on Aging, or state health department.[19] For an advance directive to be useful, it must be available and accessible. The original copies of the advance directive should be stored in a place where patients or an emergency medical team can easily find them. Patients should be encouraged to give a copy to their healthcare proxy, healthcare providers, hospital, nursing home, family, and friends. Advance directives should be updated at least annually. A continuing conversation should take place among the patient, medical providers, healthcare proxy, and loved ones to ensure that the patient's wishes are understood and that the terms of the advance directive will be honored.[19]

 Table 10.10 ▶ Living Wills and Healthcare Proxy

Living Will[a]	Healthcare Proxy
• A written statement of the healthcare that patients do and do not want in certain circumstances • Includes preferences for resuscitation as well as use of dialysis and life-sustaining treatment, do-not-hospitalize orders, and tube feeding.[17] • Desire for place of dying along with preferences for organ and tissue donation, autopsies, burial, cremation, and memorial services can be expressed as well.	• Also called durable healthcare, power of attorney is a legal document indicating the name of the person who may make healthcare decisions if the patient becomes incapacitated.[18] • Can help avoid mismatches in patient preferences and the actual care rendered • Can also grant broad authority over the patient's medical affairs, which might include coordination of care • Medical and financial power of attorney are two separate legal documents, but it is recommended that a single proxy be named • A proxy granted medical power of attorney is legally bound to follow the patient's treatment preferences, while a proxy granted financial power of attorney handles the patient's social security checks, retirement accounts, other investments, and tax returns[18]

[a]Completion of a Physician Orders for Life-Sustaining Treatment form, which has been endorsed by some states and is being developed in many others, can facilitate patient-centered care at the end of life.

Table 10.11 ▶ Treatment Options for Managing Symptoms at End of Life

Symptom	Important Points	Treatment Option
Bowel obstruction	Common in rectal, colon, pancreatic and ovarian cancer; also in peritoneal carcinomatous and malignant ascites	Dexamethasone (8 mg/24 hrs), ranitidine (200 mg/24 hrs) and octreotide (600 μg/24 hrs by infusion). Surgery is helpful if it helps with palliation; benefit must outweigh risk
Constipation and fecal impaction	Most common offenders are opioids, ondansetron and similar drugs, and calcium channel blockers	Increase fluids; Senna alone; mix 3/4 cup of prune juice, one cup of applesauce, and one cup of coarse unprocessed wheat bran mix and administer 1–2 large tablespoonful with 8 oz of water (plus milk of magnesia for added effect); magnesium citrate 30 cc every few hours until effect; Miralax; methyl naltrexone for opioid induced constipation
Cough	Chronic idiopathic cough, pleural effusion, bronchiectasis, idiopathic pulmonary fibrosis	Gabapentin; start at 300 mg daily (100 mg in frail patients) and increase to 1,800 mg/day
Depression (Chapter 22)	Underdiagnosed and untreated	CBT, psychotherapy, antidepressants very helpful; transcranial magnetic stimulation appears effective; psychostimulants not well studied
Dyspnea	Differentiate and treat cause of dyspnea if possible	Provide oxygen only if hypoxia except in patients with COPD; opioids, drug of choice; benzodiazepines (limited evidence), clonazepam is helpful
Fatigue	1. Chemotherapy-related fatigue 2. Cancer fatigue	1. American ginseng and Dexamethasone 2. Methylphenidate for 5 days, continue long term if improvement noted by patient
Hiccups	No good clinical evidence of an agent of choice	Trial of baclofen, prochlorperazine, phenothiazine, or benzodiazepines
Itching	1. Burns, hematologic malignancies, cancer, uremia 2. Liver disease/bile cholestasis	1. Gabapentin 2. Paroxetine, sertraline
Nausea and vomiting	1. Treat underlying cause 2. Chemotherapy induced 3. Constipation/opioid induced 4. Partial obstruction induced	1. Do not use Ativan, Benadryl, haloperidol 2. Serotonin or neurokinin-1 blocking drug, olanzapine very helpful 3. Antidopamine agents (e.g., haloperidol, metoclopramide) 4. Metoclopramide helps to some extent in ovarian cancer
Pulmonary secretions	Called death rattle and pooling in posterior pharynx	Scopolamine transdermal patch every 3 days; scopolamine oral or glycopyrrolate helps. Suction helps to clear secretion as needed

End-of-Life and Palliative Care

Hospice and palliative care is underutilized.[20] It is very important to identify and enroll appropriate patients into a hospice program; this will eliminate barriers to quality end-of-life care. Treatment options for managing symptoms at the end of life are presented in Table 10.11.

The most common symptom is pain. Barriers to pain management include hesitancy to report pain, use of vague terms like discomfort to report pain, comorbidities, and high cost of pain medication. Physician barriers include reluctance to prescribe opioids, lack of training in pain management and drug interactions, fear of complications and regulatory oversight. It is important to identify and quantify the symptoms that a patient is suffering. This can be accomplished by using a symptom scale such as those provided by the National Palliative Care Research Center (http://www.npcrc.org/content/25/Measurement-and-Evaluation-Tools.aspx).

Nonpharmacologic techniques for pain management include acupuncture, cognitive behavioral therapy, cold/hear and transcutaneous electrical stimulation. For a discussion of management of pain, see Chapter 20.

QUESTIONS

1. The five domains that should be addressed in the care of the elderly are patient preferences, interpreting the evidence, prognosis, clinical feasibility, and optimizing therapies and care plans.
   A. True
   B. False

2. Which one of the following is true of the common geriatric syndromes encountered in clinical primary care practice?
   A. Hyperkyphosis is resistant to attempts at extensor spinal muscle strengthening.
   B. Weight loss should be treated with prescription stimulants.
   C. Pressure ulcers are treated by performing skin care, optimizing nutrition, and repositioning.
   D. Urinary incontinence is usually the result of infection in the elderly.
   E. Fall prevention begins with routine screening for falls.

3. You are caring for a 92-year-old woman hospitalized for confusion and dehydration. On evaluation, you identify a bladder infection. Which one of the following is true of atypical presentations of illness in elderly patients?
   A. Atypical presentations are uncommon.
   B. Atypical presentations may be caused by age-related physiologic changes.
   C. A common atypical presentation of myocardial infarction is abdominal pain.
   D. The most common atypical presentation is weakness.

4. Which one of the following is true of providing mental healthcare to elderly patients?
   A. Routine screening for dementia should be conducted.
   B. Patients with dementia should be screened for behavioral and psychological symptoms.
   C. Brief (two-item) questionnaires are inaccurate for depression and anxiety screening.
   D. Medication should be provided for patients with non-Alzheimer–type dementia.
   E. Medication for depression is more effective than nonpharmacologic options.

5. You and your attending are seeing an elderly woman with terminal lung cancer who is under hospice care. She has been depressed and reports shoulder pain and difficulty with cough and fatigue. She is not taking any medications. Which one of the following is appropriate for the initial management of this patient?
   A. Treatment for depression is unlikely to be helpful.
   B. She should be given opioids for pain relief.
   C. She can be offered a trial of gabapentin for cough.
   D. She should be offered a trial of dexamethasone for fatigue.

ANSWERS

Question 1: The correct answer is A.
Care of the elderly should address five domains: (1) Patient preferences, (2) Interpreting the evidence, (3) Prognosis, (4) Clinical feasibility, and (5) Optimizing therapies and care plans.

Question 2: The correct answer is C.
Table 10.4. The National Pressure Ulcer Advisory Panel guidelines recommend performing skin care, optimizing nutrition, and repositioning at least once every 2 hours plus use of pressure redistribution devices.

Question 3: The correct answer is B.
A possible cause of atypical presentation of illness is age-related physiologic changes with loss of physiologic reserves.

Question 4: The correct answer is B.
Cognitive screening (for patients with dementia) should also include ruling out reversible causes like depression, substance abuse, endocrine disorders (relating to vitamin B12 and thyroid conditions), neoplasm, and medications (e.g., anticholinergic agents, benzodiazepine, narcotic agents, histamine H2-receptor antagonists, β blockers, and digoxin).

Question 5: The correct answer is C.
Table 10.11. For cough, patients can be given gabapentin, starting at 300 mg daily (100 mg in frail patients) and increasing to 1,800 mg/day as needed.

REFERENCES

1. Thaler M, Kole J, Rutigliano M. Team-based care optimizes outcome. *Today's Geriatric Med.* 2015;8(2):14. Available from: http://www.todaysgeriatricmedicine.com/archive/0315p14.shtml. Accessed September 18, 2016.
2. American Medical Directors Association. *Transitions of Care in the Long-Term Care Continuum Clinical Practice Guideline.* Columbia, MD: AMDA; 2010.
3. Soteriades ES. Incidence and prognosis of syncope. *N Engl J Med.* 2002;347:878–885.
4. Betancourt G, Hames E, Rivas K. Atypical presentations of common conditions in geriatric patients. *J Post-Acute and Long-Term Care Med.* 2015;16(3):B5. Available from: http://dx.doi.org/10.1016/j.jamda.2015.01.007. Accessed September 2016.
5. Limpawattana P. Atypical presentations of older adults at emergency department and associated risk factors. *Arch Gerontol Geriatr.* 2016;62:97–102.
6. Creditor MC. Hazards of hospitalization of elderly. *Ann Intern Med.* 1993;118(3):219–223.
7. *Evaluation and Management Tools (Geriatrics E&M Tools) Geriatrics Review Syllabus: A Core Curriculum in Geriatric Medicine.* 9th ed. American Geriatrics Society; 2016. Accessed September 3, 2016.

8. United States Preventive Services Task Force. Available from: http://www.uspreventiveservicestaskforce. org/Page/Document/RecommendationStatementFinal/cognitive-impairment-in-older-adults-screening. Accessed September 2016.

9. Sloane PD, Zimmerman S, Suchindran C, et al. The public health impact of Alzheimer's disease, 2000–2050: potential implications of treatment advances. *Annu Rev Public Health.* 2002;23:213–231.

10. Sloane PD, Khandelwal C, Kaufer DI. Cognitive impairment. In: Smith MA, Shimp LA, Schrager S, eds. *Lange Family Medicine Ambulatory Care and Practice.* 6th ed. New York: McGraw Hill; 2014.

11. Birks J. Cholinesterase inhibitors for Alzheimer's disease. *Cochrane Database Syst Rev.* 2006;1:CD005593.

12. McShane R, Sastre AA, Minakakran N. Memantine for dementia. *Cochrane Database Syst Rev.* 2006;5:CD003154.

13. Samuels S, Abrams R, Shengelia R, et al. Integration of geriatric mental health screening into a primary care practice: a patient satisfaction survey. *Int J Geriatr Psychiatry.* 2015;30(5):539–546.

14. American Occupation Therapy Association. Available from: http://www.aota.org/practice/productive-aging/home-mods/rebuilding-together/assessments.aspx. Accessed September 2016.

15. Durso S, Sullivan G. *Geriatrics Review Syllabus: A Core Curriculum in Geriatric Medicine.* 9th ed. American Geriatrics Society; 2016. Accessed September 3, 2016.

16. Pomidor A, ed. *Clinician's Guide to Assessing and Counseling Older Drivers.* 3rd ed. New York, The American Geriatrics Society; 2015.

17. U.S. living will registry. Available from: http://www.uslivingwillregistry.com/faq.shtm. Accessed November 2016.

18. Vanarelli D, Managing end-of-life issues. *Aging Well.* 2009;2(5):26. Available from: http://www.todaysgeriatricmedicine.com/archive/110909p26.shtml. Accessed November 2016.

19. Vanarelli D. Managing end-of-life issues. *Aging Well.* 2009;2(5):26. Available at: http://www.todaysgeriatricmedicine.com/archive/110909p26.shtml. Accessed September 2016.

20. Smith TJ. Symptom management in the older adult: 2015. *Clin Geriatr Med.* 2015;31(2):155–175.

Acute Problems: Approach and Treatment

KEY POINTS

1 ▶ Introduce yourself, focus on the patient, and listen without interruption.

2 ▶ Solicit all concerns at the start of the visit and set a visit agenda with the patient, prioritizing what should be discussed today and what might be saved for later.

3 ▶ Early in the visit, determine whether the problem is an emergency using the patient's story, signs, and symptoms; if so, alert the attending.

4 ▶ Use diagnostic testing if the diagnosis is uncertain, based on probabilities, AND if the result of the test is expected to change management.

5 ▶ Consider testing or treatment options, rank them based on best evidence, present that information to your patient, and engage them in shared decision making.

6 ▶ Causes of abdominal pain are differentiated by location, pain quality, and associated symptoms; care must be taken to identify conditions needing urgent surgical diagnosis or treatment.

7 ▶ Consider cardiac and pulmonary causes of acute shortness of breath and ask about any risk factors for venous thromboembolism; office-based examination should include pulse oximetry.

8 ▶ Most chest pain seen in primary care is musculoskeletal or gastrointestinal pain; apply a decision rule to help determine the likelihood of cardiac ischemia.

9 ▶ Dizziness can be classified into four different groups – vertigo, presyncope, disequilibrium, and lightheadedness – and can be caused by neurologic, cardiovascular, or vestibular disorders.

10 ▶ Dysuria is most often caused by urinary tract infection; these can be complicated, especially in elderly patients causing sepsis and associated confusion.

11 ▶ Fever in an infant <29 days old necessitates detailed workup for serous bacterial infection.

12 ▶ Peptic ulcer disease is the most common cause of upper gastrointestinal (GI) bleeding and diverticulosis is the most common cause of significant lower GI bleeding in older adults; upper endoscopy or colonoscopy are the initial tests for identifying the bleeding source.

13 ▶ For most patients, a careful history, vital signs, funduscopic examination, neck and neurologic examinations are sufficient for making a diagnosis of headache.

14 ▶ Leg swelling is most commonly caused by venous stasis, but a decision tool can help exclude the diagnosis of deep vein thrombosis.

15 ▶ Nausea and vomiting are common in pregnancy, with viral illness, and among patients on chemotherapy. Assess for hematemesis, dehydration, and altered mental status.

16 ▶ Most upper respiratory symptoms are caused by viruses, but the clinician should know the prevalence of influenza in their community and other risk factors for bacterial infections.

This chapter is divided into two sections. The first focuses on an approach to patients presenting with acute problems. This section will guide learners through the steps of this common visit type. Steps include recognizing emergency situations early in the encounter, focusing on the needed elements in the examination, deciding on further diagnostic testing, identifying and ranking treatment options, presenting the case to your attending, conducting shared decision-making with patients around treatment and follow-up, and documenting your findings.

The second section covers management of the common problems of abdominal pain, breathing difficulty (shortness of breath), chest pain (CP) in adults, dizziness, dysuria, fever, gastrointestinal (GI) bleeding, headache, leg swelling, nausea/vomiting, and upper respiratory symptoms, in alphabetical order. This chapter is long, and you will best learn and retain information if you read about these topics as you encounter patients with these problems.

APPROACH TO ACUTE PROBLEMS

MEETING AND GREETING THE PATIENT

> Mr. Stern, a 71-year old man, presents with abdominal pain persisting over many months. He is waiting in the room with his wife. You read in the electronic medical record that he has controlled hypertension and borderline diabetes mellitus but no other medical problems and no surgeries. He is recorded as being a "social drinker" but does not smoke.

Introductions

When introducing yourself to a new patient, begin first by directly addressing the patient, regardless of their age or capacity, and then state your name and position.

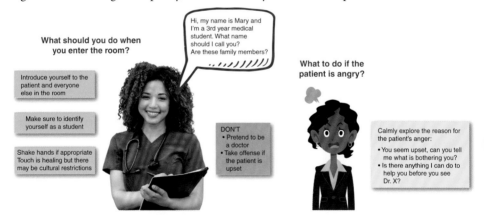

Some patients or their families will be visibly upset or angry. Reasons for this are many including the patient's current problem, family or work issues, wait time, or encounter with the nurse or receptionist among others. Rather than take offense or retreat, use the opportunity to explore the problem.

Usually the doctor or nurse will have screened the patient to be sure that he/she is comfortable with talking with a student, but not always. If the person seems hostile or refuses to talk with you, it is OK to politely exit, noting that the doctor will be in soon to see them.

Listening to the Story

A great deal can be learned by listening to patient's stories. Begin by asking the patient to tell you about the current problem. Avoid interrupting or prompting until they finish speaking.

> Sadly, one study found that residents working in primary care offices allowed patients to speak for just 12 seconds after entering the room before interrupting.[1]

Although you may feel pressured to get all the relevant facts, the patient will often tell you what you need to know without prompting, if you listen. Preparing a **short list of questions** about the "chief complaint" before entering the room can help you feel less pressured during the encounter. When the patient finishes telling you about their problem, tell them back what you heard and ask your questions to fill in any missing details such as severity, duration, or circumstances under which the symptom occurs.

> **The mnemonic FIFE can be used to understand the patient's experience**
> ▶ Feelings related to the illness (especially fears, and demonstrate empathy)
> ▶ Ideas/explanations of the cause (what do you think is happening/will help?)
> ▶ Functioning (influence on daily life, effect on the patient and others)
> ▶ Expectations of the visit/doctor (what do you hope I can do for you today?)

Soliciting collateral information from those accompanying the patient can be helpful, especially if body language tells you that the accompanying individual has something to say or that the patient may not have been entirely truthful.

If the accompanying person monopolizes the conversation, however, options include:

▶ Continue to face the patient and ask them to explain in their own words

▶ Thank the individual for their input but state that you need to hear from the patient

▶ Ask for some private time with the patient or ask your questions later, by asking others to exit the room for privacy during the examination. This is particularly important for adolescents, if you suspect abuse or bullying, or that the issue to be discussed may be of a sexual nature.

Patients often have Multiple Concerns

Soliciting those other concerns at the start of the visit—**agenda setting**—can help you and the patient prioritize what should be discussed today, and what might be saved for a future visit. The first issue that the patient presents may not actually be their main concern.[2] Presenting the list of concerns to the attending will also help ensure that the patient's most pressing issues are addressed, leading to greater satisfaction for all.

> The patient describes his pain as fairly constant aching which is sometimes severe in the left lower quadrant, especially over the last few months. His bowel movements seem normal and he hasn't noticed any blood. On prompting, his wife adds that this problem has been ongoing for over a year. She also expresses concern about his heavy alcohol use, sometimes for controlling pain. The patient is a former smoker and has not had a screening colonoscopy in 20 years.

RECOGNIZING AN EMERGENCY

Once you have enough history to begin formulating a differential diagnosis, you should determine whether the problem is an emergency.

▶ Check vital signs: noting temperature, pulse, and blood pressure (BP).
▶ **Alert attending and do a quick physical assessment of the relevant organ system** if:
  - the patient's pain is severe (e.g., the patient is pale, sweaty, grimacing)
  - pain is in the chest now
  - breathing is difficult (e.g., rapid, labored, stridor)
  - the patient has signs of stroke (FAST: **F**acial drooping, **A**rm weakness, **S**peech difficulties, and **T**ime [ongoing symptoms of recent onset])
  - swallowing is difficult (e.g., drooling), or
  - the person seems unsteady or confused, especially if hypotensive with a rapid pulse.

It is also helpful to know the location of the emergency/crash cart in your office and how emergencies should be handled (e.g., who calls for an ambulance).

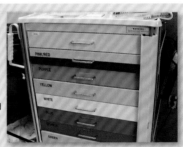

Office Crash Cart

Know where the crash cart is located and what it contains. There are no requirements for crash carts other than including material for responding to cardiac and respiratory emergencies. Contents vary from clinic to clinic.

Recommended crash cart items can be found at https://www.acls.net/acls-crash-cart.htm. Common items include:
• Airways and bag valve mask
• IV tubing and saline solution
• Angiocaths and syringes
• Monitor and defibrillator
• Medications (Epi-pen, aspirin, naloxone, atropine, and others)

Mr. Stern's vital signs are normal and he denies active bleeding from his rectum. He is not in severe pain and on initial abdominal examination, he has active bowel sounds, is moderately tender in the right lower quadrant without rebound tenderness, and there is no palpable mass. You conclude that this is not an emergency. You finish the physical examination and a rectal examination with your attending present, which is normal. You place a small amount of stool from your glove onto a test card for occult blood and exit the room.

FOCUSED HISTORY AND PHYSICAL EXAMINATION

Unlike the complete history and physical examinations performed at the beginning of medical school, examinations conducted on established patients who present for an acute visit can be less extensive and focused on the pertinent aspects of the problem at hand. It is helpful, however, to review the patient's medications, including nonprescription ones that may not have been recorded in the patient's medical record. It is also important to solicit all current concerns.

Most offices have computers in the room. Be sure to seat yourself so that the computer is not between you and the patient. Look at the patient and stop typing while the patient is speaking, especially if there is emotional content. Find ways to engage the patient: showing the screen when appropriate for recent laboratory test results or graphs of BP.

Essential aspects of the history and physical examination will be presented in each of the common problem sections in the Treatment section of this chapter. We have chosen these problems based on recommendations by the National Family Medicine Clerkship Curriculum (http://www.stfm.org/LinkClick.aspx?fileticket=upiiuNFp3Vc%3d&tabid=17603&-portalid=49) and the frequency that you might see these problems in primary care.

Approximately 928 million annual office visits (about 1/2 to primary care physicians) in 2012 (National Ambulatory Care Survey).[3] The most common acute problems were:

▶ Cough (2.8%)

▶ Knee symptoms (1.6%)

▶ Low back symptoms (1.4%)

▶ Throat symptoms (1.4%)

▶ Skin rash (1.3%)

▶ Stomach or abdominal pain (1.3%)

▶ Fever (1.2%)

▶ Otitis media or externa (1%)

DO I NEED TO DO A DIAGNOSTIC TEST?

Although this seems simple, you need a diagnostic test if the result of the test is expected to change what you do next. If the result does not change management, do not do the test!

When do you need a test?

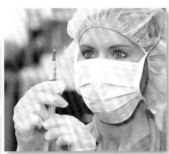

YES

Very uncertain of the diagnosis – test to narrow the differential diagnoses or wait and see if things change

Somewhat uncertain of the diagnosis – consider specific tests available and important aspects of the tests

Treatment fails – reconsider diagnosis

Aspects of a test to consider are:
• Accuracy
• Number of false positives and false negatives and the consequences of having a false result
• Invasiveness
• Cost of the test

NO

Very certain of the diagnosis – proceed to discuss treatment

Chapter 3 (*Information Mastery*) provides an overview of diagnostic test accuracy, but in general, tests that are highly specific help you rule in a disease (**Sp**in) and tests that are highly sensitive help you to rule out a disease (**Sn**out). In addition, the website *Choosing Wisely* (http://www.choosingwisely.org/about-us/) promotes discussion between patients and their healthcare providers about tests that are controversial and includes lists of tests where there are national recommendations for NOT performing the test.

Understanding Probabilities

It would be nice if the world of medicine were black and white; if we always had strong evidence from high-quality studies upon which to base our decisions. In reality, patient histories can be unclear or even contradictory, and providers must make treatment decisions based on probability rather than certainty. **Common things are common**, so for a patient with a sore throat, we know the patient likely has a virus, but we do not want to miss the 20% of patients who actually have a strep throat and might benefit from antibiotics. We do not want to treat everybody with antibiotics because that is expensive and causes the emergence of resistant organisms.

Fortunately, we often know the likelihood ratios of tests and how the results of these tests will move us along a probability threshold toward treatment or no treatment for a condition. A Likelihood Ratio (LR) is the likelihood that a given test result would be expected in a patient with the target disorder compared to the likelihood that that same result would be expected in a patient without the target disorder (See Chapter 3 for a discussion of LRs). A positive LR *over 10* is strong evidence to rule in a disease while a negative LR *less than 0.1* is strong evidence to rule out a disease.

A nomogram (http://www.cebm.net/likelihood-ratios/) can be used to easily work with these numbers to convert a pretest probability into a posttest probability (Fig. 11.1).

> **Consider a patient with sore throat**
>
> ▶ About 20% of patients with a sore throat will have streptococcal infection
>
> ▶ You would like to perform a test that:
>
>> ▶ If negative, will make strep so unlikely that you and the patient feel comfortable pursuing symptomatic treatment only OR
>>
>> ▶ If positive, you, and the patient would treat with antibiotics
>
> ▶ A rapid strep test or decision tool (Centor Score) can help move you along the probability as shown in Figure 11.1

Clinical Decision Rules

Decision rules assist in understanding how likely it is that a patient with a given clinical presentation has a disease. Validated clinical decision rules exist for many conditions such as the Centor Score for sore throat (https://www.mdcalc.com/centor-score-modified-mcisaac-strep-pharyngitis), or the Well criteria for deep vein thrombosis

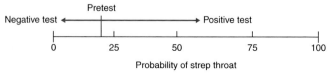

Figure 11.1 ▶ Probability diagram for patient with sore throat.

(DVT) (http://www.mdcalc.com/wells-criteria-for-dvt/). These "rules" assist in making probability estimates to guide testing and treatment. These will be highlighted when available for the conditions described below. There are many websites that can be used to access these scoring systems and some secondary sources like *Essential Evidence Plus* have built-in tools to calculate these scores.

Although you doubt that Mr. Stern has appendicitis, you recall a clinical decision tool that predicts appendicitis (LR+ of 4 with a score of 7 or more). You access the Alvarado Score (http://www.mdcalc.com/alvarado-score-for-acute-appendicitis/). Mr. Stern has none of the clinical criteria (migratory pain, anorexia, nausea/vomiting, rebound tenderness, elevated temperature) except tenderness in the right lower quadrant (2 points). Even if he had an elevated white blood count and a left shift, a score of 5 points would place him at only moderate risk of appendicitis. You suspect either diverticulitis, although pain is usually located in the left lower quadrant, or colon cancer. His stool sample tests positive for occult blood.

National Organizations

Many national organizations publish guidelines to assist in deciding whether or not to order a test. The American College of Radiology (ACR) (http://www.acr.org/quality-safety/appropriateness-criteria), for example, provides guidance on whether imaging is appropriate and which test to order.

▶ Appropriateness is represented on an ordinal scale that uses integers from 1 to 9 grouped into three categories:
  - 1, 2, or 3 are in the category "usually not appropriate" where the harms of doing the procedure outweigh the benefits
  - 4, 5, and 6 are designated "may be appropriate"
  - 7, 8, or 9 are in the category "usually appropriate" where the benefits of doing a procedure outweigh the harms or risks

▶ There is also an indication of the amount of radiation exposure that the test incurs ranging from 0 for ultrasound to 30 to 100 millisieverts (mSv) for computed tomography angiogram (CTA) of the chest, abdomen, and pelvis with contrast in an adult (annual average background radiation in the United States being 3 mSv).

The National Guideline Clearinghouse (https://www.guideline.gov/) also contains many guidelines to help determine whether and when testing is indicated and which test to choose.

You check the National Collaborating Center for Cancer, found on the clearinghouse website, which recommends colonoscopy for patients without major comorbidity, to confirm a diagnosis of colorectal cancer. ACR recommends a CT of the chest, abdomen, and pelvis for pretreatment staging of colon cancer.

Risks and Benefits of Common Tests

No test, even a simple laboratory test, is without risk. As a general rule, the more invasive the test, the more risk. However, even seemingly simple tests can incur risks, especially if repeated over time. Mammography, for example is recommended every other year by the United States Preventive Services Task Force (http://www.uspreventiveservicestaskforce.org/) for women aged 50 to 74 years. Facts about mammography are listed in Box 11.1.[4]

BOX 11.1 FACTS ABOUT MAMMOGRAPHY

Did you know?

▶ Reduction in breast cancer mortality is demonstrated with mammography, but no statistically significant reduction in all-cause mortality

▶ Cumulative rates for false-positive mammography results over 10 years are about 61% for annual and 42% for biennial screening

▶ Estimates of over diagnosis range from 11% to 22% in trials

▶ Women experience marked anxiety from a false-positive mammography test and loss of confidence from false-negative results; these feeling generally do not deter them from future screening[8]

If a Test is Needed, Where to Begin

If you need to do a test to confirm a diagnosis before treating, and you have a specific diagnosis in mind based on probability estimates or a clinical decision rule, order the most cost-effective test available. If you have several diagnoses in mind, choose the test that rules in or out the most serious of these conditions. For Mr. Stern, the most serious diagnosis that you are considering is colon cancer so you would investigate that possibility first.

CREATING A DIFFERENTIAL DIAGNOSIS

This is the fun part, where you get to put together all that you have learned from listening, talking, and examining the patient. If you have completed some initial testing, like a urinalysis or electrocardiogram (ECG), throw that information into the mix. Synthesizing information and coming up with a likely diagnosis and a list of other possible conditions that should be considered, especially if initial treatment fails, is the exciting part of medicine for many of us.

The list should not be exhaustive and, in fact, often has only one main diagnosis when the presentation is straightforward.

For Mr. Stern, considering his age, smoking, and alcohol history, his relatively benign examination and stool positive for occult blood, the most likely diagnosis is colon cancer. Additional testing is needed to confirm your suspicion. You plan to recommend colonoscopy as the first test to the attending when you present Mr. Stern.

LISTING TREATMENT OPTIONS: IDENTIFYING AND RANKING

Once you have settled on a likely diagnosis, you should consider the possible **treatment options** before discussing them with your attending and then the patient. We recommend beginning with the most likely to be helpful or, if not known, the least invasive to most invasive (lifestyle change, medication, complementary/alternative therapies, and procedures/surgery). Within those categories, you can rank options by effectiveness and cost so that you are offering the most bang for the buck. You should be able to quickly find this information by diagnosis in your secondary data source.

The **most effective treatments** are rated **A** on strength of recommendation (SOR), based on consistent, good quality patient-oriented evidence. SOR B is based on inconsistent or limited-quality, patient-oriented evidence and SOR C is based on consensus, disease-oriented evidence, expert opinion, or case series.

For example, you are seeing a 45-year-old woman with a new diagnosis of hypertension (BP 150/84 mm Hg) and a BMI of 32. Based on the Joint National Commission (JNC)-8 guidelines, her systolic BP goal is 140 mm Hg (expert opinion).[5] SOR A options include lifestyle modification and medication as shown above and discussed in Chapter 12.

Best Evidence of Effectiveness
• Life style modification (sodium restriction, exercise, weight control)
• Medication (thiazide-type diuretic, CCB, ACEI, ARB (see text))

Cost	Side effects	Patient preferences

Recommended Medications (cost: 3-mo supply):
• Thiazide-type diuretic (hydrochlorothiazide $42)
• Calcium channel blocker (CCB, diltiazem $64)
• Angiotensin-converting enzyme inhibitor (ACEI, Lisinopril $29)
• Angiotensin receptor blocker (telmisartan $51)

Costs from www.pharmacychecker.com

Of the medications shown above, none appear to have superiority for most outcomes, such as mortality. Cost information can be found on many sites, but costs differ greatly depending on whether or not the patient has insurance coverage and where they shop.

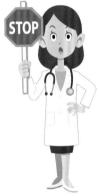

Side effects differ; diuretics can cause weakness, GI problems, and muscle spasm among others, and ACEI can cause cough, headache, and dizziness. The patient may have clear preferences and/or experience with some of the medications and may wish to check with a pharmacist before deciding.

Drug interactions can occur with many medications; be sure to **look up medications before you prescribe them** for contraindications, common side effects, and drug interactions.

PRESENTING THE CASE

When presenting the case to the attending, you want to be thorough but concise. The most important aspects are your thoughts about the patient and the data that you have collected and suggestions about the most likely diagnosis, testing if needed, and treatment options to discuss with the patient.

For Mr. Stern, presented at the beginning of this chapter, it might go like this:

▶ **History (subjective):** Mr. Stern is a 71-year-old man with controlled hypertension, borderline diabetes, and a history of alcohol use, who presents with several months of constant aching RLQ abdominal pain. Bowel movements are normal with no visible blood. He has had no surgeries. He does not smoke but his wife is concerned about his drinking. He had a screening colonoscopy 20 years ago but none since.

▶ **Examination (objective):** Mr. Stern's vital signs are normal. On abdominal examination, he is somewhat tender in the RLQ but has normal bowel sounds, no rebound, rigidity, or palpable mass. His rectal examination was benign but the stool that I tested was positive for occult blood.

▶ **Assessment:** I am most worried about a colon cancer. He could have diverticulosis. I doubt appendicitis as his Alvarado score is low, although we could get a white blood count to better assess this possibility.

▶ **Plan:** I think we should suggest a colonoscopy as soon as it can be arranged and should begin to talk with him about a possible cancer or polyp. We could also talk more with him about his **drinking.**

Discussing Treatment with the Patient

Shared Decision-Making

Although shared decision-making is discussed in Chapter 5, we will mention here that most patients prefer to be informed about their diagnosis (or likely diagnosis) and engaged in decisions about testing and treatment. Shared decision-making, which includes making the decision explicit and providing information about treatment or screening options and their associated outcomes, increases patient knowledge and confidence about their decision, and, in many situations, informed patients elect more conservative treatment options.[6,7]

Patients sometimes ask what you would do and it is fine to answer, but qualify your statement by saying that decisions involve preferences, past experience, and costs, so their input is important. This final step of the visit is usually done by or with the attending physician.

Patient Education

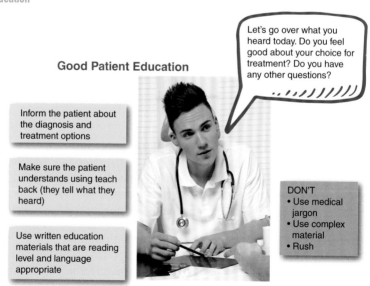

Good Patient Education

Let's go over what you heard today. Do you feel good about your choice for treatment? Do you have any other questions?

Inform the patient about the diagnosis and treatment options

Make sure the patient understands using teach back (they tell what they heard)

Use written education materials that are reading level and language appropriate

DON'T
• Use medical jargon
• Use complex material
• Rush

Opportunities for prevention should be sought during annual as well as routine visits (Chapter 7).

ENDING THE VISIT: MONITORING AND FOLLOW-UP

At the end of the visit, there should be a follow-up plan. This may include information specific to the problem, such as how long to wait before expecting to feel better or warning signs that the problem is getting worse, making the next appointment, steps for self-management, or a review of any new medications.

Be sure to ask if the patient has any other questions.

▶ If you can answer the question, do so
▶ If you cannot, but the question needs an answer now, check with the attending
▶ If the question can wait:
  • Write it down to address next time or call/email the answer
  • Have the patient ask on the patient portal, if the practice has one
  • Suggest that the patient look up the answer on a reliable website such as https://www.nih.gov/health-information.

DOCUMENTATION (AND CODING)

Most notes in ambulatory offices follow a SOAP format which stands for Subjective, Objective, Assessment, and Plan. Electronic records often have templates that are completed during the visit. You will need to check out the preferred format with your attending. If completing a traditional SOAP note, it would look a lot like the presentation above.

While as a medical student you will not likely be responsible for billing and coding your office encounters, doing so is a daily routine for family physicians. Pay attention to your attending as he/she spends time charting to get a handle on how to bill and code.

In generic terms, each problem addressed during a visit should be coded according to the International Statistical Classification of Diseases and Related Health Problems, version 10 (ICD-10). Most electronic medical records have searchable indices which help populate the appropriate ICD-10 code.

Depending on the complexity of the visit, including the number and acuity of problems addressed, time spent with the patient, and detail documenting findings in the note, physicians then assign a Current Procedural Terminology (CPT) code to the visit, which determines billing charges and payment. Most office visits are billed on a 5-level tier, with level 3 and level 4 being the most common. Table 11.1 defines these levels for established patients and the documentation which must be present to bill for each level. There are separate guidelines for billing new patient encounters, consults, preventative care visits, and many other categories not covered here.

TREATING COMMON ACUTE PROBLEMS

When possible, for the 11 common problems discussed below, treatment recommendations are based on SOR discussed in Chapter 3.

ABDOMINAL PAIN

Abdominal pain is the cause of up to 8% of all adult emergency department (ED) visits and 1.3% of adult primary care office visits.[9] While the majority are due to non–life-threatening

Table 11.1 ▶ Billing Requirements for Established Outpatient Office Visits

CPT Code	Description	History	Examination	Medical Decision-Making	Average Time
99212	Established outpatient office visit	Problem-focused • CC required • HPI: 1–3 elements • ROS: N/A • PFSH: N/A	Problem-focused, 1–5 elements	Straightforward	10 minutes
99213	Established outpatient office visit	Expanded problem-focused • CC required • HPI: 1–3 elements • ROS: pertinent • PFSH: N/A	Expanded problem-focused, 6–11 elements	Low complexity	15 minutes
99214	Established outpatient office visit	Detailed • CC required • HPI: 4+ elements (or 3+ chronic diseases) • ROS: 2–9 systems • PFSH: 1 element	Detailed, 12 or more elements	Moderate complexity	25 minutes
99215	Established outpatient office visit	Comprehensive • CC required • HPI: 4+ elements (or 3+ chronic diseases) • ROS: 10+ systems • PFSH: 2 elements	Comprehensive	High complexity	40 minutes

CC, chief complaint; CPT, current procedural terminology; HPI, history of present illness; PFSH, past family, surgical/social history; ROS, review of systems.

causes, about 10% are due to serious conditions that require immediate diagnosis and/or surgical therapy (the so-called "acute abdomen").[10] Red flags for these conditions are shown below.

Martha, a 22-year-old woman, presents with sharp, constant, nonradiating abdominal pain in her right lower quadrant (RLQ) for the past 36 hours. She feels slightly warm, and is nauseous but has not vomited; there have been no changes in her bowel habits. She denies urinary symptoms. She is sexually active with one male partner and is inconsistent with condom use; her last menstrual period was 6 weeks ago. She has had one prior uncomplicated pregnancy, and has never had any surgeries. She does not take any medications or use tobacco or alcohol.

A broad range of conditions can cause abdominal pain. The differential diagnosis can be generated in a variety of ways: by patient age or location of pain (Fig. 11.2) or by pain referral patterns (Fig. 11.3). Abdominal pain may vary in intensity and quality; pain from abdominal organs (visceral pain) is often dull and difficult to localize, whereas pain from irritation of the peritoneum (parietal pain) is sharp and focal.[11]

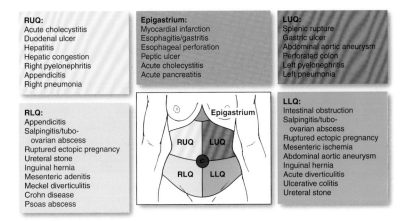

Figure 11.2 ▶ Causes of abdominal pain by location.

Steps in Evaluation

Is this an Emergency?

RLQ pain, especially in a reproductive-aged female like Martha, should prompt consideration of more serious causes such as appendicitis, ruptured ectopic pregnancy, PID, and ovarian torsion (Fig. 11.2). You check for peritoneal signs.

Are there other Red Flags for Serious Conditions?

 Clues or "red flags" about the seriousness of a patient with abdominal pain:

▶ Signs of peritoneal inflammation (guarding, rigidity)

▶ Vital sign abnormalities, especially fever, tachycardia, or hypotension

▶ Pregnant or potentially pregnant

▶ Cervical motion tenderness

▶ Abdominal pain following trauma

▶ Hematemesis, hematochezia

▶ Pain radiating to back, "tearing" pain sensation

▶ Prior abdominal surgeries

YouTube videos of tests for **peritoneal inflammation** are listed below:

▶ Rigidity (https://www.youtube.com/watch?v=2mfiGIDJfnM)

▶ Rovsing sign (https://www.youtube.com/watch?v=6I03eiLO_lU)

▶ Psoas sign (https://www.youtube.com/watch?v=n0a0PCwsVQ4)

▶ Obturator sign (https://www.youtube.com/watch?v=jV80jcnhNtA)

If you notice any of these red flags you should promptly alert your attending physician for expedited management of the patient.

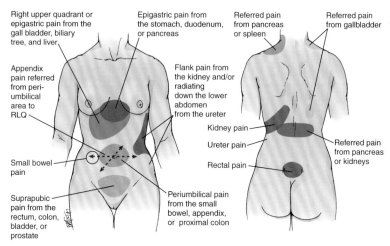

Figure 11.3 ▶ Causes of abdominal pain by referral pattern.

Martha has tachycardia and a low-grade fever. On examination, she appears uncomfortable and sweaty. Heart and breath sounds are normal. Her abdomen appears flat with normal skin color and turgor. Bowel sounds are hypoactive. There is tenderness to both light and deep palpation in the RLQ and suprapubic regions. You note voluntary guarding, with positive rebound tenderness and positive Psoas Sign on the right. On pelvic examination, she has right adnexal and cervical motion tenderness on bimanual examination. Rectal examination is normal.

Do I Need a Diagnostic Test?

It is *always* appropriate to establish pregnancy status via urine or serum testing for women of childbearing age presenting with abdominal pain. You are concerned that Martha may have a ruptured ectopic pregnancy or possibly PID. You ask your attending about obtaining a urine pregnancy test. A positive pregnancy test result influences the differential diagnosis, affects the choice of imaging studies (i.e., avoidance of modalities that confer radiation), and influences treatment decisions. Figure 11.4 outlines steps for workup of abdominal pain.

Martha's pregnancy test is positive. After discussing the likely diagnosis with Martha and your attending physician, you arrange for transport to the ED where she will undergo pelvic US. You speak with the ED physician and let her know to expect Martha's arrival by private vehicle.

Management

Initial primary care office management includes preliminary testing as indicated (e.g., CBC, urine pregnancy testing, urinalysis, plain abdominal radiography). For most patients with abdominal pain of uncertain etiology whose symptoms are severe, acute, and potentially life-threatening, immediate referral to a facility capable of accurately diagnosing and treating the cause is indicated. Martha successfully underwent surgery for an ectopic pregnancy.

For cases of abdominal pain that do not require hospital care, treatment depends on the etiology:

▶ Supportive therapy (e.g., bland diet, oral or IV rehydration for viral gastroenteritis)

▶ Dietary counseling (e.g., constipation, IBS, gluten/lactose sensitivity, GERD)

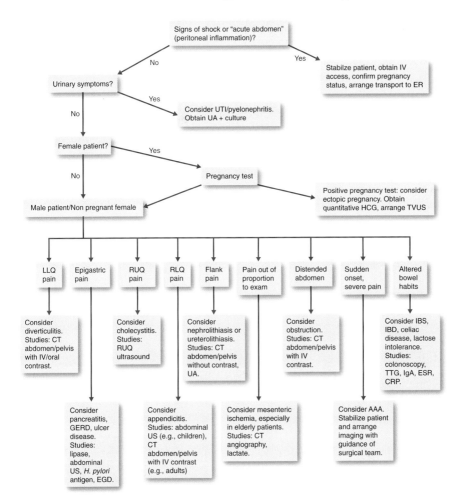

Figure 11.4 ▶ Approach to the female patient of childbearing age with abdominal pain. AAA, abdominal aortic aneurysm; CRP, c-reactive protein; CT, computed tomography; ER, emergency room; ESR, erythrocyte sedimentation rate; GERD, gastroesophageal reflux disease; HGC, human chorionic gonadotropin; IgA, immunoglobulin A; IV, intravenous; LLQ, left lower quadrant; RLQ, right lower quadrant; RUQ, right upper quadrant; TTG, tissue transglutaminase; TVUS, transvaginal ultrasound; UA, urinalysis; US, ultrasound; UTI, urinary tract infection. (Data from: Kendall JL, Moreira ME. Evaluation of the adult with abdominal pain in the emergency department. *UpToDate*. Updated January 13, 2016. Available from: http://www.uptodate.com/contents/evaluation-of-the-adult-with-abdominal-pain-in-the-emergency-department. Accessed August 2016.)

▶ Antibiotics (e.g., UTI/pyelonephritis, diverticulitis, infectious diarrhea, STI, uncomplicated PID, some cases of appendicitis)

▶ Other medications (e.g., acid suppression for GERD, antiemetics for nausea/vomiting, prokinetics for IBS, stool softeners or laxatives for constipation)

Occasionally nonurgent referral to specialty care is indicated (e.g., gastroenterology for management of IBD, OB/GYN for management of endometriosis).

BREATHING PROBLEM: SHORTNESS OF BREATH

Shortness of breath is a common concern, but what is actually meant by this term varies widely. The phrase is often used to describe a sensation of rapid breathing, air hunger, fatigue, deconditioning, or inability to take adequate breaths.

The causes of shortness of breath, or dyspnea, vary widely as well (Table 11.2). A patient's state of dyspnea reflects complex interactions between biochemical pathways of the central and peripheral nervous systems, cardiopulmonary and musculoskeletal systems, and acid–base metabolism.[12] Because proper respiratory function is critical to sustainment of life, shortness of breath must be taken seriously when encountered. This chapter will address acute dyspnea (hours to days) rather than chronic dyspnea (longer than 4 to 8 weeks). Asthma and wheezing is discussed in Chapter 12.

> Chenhua, a 55-year-old woman with a history of tobacco use, hypertension, coronary artery disease (previous stent ×1), and type 2 diabetes mellitus presents to your clinic with shortness of breath. Her symptoms began earlier today. She recently returned from a trip home to China to visit family. She describes difficulty catching her breath and mild cough but no CP. Other review of systems is negative.

Table 11.2 ▶ Differential Diagnosis of Acute Dyspnea

Category	Key Features	Possible Diagnoses
Cardiac	• *Symptoms:* arm/jaw/neck/chest pain, cough, fatigue, orthopnea, paroxysmal nocturnal dyspnea, weight gain • *Signs:* jugular venous distension; S3 or S4, cardiac rub or gallop; edema	• Acute myocardial infarction • Arrhythmia • Congestive heart failure • Coronary artery disease • Pericarditis
Lower airway	• *Symptoms:* cough, dysphagia, fever, indigestion/reflux, night sweats, pleuritic chest pain, weight loss • *Signs:* barrel chest; clubbed digits; leg swelling, redness, pain; rales or wheezing	• Asthma, COPD • GERD with aspiration • Metastatic disease • Pneumonia • Pneumothorax • Pulmonary embolism • Restrictive lung disease
Psychogenic	• *Symptoms:* Palpitations, heart racing, social or another specific phobia	• Anxiety, panic attacks • Hyperventilation
Upper airway	• *Symptoms:* Barking cough, sore throat • *Signs:* "Hot potato voice," splenomegaly, stridor	• Croup • Epiglottitis • Foreign body
Endocrine	• *Signs:* Fruity-smelling breath (ketones), pupillary changes, tachypnea	• Medications • Metabolic acidosis
Central nervous system	• *Symptom:* Muscle weakness	• Aspirin overdose • Neuromuscular disorders
Pediatric	• *Symptoms:* cough (e.g., barking) • *Signs:* accessory muscle use, drooling, stridor, tripod position, leaning forward	• Bronchiolitis, croup • Epiglottitis • Foreign body aspiration • Myocarditis

COPD, chronic obstructive pulmonary disease; GERD, gastroesophageal reflux disease.
Data from: Zoorob RJ, Campbell JS. Acute dyspnea in the office. *Am Fam Physician*. 2003;68(9):1803–1810.

Steps in Evaluation

Evaluation of patients with shortness of breath must be timely and thorough. In many cases, the process begins with telephone triage. Check to see if your clinic has a telephone protocol in place to direct patients to the hospital or emergency room instead of the clinic if they trigger certain "red flags."

Ask about **prior cardiac or pulmonary conditions** such as coronary artery disease, chronic obstructive pulmonary disease (COPD), or asthma. Chenhua has several of the risk factors for pulmonary embolism (e.g., *recent surgery or travel*, current diagnosis of cancer, *tobacco use*, oral contraceptive use, or known hypercoagulability syndrome). Review medications, ingestions, or use of illicit drugs.

Verify immunization status, especially for children. Physical examination focuses on the patient's general appearance, head and neck, chest, abdomen, and extremities.

Chenhua's vital signs are: HR 110 beats/min, RR 22 breaths/min, BP 110/75 mm Hg, Temp 98.9°F, O_2 saturation is 94% on room air. On examination, she is alert and oriented and does not appear to have increased work of breathing. Her eyes, ears, nose, mouth, throat, and neck examinations are normal. Her breath sounds are symmetric and normal with good air movement. Heart is tachycardic without murmurs, rubs, or gallops. Abdomen is nontender with normal bowel sounds. Legs are not swollen or painful.

Is this an Emergency?

Table 11.3 lists selected physical findings that suggest emergent causes of shortness of breath, as well as initial steps in stabilizing and diagnosing the patient. Although she may have a serious condition, you determine that Chenhua does not appear to be in imminent danger of respiratory or cardiac arrest.

Are there Other Red Flags for Serious Conditions?

See Table 11.3 for possible diagnoses.

Chenhua has coronary artery disease which puts her at risk for acute coronary syndrome (see section on Chest Pain, Table 11.11). Even though she does not complain of CP or other classic symptoms of myocardial infarction, these symptoms may be absent, especially in women or younger patients.[13] Although COPD is a possibility, she has not been diagnosed with this before and her symptoms began abruptly. In addition, absence of fevers or other respiratory symptoms make pneumonia or upper respiratory infection unlikely.

Like Chenhua, anyone who has acute dyspnea following recent travel should be considered to have a pulmonary embolus (PE) until proven otherwise, even in the absence of signs and symptoms of DVT (e.g., lower leg pain, redness, swelling). The Wells Criteria for PE (Table 11.4) is a clinical decision tool that can help stratify risk in this situation. Chenhua's Wells Score is at least 4.5 (PE equally likely diagnosis, HR >100). For very low-risk patients (not this case), the Pulmonary Embolism Rule-out Criteria (PERC) can help determine whether further testing for PE is needed.[14]

Do I Need a Diagnostic Test?

Office-based workup for shortness of breath is straightforward and driven by the acuity of the patient presentation.

Table 11.3 ▶ Emergent Findings, Causes, and Office Management of Acute Dyspnea

Initial Assessment	Clinical Findings Suggesting Emergency	Possible Diagnoses	Steps in Initial Management[a]
Assess airway patency and lung examination	Absent breath sounds	• Severe asthma • Pneumothorax, hemothorax • Pneumonia • Foreign body • Anaphylaxis	• Albuterol treatment • Corticosteroids for asthma • CXR • Inspect for foreign body • Suction oropharynx if obstructing blood or saliva • IM epinephrine
	Tracheal deviation	• Tension pneumothorax • Obstructing tumor	• Needle thoracotomy if tension pneumothorax suspected (do not wait for CXR to confirm)
	Stridor, drooling	• Foreign body • Croup • Epiglottitis	• Humidified air • Racemic epinephrine • Consider lateral neck x-ray for epiglottitis
	Diffuse coarse wet lung sounds	• Bronchiolitis • Acute pulmonary edema	• Suction oro/nasopharynx • Viral swab (including RSV) • IV furosemide if CHF suspected
Observe breathing	Accessory muscle use (intercostal, neck, abdominal) Tripod position Retractions, nasal flaring	• Respiratory failure imminent • Bronchiolitis (children) • COPD exacerbation	• Inhaled bronchodilators • Suction oro/nasopharynx • Viral swab • CXR
	Gasping or agonal breathing	• Cardiopulmonary arrest	• Intubation, resuscitation following ACLS guidelines
Cardiac rhythm (auscultation and ECG)	Irregular, absent p-waves, "sawtooth" pattern	• Atrial fibrillation/flutter	• Cardioversion, if hemodynamically unstable. Rate/rhythm control if stable • Assess for anticoagulation
	Wide complex tachyarrhythmia	• VT • VF	• Defibrillation if hemodynamically unstable following ACLS guidelines
	Electrical alternans, low voltage	• Cardiac tamponade • Pericardial effusion	• Alert ER/cardiology • Transport to hospital
	Narrow complex tachyarrhythmia	• SVT • AVNRT	• Attempt vagal maneuvers • Establish IV access • Adenosine • Cardioversion if hemodynamically unstable
	Heart murmur	• Aortic stenosis • Thoracic aortic dissection • Other valvulopathy	• Arrange immediate echocardiography upon transfer to hospital

Initial Assessment	Clinical Findings Suggesting Emergency	Possible Diagnoses	Steps in Initial Management[a]
Vital signs and pulse oximetry	Fever, hypoxia	• Pneumonia, PE • Viral respiratory infection	• Provide oxygen if hypoxic • CXR • Viral swab
Obtain history of cardiac or pulmonary disease, or trauma	Chest pain	• Acute coronary syndrome	• Aspirin, oxygen, nitrate, morphine, ECG, CXR
	CHF	• CHF exacerbation	• CXR, furosemide
	Tobacco use	• COPD • Lung cancer	• CXR • Steroids if indicated
	Asthma	• Asthma exacerbation	• Inhaled bronchodilators
	Chest trauma	• Pulmonary contusion • Flail chest • Pneumo or hemothorax	• CXR
	Dysphagia, elderly/frail	• Aspiration pneumonia/pneumonitis	• CXR, suction
Assess mental status	Somnolent, confused, unconscious muscle weakness	• Acute respiratory failure of any etiology • Guillain–Barré Syndrome	• Stabilize airway, breathing, circulation, arrange transport

[a]Apply oxygen, establish airway, IV access, arrange emergent ambulance transport.
ACLS, advanced cardiac life support; AVNRT, atrioventricular nodal reentrant tachycardia; CHF, congestive heart failure; COPD, chronic obstructive pulmonary disease; CXR, chest x-ray; ECG, electrocardiogram; ER, emergency room; IM, intramuscular; IV, intravenous; PE, pulmonary embolus; RSV, respiratory syncytial virus; SVT, supraventricular tachycardia; VF, ventricular fibrillation; VT, ventricular tachycardia.

Table 11.4 ▶ Wells Criteria for Pulmonary Embolism

Predictive Category	Points
Clinical signs and symptoms of DVT	3
PE #1 diagnosis, or equally likely	3
Surgery or immobilization for >3 days in the past 4 weeks	1.5
Previous DVT or PE	1.5
Heart rate >100 beats/min	1.5
Hemoptysis	1
Active cancer (treatment ongoing or within the past 6 months, or palliative treatment)	1

Scoring	Risk Group	Probability of PE
<2	Low	1.3% (95% CI, 0.5–2.7)
2-6	Moderate	16% (95% CI, 12–21)
>6	High	41% (95% CI, 29–54)

DVT, deep vein thrombosis; PE, pulmonary embolism; CI, confidence interval
Data from: Wells PS, Anderson DR, Rodger M, et al. Excluding pulmonary embolism at the bedside without diagnostic imaging: management of patients with suspected pulmonary embolism presenting to the emergency department by using a simple clinical model and d-dimer. *Ann Intern Med.* 2001;135(2):98–107. Available from: http://www.mdcalc.com/wells-criteria-for-pulmonary-embolism-pe/.

▲▲▲ Table 11.5 ▸ Common ECG Findings for Selected Causes of Dyspnea

Diagnosis	EKG Findings	Examples
Myocardial infarction	ST segment elevation or depression T wave inversion New left bundle branch block	http://lifeinthefastlane.com/ecg-library/ myocardial-ischaemia/
Pulmonary embolism	S wave in lead I, q-wave in lead III, T wave inversion in lead III	http://lifeinthefastlane.com/ecg-library/ pulmonary-embolism/
Pericardial effusion/ cardiac tamponade	Electrical alternans	http://lifeinthefastlane.com/ecg-library/ electrical-alternans/
Pericarditis	Concave ST segment elevation and PR depression	http://lifeinthefastlane.com/ecg-library/ basics/pericarditis/
Atrial fibrillation/flutter	Absent p waves, irregularly irregular rhythm, "sawtooth" pattern with variable A-V block	http://lifeinthefastlane.com/ecg-library/ atrial-fibrillation/ http://lifeinthefastlane.com/ecg-library/ atrial-flutter/
Supraventricular tachycardia	Regular narrow-complex tachycardia	http://lifeinthefastlane.com/ecg-library/ svt/
Ventricular tachycardia	Wide-complex tachycardia, extreme axis deviation, fusion beats	http://lifeinthefastlane.com/ecg-library/ ventricular-tachycardia/

All patients should have vital signs including pulse oximetry. If there is time to complete office testing, a complete blood count (CBC) can help establish infection (elevated white blood cells or neutrophilia) or anemia (low hemoglobin) as potential causes of shortness of breath. Most adults presenting with shortness of breath should have an ECG, which can help diagnose acute coronary syndrome, PE, cardiac tamponade, or cardiac arrhythmia (Table 11.5).

Chest radiography is a useful office tool that helps rule in or out many etiologies of dyspnea including pneumonia, bronchitis, congestive heart failure, aspiration, foreign body, COPD, aortic dissection, or malignancy. The specificity of chest radiography is low, so it should be used as a confirmatory step when possible.

Spirometry can be obtained in the clinic or in pulmonary function laboratories to diagnose obstructive or restrictive lung processes (see http://www.aafp.org/afp/2004/0301/ p1107.html for spirometry interpretation). More advanced testing such as arterial blood gas measurement, D-dimer, cardiac biomarkers (e.g., troponin), or imaging studies (e.g., CT angiography of the chest, venous Doppler ultrasonography, or ventilation-perfusion scans) are routinely performed in the hospital/emergency department setting.

Chenhua's probability of either acute coronary syndrome or PE is moderate-to-high. You obtain office ECG and CXR, which are normal. You elect to send her to the emergency department for further tests to rule out these serious conditions.

Management

The following includes suggested management for selected causes of shortness of breath, along with the SOR rating, if available:

▸ Pneumonia (SOR A): antibiotics; steroids if inpatient

▶ Bronchitis (SOR C): antitussives in patients >6 years (SOR B): inhaled beta agonists for wheezing, inhaled corticosteroids, echinacea, pelargonium, dark honey in children over age 2 years[15]

▶ COPD exacerbation (Chapter 12)[16]

▶ Asthma exacerbation (Chapter 12)

▶ PE (SOR A): anticoagulation[17]

▶ Congestive heart failure exacerbation (Chapter 12)[18]

▶ Croup (SOR A): corticosteroids, nebulized epinephrine for moderate–severe croup[19]

▶ Viral upper respiratory infection: see section below.[20]

CHEST PAIN IN ADULTS

Chest pain (CP) is discomfort or pain experienced anywhere along the front of the body between the neck and the upper abdomen. The pain can be acute (<72 hours), subacute (3 days to a month), or chronic (more than a month) and is caused by many non–life-threatening and life-threatening conditions shown in Table 11.6. About 1% of primary care office visits are CP.[21]

Raj is a 40-year-old man, who presents with CP that has been occurring off and on for the past week. He denies shortness of breath, diaphoresis, or radiation of pain. He has been working out in the gym to get into shape and during the workout experienced sharp, stinging pain; the pain did not worsen with exercise. He has no medical problems and is a nonsmoker and a social drinker. Family history is significant for heart disease in his dad who had bypass surgery last year at age 70 years. He is worried about his heart.

Steps in Evaluation

Is this an Emergency?

The probability that Raj has acute cardiac ischemia, based on the frequencies in Table 11.6, is low. On the other hand, this is the most likely of the life-threatening diagnoses. Look for typical patterns of the life-threatening illnesses and apply a decision rule to help determine the likelihood of cardiac ischemia/coronary artery disease (CAD). If you suspect ischemia, follow the rapid evaluation scheme shown in Table 11.7, alert your attending, and request an ECG.

The remainder of Raj's history was benign and he has no pain with inspiration. Vital signs are normal. On examination, his heart and lungs are normal and he has reproducible CP on palpation.

Raj meets none of the criteria in Table 11.7 except worry that the pain is cardiac; his score of 1 makes it unlikely that his pain is cardiac. A similar decision rule, the Emergency Department Assessment of Chest Pain, can be used to determine which stable adult patients are at low risk of a major cardiac event; it can be accessed at http://www.mdcalc.com/emergency-department-assessment-chest-pain-score-edacs/. Raj's score using this system is +2, again placing him at low risk for cardiac CP.

Are there Other Red Flags for Serious Conditions?

Red flags can help you determine next steps in the evaluation. If no red flags, proceed with a complete evaluation presented in Table 11.8.

Table 11.6 ▶ Causes of Chest Pain in Primary Care

Life-Threatening Conditions		Non–Life-Threatening Conditions	
Condition (Frequency)[a]	Key Features	Condition (Frequency)[b]	Key Features
Acute cardiac ischemia, myocardial infarction (1.5–2%)	Dull, squeezing pain CP, chest heaviness, can radiate to shoulder, arm, jaw/neck Diaphoresis, palpitations, pallor, dyspnea also occur	Musculoskeletal pain (36%) (includes costochondritis)	Tenderness to palpation, stinging pain, localized muscle tension, no cough
Aortic dissection (<1%; 6/100,000 people)	Major risk factors: smoking and hypertension Sudden onset, severe CP with tearing quality, jaw pain, syncope	Gastrointestinal pain (19%) (includes GERD)	Burning CP, reflux, N/V, bad breath, dysphagia
Pneumothorax (<1%; 7–37/100,0000 people)	Reduced breath sounds and ipsilateral chest expansion, hyperresonant percussion. Tracheal shift away from the affected side: tachycardia, tachypnea, and hypotension occur in tension pneumothorax	Nonspecific chest pain (16%)	Does not fit the other patterns
Pulmonary Embolism (<1%; 60–70/100,000 people)	Major risk factor: VTE Sudden-onset or worsened dyspnea, tachypnea or sharp chest pain. Cough, hemoptysis, and syncope less common	Stable angina (11%)	History of angina and CAD with usual CP
Esophageal rupture (3/100,000 people)	Chest, neck or back pain, vomiting, subcutaneous emphysema, hematemesis, dysphagia, dyspnea	Psychosocial pain (7%)[c]	Features of anxiety and/or depression (Chapter 22)
		Pulmonary pain (5%) (includes infection and neoplasm)	Sharp CP worsens with breathing, cough or sneeze
		Nonischemic cardiac pain (4%) (includes pericarditis and MVP)	Varies—can be pleuritic or sharp with dyspnea, fatigue, and palpitations

[a]Information on frequencies from: http://circ.ahajournals.org/content/127/20/2031 (aortic dissection); http://www.uptodate.com/contents/primary-spontaneous-pneumothorax-in-adults (pneumothorax); http://www.ncbi.nlm.nih.gov/pmc/articles/PMC3718593/ (pulmonary embolism); and http://emedicine.medscape.com/article/425410-overview#a5 (esophageal rupture). Accessed September 2016.
[b]Information on frequencies from: Klinkman MS, Stevens D, Gorenflo DW. Episodes of care for chest pain. *J Fam Pract*. 1994;38:344–352.
[c]A single question "In the past four weeks, have you had an anxiety attack (suddenly feeling fear or panic)? Has a LR+ of 4.2 for an anxiety state/panic disorder. Information from: Löwe B, Gräfe K, Zipfel S, et al. Detecting panic disorder in medical and psychosomatic outpatients: comparative validation of the Hospital Anxiety and Depression Scale, the Patient Health Questionnaire, a screening question, and physicians' diagnosis. *J Psychosom Res*. 2003;55(6):515–519.
CAD, coronary artery disease; CP, chest pain; N/V, nausea/vomiting; GERD, gastrointestinal reflux disease; MVP, mitral valve prolapse; VTE, venous thromboembolism.

Table 11.7 ▶ Decision Rule for Chest Pain from Ischemia

Decision Rule[11]

Variable Points
Man aged 55 years or older OR woman age 65 years or older 1
Known coronary artery or cerebrovascular disease 1
Pain not reproducible with palpation 1
Pain worse with exercise 1
Patient thinks that the pain is cardiac 1

If the patient has 0 or 1 points, it is very unlikely to be cardiac
• **Evaluate** for other causes

If the patient has 2–3 points, it is unlikely to be cardiac
• **Request** an ECG, if abnormal, see below
• If normal or nonspecific changes, discuss cardiology evaluation, troponin, or stress testing with the attending

If the patient has 4 or 5 points, the LR+ is 11.2 for ischemia
• **Alert** the attending, provide oxygen and an aspirin
• The attending may decide to do an ECG or arrange immediate **transport** to the emergency department

 Clues or "red flags" about the seriousness of the problem are:

▶ Hypotension, pulmonary edema, oliguria (MI)

▶ Tachycardia, tachypnea, hypoxia (PE)

▶ New systolic murmur (ruptured papillary muscle)

▶ Arrhythmia or CP in young person (cocaine)

▶ Mediastinal widening on CXR (aortic dissection)

 Table 11.8 ▶ Key Elements of the History and Physical Examination of the Patient with Chest Pain

Rapid Evaluation for Potential Acute Coronary Syndrome

History
• Onset and character of pain
• Prior history of coronary artery disease

ECG within 10 minutes of presentation (findings in descending order of importance)
• ST segment elevation or depression of >1 mm in at least two consecutive leads
• Q waves in at least two leads, not including aV_R, not known to be old
• T-wave hyperacuity or inversion in at least two leads, not including aV_R
• New bundle-branch block

Complete Evaluation

History
• Anxiety symptoms (choking feeling, fear, light-headedness, paresthesias)
• Nighttime symptoms
• Previous episodes, age at onset
• Tachycardia
• Acid regurgitation, heartburn
• Relationship to activity
• Relationship to respiration
• Cardiac risk factors (hypertension, diabetes, smoking, family history, hyperlipidemia)
• Claudication
• Use of cocaine
• Thromboembolic risk factors (recent fracture or immobilization, hypercoagulable states, history of DVT or PE)

(continued)

Table 11.8 ▶ Key Elements of the History and Physical Examination of the Patient with Chest Pain *(Continued)*

Physical examination
- Blood pressure
- Oxygenation assessment (respiratory effort, color, pulse oximetry or arterial samplings if indicated)
- Heart murmur
- Third, fourth heart sounds
- Pulmonary edema (dyspnea, bilateral rales)
- Stigmata of vascular disease (bruits, diminished pulse, arterial changes or AV nicking on retinal examination, skin changes, or ulcerations of lower extremities)

aV$_R$, augmented vector right; AV, arteriovenous; DVT, deep vein thrombosis; PE, pulmonary embolism.

Do I Need a Diagnostic Test?

The algorithm shown in Figure 11.5 below can help you determine if other testing is needed—either now or later—to rule out a life-threatening illness. If you decide, based on your complete evaluation of the patient, that the condition is likely musculoskeletal, GI, or psychological, you can often proceed to treatment.

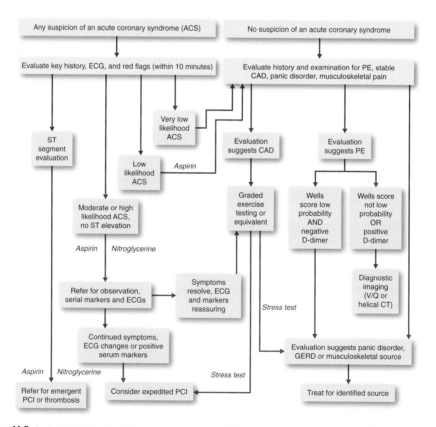

Figure 11.5 ▶ Approach to the patient with chest pain. CAD, coronary artery disease; ECG, electro-cardiogram; GERD, gastroesophageal reflux disease; PCI, percutaneous coronary intervention.

Raj does not have any red flags for other illnesses. You believe that his new exercise routine with weights may have resulted in pulled intercostal muscles causing the pain. You suggest that he change up his routine and use lower weights or strengthen different muscle groups; consultation with a trainer might be helpful. After discussion with Raj who is quite worried, the attending also orders a stress test to rule out CAD.

Management

The following list includes possible diagnoses for CP and suggested management along with the SOR rating:

▶ Coronary artery disease (Chapter 12)

▶ GERD (SOR B): diet and lifestyle modification, weight loss, antacids, H2 blockers, proton pump inhibitors, sucralfate, surgery

▶ Musculoskeletal pain (SOR C): NSAIDs

▶ Panic (SOR A): cognitive behavioral therapy, benzodiazepine short-term, tricyclic antidepressant or selective serotonin reuptake inhibitor

DIZZINESS

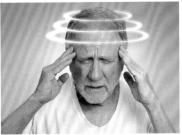

Dizziness is the chief complaint in about 3% of all primary care visits.[22] Most causes are benign but it is important to rule out serious causes. In most cases (80%), the history and physical examination identifies the cause. Common causes are listed in Table 11.9.

Mr. Polk, aged 62 years, presents with dizziness. He says that when he turned over in bed this morning, the room started spinning. He was unable to walk to the bathroom and has vomited twice. This has never happened to him before. He describes having a cold last week, but the symptoms resolved. He has some tinnitus in the left ear but is otherwise healthy.

What do you mean by dizziness? Four different types of dizziness:

▶ Vertigo—False sensation that the body or the environment is moving. Due to an imbalance of tonic vestibular signals; usually arises from the inner ear, middle ear, brainstem, or cerebellum. People describe it as the "room is spinning."

▶ Presyncope—Feeling of lightheadedness or faintness, as though one were about to pass out. Usually reflects cerebral hypoperfusion and has a cardiovascular origin, such as orthostatic hypotension (often from medication), arrhythmia, or congestive heart failure.

▶ Disequilibrium—A feeling of unsteadiness or imbalance primarily felt in the lower extremities. Most prominent when standing or walking and relieved by sitting or lying down. Any disturbance of the motor control system (vision, vestibulospinal, proprioceptive, somatosensory, cerebellar, or motor function) can lead to disequilibrium.

▶ Other: May include swimming or floating sensations, vague light-headedness, or feelings of dissociation. This feeling may be difficult for the patient to describe. Virtually any type of dizziness can be responsible for such symptoms.

Table 11.9 ▶ Common Causes of Dizziness

Type of Dizziness	Potential Cause	
Vertigo (45–54%)	• Acoustic neuroma (associated with hearing loss) • Acute labyrinthitis (recent viral illness, associated hearing loss) • Acute vestibular neuritis (constant, can last days to weeks) • Benign positional paroxysmal vertigo (BPPV) (episodic) • Cerebrovascular disease (TIA, CVA, cerebellar tumor, migraine, MS) • Cervical vertigo • Cholesteatoma • Drug induced (new medications) • Head trauma (concussion or whiplash injury) • Herpes zoster oticus (Ramsay Hunt syndrome) • Meniere disease (associated with hearing loss) • Psychological	
Presyncope (up to 14%)	• Arrhythmias • Carotid artery stenosis	• MI • Orthostatic hypotension
Disequilibrium (up to 16%)	• Balance problems • CVA, TIA • Gait disturbances • Medication related	• Parkinson disease • Peripheral neuropathy • Poor vision
Other (lightheadedness) (about 10%)	• Alcohol and other drug use • Head trauma (concussion or whiplash injury)	• Hyperventilation • Panic disorder

CVA, cerebrovascular disease; MI, myocardial infarction; MS, multiple sclerosis; TIA, transient ischemic attack.

During the physical examination of the dizzy patient, try to reproduce the dizziness. Perform the following:

▶ **Measure BP**—look for hypotension or orthostatic hypotension (decrease in systolic BP of 20 mm Hg, decrease in diastolic BP of 10 mm Hg, or increase in pulse of 20 to 30 beats per minute from supine to standing positions)

▶ **Dix–Hallpike maneuver.** This is performed on a flat examination table, watching the patient's eyes for 30 seconds looking for nystagmus. Sensitivity of the Dix–Hallpike maneuver for posterior semicircular canal benign positional paroxysmal vertigo (BPPV) is 50% to 88%.[22,23] If the patient has a history compatible with BPPV and the Dix–Hallpike maneuver is negative, a supine roll test should be performed to assess for lateral semicircular BPPV.

▶ **Careful cardiac examination**—look for murmurs or arrhythmias

▶ **Ear examination**—look for otitis media (OM), cholesteatoma, and OM with effusion (see Earache)

▶ **Ocular examination**—look for nystagmus, equal pupillary reactions

▶ **Neurologic examination**—a positive Romberg test indicates a possible vestibular or cerebellar lesion

Mr. Polk looks uncomfortable. His vital signs are normal. He has resting horizontal nystagmus toward the right side, normal cranial nerves, and a negative Dix–Hallpike maneuver. His ear examination is normal.

Steps in Evaluation

Is this an Emergency?

Patients with severe symptoms from any cause may need hospitalization for IV fluids and supportive care if unable to eat or drink. If stroke or a transient ischemic attack is suspected as the cause of acute dizziness, hospital evaluation is important. ECG evidence of arrhythmia is a reason for further evaluation in the emergency department. Mr. Polk does not appear severely dehydrated or in need of emergency care.

Are there Other Red Flags for Serious Conditions?

 Clues or "red flags" in patients with dizziness:

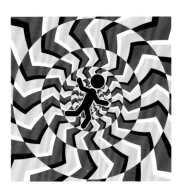

▶ Neurologic abnormalities (consider CVA, intracranial process)

▶ Unilateral hearing loss (consider labyrinthitis or acoustic neuroma)

▶ Hypotension (consider MI, arrhythmia, CHF)

▶ Falling or inability to walk (consider CVA, intracranial lesion, or hemorrhage)

Do I Need a Diagnostic Test?

If possible, consider additional testing based on the type of dizziness described by the patient as shown in Figure 11.6. For example, 93% of patients who present with vertigo have BPPV, acute vestibular neuritis, or Meniere disease.[22]

Management

Management of patients with dizziness is outlined in Table 11.10.

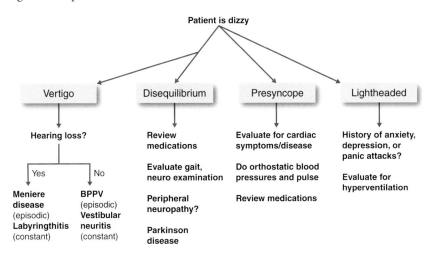

Figure 11.6 ▶ Approach to the patient with dizziness. (Data from: Post RE, Dickerson LM. Dizziness: a diagnostic approach. *Am Fam Physician*. 2010;82(4):361–368.)

Table 11.10 ► Key Features, Diagnostic Tests and Treatment for Patients with Dizziness

Common Causes	Key Features	Diagnostic Test	Treatment
Vertigo			
BPPV	Episodic, vertigo, precipitated with movement	Positive Dix–Hallpike maneuver	Supportive (assess fall risk, home support, CNS disorders, and impaired mobility or balance)[a] Epley,[b] antiemetic[c]
Labyrinthitis (vestibular neuritis)	Constant, vertigo, often previous infection	Negative Dix–Hallpike maneuver	Supportive, possible antiviral, antiemetic[c]
Meniere disease (increased endolymphatic fluid in inner ear)	Hearing loss, vertigo, tinnitus, ear fullness; episodic, usual onset ages 20–50 years	Clinical evaluation, exclusion of other causes of vertigo, may do MRI to exclude acoustic neuroma	Supportive, low-quality evidence supports diuretic use to improve vertigo, but not hearing[d]
Disequilibrium			
Balance or gait disturbance	Symptoms of disequilibrium, history of falling	Careful neurologic examination, evaluate gait	Treat underlying neurologic disorder, PT for gait training
Presyncope			
Arrhythmia	Palpitations	Abnormal cardiac examination, abnormal ECG or Holter monitor	Based on type of arrhythmia
Orthostatic hypotension	Often positional symptoms	Orthostatic blood pressures and pulse	Review medications
Lightheadedness			
Anxiety, depression, panic disorder	Symptoms of lightheadedness	Hyperventilation simulation	Breathing control exercises, β-blockers, antianxiety treatment

[a]American Academy of Otolaryngology—head and neck surgery. Benign Paroxysmal Positional Vertigo. Available at, www. aafp.org/patient-care/clinical-recommendations/all/vertigo.html. Accessed August 2016.
[b]Epley maneuver (particle repositioning maneuver) for patients with posterior canal BPPV: https://www.youtube.com/watch?v=9SLm76jQg3g.
[c]Anti-emetics include anticholinergics (e.g., scopolamine), antihistamines (e.g., meclizine), cannabinoids (e.g., dronabinol), 5-HT$_3$ receptor antagonists (e.g., ondansetron), and phenothiazines (e.g., chlorpromazine) (among others).
[d]Crowson MG, Patki A, Tucci DL. A systematic review of diuretics in the medical management of Meniere's disease. *Otolaryngol Head Neck Surg.* 2016;154(5):824-834.
BPPV, benign paroxysmal positional vertigo; CNS, central nervous system; PT, physical therapy.

You diagnose Mr. Polk with probable viral labyrinthitis. Your attending prescribes meclizine and asks him to come back in 3 to 5 days if he is no better.

DYSURIA

Dysuria is pain or discomfort associated with urination that is usually described as burning or stinging and localized to the urethra and meatus. Occasional irritative voiding symptoms are reported by 3% of adults older than 40 years.[24]

Table 11.11 ▶ Differential Diagnosis of Dysuria in Otherwise Healthy Women and Men

Diagnosis	Frequency	Distinguishing Symptoms and Signs
Women of Reproductive Age		
Lower tract UTI[a]	Very common	Nocturia, cloudy or malodorous urine
Vaginitis	Common	Vaginal discharge, perineal pruritus
Upper tract UTI	Uncommon	Fever, flank pain, CVA tenderness
Urethritis	Uncommon	Fever, urinary frequency, urethral discharge
Perineal trauma	Uncommon	Evidence of trauma and tenderness on examination
Interstitial cystitis	Uncommon	Frequency and urgency for 6 months with negative workup
Older Women		
Vaginal atrophy	Common	Vaginal mucosal atrophy on examination
Men		
Prostatitis	Common	Hesitancy, urgency with decreased urine flow, tender prostate
Urethritis	Uncommon	Urethral discharge, dysuria localized to penis

CVA, Costovertebral angle; UTI, urinary tract infection.
[a]Among children, 5% to 8% of girls and 1% to 2% of boys have a symptomatic UTI during childhood.[25]

Camila is a 27-year-old Hispanic woman who presents with recurrent bladder pain, dysuria, and urinary frequency. She was treated last month for a urinary tract infection (UTI) with nitrofurantoin based on dipstick presence of leukocyte esterase in the office, and once again 2 weeks ago over the telephone with Bactrim.

The causes of dysuria are listed in Table 11.11. The most common cause is UTI in women; about half of women will have a UTI in their lifetime.

Steps in Evaluation

Is this an Emergency?

A complicated urinary tract or kidney infection can result in sepsis. This can present in the elderly as mental status changes such as confusion. In general, patients who are septic appear ill, are febrile, and have tachycardia, tachypnea, and hypotension.

Are there Other Red Flags for Serious Conditions (in this case pyelonephritis)?

 Clues or "red flags" for a complicated infection are:

▶ Male gender, infant, or elderly person

▶ Symptoms for more than 7 days

▶ Immunosuppression or diabetes

▶ Episode of pyelonephritis in the past year

▶ Hematuria

▶ Known anatomic abnormality

▶ Fever or flank pain

Do I Need a Diagnostic Test?

Although typical signs and symptoms of an UTI, including dysuria, urgency, frequency, nocturia, and malodorous or cloudy urine are common, no single element has a high likelihood ratio for UTI. In addition, sexually transmitted infections (STIs) can cause these symptoms, especially in males, so a nucleic acid amplification test (NAAT) may be needed.

In a woman, however, the combination of dysuria and urinary frequency without vaginal discharge or irritation yielded a very high likelihood of UTI (LR+ 24.6).[26] This is justification for treating a woman, especially one with a prior history of UTI, empirically or over the telephone as was done for Camilla.

Physical examination in adults is focused on detecting suprapubic tenderness (UTI or cystitis), flank pain (LR+ pyelonephritis), and, in men or trans women, penile discharge (STI) and a rectal examination (prostatitis). If other symptoms such as rash or joint pain are present, examine these areas.

The **single best test** is a urinalysis—the presence of 10 bacteria per high power field has a LR+ of 85. A urine dipstick showing both nitrites and leukocytes is also highly predictive of an UTI.[27] An initial approach is shown in Figure 11.7.

Your examination of Camila is remarkable only for suprapubic tenderness. Her urinalysis is normal although you have retained the specimen to send for culture. She has no red flags in her history and is in a monogamous sexual relationship.

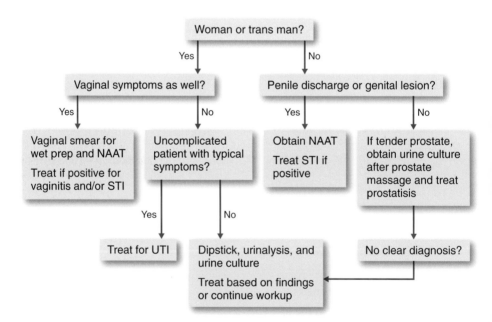

Figure 11.7 ▶ Initial approach to the patient with dysuria. NAAT, nucleic acid amplification test; STI, sexually transmitted disease; UTI, urinary tract infection.

Differential Diagnosis

If the diagnosis is still unclear after the focused history, physical examination and initial testing, diagnostic considerations include:[27]

▶ Bladder or topical irritant, including drugs (e.g., diuretics)

▶ Chronic constipation

▶ Endometriosis

▶ Hyperglycemia

▶ Interstitial cystitis/bladder pain syndrome

▶ Obstruction (e.g., prostate, urethral stricture)

▶ Overactive bladder

▶ Urethral diverticulum

▶ Urethritis

For Camila, with a normal urinalysis, you need to conduct additional history for potential bladder irritants (you find none), ask specifically about incontinence (often seen with overactive bladder but not present in her case), assess her menstrual history (normal with a recent period), and consider NAAT testing for STI. Camila agrees to a NAAT test, which is negative.

Management

▶ Infection

- UTI (SOR A): antibiotic, in consideration of community resistance patterns. (SOR C): cranberry juice and increased fluids; in children under age 2 years or older with recurrent infection or an episode of pyelonephritis, consider imaging for vesicoureteral reflux
- Pyelonephritis: (SOR A): antibiotics

▶ Interstitial cystitis (SOR C): confirm with bladder filling test and cystoscopy; lifestyle modification, bladder training, pain control

▶ Irritant (SOR C): remove when possible

▶ Overactive bladder (SOR C): lifestyle intervention. (SOR B): pelvic floor muscle and bladder training, medication.[28]

▶ Prostatitis (acute) (SOR A): antibiotic. (SOR B): NSAID

▶ STI (SOR A): antibiotics, based on most recent Centers for Disease Control guideline

▶ Urethritis (SOR A): antibiotic or antifungal

▶ Vaginitis (infectious): (SOR A) based on etiology—antibiotic or antifungal

▶ Vaginitis (atrophic): (SOR A): topical estrogen. (SOR C): lubricant

Pyridium, a local anesthetic, can be used for severe dysuria. Referral may be needed for diagnosis or treatment of complicated cases.

After discussing possible causes for her dysuria with you and the attending, Camila states that she does not want anything for her symptoms but would like a diagnosis. If her culture is negative, she will be referred to a urologist for further evaluation for possible interstitial cystitis.

FEVER

Fever is a sign most commonly associated with infectious processes, but can also be caused by inflammatory/connective tissue diseases, malignancy, medications, or hereditary conditions. Fevers also cause headache, muscle aches (myalgia), chills or rigors, and sweating. Treating these symptoms with antipyretic medications is simple compared to the sometimes challenging task of diagnosing a fever's underlying cause.

Definitions

▶ **Fever:** Elevation in core body temperature above the normal range for an individual. Most sources define fever as core temperature ≥38°C (100.4°F); others list 38.3°C (101°F) as the threshold. Development of fever is a controlled process governed by the thermoregulatory center in the hypothalamus.

▶ **Hyperthermia:** Elevated core body temperature not regulated by the hypothalamus; results in loss of the body's ability to lose heat. Hyperthermia may be exogenous (e.g., heat stroke) or caused by endogenous factors (e.g., medications or hyperthyroidism).

▶ **Hyperpyrexia:** Very high fever (>41.5°C; 106.7°F), often caused by intracerebral hemorrhage.[29]

▶ **Fever of unknown origin (FUO):** Prolonged febrile illness (opinions vary on fever duration; generally accepted as >1 to 3 weeks) without an established etiology despite dedicated laboratory and imaging evaluation.[30]

▶ **Fever without a source (FWS):** Specific to children between 3 and 36 months of age with fever <7 days, this term is used if the cause of the fever cannot be identified based on history and physical examination alone.[31]

> Sadie is a 2-and-a-half-month-old girl who presents with her father, who reports she has had fevers for the past 3 days. She has not had any rashes, runny nose, discolored urine, cough, or signs of discomfort. She is slightly fussier than usual but has been feeding (breast milk) well and urinating and stooling normally. There have been no sick contacts. She does not attend daycare. She is up to date on her immunizations. Her birth history is unremarkable, with no history of prematurity or previous infections.

The differential diagnosis for fever is shown in Table 11.12.

Steps in Evaluation

Is this an Emergency?

Fever is usually not an emergency when caused by connective tissue disorders or malignancies. Exceptions include febrile neutropenia and giant cell (temporal) arteritis. Drug-induced fever may be an emergency, as in serotonin syndrome or malignant hyperthermia. Sadie has none of these problems.

Table 11.12 ▶ Differential Diagnosis for Fever

INFECTIOUS
Upper respiratory/HEENT:
- Cerebral abscess, meningitis
- Dental abscess
- Epiglottitis
- Mononucleosis
- Otitis media
- Septal/preseptal cellulitis
- Sinusitis
- Strep throat
- Viral URI

Lower Respiratory:
- Aspiration
- Cystic fibrosis
- Fungal infection
- Influenza
- Pneumonia
- Tuberculosis

Cardiovascular:
- Endocarditis
- Pericarditis

Abdominal/Pelvic:
- Appendicitis
- Cholecystitis/cholangitis
- Diverticulitis
- Infectious diarrhea *(Clostridium difficile, E. coli, Shigella, Campylobacter, Yersinia, Giardia, Cryptococcus, Cryptosporidium)*
- Omphalitis
- Typhlitis
- Viral hepatitis

Genitourinary:
- Epididymitis
- Pelvic inflammatory disease/ salpingitis/cervicitis
- Prostatitis
- Urinary tract infection/ pyelonephritis

Musculoskeletal/Soft Tissues:
- Cellulitis/abscess
- Osteomyelitis
- Septic arthritis

Miscellaneous:
- CMV
- Herpes simplex virus
- HIV/AIDS
- Lyme disease/tick-borne illness
- Pediatric viral exanthem
- Tropical diseases (e.g., Zika, dengue, yellow fever, chikungunya, malaria, leishmaniasis, filariasis)

MALIGNANCY
- Atrial myxoma
- Colon cancer
- HCC
- Kaposi sarcoma
- Leukemia
- Lymphoma
- Multiple myeloma
- Osteosarcoma
- Renal cell carcinoma

MISCELLANEOUS
- Factitious fever
- Familial Mediterranean fever
- Pulmonary embolism
- Neuroleptic malignant syndrome
- Thyroid disorder

MEDICATIONS
- Allopurinol
- Atropine
- Carbamazepine
- Clozapine
- Dantrolene
- Haloperidol
- Heparin
- Minocycline
- Nitrofurantoin
- Phenobarbital
- Phenytoin
- Primidone
- SSRIs
- Succinylcholine
- Zonisamide

RHEUMATOLOGIC/CONNECTIVE TISSUE DISEASE
- Autoimmune hepatitis
- Behcet disease
- Cryoglobulinemia
- Giant cell (temporal) arteritis
- Granulomatosis with polyangiitis
- Inflammatory bowel disease
- Juvenile rheumatoid arthritis
- Polyarteritis nodosa
- Sarcoidosis
- SLE
- Vasculitis

AIDS, acquired immune deficiency syndrome; CMV, cytomegalovirus; HCC, hepatocellular carcinoma; HEENT, head/eyes/ears/nose/ throat; HIV, human immunodeficiency virus; SLE, systemic lupus erythematosus; SSRIs, selective serotonin reuptake inhibitors; URI, upper respiratory infection.
Data from: Allen CH. Fever without a source in children 3 to 36 months of age. *UpToDate.* Updated Feb 2, 2016. Available from: https:// www-uptodate-com.ezproxy.library.wisc.edu/contents/fever-without-a-source-in-children-3-to-36-months-of-age?source=search_ result&search=fever±without±a±soucre&selectedTitle=1~150. Accessed September 4, 2016 (and other sources).

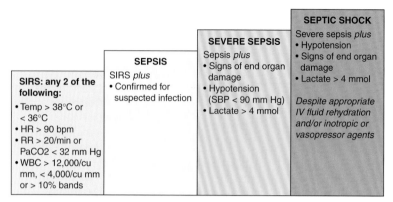

Figure 11.8 ▶ Definitions of SIRS, sepsis, severe sepsis, and septic shock (adults). HR, heart rate; IV, intravenous; PaCO₂, alveolar pressure of carbon dioxide; RR, respiratory rate; SBP, systolic blood pressure; SIRS, systemic inflammatory response syndrome; WBC, white blood cell count. (Definitions based on Levy MM, Fink MP, Marshall JC, et al. 2001 SCCM/ESICM/ACCP/ATS/SIS. International Sepsis Definitions Conference. *Crit Care Med.* 2003;31:1250–1256.)

While most infectious fevers are not life-threatening, infection can progress to sepsis, a syndrome in which the body's inflammatory response to infection becomes dysregulated, leading to organ dysfunction and possible death.[32] Sepsis develops on a continuum, beginning with systemic inflammatory response system (SIRS) and ending with septic shock (Fig. 11.8).

The SIRS criteria above are sensitive (69%) but not specific (37%).[33] A newer clinical assessment tool, the Quick Sequential Organ Failure Assessment (qSOFA), is increasingly used to rapidly identify patients with sepsis who are at risk for poor outcomes.[34–36] qSOFA is less sensitive but more specific; therefore, it is more useful as a prognostic tool than a diagnostic tool.

qSOFA Criteria: ≥2 criteria suggest risk of poor outcome

▶ Hypotension (systolic blood pressure <100 mm Hg)

▶ Altered Mental Status (Glasgow Coma Score <13)

▶ Tachypnea (Respiratory rate >22 breaths/min)

Are there Other Red Flags for Possible Sepsis?

 Clues or "red flags" for possible sepsis:

Pediatric[37]

▶ Parental concerns or physician instinct

▶ Changes in crying pattern, drowsiness, moaning, inconsolability, unconsciousness

▶ Pulmonary rales, rapid breathing, shortness of breath, or decreased breath sounds

▶ Cyanosis, decreased skin turgor, hypotension, meningeal signs, petechial rash, seizures

▶ Age <3 months (especially age <1 month)

Adult or Child[38]

▶ Febrile neutropenia (fever plus absolute neutrophil count, ANC, <500 per mm^3). This condition contributes to 50% of deaths from leukemia, lymphoma, and solid tumors[39]

▶ Meningeal signs

▶ SIRS or sepsis syndrome present

Meningeal signs include Kernig's Sign: https://www.youtube.com/watch?v=rJ-5AFuP3YA and Brudzinski's Sign: https://www.youtube.com/watch?v=jO9PAPi-yus.

Sadie's temperature is 38.2°C (100.8°F). Her heart rate is 110 bpm and her respiratory rate is 28 breaths/min. She appears well-hydrated but tired. Her skin turgor is normal and capillary refill is <2 seconds. She has no rashes. Her lungs are clear, and abdomen is nontender. Her diaper is wet with clear yellow urine. She does not have any signs of meningeal irritation. Other examination is unremarkable.

Do I Need a Diagnostic Test?

As you can see from Table 11.12, the differential diagnosis for causes of fever is quite *broad* (Table 11.12 is not even an exhaustive list). Obtaining laboratory and imaging tests for all etiologies is impractical and uneconomical. However, there are certain classes of patients in whom certain empiric testing is indicated. These include toxic-appearing adults and children, infants (Fig. 11.9), and neutropenic or otherwise immune-compromised patients. Given Sadie's age (75 days), you obtain a CBC with differential and urinalysis with culture. WBC are 8,000/mm^3 without increased neutrophil percentage. Urinalysis is normal.

Patients with febrile neutropenia should have CBC with differential, comprehensive metabolic panel, serum lactate, and blood cultures drawn. Depending on their age and risk stratification (not covered in this text), they should be given empiric anti-infective agents covering opportunistic bacterial and fungal infections. The decision to admit to the hospital depends on clinical symptoms and overall risk of serious infection.[38]

When the source of fever remains uncertain, additional testing to consider (for both children and adults) includes[40,41]:

▶ Cultures: blood, stool (with stool toxins and fecal leukocyte count)

▶ Labs: antinuclear antibody, CBC with differential, C-reactive protein, erythrocyte sedimentation rate, heterophile antibody test, HIV testing. influenza and other viral testing, lactate, Lyme antibody, rheumatoid factor

▶ Procedures: lumbar puncture

▶ Serum protein electrophoresis

▶ Tuberculin skin test or Quantiferon Gold Test

▶ Urinalysis with culture

Imaging does not necessarily improve diagnostic accuracy with FUO. In one study of 73 adult patients, the following false positive rates were shown:[33]

▶ Chest radiograph—false positive rate 11%

▶ Chest CT—17%

▶ Abdominal CT—28%

▶ Positron emission tomography (PET) scan—14%

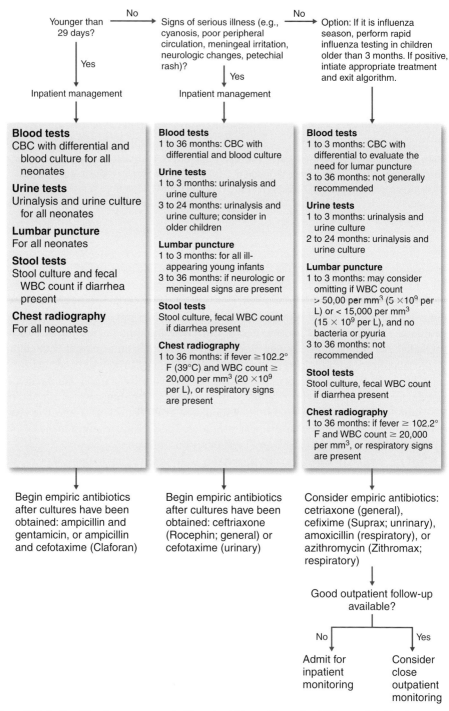

Figure 11.9 ▸ Algorithm for management of fever in children <36 months. CBC, complete blood count; WBC, white blood cell. (From: Hamilton JL, John SP. Evaluation of fever in infants and young children. *Am Fam Physician.* 2013;87(4):254–260. http://www.aafp.org/afp/2013/0215/p254.html)

Since Sadie appears well and does not have localizing signs of infection, and you have confidence in her parents' judgment and ability to follow up, you administer a dose of empiric ceftriaxone in the office and arrange for her parents to bring her in the next day for re-check. You advise her parents to give weight-appropriate doses of acetaminophen to reduce her fever and discomfort.

Management

Treatment of fever depends on the etiology. Antipyretics can improve patient comfort. Acetaminophen (15 mg/kg/dose, max dose 60 mg/kg/24 hrs in children) or ibuprofen (10 mg/kg/dose, maximum dose 40 mg/kg/24 hrs in children) are effective choices to reduce fever and pain. Ibuprofen and other NSAIDs should be used with caution in patients with coronary artery disease, risk of GI bleeding, or renal disease. Aspirin (acetylsalicylic acid) should not be used in children due to risk of Reye syndrome, an acute noninflammatory encephalopathy and hepatopathy.

The following list details on management for various etiologies of fever, along with SOR, if known:

▶ Bacterial infection (SOR A): antibiotics

▶ Influenza (SOR C): antiviral therapy[41]

▶ Malignancy: surgery, chemotherapy, radiation, or biologic therapy as appropriate

▶ Inflammatory/Connective Tissue disorder (SOR B): anti-inflammatory agents (e.g., NSAIDs, corticosteroids, disease-modifying antirheumatic drugs, biologic drugs)

▶ Drug fever (SOR C): removal of offending agent, supportive therapy, benzodiazepines for serotonin syndrome.[42] (SOR C): dantrolene for malignant hyperthermia (SOR C)

GASTROINTESTINAL BLEEDING

GI bleeding refers to bleeding from any part of the GI tract, regardless of patient symptoms. Bleeding occurring proximal to the ligament of Treitz (duodenojejunal junction) is considered upper GI (UGI) bleeding (associated with **hematemesis** [vomiting blood] or **melena** [black, tarry stool]). UGI bleeding is approximately five times more common than lower GI (LGI) bleeding (associated with **hematochezia** [passing fresh blood through the rectum] or "currant jelly stool" [combination blood, mucus, and stool]).

Many of the causes, identifying features, and diagnostic tests for GI bleeding are listed in Table 11.13.

Of the UGI causes, peptic ulcer disease (PUD) is the most common.[43] Risk factors include medications (nonsteroidal anti-inflammatory drugs [NSAIDs], clopidogrel, warfarin, serotonin reuptake inhibitors [SSRIs], corticosteroids), alcohol, *Helicobacter pylori* infection, and excess acid production.

Of the LGI causes, diverticulosis is the most common cause of significant LGI bleeding in older adults.[43] However, colon cancer should be considered in any older adult with unexplained anemia or lower GI bleeding. As you may recall from part 1 of this chapter, Mr. Stern, the 71-year-old man who was a former smoker and current alcohol drinker, had

Table 11.13 ▶ Selected Causes of Gastrointestinal Bleeding

Condition	Key Features	Diagnostic Test
Upper GI Bleeding		
Gastritis or esophagitis	Epigastric pain, current medication[a] or alcohol use	Upper endoscopy
Gastric cancer	Rare (more common in Japanese patients), smoker, pesticide exposure, N/V, postprandial fullness, weight loss	CEA (elevated in about half), upper endoscopy
Peptic ulcer disease	Current medication[a] or alcohol use, epigastric pain, dyspeptic symptoms (belching, bloating, and distention)	*H. pylori* stool or breath test; upper endoscopy, if red flags, anemic, or persistent
Mallory–Weiss tear	Forceful coughing, vomiting, or retching; can be a complication of endoscopic procedures	Most spontaneously resolve, esophagogastroduodenoscopy especially if active bleeding
Varices (esophageal or gastric)	History of liver disease, excessive alcohol use, sign of portal hypertension (e.g., ascites, lower extremity edema, splenomegaly) or cirrhosis (e.g., spider nevi, fatigue, N/V, pruritus, jaundice)	LFTs, hepatitis panel, antimitochondrial antibodies (primary biliary cirrhosis) Ultrasound (liver, biliary tree), endoscopy, liver biopsy
Lower GI Bleeding: Adult		
Colitis (infection, inflammation, radiation, or ischemia)	Crampy abdominal pain, diarrhea, tenesmus (urgency with a feeling of incomplete evacuation), passage of mucus, extraintestinal manifestations with IBD[b]	Stool culture or colonoscopy with biopsy or CT enterography (add tagged RBC nuclear scan?)
Diverticulitis/osis	Abdominal pain/abrupt painless bleeding; most diverticular bleeding spontaneously resolves	None or colonoscopy
Hemorrhoids	Pain, itching, protruding rectal "mass"	Rectal examination, anoscopy
Tumor or polyp	Older age, no symptoms or cramps, weight loss, change in bowel habits, obstruction (malignancy); family history (polyp; common [30% of adults], but <5% bleed)[c]	Colonoscopy or barium enema
Vascular ectasias	Painless chronic bleeding, anemia	Colonoscopy; possible radionuclide scan or angiography
Lower GI Bleeding: Child		
Anal fissure	Visible crack, painful defecation	None (visual)
Colitis (infection, inflammation, allergy)	Crampy abdominal pain, diarrhea	Stool culture or colonoscopy as above
Intussusception[d]	Second most common cause of bleeding; severe abdominal pain, vomiting	Air contrast enema or barium enema (may resolve problem)
Meckel diverticulum (congenital pouch in small intestine)	Most common cause of significant LGI bleeding in children; severe abdominal pain, obstruction (N/V)	Colonoscopy, technetium scan

Condition	Key Features	Diagnostic Test
Polyps (juvenile)	Usually benign	Colonoscopy, monitoring
Rectal foreign bodies	Often with diarrhea, onset 6–12 hours after ingestion, fever, cramping	No test needed; remove

[a]Nonsteroidal anti-inflammatory drug, warfarin, clopidogrel, aspirin, selective serotonin reuptake inhibitors, bisphosphonate, corticosteroid, alcohol.
[b]Extraintestinal manifestations (present in up to 40% with IBD) include skin (e.g., erythema nodosum), rheumatologic (e.g., arthritis), ocular (e.g., iritis), hepatobiliary (e.g., primary sclerosing cholangitis), cardiovascular (e.g., deep vein thrombosis), bone (e.g., osteoporosis), and renal (e.g., obstructive uropathy).
[c]Mayer R. Gastrointestinal tract cancer. In: Kasper DL, Braunwald E, Fauci AS, Hauser SL, Longo DL, Jameson, JL, eds. *Harrison's Principles of Internal Medicine*, 16th ed. New York, NY: McGraw-Hill Companies Inc.; 2005:523–533.
[d]Involution of one segment of bowel into another segment.
CT, computed tomography; IBD, inflammatory bowel disease; LFTs, liver function tests; N/V, nausea, vomiting; PPI, proton pump inhibitor; SOR, strength of recommendation.

heme-positive stool, raising concern about colon cancer. Following the history and initial examination consisting of inspection, an abdominal and rectal examination (checking stool, if present on the examining glove, for blood), continue with the next steps.

Steps in Evaluation

Is this an Emergency?

Active bleeding or severe blood loss can be medical emergencies. You cannot always judge severity by the hemoglobin/hematocrit level so look for physical signs of:

▷ Rapid pulse (β-blockers can mask tachycardia normally associated with hemodynamic instability)

▷ Low BP (supine hypotension represents a 40% blood loss)[43]

▷ Orthostasis (rise in pulse by 20 beats/minute and a fall in systolic BP by 20 mm Hg when standing)

▷ Dizziness or confusion

In addition, several of the causes of bleeding can also result in bowel perforation. Look for peritoneal signs on abdominal examination (rebound, rigidity). If you are concerned about any of these, alert your attending.

Are there Other Red Flags for Serious Conditions?

 Clues or "red flags" in patients with GI bleed:

▶ Child with severe pain and vomiting (Meckel diverticulum or intussusception)

▶ Severe pain/tenderness, peritoneal signs (bowel perforation)

▶ Coughing, vomiting, retching prior to bleed (Mallory–Weiss tear)

▶ History of atherosclerotic disease (ischemic colitis)

▶ High-risk medications (e.g., peptic ulcer disease)

▶ Weight loss (malignancy)

Do I Need a Diagnostic Test?

Unless the cause of bleeding is obvious (anal fissure, external hemorrhoid), minor and resolves with treatment (gastritis) or infectious and resolves with treatment (infectious colitis), additional testing will likely be needed to rule out malignancy and confirm a diagnosis before treatment. The usual tests are shown in Table 11.13. Mr. Stern was referred for colonoscopy.

If upper endoscopy or colonoscopy fail to identify the bleeding source, other tests that can be considered include technetium red cell scan (highly sensitive and detects bleeding at a rate of 0.1 to 0.5 mL/minute), angiography (considered in patients with emergent bleeding), video capsule endoscopy, or double-balloon enteroscopy.

> Mr. Stern is on your schedule for follow up. You review his chart and see that he had surgery for a right-sided colon cancer. He reports that things moved pretty quickly after the colonoscopy that you suggested demonstrated a cancer. His surgery went well, although his cancer is stage C and he will need chemotherapy. He thanks you for your help in his care and you encourage him to follow-up during his treatment as needed.

Management

Management of common causes of GI bleeding in adults is displayed in Table 11.14.

Treatment for common causes of **lower GI bleeding in children** include the following:

▶ Anal fissure (SOR C): symptomatic treatment, treat constipation

▶ Colitis (infant) (SOR C): remove allergen, if identified; see treatment for adults above

▶ Intussusception (SOR C): enema may resolve problem or surgery

▶ Meckel diverticulum (SOR C): surgery (excision of abnormal section)

Table 11.14 ▶ Management of Common Causes of Gastrointestinal Bleeding in Adults

Condition	Treatment	Comment
Upper GI Source		
Gastritis or esophagitis	• Remove trigger if possible • Antacid, PPI, or histamine-2 blocker (SOR C)	
Peptic ulcer disease	• Remove trigger if possible • Eradicate *H. pylori* plus PPI for 4–8 weeks if ulcer on endoscopy (SOR A)	For those without ulcer, use PPI or H2 blocker (SOR B)
Mallory–Weiss tear	• Contact thermal treatment, sclerotherapy, esophageal balloon tamponade or clips, endoscopic band ligation are options	Angiographic embolization has been used in adults
Varices	• Treat cause[a] • Nutritional support • Control ascites (salt/fluid restriction, gentle diuresis, shunting, liver transplant) • Nonselective beta-blockers or endoscopic variceal ligation to prevent hemorrhage in patients with medium to large varices (SOR A)	Authors of a Cochrane review found significant bleeding reduction from banding ligation over nonselective beta-blockers in patients with esophageal varices, but no effect on mortality.[44]

Condition	Treatment	Comment
Lower GI source: Adult		
Colitis	• Antibiotics if infectious (SOR A) • Inflammatory bowel disease, depending on severity: oral aminosalicylates, topical mesalamine or steroids, oral or intravenous steroids, infliximab, colectomy (SOR A)	
Diverticulitis	• Antibiotics (SOR A) • Bowel rest (no food/drink or clear liquids only) (SOR C) • Analgesics • Surgery if complication such as perforation	For bleeding diverticula, epinephrine injection or electrocautery can be done via colonoscopy.[45]
Hemorrhoids	• Dietary fiber[46] • Avoid constipation (diet, stool softener, adequate fluids) • *External hemorrhoids* (distal to the dentate line), based on severity: symptomatic treatment (sitz bath, topical steroids), surgery • *Internal hemorrhoids* (above dentate line), based on severity: sclerotherapy, rubber band ligation (SOR C); hemorrhoidectomy; infrared photocoagulation, bipolar electrocautery, staples, laser therapy (SOR A)	Most external hemorrhoids resolve but about half recur within 5 years
Tumor/polyp	• Removal if solitary; other based on type	

[a]Causes include: alcohol/trigger medication avoidance, antiviral therapy [hepatitis], ursodeoxycholic acid [primary biliary cirrhosis].

HEADACHE

Headache is pain or discomfort perceived in the head. Headache is a common reason for visit in primary care settings. Based on data from the 2012 National Health Interview Survey, 14.2% of US adults of ages 18 or older reported having migraine or severe headache in the previous 3 months.[47] The estimated lifetime prevalence of headache is 66%: 46% to 78% for tension-type headache, 14% to 16% for migraine, and 0.1% to 0.3% for cluster headache.[48]

Havier is a 27-year-old medical student who presents with headache that has been fairly continuous for the past few days. The pain is not severe but is interfering with his ability to work and study. Now that he is in his 4th year of school, he is less stressed and has been trying to follow his own advice to patients to eat better and exercise more so this headache is completely puzzling to him. He does not smoke or drink alcohol and is basically healthy. His mother had migraine headaches but her headaches were unilateral and throbbing.

The formal classification and full list of headache types categorized by the International Headache Society can be found at http://www.ihs-klassifikation.de/en/02_klassifikation/06_glossar/. Headaches are divided into primary, secondary, and a third category of "cranial neuralgias, central and primary facial pain, and other headaches." The differential diagnosis for patients presenting in primary care with headache is shown in Table 11.15.

Table 11.15 ▶ Differential Diagnosis for Patients Presenting with Headache

Disorder	Key Features	Prevalence[a]
Primary Headache		
Tension-type	Mild–moderate bilateral headband-like pain	38.3% (2.2% for chronic)
Migraine	Intense pain, photophobia, often unilateral, throbbing; neurologic complaints are common	13%
Cluster	Series of intense, unilateral headaches often with concurrent lacrimation, rhinorrhea, and ptosis; more common in men	53/100,000 persons (95% CI 26–95) lifetime prevalence
Chronic daily headache disorder	Headache occurs 15 or more times/month. Long duration group (average duration >4 hrs/day) includes chronic migraine, transformed migraine, chronic tension-type headache, hemicrania continua, and new daily persistent headache	3–5% of the population
Secondary Headache		
Infection-related		
Viral syndrome	Fever, myalgia, cough	Common[b]
Encephalitis	Fever, mental status changes	Rare
Meningitis	Fever, stiff neck, toxic appearance, purpuric rash	Rare
Withdrawal from a substance (caffeine, alcohol, opiates)	Associated with cessation of substance	Common
Disorder of homeostasis		
Fasting	Appropriate history, ketosis	Common
Hypoxia/hypercapnia	Color change, air hunger, abnormal blood gas	Uncommon
Dialysis	End-stage renal disease on dialysis	Rare
Attributed to cranial structure (eye, sinus)		
Sinusitis	Pain behind the eyes, nasal purulence/obstruction	Common
Cervical spine OA TMJ disease	Joint pain, neck pain	Uncommon
	Pain over TMJ and with chewing	Uncommon
Psychiatric		
Somatic symptom D	Often multiple symptoms, feeling overwhelmed, affects work, more common in women	Common
Trauma-associated	History of head trauma	Uncommon
Ophthalmologic (glaucoma, strain)	Vision disturbance, pain around the eye, conjunctival irritation	Uncommon

Disorder	Key Features	Prevalence[a]
Vascular		
Stroke or TIA	Neurologic signs, confusion	Uncommon
Subarachnoid	Sudden onset, severe ± focal neurologic findings	Rare
Subdural	Older age, history of trauma	Rare
Arteritis	Older age, muscle aches, pain over artery	Rare
Nonvascular intracranial		
Cerebral spinal fluid disorder	LP-related, high or low pressure	Rare
Inflammatory	Aseptic meningitis, neurosarcoidosis	Rare
Malignancy	Neurologic impairment, seizure, cancer history	Rare
Cranial Neuralgias and Other Headaches		
Trigeminal neuralgia	Extreme sudden, burning pain lasting seconds to minutes in distribution of trigeminal nerve[c]	Rare

[a]Data from Robbins MS, Lipton RB. The epidemiology of primary headache disorders. *Semin Neurol.* 2010;30:107–119.
[b]Common cause of headache in primary care setting, uncommon <5% but >1%; rare <1%.
[c]Fifth cranial nerve with three branches: ophthalmic branch supplies sensation to most of the scalp, forehead, and front of the head; maxillary branch supplies sensation to the cheek, upper jaw, top lip, teeth, gums, and side of the nose; mandibular branch supplies sensation to the lower jaw, teeth, gums, and bottom lip.
CI, confidence interval; CSF, cerebrospinal fluid; D, disorder; LP, Lumbar puncture; OA, osteoarthritis; TIA, transient ischemic attack; TMJ, temporomandibular joint.

Risk factors for chronic daily headache include female gender, obesity, habitual snoring, head or neck injury, and caffeine consumption.[48] Interestingly, the medications used to treat episodic headaches (including nonprescription analgesics and opioids) are implicated in the transformation of episodic to chronic headaches.

Steps in Evaluation

Is this an Emergency?

The two headache emergencies are meningitis/encephalitis and intracranial bleed. Suspect these if a patient exhibits the symptoms displayed in Table 11.15. If you suspect these conditions, immediately alert your attending. In cases of meningitis, immediate antibiotic treatment can be life-saving.

Are there Other Red Flags for Serious Conditions?

 Clues or "red flags" in patients with headache:

▶ Sudden onset and severe (bleed)
▶ Onset after age 50 years (tumor)
▶ Headache accompanied by fever or mental status changes (infection)
▶ Focal neurologic findings (intracranial disorder or migraine)
▶ Change in headache characteristics or intensity (intracranial disorder)
▶ Progressive worsening despite treatment (intracranial disorder)

Do I Need a Diagnostic Test?

For most patients a careful history, vital signs, funduscopic examination (papilledema), neck (stiffness), and neurologic examination (strength, sensation, cerebellar, and cranial nerve function) are sufficient for making a diagnosis. Note any focal or lateralizing signs.

▸ Examine the skin for rashes and neck for stiffness in patients who appear ill (meningitis).

▸ Examine the head, eyes, ears, nose, and throat if the history suggests vision change, ear pain, sore throat, or other symptoms in those regions (infectious).

▸ If the history is suggestive (Table 11.15), palpate the temporal artery or auscultate the neck and orbit for bruits (temporal arteritis), and assess the temporomandibular joint (TMJ dysfunction).

Imaging is considered in patients with red flag signs and symptoms noted above. ACR states that imaging is usually not appropriate (rated 4) in patients with chronic headache without new features and with a normal neurologic examination.[49] ACR recommendations (rating [1 to 3 usually not appropriate, 4 to 6 may be appropriate; 7 to 9 usually appropriate]) are shown in Table 11.16.

It should be noted that individual alarm features do not have high likelihood ratios for pathology (focal findings [LR+ 3.0-4.2], abrupt onset [LR+ 2.5]).[50]

Additional help can be found in a guideline developed by the National Clinical Guideline Center for the National Institute for Health and Clinical Excellence at (https://www.guideline.gov/summaries/summary/38444/headaches-diagnosis-and-management-of-headaches-in-young-people-and-adults).

Management

Avoid headache triggers (Table 11.17)

On further questioning, you learn that Havier very recently stopped drinking coffee throughout the day – from about 6–8 cups of coffee a day to 1 in the morning. His vital signs are normal as is a funduscopic and neurologic examination. You and the attending concur that his headache is likely from caffeine withdrawal.

Table 11.16 ▸ American College of Radiology Imaging Recommendations

Headache Type	Recommendation
Sudden onset, severe	Head CT without contrast (9) or with contrast (8) or MRA head without and with IV contrast (7), arteriography cervicocerebral (7) or MRI head without IV contrast
Chronic with new feature or neurologic finding	MRI head with out and with IV contrast (8) or MRI head without contrast (7) or CT head without contrast (7)
Trigeminal autonomic origin	MRI head without and with IV contrast (8) or MRI head without contrast (7)

Data from: American College of Radiology *ACR Appropriateness Criteria*, 1996 (updated 2013), https://acsearch.acr.org/docs/69482/Narrative/

Table 11.17 ▶ Common Headache Triggers

Categories of Triggers	Specific Triggers	Comments
Alcoholic beverages	Tyramine in red wines, sulfites in white wines, dehydration, "hangover."	Variable response
Caffeine and/or caffeine withdrawal	May be related to changes in vasomotor tone.	Headaches are worse on weekends in patients who drink a lot of caffeine at work
Food additives	MSG, aspartame, tyramine (e.g., found in aged cheeses, some red wines, smoked fish), sodium nitrite (found in processed meats).	Food diaries may be helpful, as may food challenges
Foods	Chocolate, fruits, dairy, onions, beans, nuts.	As above
Environmental changes	Light, odors (perfume, paint, etc.), travel, abrupt changes in weather or altitude.	May present as nasal "stuffi-ness" (sinus symptoms)
Lifestyle factors	Insufficient, excessive, disrupted, or irregular sleep; tobacco or alcohol use; fasting; physical activity; head injury; schedule changes; stress or release from stress; anger; or exhilaration.	Very common. Some people increase tobacco or alcohol use to try to alleviate headaches, thereby contributing to the problem.
Hormone changes, or addition of estrogen-containing medication	Timing of headache with menses or change/addition of hormones.	Headaches may worsen or improve

▶ Primary headache—Key therapies along with their SOR ratings are shown in Table 11.18. The Cochrane library is an excellent resource for information on headache treatment (http://www.cochranelibrary.com/topic/Neurology/Headache%20%26%20 migraine/).

Table 11.18 ▶ Key Therapies for Chronic Headache

Target Condition and Intervention	Strength of Recommendation	Comments and Cautions
Acute Migraine		
Intranasal sumatriptan	A	Can use when patient unable to tolerate oral medications
Subcutaneous sumatriptan (4–6 mg)	A	Most effective for pain-free at 2 hours
Oral sumatriptan	A	Other triptan preparations available; all equally effective and can be used in children
APAP/ASA/caffeine	A	First-line treatment for acute migraine
NSAID	B	Can be administered to children
Butorphanol nasal spray	A	Rescue treatment, higher abuse potential; oral opiate combinations are another alternative
Dihydroergotamine nasal spray	A	For more severe migraine

(continued)

Table 11.18 ▶ Key Therapies for Chronic Headache *(Continued)*

Target Condition and Intervention	Strength of Recommendation	Comments and Cautions
Migraine Prevention		
Antiepileptic (topiramate, valproate)	A	Weigh adverse effect risk versus benefit in decision to treat
Propranolol	A	Caution in cases of asthma or COPD
Amitriptyline	B	Titrate to effect and side effect tolerability (range 10–150 mg/kg)
Tension-type Headache		
Acetaminophen (1 g)	A	Small benefit for pain-free at 2 hours
NSAID (e.g., 400 mg ibuprofen)	A	Works on a small number of people
Amitriptyline	A	Titrate to effect and side effect tolerability (range 10–150 mg/day)
Spinal manipulation Low risk of side effects	C	Manual therapy with the best evidence
Cranial electrotherapy	C	Less studied, but low likelihood of side effects
Cluster Headaches		
High-flow oxygen	B	Can be used in combination with a triptan
Sumatriptan	A	Administered subcutaneous, orally, or intranasal
Verapamil	A	Used for prophylaxis in doses of 120–160 mg PO three times daily
Chronic Daily Headache		
Amitriptyline	A	Start with 10 mg orally at bedtime; can titrate up to 75 mg
Screen for medication overuse	A	Medication overuse is a common cause of chronic headache

APAP, acetaminophen; ASA, acetylsalicylic acid; NSAID, nonsteroidal anti-inflammatory drug.
From: Coeytaux RR, Kaufman JS, Chao R, et al. Four methods of estimating the minimal important difference score were compared to establish a clinically significant change in Headache Impact Test. *J Clin Epidemiol.* 2006; 59(4):374–380; Brønfort G, Nilsson N, Haas M, et al. Non-invasive physical treatments for chronic/recurrent headache. *Cochrane Database Syst Rev.* 2004(3):CD001878; Silberstein SD. Practice parameter: evidence-based guidelines for migraine headache (an evidence-based review): report of the Quality Standards Subcommittee of the American Academy of Neurology. *Neurology.* 2000;56(1):142; Fogan L. Treatment of cluster headache. A double-blind comparison of oxygen v air inhalation. *Arch Neurol.* 1985;42:362–363; Van Vliet JA, Bahra A, Martin V, et al. Intranasal sumatriptan in cluster headache: randomized placebo-controlled double-blind study. *Neurology.* 2003;60:630–633; Leone M, Amico D, Frediani F, et al. Verapamil in the prophylaxis of episodic cluster headache: a double-blind study versus placebo. *Neurology.* 2000;54:1382–1385; Stephens G, Derry S, Moore RA. Paracetamol (acetaminophen) for acute treatment of episodic tension-type headache in adults. *Cochrane Database Syst Rev.* 2016;(6):CD011889; Derry S, Wiffen PJ, Moore RA, et al. Ibuprofen for acute treatment of episodic tension-type headache in adults. *Cochrane Database Syst Rev.* 2015;(7):CD011041; Law S, Derry S, Moore RA. Triptans for acute cluster headache. *Cochrane Database Syst Rev.* 2013;(7):CD008042; Derry CJ, Derry S, Moore RA. Sumatriptan (all routes of administration) for acute migraine attacks in adults - overview of Cochrane reviews. *Cochrane Database Syst Rev.* 2014;(5):CD009108; Linde M, Mulleners WM, Chronicle EP, et al. Topiramate for the prophylaxis of episodic migraine in adults. *Cochrane Database Syst Rev.* 2013;(6):CD010610; Bennett MH, French C, Schnabel A, et al. Normobaric and hyperbaric oxygen therapy for the treatment and prevention of migraine and cluster headache. *Cochrane Database Syst Rev.* 2015;(12):CD005219.

- To prevent migraines, if frequent, avoid fatigue and stress and use a medication shown in Table 11.18. Adding acupuncture to symptomatic treatment of attacks can reduce headache frequency.[51]

▶ Secondary headache—Treat cause and provide pain relief

Provide ongoing monitoring for patients with chronic headache to ensure that their headache are controlled or adequately prevented. Headache diaries can be useful for monitoring (http://www.headaches.org/2007/11/16/headache-diary-can-help-doctor-help-you/). With the likely diagnosis of caffeine-withdrawal headache, Havier can be advised to resume caffeine and gradually decrease the amount or remain off caffeine. He can use pain medication until his headache resolves.

LEG SWELLING

Leg swelling, or edema, is a common problem in family medicine. Edema is caused by accumulation of fluid in the intracellular tissue, caused by a disruption of the equilibrium between the capillary hydrostatic pressure and the oncotic pressure gradient across the capillary.

Ms. Ramirez, a 53-year-old woman with a history of hypertension and sleep apnea, comes in because of bilateral lower leg swelling for the last 2 weeks. It is better in the morning when she gets up, but worsens during the day. She has no systemic symptoms (fever, chills, shortness of breath) but hasn't been using her continuous positive airway pressure (CPAP) machine lately because she doesn't like her mask. On examination, she has 2+ edema in the pretibial area of both lower legs and her weight is up 4 lb from her last visit (BMI 31). There is minimal erythema on both legs, but worse on the right.

Taking a history

▶ Is the edema unilateral or bilateral (local vs. systemic disease)?

▶ How long has it been going on (<72 hours labeled acute, >72 hours chronic)?

▶ Does it get better with elevation?

▶ Other systemic symptoms (e.g., shortness of breath, fever, chills)?

▶ Any new medications (e.g., calcium channel blockers, beta blockers, steroids, NSAIDs)?

▶ Weight loss (think about malnutrition)?

▶ Jaundice or ascites (think about liver disease)?

▶ Decreased urine output (think about renal failure)?

Causes of leg edema are shown in Table 11.19.

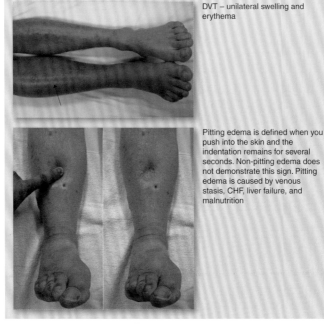

DVT – unilateral swelling and erythema

Pitting edema is defined when you push into the skin and the indentation remains for several seconds. Non-pitting edema does not demonstrate this sign. Pitting edema is caused by venous stasis, CHF, liver failure, and malnutrition

From James Heilman, MD, Wikipedia.

Based on the clinical presentation, Ms. Ramirez likely has venous stasis. Venous stasis is the most common cause of edema in the adult population, affecting up to 30%.[52] In venous stasis, interstitial fluid extravasates into the surrounding tissues. The edema of venous stasis improves with elevation and worsens with dependency. It is also possible that Ms. Ramirez has edema associated with uncontrolled sleep apnea. Edema associated with systemic disease that causes decreased plasma oncotic pressure does not vary with dependency. Either can cause leg ulceration.

Table 11.19 ▶ Causes of Leg Edema

Diagnosis	Key Features	Diagnostic Test
Unilateral Edema		
Cellulitis	Pain, erythema, systemic signs of infection	None or WBC
Compartment syndrome	Pain, history of injury or overuse, tender over muscle	None
Complex regional pain syndrome type 1 (reflex sympathetic dystrophy)	Localized pain, may see decreased hair growth, often with history of injury or trauma	None
DVT	Unilateral, usually acute, painful, associated erythema, risk factors	Doppler ultrasound, D-dimer
Lymphedema	Associated with cancer or radiation or trauma	None
Ruptured Baker cyst	Tender behind knee, may see bruising	Ultrasound, MRI
Ruptured gastrocnemius muscle	Tender posteriorly, may see ecchymosis or bulge over muscle.	None or Ultrasound

Diagnosis	Key Features	Diagnostic Test
Bilateral		
Allergic reaction (angioedema)	Timing to exposure/ingestion	None
Lymphedema	Associated with cancer, radiation, or trauma	None
Medication-related	History of medication use[a]	None
Pregnancy or premenstrual-related	History, timing in menstrual cycle, visible pregnancy	Pregnancy test
Systemic causes		
CHF	History of HD, fatigue, dyspnea, rales	BNP, CXR, echo
Kidney disease	History of kidney disease	BUN, creatinine
Liver disease	History of alcoholism, jaundice, ascites	LFT, albumin (low)
Malnutrition	Poor diet, cachectic	Protein, albumin
Pulmonary HTN	Heart or lung disease, CP, SOB, exercise intolerance	Right heart catheter
Sleep apnea	Snoring, obesity	Sleep study
Venous stasis	Common in patients over age 50 years, may start unilaterally, ulcerations	None

[a]Medications causing edema include beta blockers, calcium channel blockers, chemotherapy agents, hormones (testosterone, estrogen, progesterone, steroids), MAO inhibitors, NSAIDs (Celebrex, ibuprofen), trazodone.
BNP, beta natriuretic peptide; BUN, blood urea nitrogen; CHF, congestive heart failure; CP, chest pain; CXR, chest x-ray; DVT, deep vein thrombosis; echo, echocardiogram; HD, heart failure; HTN, hypertension; LFT, liver function tests; SOB, shortness of breath; WBC, white blood count.
Data from: Trayes KP, Studdiford JS, Pickle S, et al. Edema: diagnosis and management. *Am Fam Physician*. 2013;88(2):102–110; Ely JW, Osberoff JA, Chambliss ML, et al. Approach to leg edema of unclear etiology. *J Am Board Fam Med*. 2006;19(2):148–160.

Steps in Evaluation

Is this an Emergency?

The most serious conditions involving isolated leg edema are those potentially requiring hospital evaluation—DVT, which places patients at risk of PE, and cellulitis or deep ulceration, which places patients at risk of sepsis. Allergic reactions can cause diffuse swelling and can also be an emergency, especially if there is evidence of anaphylaxis or any restriction in upper airway patency. If you suspect any of these, notify your attending. Although DVT is unlikely based on Ms. Ramirez presentation, application of a decision rule might be helpful.

Are there Other Red Flags for Serious Conditions?

Clues or "red flags" about a more serious condition associated with leg edema include:

Clues or "red flags" indicating a serious condition in patients with leg edema:

▸ Acute onset (DVT, cellulitis, worsening systemic disease)
▸ Clinical suspicion of systemic disease
▸ Difficulty breathing
▸ History or suspicion of pelvic malignancy
▸ Symptoms of sleep apnea

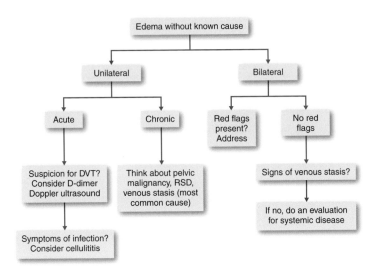

Figure 11.10 ▶ Approach to patients with leg edema.

Do I Need a Diagnostic Test?

An approach to patients with leg edema is shown in Figure 11.10.

Decision-support tools can be used to help determine the need for additional testing. Prediction scores for the pretest probability of DVT such as the Hamilton score and the AMUSE (Amsterdam Maastricht Utrecht Study on thromboembolism) can be used, but the Wells score is used the most (see section above on Breathing; Shortness of Breath or access with http://www.mdcalc.com/wells-criteria-for-dvt/).[53]

AAFP/ACP recommendations for diagnosis of venous thromboembolism in primary care[54]:

▶ Use a validated clinical prediction rule to estimate pretest probability of DVT

▶ In appropriately selected patients with low pretest probability of DVT, obtaining a high-sensitivity D-dimer is a reasonable option; if negative, low likelihood of DVT

▶ Outpatient ultrasound for patients with intermediate to high pretest probability of DVT

Ms. Ramirez has a Wells score of –2, making DVT highly unlikely. You encourage her to see the sleep doctor to refit her mask and order some laboratory tests (shown below) to exclude other medical illnesses causing her edema.

Evaluation for systemic disease causing leg edema

▶ CBC (looking for anemia)

▶ Urinalysis (looking for protein, nephrotic syndrome causes edema)

▶ BMP (looking for elevated creatinine or electrolyte abnormalities)

▶ TSH (hypothyroidism can cause pretibial edema)

> ▸ LFTs and albumin (hepatic disease can cause edema)
> ▸ Suspicious for cardiac disease? Consider ECG, echocardiogram
> ▸ Suspicious for pelvic malignancy or lymphedema? Consider a pelvic CT
>
> BMP, basic metabolic panel; CBC, complete blood count; CT, computed tomography; ECG, electrocardiogram; LFT, liver function tests; TSH, thyroid-stimulating hormone.

Ms. Ramirez comes back 2 weeks later. She has been using her CPAP every night but still has edema. Her laboratory tests, including thyroid studies and a beta natriuretic peptide, were all negative and she continues to feel well otherwise. You diagnose her with venous stasis and recommend compression stockings (Fig. 11.11), elevation of her legs, and encourage her to lose weight.

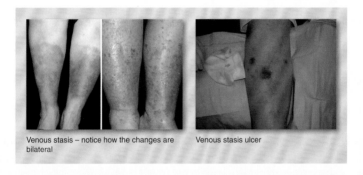

Venous stasis – notice how the changes are bilateral

Venous stasis ulcer

Ms. Ramirez comes back 6 months later for a physical. She brought in her new compression stockings that she bought online. She has been exercising and has lost 8 lb and continues to wear her CPAP every night. Her edema is much improved.

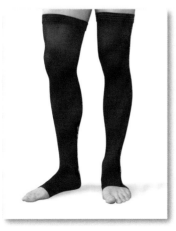

Compression stockings are specialized hosiery that provide leg compression. They come in different amounts of compression (usually 15–20 mm Hg, 20–30 mm Hg, and 30–40 mm Hg), different lengths (knee high or thigh high), and in a variety of colors and patterns

Figure 11.11 ▸ Compression stockings.

Management

Management options for common causes of leg edema are:

▶ Localized:
- DVT: anticoagulation (SOR A): anticoagulation
- Cellulitis (SOR A): antibiotics

▶ Systemic:
- CHF (Chapter 12)
- Liver failure: compression, treatment of underlying liver condition
- Malnutrition (SOR C): protein supplementation and improved diet
- Pregnancy or premenstrual-related (SOR C): reassurance, elevation, compression
- Pulmonary hypertension: CPAP, medical treatment of pulmonary hypertension
- Renal disease: compression, treat underlying kidney disease
- Venous stasis (SOR C): elevation, compression, weight loss, exercise.

NAUSEA AND VOMITING

Nausea is a subjective sensation of unease and discomfort in the upper stomach accompanied by an involuntary urge to vomit. Vomiting is the rapid, forceful evacuation of gastric contents in a retrograde fashion from the stomach up to and out of the mouth.

Nausea and vomiting are common in certain conditions. Among pregnant women in one study, nausea was reported by 74% and vomiting by 51%.[55] Among patients on chemotherapy, 70% to 80% experience nausea and/or vomiting.[56] In 2006, vomiting was the eighth highest cause of emergency room visits in the United States.[57] Conditions that are associated with nausea and vomiting are listed in Table 11.20. They can be grouped under infectious or inflammatory, neurologic, obstructive, situational, and other conditions.

> Ayisha, a 6-year-old girl, presents with a 1-day history of nausea and vomiting. Her father states that she is refusing to drink liquids or eat anything because of continued nausea. She hasn't urinated since early this morning. She reports that her stomach was hurting earlier but not so much now. She looks tired but not terribly ill and smiles when you tell her a joke. She has had no diarrhea or hematemesis.

Steps in Evaluation

Is this an Emergency?

Emergencies in patients with nausea and vomiting occur when there is hematemesis (vomiting blood), causing shock if enough blood is lost, or an electrolyte disturbance (usually hypokalemia or metabolic alkalosis [urine chloride <20 mEq/L]) causing muscle weakness or altered mental status.

▶ If this is suspected, usually the patient will be transferred to the emergency department.

▶ **Labs to consider:** serum electrolytes; creatinine; blood urea nitrogen; glucose; spot urine measurement of sodium, potassium, chloride, creatinine; and ECG.

▶ ECG in hypokalemia may show flat or inverted T waves, U-wave formation, and ST-segment depression.

Table 11.20 ► Causes, Key Features, and Initial Testing for Nausea and Vomiting

Condition	Key Features	Diagnostic Test
Infectious/Inflammatory		
Appendicitis	Pain starts at umbilicus then RLQ, fever	None or ultrasound or CT
Cholecystitis	RUQ pain, positive Murphy's sign	Ultrasound
Gastroenteritis, bacterial	Bloody diarrhea, abdominal cramping	Stool WBCs and culture
Gastroenteritis, viral	Watery diarrhea, fever, headache, abdominal cramping, self-limited	None needed
Hepatitis	Fever, jaundice, weakness	Liver function test
Nonulcer dyspepsia	Epigastric pain, postprandial fullness, bloating	*H. pylori* stool or breath test; endoscopy, if red flags or persistent
Pancreatitis	LUQ pain radiating to back	Elevated lipase
Neurologic		
Inner ear disorders (including acute labyrinthitis, BPV)	Vertigo, nystagmus, postural instability	No test needed
Intracranial disorder	Morning projectile vomiting without nausea, focal neurologic deficit	Head CT or MRI, Urgent referral
Migraine	Photophobia, aura, throbbing headache	No test needed
Obstructive		
Gastroparesis	Insidious, more than 1 hour after meals, partial food digestion	Numerous options such as endoscopy, CT or MR enterography, gastric emptying
Mechanical obstruction	Vomiting within one hour of meal ingestion, distension, hypo or hyperactive bowel sounds	X-ray, CT scan
Situational		
Alcohol poisoning	Alcohol ingestion, confusion, seizures	Blood alcohol level
Food poisoning	Often with diarrhea, onset 6–12 hours after ingestion, fever, cramping	No test needed
Medications	Recent change or addition of medications, hormones, opiates, among *many* others	No test needed; time, elimination
Pregnancy	Missed menstrual period, morning occurrences	Urine/serum pregnancy test
Other		
Cyclic vomiting syndrome	Improves with sleep, no prodrome, average length: 6 days per episode	No test needed
Malignancy	Fever, palpable mass, fecal blood, tenderness, weight loss, jaundice	Colonoscopy, CT scan
Myocardial infarction	Chest pain (see above), ST elevation on ECG	Elevation in troponin
Psychiatric disease including eating disorder	History of psychiatric illness, habitual postprandial symptoms	Screening test and apply DSM5 criteria

BPV, benign positional vertigo; CT, computed tomography; DSM, diagnostic and statistical manual; ECG, electrocardiogram; LUQ, left upper quadrant; RUQ, right upper quadrant; WBC, white blood cells.

Are there Other Red Flags for Serious Conditions?

 Clues or "red flags" about the seriousness of the problem are:

▶ Dehydration (e.g., sunken eyes, reduced skin turgor, tachycardia)

▶ Deterioration or altered mental status (e.g., lethargic, irritable)

▶ Hematemesis

For Ayisha, the most important consideration is dehydration, although this would be more concerning if she also had diarrhea.

ASSESSING DEHYDRATION

Mild to Moderate	Severe
▶ Fatigue, weak, dizzy	▶ Irritable or confused
▶ Dry mouth	▶ Fever, sunken eyes
▶ Dry skin	▶ Poor skin turgor
▶ Constipation	▶ Poor capillary refill
▶ Low urine output	▶ Tachycardia, tachypnea
▶ Few tears	▶ Little or no urine output
▶ Headache	▶ No tears
▶ Muscle cramps	▶ Hypotension
	▶ Altered consciousness

The most useful individual signs for identifying dehydration in children are prolonged capillary refill time, abnormal skin turgor, and abnormal respiratory pattern.[58] Factors in one study that predicted dehydration with a fluid deficit of at least 5% were at least two of: capillary refill time of >2 seconds, absence of tears, dry mucous membranes, and ill general appearance.[59]

Ayisha's vital signs are normal with the exception of a low-grade fever. Her mouth is dry but she has adequate skin turgor and normal capillary refill. You determine that she is mildly dehydrated. You think that she could drink fluids if the nausea could be controlled but plan to discuss use of IV fluids in the office with your attending.

Do I Need a Diagnostic Test?

Additional testing is based on the suspected cause of the nausea and vomiting; these are listed in Table 11.20. If the problem has been severe or persistent, also evaluate for any complications including malnutrition, electrolyte imbalance, and vitamin deficiencies. Ayisha has only had her symptoms for 1 day and laboratory testing at this time is not likely needed.

Management

Management is based on the cause (Tables 11.21 and 11.22). The following list includes management of the most common conditions, along with the SOR rating. Conditions such as appendicitis, cholecystitis, intracranial cranial disorder, mechanical obstruction, and malignancy likely require referral.

Table 11.21 ▶ Management of Common Causes of Nausea and Vomiting

Condition	Treatment
Infectious/Inflammatory	
Appendicitis, chole-cystitis, pancreatitis	• Treat underlying disorder • Medication to control symptoms (see Table 11.22) • Bowel rest
Gastroenteritis	• Treat symptoms with fluid/medication • If bacterial, antibiotics (SOR A)
Nonulcer dyspepsia	• Antacid or antisecretory therapy (proton-pump inhibitors or H2-receptor antagonists) (SOR A) • Eradicate *H. pylori* if present (SOR C)
Neurologic	
Inner ear disorder	• Avoid head movement • Medication (e.g., meclizine) (SOR B) • Epley maneuver[a] or Cawthorne exercises[b] for BPV (SOR A)
Migraine headache	• See section on headache above
Situational	
Pregnant	• Consider wrist bands, ginger ale or ginger capsules (SOR B) • Pyridoxine/B_6 (25 mg 2–3 times daily) PLUS doxylamine (10 mg daily) (SOR A)
Other	
Cyclic nausea and vomiting	• Avoid triggers when known (SOR C) • Assess and treat for depression, • Anti-nausea medications (Table 11.22)
Eating disorder	• Cognitive behavioral therapy (bulimia nervosa and binge-eating disorder) (SOR B) • Antidepressant (anorexia nervosa) (SOR C)

[a]https://www.youtube.com/watch?v=IlvUbxEoadQ
[b]https://www.youtube.com/watch?v=IdALQB0qQ2I
BPV, benign positional vertigo.

Ayisha is prescribed prochlorperazine per rectum and her father is instructed to administer small amounts of an oral electrolyte solution as tolerated. Her father calls back several hours later to report that she seems better and is able to take small amounts of liquid now. He will follow up if the problem persists.

Table 11.22 ▶ Common Medications That Help Control Nausea and Vomiting

Drug	Dose	Common Side Effects	Comments
Dimenhydrinate (Dramamine)	Oral: 50–100 mg every 4–6 hours (adult); 12.5–25 mg every 6–8 hours (child)	Fatigue, headache, palpitations, blurred vision	
Meclizine (Antivert, Bonine)	Oral: 25 mg up to 4 times daily (adult or child)	Dizziness, drowsiness, rash, swelling, palpitations	

(continued)

Table 11.22 ▶ Common Medications That Help Control Nausea and Vomiting *(Continued)*

Drug	Dose	Common Side Effects	Comments
Metoclopramide (Reglan)	Oral: 10–20 mg before meals and at bedtime	Drowsiness, dystonic/ extrapyramidal symptoms, cardiac abnormalities	Multiple drug interactions
Ondansetron[a] (Zofran)	1.6–4 mg every 8 hours (child)	Headache, fever, palpitations, weakness, dizziness, confusion	Primarily for chemo or postop N/V, multiple drug interactions
Prochlorperazine (Compazine)	Oral: 5–10 mg every 6–8 hours as needed; peds: IM: 5–10 mg every 3–4 hours PR: 25 mg every 12 hours	Drowsy, dizziness, dry mouth, rash, tinnitus, nausea, extrapyramidal reactions	Multiple drug interactions Do not use in children <age 2 years or <9 kg
Promethazine (Phenergan)	Oral, IM, PR: 12.5–25 mg every 4–6 hours as needed	Bleeding (many sites), headache, palpitations	Do not use in children under age 2 years
Scopolamine (Transderm Scop)	Apply patch 4 hours before exposure and every 3 days as needed	Dry mouth, rash, drowsiness, blurred vision, urinary retention	Avoid in narrow angle glaucoma or with potassium use
Trimethobenzamide (Tigan)	Oral: 300 mg every 6–8 hours	Dizziness, drowsiness, extrapyramidal symptoms, depression	

[a]When given as chemo prophylaxis, IV 0.15 mg/kg/dose three times daily.

UPPER RESPIRATORY SYMPTOMS

It is January and you are seeing Molly, a healthy 27-year-old presenting with sore throat. She describes having a low-grade fever (100.3°F), nasal congestion, and a cough with body aches for 4 days. She is here because she is not getting better. People at work are also sick. She did not get a flu shot this year.

Common causes of upper respiratory tract symptoms in primary care are shown in Table 11.23.

Steps in Evaluation

Is this an Emergency?

The primary emergency in (pediatric) patients with URI symptoms is epiglottitis. Suspect epiglottitis if a child is febrile, drooling, looks toxic and has a sore throat.

Another emergency is pneumonia associated with sepsis. Suspect if the patient has cough, fever, and is short of breath and hypoxic or has unstable vital signs.

Secondary (or referred) ear pain comes from an extrinsic source such as the jaw, cranial nerves, or neck; physical examination is often unremarkable. While most secondary ear pain is due to nonemergencies such as dental pain (38%), TMJ disorders (35%), cervical spine pain (8%), and cranial neuralgias (5%),[60] ear pain can be a symptom of myocardial infarction (MI) or temporal arteritis. Suspect MI if the patient has a history of, or risk factors for, coronary artery disease and angina; suspect temporal arteritis in older patients with associated temporal pain and an elevated erythrocyte sedimentation rate.

Table 11.23 ▶ Common Causes of Upper Respiratory Symptoms

Symptom	Cause
Cough	• Allergic rhinitis • Asthma • Bronchiolitis • Bronchitis • GERD • Influenza • Pneumonia • Viral URI
Earache	• Otitis externa • Otitis media • Otitis media with effusion
Nasal congestion	• Allergic rhinitis • Bacterial sinusitis • Foreign body (usually unilateral, purulent nasal discharge; often seen in children) • Influenza • Viral URI
Sore throat	• Epiglottitis • GERD • Group A streptococcal infection • Influenza • Infectious mononucleosis • Peritonsillar abscess • Viral pharyngitis • Vocal strain

GERD, gastroesophageal reflux disorder; URI, upper respiratory tract infection.

Are there Other Red Flags for Serious Conditions?

 Clues or "red flags" indicating a serious condition in patients with URI symptoms:

▶ Severe sore throat with uvula deviation (peritonsillar abscess)

▶ Increased breathing effort, including use of accessory muscles (https://www.youtube.com/watch?v=bzV1C44IPBc) (impending respiratory failure)

▶ Silent, diminished, or unilateral breath sounds (pneumonia, pneumothorax, foreign body)

▶ Difficulty swallowing, with stridor (epiglottis)

▶ Long-duration of hoarseness (laryngeal cancer or vocal cord nodule)

▶ Long-duration cough or hemoptysis (lung cancer, tuberculosis)

▶ High fever (>101°F) in a child (sepsis, meningitis)

▶ Seventh cranial nerve palsy, diabetes, immunocompromised, unilateral hearing loss (malignant otitis externa)

▶ Mastoid process tenderness (mastoiditis)

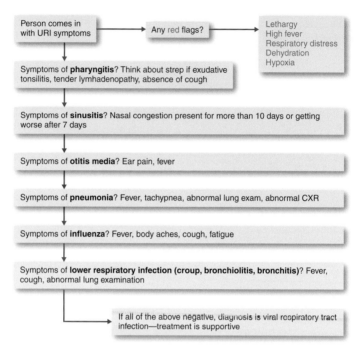

Figure 11.12 ▶ Approach to a person with respiratory symptoms.

Pneumonia and influenza can also be serious, especially in an older person. Molly is a young person primarily at the office because of persistent symptoms, not severe ones, so pneumonia is unlikely. The diagnostic approach shown in Figure 11.12 can help you to determine whether these conditions are present.

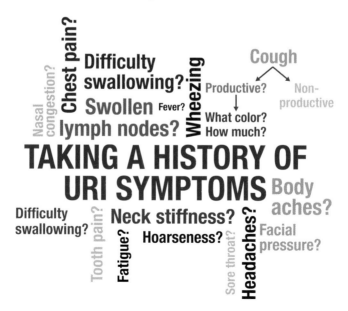

Do I Need a Diagnostic Test?

Decision rules can be helpful in determining the likelihood of a particular diagnosis and whether to perform a diagnostic test. Examples below are the Centor score for group A β-hemolytic strep (GABS) and the Heckerling clinical decision tool for community-acquired pneumonia.

On examination, Molly has some tender cervical lymph nodes and her tonsils are erythematous, mildly swollen, with no exudate. Her lungs are clear. Your differential includes viral URI, influenza, and strep pharyngitis.
    You calculate a Centor score of 1, so her likelihood of having strep pharyngitis is 5% to 10%. You do not do a rapid strep antigen screen. You quickly check the CDC website for the prevalence of influenza in your area and it is very low. You diagnose Molly with a viral URI, recommend supportive therapy, and ask her to call back if she is no better in 3 to 5 days.

Centor Score for determining likelihood GABS infection vs. viral pharyngitis

▶ +1 Point for age 3–14 years

▶ −1 point for age >45 years

▶ +1 point for exudative tonsillitis

▶ +1 point for tender cervical lymphadenopathy

▶ +1 point for absence of cough

Probability of GBBS is calculated based on score. https://www.mdcalc.com/centor-score-modified-mcisaac-strep-pharyngitis

---

Molly comes back the following week; her mother is also here for her own appointment. Molly's fevers, body aches, and sore throat have resolved, but she continues to have nasal congestion and facial pain. Her examination is normal except for edematous and erythematous nasal turbinates with purulent nasal discharge.

About one in eight adults in the United States are diagnosed with sinusitis annually (~30 million cases per year). Acute bacterial sinusitis is diagnosed as follows[62,63]:

▶ Symptoms: purulent nasal drainage, nasal obstruction, facial pain or fullness, and fever

▶ Symptoms lasting for over 10 days with no improvement (for up to 10 days, consider viral sinusitis more likely)

▶ Subacute sinusitis: symptoms >4 weeks but <12 weeks

▶ Chronic sinusitis: symptoms last >12 weeks

Molly has now been sick for 12 days. You diagnose her with acute bacterial sinusitis and recommend a course of amoxicillin. She calls back the following week to let you know that she is finally better.
    Molly's mother, Heather is next on your schedule. She got sick at the same time as Molly. She has persistent cough and intermittent fevers. She is 53 years old, healthy and a nonsmoker. She has a temperature of 100.2°F, crackles in her right lower lung, and decreased breath sounds. You suspect community-acquired pneumonia (CAP) and use the Heckerling Clinical Decision Tool to help determine the likelihood of CAP.

Heckerling Clinical Decision Tool for community-acquired pneumonia in adults

► 1 point for each of the following: temperature >100°F, presence of asthma, pulse over 100 beats per minute, crackles, decreased breath sounds

► Likelihood of pneumonia increases with increasing points. A score of 5 is associated with a 47% likelihood of diagnosing pneumonia in a primary care visit.

https://www.easycalculation.com/medical/pneumonia-clinical-prediction-heckerling.php

Heather has a Heckerling score of 3 which signifies a 27% likelihood that she has pneumonia. You decide to treat her with outpatient antibiotics with a macrolide (http://www.thoracic.org/statements/resources/mtpi/idsaats-cap.pdf). She recovers uneventfully.

Eighty-five percent of cases of community acquired pneumonia are caused by **streptococcus pneumonia**, **Haemophilus influenza**, or **Moraxella catarrhalis**. Table 11.24 reviews common causes of URI symptoms, potential tests, and treatments.

Management

Initial treatment for common causes of URI are shown in Table 11.24. With respect to earache, it is important to distinguish between acute otitis media (AOM) and otitis media with effusion (OME) (Table 11.25). OME may last for months and is often mistaken for AOM, leading to unnecessary prescription of antibiotics.[64] OME can cause damage to the TM

Table 11.24 ► Common Causes of URI Symptoms with Key Features, Diagnostic Tests and Treatment

Common Cause	Key Features	Diagnostic Test	Treatment
Bacterial sinusitis	Nasal congestion, purulent nasal discharge, symptoms for more than 10 days or getting worse after 7 days	Physical examination	Antibiotics. First-line includes amoxicillin, amoxicillin/clavulanate
Bronchitis	Cough, possibly other URI symptoms	Physical examination	Inhalers
Influenza	Fever, cough, body aches, fatigue, sore throat	Influenza rapid antigen test, knowledge of local prevalence	Antiviral treatment if present within 72 hours of symptoms, otherwise supportive care
Otitis media	Ear pain, URI symptoms	Physical examination, pneumatoscopy[a]	Watchful waiting for children over age 2 years with uncomplicated unilateral acute otitis media, antibiotics, tympanostomy tubes[b]
Pneumonia	Fever, cough, abnormal lung examination	CXR	Antibiotics: First-line includes azithromycin, clarithromycin, doxycycline; consider levofloxacin, moxifloxacin, or Augmentin if comorbidities
Strep pharyngitis	Sore throat, exudative tonsillitis, tender cervical lymph nodes, absence of cough	Centor score, rapid strep antigen test or strep culture	Antibiotics: First-line includes PCN amoxicillin, cephalexin, azithromycin, or clindamycin (if PCN allergic)

Common Cause	Key Features	Diagnostic Test	Treatment
Viral URI	Cough, nasal congestion, sore throat, low-grade fever	None; diagnosis of exclusion	Supportive care, nonprescription remedies for adults

[a]Pneumatoscopy is pneumatic insufflation of the ear to determine TM mobility and improve accuracy of diagnosis of otitis media or effusion (Ely JW, Hansen MR, Clark EC. Diagnosis of ear pain. *Am Fam Physician.* 2008;77(5):621–628).
[b]Tympanostomy tubes are indicated in children with acute otitis with >3 episodes within 6 months, >4 episodes within 12 months, recurrence on antibiotic prophylaxis or multiple drug allergies, and in children with otitis media with effusion who have acute or threatened hearing loss, structural damage to the tympanic membrane; persistent effusion (>3 months bilateral or >6 months unilateral; or associated symptoms of vertigo, ear pain or tinnitus).
CXR, chest x-ray; PCN, penicillin; URI, upper respiratory tract infection.
Data from: Aring AM, Chan MM. Current concepts in adult acute rhinosinusitis. *Am Fam Physician.* 2016;94(2):97–105; Kalra MG, Higgins KE, Perez, ED. Common questions about streptococcal pharyngitis. *Am Fam Physician.* 2016;94(1):24–31; Rosenfeld RM, Piccirillo JF, Chandrasekhar SS, et al. Clinical practice guideline (update): adult sinusitis executive summary. *Otolaryngol Head Neck Surg.* 2015;152(4):598–609.

as well as language delay in preverbal children; if diagnosed, serial observation to ensure proper speech development and TM appearance is necessary.

If initial treatment fails, the patient is encouraged to return for reassessment. Cough, however, can last several weeks and is not of concern unless the symptoms are worse or the cough is productive (mucus).

Influenza

Those at higher risk of influenza complications for whom antiviral treatment might be indicated are listed in Box 11.2. Antiviral treatment is only effective if it is started within 72 hours of symptom onset. It shortens the course and lessens the severity of the influenza infection. Antivirals for influenza are displayed in Table 11.26.

Table 11.25 ▶ Features of Acute Otitis Media (AOM) and Otitis Media with Effusion (OME)

AOM	OME	Cholesteatoma
• Moderate–severe TM bulging • Mild TM bulging with pain <48 hours • New otorrhea not from otitis externa • Pain, irritability and fever (child)	• Often follows AOM • Mild hearing loss • Absence of signs of acute illness • Air/fluid level, bubbles or cloudy TM	• Abnormal skin growth in middle ear • Can follow infections • No symptoms; hearing loss occurs with time

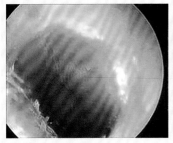 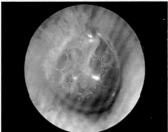 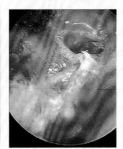

Acute otitis media in the left ear of a 15-month-old patient with marked erythema and bulging of the tympanic membrane. The malleus and light reflex are not visible.[a]

Otitis media with effusion (OME) in the right ear. Note multiple air–fluid levels in this slightly retracted, translucent, nonerythematous tympanic membrane.[b]

Primary acquired cholesteatoma with debris removed from the attic retraction pocket.[a]

Images courtesy of William Clark, MD[a] and Frank Miller, MD[b]

BOX 11.2 PERSONS WITH SUSPECTED INFLUENZA RECOMMENDED FOR ANTIVIRAL TREATMENT

▶ Children aged <2 years

▶ Adults aged 65 years and older

▶ Persons with chronic illness[a]

▶ Persons with immunosuppression, including that caused by medications or by HIV infection

▶ Pregnant women or postpartum (within 2 weeks after delivery)

▶ Persons aged <19 years who are receiving long-term aspirin therapy

▶ American Indians/Alaska Natives

▶ Persons who are morbidly obese (body mass index 40 or more)

▶ Residents of nursing homes and other chronic care facilities

[a]Illnesses include pulmonary (including asthma), cardiovascular (except hypertension alone), renal, hepatic, hematologic (including sickle cell disease), and metabolic disorders (including diabetes mellitus), or neurologic and neurodevelopment conditions (including disorders of the brain, spinal cord, peripheral nerve, and muscle, such as cerebral palsy, epilepsy [seizure disorders], stroke, intellectual disability [mental retardation], moderate to severe developmental delay, muscular dystrophy, or spinal cord injury) Data from Erlikh IV, Abraham S, Kondamudi VK. Management of influenza. *Am Fam Physician*. 2010;82(9): 1087–1095.

Important sites to check about influenza:

▶ **General Information:** http://www.cdc.gov/flu/professionals/index.htm

▶ **Epidemiology:** State health department, CDC (http://www.cdc.gov/flu/), or WHO (http://www.who.int/influenza/surveillance_monitoring/en/) for information on prevalence of influenza, types, and match with vaccines.

▶ The CDC compiles a **weekly flu** report that covers positive tests, hospitalizations, and state by state information (http://www.cdc.gov/flu/weekly/).

▶ **Vaccine recommendations:** new recommendations advise AGAINST using nasal immunization (http://www.cdc.gov/flu/about/season/flu-season-2016-2017.htm)

Table 11.26 ▶ Antiviral Agents for Influenza

Antiviral Agent	Activity Against	Use	Recommended For	Not Recommended For
Oseltamivir (Tamiflu)	Influenza A & B	Treatment Chemoprophylaxis	Any age Over age 3 months	NA
Zanamivir (Relenza)	Influenza A & B	Treatment Chemoprophylaxis	7 years and older 5 years and older	People with underlying respiratory disease (e.g., COPD)
Peramivir (Rapivab)	Influenza A & B	Treatment Chemoprophylaxis	18 years and older NA	NA

Data from: Centers for Disease Control and Prevention: Influenza Antiviral Medications: Summary for Clinicians, http://www.cdc.gov/flu/professionals/antivirals/summary-clinicians.htm.

As part of treatment decisions, you need to decide when a patient requires **hospitalization**. In addition to looking for clues of a serious illness, listed above, you can use a decision tool to help access condition severity, such as CURB-65.[65]

Your patient has pneumonia. Should you admit them?

CURB-65 severity scale (http://www.mdcalc.com/curb-65-severity-score-community-acquired-pneumonia/)

▶ Uses a combination of factors to determine whether inpatient treatment is required:

▶ Confusion

▶ BUN >19 mg/dL

▶ RR >30 breaths per minute

▶ SBP <90 mm Hg or DBP <60 mm Hg

▶ Age >65 years

QUESTIONS

1. Which one of the following should occur early in the visit with a patient with an acute medical problem?
   A. Solicit a complete history, including a family and social history.
   B. Perform a complete physical examination.
   C. Determine whether the problem is an emergency.
   D. Determine whether you need to order a laboratory test based on the differential diagnosis.
   E. Check to see if there is a relevant guideline about the problem.

2. You are seeing a 3-year-old child with an earache. Based on your evaluation, you have decided that he has an acute ear infection. Which one of the following is true of providing treatment for this patient?
   A. Prescribe antibiotics.
   B. Recommend watchful waiting before prescribing antibiotics.
   C. List the possible treatment options and have the parent choose one.
   D. Provide information about the diagnosis and engage the parent in the treatment decision.

3. You are seeing a 48-year-old woman with abdominal pain. You determine that she does not have an acute abdomen. Her pain is localized to the left lower quadrant. Her bladder and bowel habits have been normal. A pregnancy test is negative. Which one of the following is the likely cause of her pain?
   A. Diverticulitis
   B. Peptic ulcer disease
   C. Nephrolithiasis
   D. Cholecystitis
   E. Celiac disease

4. Which one of the following should be the first test to perform in an adult patient presenting to the office with acute dyspnea and stable vital signs?
   A. Pulse oximetry
   B. Spirometry

C. Electrocardiogram

D. Chest X-ray

5. You are seeing a 58-year-old woman with chest pain occurring with exercise. She has a history of hypertension but is otherwise well. Her examination is normal with no chest pain to palpation. She scores 2 points (not low probability of cardiac etiology) on a chest pain decision rule. An office electrocardiogram is normal. Which one of the following is the suggested management?

A. Reassurance and monitoring

B. Order a stress test

C. Provide nitroglycerin and obtain serial markers

D. Refer her to a cardiologist for invasive testing

E. Manage her for cardiac ischemia with a nitrate and beta blocker

6. You are seeing a 48-year-old man who you diagnose with benign positional paroxysmal vertigo based on his history and a positive Dix–Hallpike maneuver. Which one of the following is the suggested treatment?

A. Physical therapy for balance training

B. Supportive care and the Epley maneuver

C. An antiviral medication

D. A diuretic

E. A beta-blocker

7. A 28-year-old woman calls the office and reports that she has had dysuria and urinary frequency for the past 12 hours. She has no known medical problems but has had one urinary tract infection (UTI) 2 years ago. She is not febrile and has no vaginal symptoms. Which one of the following is true regarding management of this patient's likely UTI?

A. She should come to the office for evaluation.

B. She should start cranberry juice.

C. She should bring in a urine sample to confirm UTI.

D. She should be treated for a presumptive urinary tract infection.

E. She should be screened for sexually-transmitted infections before UTI treatment.

8. Which one of the following is a "red flag" sign for sepsis in an adult patient presenting with fever?

A. Excessive thirst

B. Meningeal signs

C. High temperature (above 103°F) alone

D. Drowsiness

E. Bradycardia

9. You are seeing an elderly man in the office with anemia. He reports no pain or other symptoms. He does not currently smoke or drink alcohol. His stool is positive for occult blood but rectal examination is normal. Which one of the following is the likely etiology of gastrointestinal bleeding in this patient?

A. Gastric cancer

B. Esophageal varices

C. Hemorrhoids

D. Vascular ectasia

E. Colitis

10. Which one of the following is true of headaches (HA)?
    A. The four types of primary HAs are migraine, tension, cluster and chronic daily HA.
    B. Withdrawal HA is one of the HA emergencies.
    C. Risk factors for chronic daily HA include being male and alcohol consumption.
    D. A head CT should be ordered for a patient with new onset headache.
    E. Amitriptyline is helpful for cluster headaches.

11. Which one of the following would make you consider a venous thromboembolism in a patient with leg swelling?
    A. Unilateral with painful erythema and fever.
    B. Unilateral, acute, with history of leg trauma.
    C. Decreased hair growth and history of trauma.
    D. Tenderness and bruising behind the knee.

12. Which one of the following should be considered in a patient with nausea and vomiting due to pancreatitis?
    A. Obtain liver function tests to confirm.
    B. Provide a proton pump inhibitor.
    C. Provide antibiotics.
    D. Provide bowel rest and medication for symptom control.

13. You are seeing a 6-year-old girl in the emergency room with a 2-day history of upper respiratory symptoms. Which one of the following should lead you to believe that this is an emergency and not just a respiratory tract infection?
    A. The child's temperature is 103°F.
    B. The child is drooling.
    C. The child has bilateral ear pain with drainage.
    D. The child has a barking cough.
    E. The child is wheezing.

ANSWERS

Question 1: The correct answer is C.
Key point 3. Early in the visit, determine whether the problem is an emergency using the patient's story, signs and symptoms; if so, alert the attending. Once you have enough history to begin formulating a differential diagnosis, you should determine whether the problem is an emergency.

Question 2: The correct answer is D.
Most patients prefer to be informed about their diagnosis (or likely diagnosis) and engaged in decisions about testing and treatment. Shared decision-making, which includes making the decision explicit and providing information about treatment or screening options and their associated outcomes, increases patient knowledge and confidence about their decision, and, in many situations, informed patients elect more conservative treatment options.

Question 3: The correct answer is A.
In a woman who is not pregnant and has no urinary symptoms, consider diverticulitis as the source of left lower quadrant pain.

Question 4: The correct answer is A.
Office-based workup for shortness of breath is straightforward and driven by the acuity of the patient presentation. All patients should have vital signs obtained, including pulse oximetry.

Question 5: The correct answer is B.

Table 11.7 and Figure 11.5. If a patient has 2 to 3 points on the decision rule for chest pain from ischemia and normal or nonspecific changes on ECG, discuss evaluation, troponin, or stress testing. (From the figure, when your evaluation suggests coronary artery disease, obtain graded exercise testing or its equivalent.)

Question 6: The correct answer is B.

Table 11.10. For patients with benign positional paroxysmal vertigo, provide supportive care (assess fall risk, home support, CNS disorders and impaired mobility or balance), teach the Epley maneuver and offer an antiemetic drug.

Question 7: The correct answer is D.

Figure 11.7. For a woman with dysuria, no vaginal symptoms and a prior history of a UTI, treat for UTI if her symptoms are typical of uncomplicated UTI.

Question 8: The correct answer is B.

Other Red Flags for possible sepsis in an adult patient include febrile neutropenia (fever plus absolute neutrophil count, ANC, <500 per mm³), meningeal signs (Kernig sign and Brudzinski sign), and Systemic Inflammatory Response System or Sepsis syndrome present.

Question 9: The correct answer is D.

Table 11.3. In a patient with anemia and painless chronic lower gastrointestinal bleeding, consider vascular ectasia. Obtain colonoscopy and possibly a radionuclide scan or angiography.

Question 10: The correct answer is A.

Table 11.15. HAs are divided into primary, secondary, and a third category of "cranial neuralgias, central and primary facial pain, and other headaches." The four types of primary HAs are migraine, tension, cluster, and chronic daily HA.

Question 11: The correct answer is B.

Table 11.19. Consider deep vein thrombosis in a patient with unilateral leg edema that is usually acute, painful, with associated erythema, and risk factors.

Question 12: The correct answer is D.

Table 11.21. Management of patients with appendicitis, cholecystitis, or pancreatitis include treating the underlying disorder, medication for symptoms, and bowel rest.

Question 13: The correct answer is B.

The primary emergency in (pediatric) patients with URI symptoms is epiglottitis. Suspect epiglottitis if a child is febrile, drooling, looks toxic, and has a sore throat.

REFERENCES

1. Rhoades DR, McFarland KF, Finch WH, et al. Speaking and interruptions during primary care office visits. *Fam Med.* 2001;33(7):528–532.
2. Baker LH, O'Connell D, Platt FW. What else? Setting the agenda for the clinical interview. *Ann Intern Med.* 2005;143(10):766–770.
3. National Ambulatory Medical Care Survey. State and National Summary Tables. Table 11. Based on A Reason for Visit Classification for Ambulatory Care (RVC) defined in the 2012 National Ambulatory Medical care Survey Public Use Data File documentation. 2012. Available from: ftp://ftp.cdc.gov/pub/Health_Statistics/NCHS/Dataset_Documentation/NAMCS/doc2012.pdf. Accessed August 15, 2016.
4. Nelson HD, Cantor A, Humphrey L, et al. Screening for Breast Cancer: A Systematic Review to Update the 2009 U.S. Preventive Services Task Force Recommendation [Internet]. Rockville (MD): Agency for Healthcare Research and Quality (US); 2016 Jan. Report No.: 14-05201-EF-1. Available from: U.S. Preventive Services Task Force Evidence Syntheses, formerly Systematic Evidence Reviews. Accessed August 15, 2016.

5. James Pa, Oparil S, Carter BL, et al. 2014 evidence-based guideline for the management of high blood pressure in adults. Report from the panel members appointed to the eighth Joint National Committee (JNC 8). *JAMA*. 2014;311(5):507–520.

6. Stacey D, Légaré F, Col NF, et al. Decision aids for people facing health treatment or screening decisions. *Cochrane Database Syst Rev*. 2014;(1):CD001431.

7. Elwyn G, Frosch D, Thomson R, et al. Shared decision making: a model for clinical practice. *J Gen Intern Med*. 2012;27(10):1361–1367.

8. Health Quality Ontario. Women's Experiences of Inaccurate Breast Cancer Screening Results: A Systematic Review and Qualitative Meta-synthesis. *Ont Health Technol Assess Ser*. 2016;16(16):1–22.

9. Roskos SE. Abdominal pain (adult). *Essential Evidence Plus*. Updated April 19, 2016. Available from: http://www.essentialevidenceplus.com.ezproxy.library.wisc.edu/content/eee/162. Accessed August 15, 2016.

10. Viniol A, Keunecke C, Biroga T, et al. Studies of the symptom abdominal pain—a systematic review and meta-analysis. *J Fam Pract*. 2014;31:517–529.

11. Leung AK, Sigalet DL. Acute abdominal pain in children. *Am Fam Physician*. 2003;67(11):2321–2326.

12. Parshall MB, Schwartzstein RM, Adams L, et al., American Thoracic Society Committee on Dyspnea. An official American Thoracic Society statement: update on the mechanisms, assessment, and management of dyspnea. *Am J Respir Crit Care Med*. 2012;185(4):435–452.

13. Canto JG, Rogers WJ, Goldberg RJ, et al. Association of age and sex with myocardial infarction symptom presentation and in-hospital mortality. *JAMA*. 2012;307(8):813–822.

14. Kline JA, Courtney DM, Kabrhel C, et al. Prospective multicenter evaluation of the pulmonary embolism rule-out criteria. *J Thromb Haemost*. 2008;6(5):772–780.

15. Albert RH. Diagnosis and treatment of acute bronchitis. *Am Fam Physician*. 2010;82(11):1345–1350.

16. Evensen AE. Management of COPD exacerbations. *Am Fam Physician*. 2010;81(5):607–613.

17. Ramzi DW, Leeper KV. DVT and pulmonary embolism: Part II. Treatment and prevention. *Am Fam Physician*. 2004;69(12):2841–2848.

18. Chavey WE, Bleske BE, Van Harrison R, et al. Pharmacologic management of heart failure caused by systolic dysfunction. *Am Fam Physician*. 2008;77(7):957–964.

19. Zoorob R, Sidani M, Murray J. Croup: an overview. *Am Fam Physician*. 2011;83(9):1067–1073.

20. Fashner J, Ericson K, Werner S. Treatment of the common cold in children and adults. *Am Fam Physician*. 2012;86(2):153–159.

21. McConaghy JR, Oza RS. Outpatient diagnosis of acute chest pain in adults. *Am Fam Physician*. 2013;87(3):177–182.

22. Post RE, Dickerson LM. Dizziness: a diagnostic approach. *Am Fam Physician*. 2010;82(4):361–368.

23. Labuguen RH. Initial evaluation of vertigo. *Am Fam Physician*. 2006;73:244–251, 254.

24. Michels TC, Sands JE. Dysuria: evaluation and differential diagnosis in adults. *Am Fam Physician*. 2015;92(9):778–786.

25. Stark H. Urinary tract infections in girls: the cost-effectiveness of currently recommended investigative routines. *Pediatr Nephrol*. 1997;11(2):174–177; discussion 180–181

26. Brent S, Nallamothu BK, Simel DL, et al. Does this woman have an acute uncomplicated urinary tract infection? *JAMA*. 2002;287(20):2701–2710.

27. Guralnick ML, O'Connor RC, See WA. Assessment and management of irritative voiding symptoms. *Med Clin North Am*. 2011;95(1):121–127.

28. Arnold J, McLead N, Thani-Gasalam R, et al. Overactive bladder syndrome. *Am Fam Physician*. 2012;41(11):878–883.

29. Dinarello CA. Thermoregulation and the pathogenesis of fever. *Infect Dis Clin North Am*. 1996;10:433–449.

30. Stevceva L. Fever of unknown origin. *Essential Evidence Plus*. Updated May 26, 2016. Available from: http://www.essentialevidenceplus.com.ezproxy.library.wisc.edu/content/eee/308. Accessed September 4, 2016.

31. Allen CH. Fever without a source in children 3 to 36 months of age. *UpToDate*. Updated Feb 2, 2016. Available from: https://www-uptodate-com.ezproxy.library.wisc.edu/contents/fever-without-a-source-in-children-3-to-36-months-of-age?source=search_result&search=fever±without±a±soucre&selectedTitle=1~150. Accessed September 4, 2016.

32. Levy MM, Fink MP, Marshall JC, et al. 2001 SCCM/ESICM/ACCP/ATS/SIS. International Sepsis Definitions Conference. *Crit Care Med*. 2003;31:1250–1256.

33. Jaimes F, Garces J, Cuervo J, et al. The systemic inflammatory response syndrome (SIRS) to identify infected patients in the emergency room. *Intensive Care Med*. 2003;29:1368–1371.

34. Singer M, Deutschman CS, Seymour CW, et al. The third international consensus definitions for sepsis and septic shock (Sepsis-3). *JAMA*. 2016;315(8):801–810.

35. Seymour CW, Liu VX, Iwashyna TJ, et al. Assessment of clinical criteria for sepsis (Sepsis-3). *JAMA*. 2016;315(8):762–774.

36. Shankar-Hari M, Phillips GS, Levy ML, et al. Developing a new definition and assessing new clinical criteria for septic shock (Sepsis-3). *JAMA*. 2016;315(8):775–787.

37. Van den Bruel A, Haj-Hassan T, Thompson M, et al; European Research Network on Recognising Serious Infection Investigators. Diagnostic value of clinical features at presentation to identify serious infection in children in developed countries: a systematic review. *Lancet*. 2010;375(9717):834–845.

38. Higdon ML, Higdon JA. Treatment of oncologic emergencies. *Am Fam Physician*. 2006; 74(11):1873–1880.

39. Viscoli C. The evolution of the empirical management of fever and neutropenia in cancer patients. *J Antimicrob Chemother*. 1998;41(suppl D):S65–S80.

40. Bleeker-Rovers CP, Vos FJ, de Kleijn EM, et al. A prospective multicenter study on fever of unknown origin: the yield of a structured diagnostic protocol. *Medicine (Baltimore)*. 2007;86(1):26–38.

41. Erlikh IV, Abraham S, Kondamudi VK. Management of influenza. *Am Fam Physician*. 2010;82(9):1087–1095.

42. Ables AZ, Nagubilli R. Prevention, recognition, and management of serotonin syndrome. *Am Fam Physician*. 2010;81(9):1139–1142.

43. Contratto EC, Jennings MS. Gastrointestinal bleeding. In: Smith MA, Shimp LA, Schrager S (eds). *Lange Family Medicine Ambulatory Care and Practice*. 6th ed. New York: McGraw Hill; 2014.

44. Gluud LL, Krag A. Banding ligation versus beta-blockers for primary prevention in esophageal varices in adults. *Cochrane Database Syst Rev*. 2012;(8):CD004522.

45. Wilkins T, Baird C, Pearson AN, et al. Diverticular bleeding. *Am Fam Physician*. 2009; 80(9):977–983.

46. Alonso-Coello P, Guyatt G, Heels-Ansdell D, et al. Laxatives for the treatment of hemorrhoids. *Cochrane Database Syst Rev*. 2005(4):CD004649.

47. Burch RC, Loder S, Loder E, et al. The prevalence and burden of migraine and severe headache in the United States: updated statistics from government health surveillance studies. *Headache*. 2015;55(2):356.

48. Robbins MS, Lipton RB. The epidemiology of primary headache disorders. *Sem Neurol*. 2010; 30(2):107–119.

49. American College of Radiology Appropriateness Criteria (Neurologic: Headache). Available from: https://acsearch.acr.org/list. Accessed September 2016.

50. Aygun D, Bildik F. Clinical warning criteria in evaluation by computed tomography the secondary neurological headaches in adults. *Eur J Neurol*. 2003;10(4):437–442.

51. Linde K, Allais G, Brinkhaus B, et al. Acupuncture for the prevention of episodic migraine. *Cochrane Database Syst Rev*. 2016;(6):CD001218.

52. Ely JW, Osheroff JA, Chambliss ML, et al. Approach to leg edema of unclear etiology. *J Am Board Fam Med*. 2006;19(2):148–160.

53. Wilbur J, Shian B. Diagnosis of deep venous thrombosis and pulmonary embolism. *Am Fam Physician*. 2012;86(10):913–919.

54. Qaseem A, Snow V, Barry P, et al. Current diagnosis of venous thromboembolism in primary care: a clinical practice guideline from the American Academy of Family Physicians and the American College of Physicians. *Ann Fam Med*. 2007;5:57–62.

55. Lacroix R, Eason E, Melzack R. Nausea and vomiting during pregnancy: A prospective study of its frequency, intensity, and patterns of change. *Am J Obstet Gynecol*. 2000;182:931–937.

56. Naeim A, Dy SM, Lorenz KA, et al. Evidence-based recommendations for cancer nausea and vomiting. *J Clin Oncol*. 2008;26(23):3903–3910.

57. Pitts SR, Niska RW, Xu J, et al. National hospital ambulatory medical care survey: 2006 Emergency department summary. *Natl Health Stat Report*. 2008;7:1–38.

58. Canavan A, Arant BS. Diagnosis and management of dehydration in children. *Am Fam Physician*. 2009;80(7):692–696.

59. Gorelick MH, Shaw KN, Murphy KO. Validity and reliability of clinical signs in the diagnosis of dehydration in children. *Pediatrics*. 1997;99(5):E6.

60. Leung AK, Fong JH, Leong AG. Otalgia in children. *J Natl Med Assoc*. 2000;92(5):254–260.

61. Harmes KM, Blackwood RA, Burrows HL, et al. Otitis media: diagnosis and treatment. *Am Fam Physician*. 2013;88(7):435–440.

62. Aring AM, Chan MM. Current concepts in adult acute rhinosinusitis. *Am Fam Physician*. 2016;94(2):97–105.

63. Rosenfeld RM, Piccirillo JF, Chandrasekhar SS, et al. Clinical practice guideline (update): adult sinusitis executive summary. *Otolaryngology, Head and Neck Surg*. 2015;152(4):598–609.

64. Harmes KM, Blackwood RA, Burrows HL, et al. Otitis media: diagnosis and treatment. *Am Fam Physician*. 2013;88(7):435–440.

65. Ebell MH. Predicting pneumonia in adults with respiratory illness. *Am Fam Physician*. 2007;76(4):560–562.

Approach to Common Chronic Problems

KEY POINTS

1 ▶ The chronic care model espouses a multidisciplinary approach to care that includes community resources as well as self-management training for patients to efficiently manage chronic disease.

2 ▶ Asthma management focuses on reducing impairment and risk by managing symptoms with short- and long-acting medications, reducing risk factors, and using tools to reduce serious exacerbations.

3 ▶ Diagnose chronic obstructive pulmonary disease with spirometry and treat based on GOLD group—considering symptoms, exacerbation frequency, and severity.

4 ▶ Reduce mortality of coronary artery disease with ACE-inhibitors, aspirin, beta blockers, statins, smoking cessation, influenza vaccination, and management of diabetes and hypertension.

5 ▶ Diabetes treatment goals are to prevent hyper and hypoglycemia and reduce complications by controlling risk factors and comorbidities.

6 ▶ Heart failure treatment aims to improve quality of life by preventing hospitalizations through symptom management, diet and exercise, and prevent progression through mitigating comorbid conditions and smoking cessation.

7 ▶ Hyperlipidemia treatment is based on 10-year risk of an acute cardiovascular event; low-density lipid levels are directly related to atherosclerotic cardiovascular disease (ASCVD) risk.

8 ▶ Hypertension is a major risk factor for ASCVD and is initially treated with diuretics and ACE-inhibitors for most, and diuretics and calcium channel blockers for African American patients.

9 ▶ Screen patients with obesity for comorbid conditions such as hypertension and discuss diet and exercise; offer medication or surgery to those with comorbid conditions or treatment.

10 ▶ All women should be screened for osteoporosis at age 65 years with a treatment goal of preventing hip fracture.

Ms. Potts is a 57-year-old woman with diabetes, hypertension (HTN), and hyperlipidemia. She is obese with a BMI of 36. She presents today to talk about management. She is currently on metformin 2,500 mg daily for her diabetes. You introduce yourself as a medical student who wants to talk about her diabetes. When asked if she monitors her blood sugar, she tells you that her glucose monitor broke and the test strips are expensive. She is a former smoker.

THE CHRONIC CARE MODEL

Taking care of people with chronic disease is an important task in primary care. What happens in the clinic with the provider, however, is only a small part of successful chronic disease management. In your brief interview with Ms. Potts, you have already discovered that she has multiple, related medical problems, she has no means to monitor her diabetes, she was able to quit smoking, and she has difficulty with expenses.

Facts About Chronic Diseases[1]:

▶ About 90% of people over age 65 years have at least one chronic illness

▶ Chronic illness care accounts for almost three-fourths of all healthcare expenditures annually in the United States

▶ Primary care providers do not have adequate time or infrastructure to manage all chronic illness

▶ Seven of the top 10 causes of death are related to chronic diseases

▶ About one in four people with a chronic disease has a daily activity limitation

---

The chronic care model provides a guide for healthcare organizations to use a multidisciplinary approach that includes community resources as well as self-management training for patients to efficiently manage chronic disease. Table 12.1 shows the six different aspects of successful chronic disease care.[1]

GENERAL APPROACH TO A VISIT FOR A CHRONIC PROBLEM

Before seeing the patient, it is helpful to review the medical record for information about the patient, their medications, history of the disorder, recent management plan or laboratory data, and any evidence of disease (e.g., hemoglobin A1C for diabetes, diabetic neuropathy), complicating factors (e.g., blood pressure [BP]), or symptom control (e.g., hypoglycemic episodes) (Chapter 4).[2] In your review of Ms. Pott's vital signs, her BP is well controlled at 124/78 mm Hg but she has gained 10 lb in the last 6 months. Her last HgA1c was 8.6 and her cholesterol is elevated. Use the information on introductions, listening, and agenda setting from Chapter 11, Part 1 to begin the visit.

Greeting (see Chapter 11, Part 1) and History Taking

What is Included in a Chronic Disease Follow-up Visit?

History

▶ Assessment of **how the patient is doing** today, both physically and emotionally. How does their disease affect their daily life?

▶ Obtain **relevant disease history:** duration, how it was diagnosed, prior treatments

▶ Review any **self-monitoring** data (e.g., home glucose monitoring)

▶ Review **medications** (side effects, adherence; see below)

▶ If the patient is not taking all prescribed medications, ask why (e.g., cost, side effects, fear of long-term effects)

▶ Are medication refills needed?

▶ Review disease control with the patient (e.g., hemoglobin A1C)

▶ Ask about any visits with other health providers/specialists.

▶ Review **schedule of testing**

Physical Examination

▶ How much to do? Usually related to the disease process

▶ For example, in someone with hypertension, listen to the heart and lungs, check for carotid bruits, and look at retinas. In someone with diabetes, check feet due to risk for neuropathy

Do you check your blood sugars?
Let's look at them today.
How does diabetes affect your life?

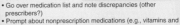

Medication Review

• Review any medications brought in
• Ask about dose, missed or fewer doses to reduce cost, and when meds are taken
• Ask about medication concerns/effectiveness
• Go over medication list and note discrepancies (other prescribers?)
• Prompt about nonprescription medications (e.g., vitamins and supplements are not always considered "medications")
• Check for any potential drug interactions

Table 12.1 ▶ Aspects of Successful Chronic Disease Management

Healthcare Organizations

• Priority of chronic disease management within the organization and payers
• Reimbursement environment supportive of chronic disease care and management
• Awards for chronic care quality
• Support for team-based care

Decision Support

• Evidence-based clinical practice guidelines available and optimally integrated into daily care
• Specialty support via phone or electronic consults
• Physician champions supporting practice teams in following of clinical guidelines

Delivery System Redesign

• Redesign of primary-care practice
• Practice teams with specific duties
• Attempt to separate acute care from chronic disease care
• Support of nonphysician staff to support patient self-management of disease
• Routine laboratory orders
• Scheduled, regular visits

Clinical Information Systems

• Electronic reminders to help clinical teams follow practice guidelines
• Electronic feedback to physicians informing them about their practice outcomes
• Registries to keep track of all patients with chronic diseases, which can help at the individual and population levels

Self-management Support

• Empower patients and their families to participate in the management of their chronic disease
• Provide tools to help patients manage their disease and referrals to community resources

Ms. Potts tells you that she is unable to afford healthy food so she has been going to the food pantry and most of the food there is heavy on carbohydrates. She does not do any exercise. Her physical examination is otherwise normal.

Management

▶ If disease is not controlled, **discuss treatment options** such as lifestyle modification, adding medications or increasing doses using motivational interviewing (Chapter 5)

▶ Consider **needed prevention** (e.g., diabetic eye examinations in people with diabetes or pneumonia vaccine in people with asthma)

▶ **Consider referral** to community resources, case management

▶ Discuss **follow-up plan**

▶ **Documentation** (progress note, charts of blood pressures or graphs of blood sugars)

▶ End visit by asking the patient to set one or more **SMART goals** (specific, measurable, realistic, and time-bound) for managing their disease

For instance, "I will lose 5 pounds in the next 2 months."

Treatment options: You talk to Ms. Potts about the possibility of adding exercise and working on her weight versus starting a second oral agent like glipizide for better blood sugar control and a statin for lowering cholesterol (Decision Support). You write a prescription for a new glucometer and discuss episodic versus daily use.

Referral: You also introduce her to the Nurse Care Coordinator at your clinic who will help her obtain the new glucometer and test strips and provide ongoing support (Self-Management Support and Delivery System Redesign).

You also provide Ms. Potts with information about a free exercise class for people with diabetes at the senior center and about a diabetic diet as well as a referral to a nutritionist to help her find healthy foods at the pantry (Community Resources and Self-Management Support).

Follow-up plan and prevention: Finally, you review when she should come back for follow-up, when she needs more laboratory tests and an eye examination, and have her schedule a time with the Nurse Care Coordinator (Delivery System Redesign).

SMART goals: You end the visit by asking what goals she wants to set before her next visit. She says that she wants to go to the free exercise class twice a week and wants to lose some of the 10 lb before her next appointment in 3 months (Self-Management Support).

COMMON CHRONIC PROBLEMS IN PRIMARY CARE

In this chapter, we will discuss asthma, chronic obstructive pulmonary disease (COPD), coronary artery disease (CAD), type 2 diabetes mellitus (DM), heart failure (HF), hyperlipidemia, HTN, obesity, and osteoporosis (OP). While this is not a complete list of chronic problems, these are the ones that you are most likely to see in the Family Medicine clinic. Discussions of other common chronic problems seen in primary care can be found in Chapters 10, 15 to 17, and 20 to 23. We recommend that you read the sections of this chapter as you encounter patients with these problems.

The **most effective treatments** are rated strength of recommendation (SOR) A, based on consistent, good-quality patient-oriented evidence. SOR B is based on inconsistent or limited-quality, patient-oriented evidence and SOR C is based on consensus, disease-oriented evidence, expert opinion, or case series. For more information about the Strength of Reference Taxonomy evidence-rating system, see http://www.aafp.org/afpsort.xml.

Asthma

Asthma is a chronic inflammatory condition marked by intermittent bronchial hyperres-ponsiveness causing airflow obstruction. This obstruction manifests as clinical symptoms of wheezing, cough, shortness of breath, and chest tightness, though the presentation varies from person to person and depending on disease severity.[3]

Asthma "exacerbations" are often triggered by environmental allergens (e.g., mold, animal dander, pollens, insects), airborne irritants (e.g., cigarette or wood smoke, noxious chemicals, dust), activity (exercise), or infectious causes (e.g., upper respiratory viruses, pneumonia). The term "reactive airway disease" is sometimes used synonymously with asthma, but should refer only to young children with asthma-like symptoms who do not yet have a formal diagnosis of asthma.[4]

> Haley, a 14-year-old girl with asthma, is in your clinic for a general checkup. She reports get-ting up 3 to 4 nights a week to use her albuterol inhaler, including early this morning. She also wheezes at least 3 to 4 times a week when she runs in gym class or pets her neighbor's cats. Her only current medication is inhaled albuterol. She feels well today. Her father smokes cigarettes.

How Common is Asthma?

Asthma is quite common, affecting about 9% of all children and 7% of all adults in the United States. Risk factors for asthma include lower socioeconomic status, black or African American race, Puerto Rican heritage, and male gender. Compared with other races, Blacks have disproportionately higher rates of emergency department visits, hospitalizations, and mortality due to asthma.[5]

How to Assess Severity/Control

Asthma is classified according to level of impairment and risk. Table 12.2 defines the clas-sification scheme for children >12 years of age and adults. You would use this scheme to classify Haley's asthma; with her 3 to 4 times nighttime awakenings each week, she likely has moderate, persistent asthma. Similar schemata are used for younger children (tables found at http://www.nhlbi.nih.gov/files/docs/guidelines/asthgdln.pdf).

The most severe form of asthma is severe continuous bronchospasm, known as status asthmaticus. The physical findings are noted below. Please see Figure 12.1 for management principles.

Physical Examination Findings in Status Asthmaticus

▶ Tachycardia (>120 beats/min) and tachypnea (>30 breaths/min)[a]

▶ Use of accessory respiratory muscles

▶ Pulsus paradoxus (inspiratory decline in SBP >10 mm Hg)

(continued)

▶ Wheezing; absence/decreased wheezing can indicate worsening obstruction

▶ Mental status changes: usually due to hypoxia and hypercapnia; these constitute an indication for urgent intubation

▶ Paradoxical abdominal and diaphragmatic movement on inspiration; indicates diaphragmatic failure and possible respiratory crisis

[a]Involves measuring FEV1 and FVC before and after administration of a bronchoconstricting medication, such as methacholine. Decrease in FEV1 by >20% with 8 mg/mL methacholine is considered a positive test

Table 12.2 ▶ Classification of Asthma in Adults and Children Less Than 12 Years of Age

Components of Severity		Intermittent	Severity		
			Persistent		
			Mild	Moderate	Severe
Impairment Normal FEV_1/FVC: 8–19 years 85% 20–29 years 80% 40–59 years 75% 60–80 years 70%	Symptoms	≤2 days/week	>2 days/week, but not daily	Daily	Throughout the day
	Nighttime awakenings	≤2 times/month	3–4 times/month	>1 time/week, but not nightly	Often 7 times/week
	Short-acting β_2-agonist used for symptom control (not for prevention of EIB)	≤2 days/week	>2 days/week, but not >1 time/day	Daily	Several times per day
	Interference with normal activity	None	Minor limitation	Some limitation	Extremely limited
	Lung function	• Normal FEV_1 between exacerbations • FEV_1 >80% predicted • FEV_1/FVC normal	• FEV_1 ≥80% predicted • FEV_1/FVC normal	• FEV_1 >60%, but ≥80% predicted • FEV_1/FVC reduced 5%	• FEV_1 ≥60% predicted • FEV_1/FVC reduced 5%

EIB, exercise-induced bronchospasm; FEV_1, forced expiratory volume in 1 second; FVC, forced vital capacity.
From National Asthma Education and Prevention Program: Expert panel report III: *Guidelines for the diagnosis and management of asthma*, p 74. Bethesda, MD: National Heart, Lung, and Blood Institute, 2007. (NIH publication no. 08–4051) www.nhlbi.nih.gov/guidelines/asthma/asthgdln.htm.

Assess Severity

• Patients at high risk for a fatal attack require immediate medical attention after initial treatment.
• Symptoms and signs suggestive of a more serious exacerbation such as marked breathlessness, inability to speak more than short phrases, use of accessory muscles, or drowsiness should result in initial treatment while immediately consulting with a clinician.
• Less severe signs and symptoms can be treated initially with assessment of response to therapy and further steps as listed below.
• If available, measure PEF—values of 50–79% predicted or personal best indicate the need for quick-relief medication. Depending on the response to treatment, contact with a clinician may also be indicated. Values below 50% indicate the need for immediate medical care.

Initial Treatment

• Inhaled SABA: up to two treatments 20 minutes apart of 2–6 puffs by metered-dose inhaler (MDI) or nebulizer treatments.
• Note: Medication delivery is highly variable. Children and individuals who have exacerbations of lesser severity may need fewer puffs than suggested above.

Good Response

No wheezing or dyspnea (assess tachypnea in young children).

PEF ≥80% predicted or personal best.

• Contact clinician for follow-up instructions and further management.
• May continue inhaled SABA every 3–4 hours for 24–48 hours.
• Consider short course of oral systemic corticosteroids.

Incomplete Response

Persistent wheezing and dyspnea (tachypnea).

PEF 50–79% predicted or personal best.

• Add oral systemic corticosteroid.
• Continue inhaled SABA.
• Contact clinician urgently (this day) for further instruction.

Poor Response

Marked wheezing and dyspnea.

PEF <50% predicted or personal best.

• Add oral systemic corticosteroid.
• Repeat inhaled SABA immediately.
• If distress is severe and nonresponsive to initial treatment:
 —Call your doctor AND
 —PROCEED TO ED;
 —Consider calling 9–1–1 (ambulance transport).

• To ED.

Figure 12.1 ▶ Algorithm for home management of acute asthma exacerbations. ED, emergency department; MDI, metered-dose inhaler; PEF, peak expiratory flow; SABA, short-acting β2-agonist (quick-relief inhaler). (Adapted from the National Heart Lung and Blood Institute. National Asthma Education and Prevention Program. Expert panel report 3: Guidelines for the diagnosis and management of asthma; 2007:382. http://www.nhlbi.nih.gov/guidelines/asthma/asthgdln.htm and https://www.nhlbi.nih.gov/files/docs/guidelines/asthgdln.pdf.)

BOX 12.1 THE ASTHMA CONTROL TEST (ACT) AND THE CHILDHOOD ACT

ACT https://www.asthma.com/additional-resources/asthma-control-test.html

Childhood ACT https://www.asthma.com/additional-resources/childhood-asthma-control-test.html

A variety of clinical assessment tools can be used by patients and health practitioners to determine asthma impairment and risk. The Asthma Control Test (ACT) and the Childhood ACT(tm) are two such validated questionnaires (Box 12.1).[6,7]

Peak expiratory flow (PEF) can help measure degree of airway obstruction.

> You ask Haley to fill out an Asthma Control Test (adult version). Her score is 13, out of a possible 25. Scores of 19 or less indicate poor asthma control. Her PEF today is normal.

Diagnostics

Certain elements of a patient's history suggest asthma:

▶ Cough, especially at night

▶ Recurrent difficulty breathing or chest tightness

▶ Symptoms worsened by exercise, viral infections, exposure to fur-bearing animals, molds, smoke, pollen, dust mites, airborne chemicals or dusts, menstrual cycles, strong emotional expressions (e.g., laughing or crying), or changes in weather

▶ Wheezing (http://www.easyauscultation.com/wheezing)—continuous high-pitched whistling that occurs when air flows through narrowed airways (lack of wheezing does not exclude asthma)

Measurement of **PEF rate** (often referred to as peak flow) is a useful and economic office-based test which can help confirm asthma, COPD, or other obstructive causes of wheezing. https://www.youtube.com/watch?v=6oKupWgDu80. Although Haley's test is normal today, she has known asthma that, in the past, was confined to response to triggers such as pet exposure and exercise, and she used her inhaler this morning.

Pulmonary function testing (spirometry) is required for formal diagnosis of asthma.[8,9]

▶ Measures forced expiratory volume in 1 second (FEV1) and forced vital capacity (FVC)

▶ Asthma is frequently marked by reduced FEV1/FVC ratio (Table 12.2)

▶ Improvement in FEV1 by >12% after administration of a short-acting bronchodilator demonstrates reversibility of airway obstruction

▶ If there is no baseline obstruction but asthma is suspected, bronchoprovocation testing can be performed

Wheezing is a common cause of office visits for children and adults, with prevalence up to 26% among 2- to 3-year olds, 13% among 9- to 11-year olds, and 16% among adults in the United States.[10,11] Depending on the cause, wheezing can be a minor annoyance (e.g.,

Table 12.3 ▶ Diagnostic Evaluation of Selected Causes of Wheezing in Adults and Children

Cause of Wheezing	Presentation	Steps in Evaluation
Asthma	Wheezing episodes triggered by URI, allergies, exercise + response to bronchodilator	PFT with bronchodilators, exercise or methacholine challenge testing, allergy testing
Bronchiolitis	Rhinitis, cough, pediatric patient	RSV/influenza/viral testing; CXR
CHF	History of cardiac disease, leg swelling or weight gain, chronic cough	CXR, BNP, echocardiography, ECG
COPD	History of smoking, chronic cough, recurrent wheezing	PFT with bronchodilators and DLCO, CXR, alpha-1-antitrypsin testing if nonsmoker
Foreign body aspiration	Sudden onset wheezing	CXR (2 views), bronchoscopy
GERD	Association with food/eating, worse at night, acid taste in mouth, "burning" chest/epigastric pain	Trial H2 blocker or PPI therapy, esophagogastroduodenoscopy if alarm symptoms
Immune deficiency	Frequent recurrent infections	Immune testing, immunoglobulin therapy
Pulmonary embolism (PE)	Sudden onset after travel, surgery, immobilization, or malignancy	D-dimer, CT chest angiography, V/Q study, MR angiography
Tumor	Weight loss, night sweats, no response to bronchodilator	CXR, CT chest, bronchoscopy
Vocal cord dysfunction	Inspiratory wheezing or stridor, no bronchodilator response	Laryngoscopy

BNP, B-type natriuretic peptide; CHF, congestive heart failure; COPD, chronic obstructive pulmonary disease; CT, computed tomography; CXR, chest x-ray; DLCO, diffusion capacity of the lungs for carbon monoxide; ECG, electrocardiogram; GERD, gastroesophageal reflux disease; MR, magnetic resonance; PFT, pulmonary function testing; PPI, proton-pump inhibitor; RSV, respiratory syncytial virus; URI, upper respiratory infection; V/Q, ventilation–perfusion.
Data from Dorkin HL. Noisy breathing. In: Loughlin GM, Eigen H, eds. *Respiratory Disease in Children: Diagnosis and Management.* Williams and Wilkins; 1994:171 and Fakhoury K. Approach to wheezing in children. *UpToDate.* Updated November 18, 2015.

during uncomplicated upper respiratory infection) or a sign of impending catastrophe (e.g., anaphylaxis or status asthmaticus). The differential diagnosis and evaluation for causes of wheezing is shown in Table 12.3.

Treatment Goals

▶ Reduce impairment

- Prevent coughing, breathlessness, night-time awakening
- Minimize need for short-acting bronchodilator therapy
- Maintain (near) "normal" pulmonary function
- Maintain normal activity levels at home, work, and play (e.g., sports)

▶ Reduce morbidity and mortality

- Prevent emergency room visits and hospitalizations
- Prevent loss of lung function
- Minimize adverse medication side effects
- Minimize need for oral corticosteroids
- Address concurrent tobacco use

Treatment Options

For acute asthma-induced wheezing, the initial step is to determine severity based on PEF. For mild or moderate cases, initial treatment is with a bronchodilator like albuterol. There is no clinical benefit of using a nebulizer over a metered dose inhaler in patients who are able to comply with dosing instructions.[12] Haley is not having an acute episode today.

Follow the algorithm in Figure 12.1 for patients with an acute exacerbation of asthma. Treatments for chronic asthma include long-term control medications as well as short-term "rescue" medications (Table 12.4). Haley has only been prescribed a rescue medication, albuterol, that is no longer sufficient for her needs.

Table 12.4 ► Pharmacotherapy for Management of Asthma

		Short-Acting Rescue Medications		
Drug Class	Mechanism of Action	Adverse Effects	Warnings, Contraindications	Examples
Short-acting beta agonists (SABAs)	• Relaxation of airway smooth muscles • Inhibits cyclic AMP	Hypokalemia, tachycardia	Hypersensitivity	• Albuterol • Levalbuterol • Pirbuterol
Anticholinergics	• Inhibits muscarinic cholinergic receptors • Decreases mucous gland secretion • Reduces vagal tone of airways	Dry mouth, paradoxical bronchospasm	Hypersensitivity	• Ipratropium
Systemic corticosteroids	• Block late-phase reaction to allergen • Reduce airway hyper responsiveness • Inhibit inflammatory cell migration and activation	Immune system impairment, hyperglycemia, OP, peptic ulcer, skin thinning, weight gain	Use with caution in patients with immune compromise, adrenal suppression	• Dexamethasone • Methylprednisolone • Prednisolone • Prednisone
		Long-Acting Control Medications		
Corticosteroids (inhaled; ICS)	• Block late-phase reaction to allergen • Reduce airway hyperresponsiveness • Inhibit inflammatory cell migration and activation	Immune system impairment, hyperglycemia, OP, peptic ulcer, skin thinning, weight gain	Use with caution in patients with immune compromise, adrenal suppression	• Beclomethasone • Budesonide • Flunisolide • Fluticasone • Mometasone • Triamcinolone
Long-acting beta agonists (LABAs)	• Relaxation of airway smooth muscles • Inhibits cyclic AMP	Hypokalemia, tachycardia	Not for monotherapy; slightly increased risk (rare) of severe asthma exacerbations leading to death	• Formoterol • Salmeterol

	Long-Acting Control Medications			
Drug Class	**Mechanism of Action**	**Adverse Effects**	**Warnings, Contraindications**	**Examples**
Cromolyn sodium	• Stabilizes mast cells • Interferes with chloride channel function	Dizziness, flushing, tachycardia	Hypersensitivity	• Cromolyn sodium • Nedocromil
Leukotriene modifiers, 5-lipoxygenase inhibitors (LTRAs)	• Inhibit 5-lipoxygenase and leukotriene receptors	Behavioral disturbance, eosinophilia, and vasculitis	Hypersensitivity	• Montelukast • Zafirlukast • Zileuton
Methylxanthines	• Inhibit phosphodiesterase • Reduce airway inflammation	Nausea, seizures, tachycardia, vomiting	Use with caution in patients with seizure disorder, cardiac disease, hyperthyroidism	• Theophylline
Immune modulators	• Prevents binding of IgE to basophil and mast cell receptors	Anaphylaxis, fever, arthralgia, rash, TIA, stroke	Hypersensitivity	• Omalizumab

AMP, adenosine monophosphate; IgE, immune globulin E; OP, osteoporosis; TIA, transient ischemic attack.
Adapted from National Asthma Education and Prevention Program: Expert panel report III: *Guidelines for the diagnosis and management of asthma.* Bethesda, MD: National Heart, Lung, and Blood Institute, 2007. (NIH publication no. 08–4051) www.nhlbi.nih.gov/guidelines/asthma/asthgdln.htm.

Figure 12.2 outlines the stepwise application of controller and rescue asthma medications for children >12 years of age and adults.

Based on her symptoms, Haley likely has moderate persistent asthma inadequately controlled on albuterol alone. You decide to step up her management by adding fluticasone, a low-dose inhaled corticosteroid.

Secondary Prevention

If allergens are suspected or known triggers of a patient's asthma, education about preventative measures can reduce frequency and severity of symptoms. For Haley, as her symptoms frequently occur at night, consider changes in bedding or her bedroom; her father's smoking is likely another trigger. Preventive measures include[13]:

➤ Placing pillows and bedding in dust mite-proof covers
➤ Washing bedding weekly with hot water (temperature >130°F)
➤ Vacuuming bedrooms with HEPA filter
➤ Placing children's soft toys in the freezer or hot washing regularly
➤ Removing carpets and upholstered furniture from households
➤ Washing window curtains regularly in hot water
➤ Using a dehumidifier to keep home humidity between 30% and 50%

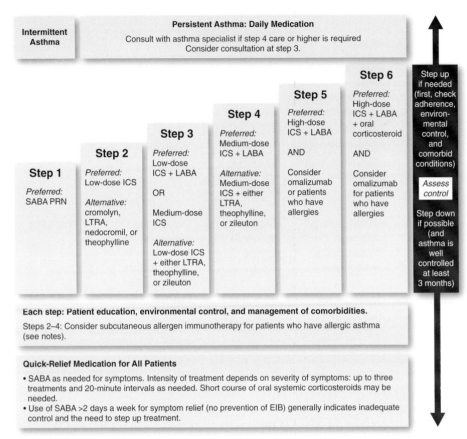

Figure 12.2 ▶ Stepwise approach for management of asthma in youths and adults. EIB, exercise-induced bronchospasm; ICS, inhaled corticosteroid; LABA, long-acting inhaled β2-agonist; LTRA, leukotriene receptor antagonist; SABA, short-acting inhaled β2-agonist. (From: National Heart, Lung, and Blood Institute, National Asthma Education and Prevention Program. Expert Panel Report 3: Guidelines for the Diagnosis and Management of Asthma. Bethesda, MD; 2007:305. [NIH publication no. 08–4051] www.nhlbi.nih.gov/guidelines/asthma/asthgdln.htm and https://www.nhlbi.nih.gov/files/docs/guidelines/asthgdln.pdf.)

▶ Removing mold from the home (washing with bleach or professional removal)
▶ Removing cockroaches
▶ Considering relocating pets if animal allergies present
▶ Avoid exposure to wood-burning stoves, unvented heaters
▶ Smoking cessation

Patients with asthma who require daily medication should be referred to an allergist immunologist for allergy testing and consideration of immunotherapy.[14]

Monitoring/Case Management

Effective asthma care hinges on patient education, which is critical to reducing impair ment and risk. Among other topics of education, healthcare practitioners should discus and create individualized Asthma Action Plans for patients with asthma, especially children (For example, http://www.aafa.org/page/asthma-treatment-action-plan.aspx). Your attending may have an action plan that the office uses.

> After prescribing the new inhaled corticosteroid, you spend time with Haley and her parents reviewing her medications, their proper administration, and asthma risk reduction. You suggest referral to an allergist given Haley's probable cat allergy and counsel her father about tobacco cessation strategies. You send Haley home with an updated Asthma Action Plan for home and for school.

Chronic Obstructive Pulmonary Disease

> Eugenia is a 72-year-old long-time smoker accompanied by her husband who notes that she is having more difficulty playing cards as "she can't seem to remember the plays." She has a chronic cough but otherwise states that she feels "just fine." As you talk with her, you note that her lips are blue and she has difficulty speaking in full sentences. On exam, her lungs are clear although hyperresonant, and she has bilateral peripheral edema and hepatomegaly.

COPD is a chronic lung disorder characterized by progressive, nonreversible airflow limitation. It is usually caused by smoking. The airflow limitation is associated with an abnormal inflammatory response in the lung to noxious particles or gases.

An acute exacerbation of COPD is defined as an acute event characterized by a worsening, beyond daily variation, of the patient's respiratory symptoms. These exacerbations negatively affect quality of life and are associated with accelerated decline of lung function and increased mortality.

Many groups have defined the parameters of COPD including the British Thoracic Society, European Respiratory Society, Global Initiative for Chronic Obstructive Lung Disease (GOLD), and American Thoracic Society. In this section, we will use the GOLD classifications.[15]

How Common is COPD?

Estimated prevalence of COPD in US adults is about 15.7 million cases, or 6.4% of the population (2014).[16] Prevalence varies by state with the highest prevalence rates clustered along the Ohio and lower Mississippi Rivers. Alpha-1 antitrypsin deficiency, an uncommon cause of COPD, affects 1 in 1600 to 5000 individuals.[17] The Centers for Disease Control and Prevention lists chronic lower respiratory disease as the third leading cause of death in 2013 with 149,205 attributed deaths.[18]

How to Assess Severity/Control

The most recent GOLD report classifies patients into four categories (A–D) in addition to a **severity classification**:

▶ GOLD 1: mild, FEV_1 ≥80% predicted

▶ GOLD 2: moderate, FEV_1 less than 80% but ≥50% predicted

▶ GOLD 3: severe, FEV_1 less than 50% but ≥30%

▶ GOLD 4: very severe, FEV_1 <30% predicted (the latter based on postbronchodilator FEV1). This classification system can be used to guide treatment as shown below:

Group A: severity class 1 or 2 and/or few symptoms, 0–1 exacerbations/year

Group B: severity class 1 or 2 and/or more symptoms, 0–1 exacerbations/year

Group C: severe impairment (class 3 or 4) and/or few symptoms, 2 or more exacerbations/year

Group D: severe impairment (class 3 or 4) and/or more symptoms, 2 or more exacerbations/year

---

The BODE index (**B**ody mass index, degree of airflow **O**bstruction, **D**yspnea as measured on the Modified Medical Research Council (MRC) Dyspnea Scale, and **E**xercise capacity measured using the 6-minute walk distance) can be used to predict risk of hospitalization and death in patients with COPD (http://reference.medscape.com/calculator/bode-index-copd). Four-year survival with 0 to 2 points is 80% but only 18% with a score of 7 to 10 points.

Diagnostics

▶ Diagnose COPD with **spirometry** showing persistent airflow limitation.

▶ Suspect COPD in patients with chronic and progressive **dyspnea, cough,** and **sputum production** and a history of exposure to disease risk factors. Eugenia, as a long-time smoker, likely has COPD. On examination, her lungs are clear, although hyperresonant, and she has bilateral peripheral edema and hepatomegaly.

▶ Other signs and symptoms include hyperinflation of the chest with increased anterior-posterior diameter; use of accessory muscles of respiration; pursed-lip breathing; and symptoms of right-sided HF as demonstrated during Eugenia's examination.

▶ As the disease progresses, look for reduced exercise capacity, fatigue, and dyspnea at rest.

▶ Respiratory failure can lead to right-sided HF (cor pulmonale) as noted in the case; signs of right-sided HF are elevated jugular venous pressure, hepatomegaly, and peripheral edema.

▶ Other tests to consider are shown in Table 12.5. Eugenia's oxygen saturation is 74%, which improves to 92% with supplemental oxygen.

The **differential diagnosis** of COPD includes:

▶ Asthma: airway obstruction is reversible

▶ Congestive HF: improves with diuresis, normal spirometry

▶ Bronchiectasis: may have hemoptysis, history of infection, CT confirms

▶ Tuberculosis: positive TB test and/or sputum, typical chest x-ray features

> You discuss with Eugenia and her husband the likely diagnosis of COPD with right-sided HF and advise smoking cessation and the need for home oxygen, at least for now. The patient agrees to hospitalization for improvement of HF and additional tests.

Treatment Goals

Optimize function and limit disease progression.

Table 12.5 ▶ Tests to Consider in Patients with Chronic Obstructive Pulmonary Disease

Test	Indication	Comment
Alpha 1-antitrypsin level	Patient with COPD younger than age 50 years with positive family history and minimal smoking history	
Arterial blood gas	GOLD 3 or 4 or clinical signs of respiratory failure or heart failure	Helps determine if oxygen is needed
Chest x-ray (CXR)	GOLD 2 or higher to excluding other diagnoses and establishing the presence of comorbidities (e.g., heart failure)	Also performed in acute exacerbation to rule out pneumonia
Computed tomography	To investigate symptoms that are disproportionate to spirometry findings, to assess abnormalities identified on CXR	Also performed for patients who are surgical candidates
Echocardiogram	If features of right-sided heart failure present	

Data from: Global Strategy for the Diagnosis, Management and Prevention of COPD, Global Initiative for Chronic Obstructive Lung Disease (GOLD) 2016. Available from: http://goldcopd.org/. Accessed October 2016.

Treatment Options

The most important step for patients with COPD is to quit smoking. This can result in dramatic improvement in symptoms over time and lowers all-cause mortality (SOR A).[19] Exercise and pulmonary rehabilitation can reduce symptoms while vaccination can prevent serious illness and possibly reduce mortality.[15] Other medications are shown in Table 12.6 and are based on GOLD group.

Table 12.6 ▶ Treatment Options for Patients with Chronic Obstructive Pulmonary Disease

GOLD Group	Treatment (SOR)
All stages	Smoking cessation
	Exercise and pulmonary rehabilitation
	Influenza and pneumococcal vaccination
GOLD A	Short-acting inhaled bronchodilators (SOR C)
GOLD B	Long-acting inhaled bronchodilator (beta)-agonist ([LABA] or muscarinic anticholinergic [LAMA]) (SOR A for symptom improvement)
GOLD C	Combination LABA/ICS (SOR A for symptoms; may reduce exacerbations)
	Combination LABA/LAMA as alternative (SOR A improves symptoms and reduces exacerbations without increasing risk of pneumonia)
GOLD D	As for GOLD C PLUS oxygen (15–20 hrs/day)[a] (SOR A for improved survival if PaO_2 <55 mm Hg)

[a]Indications: resting PaO_2 ≤60 mm Hg (8 kPa) with evidence of peripheral edema, polycythemia (hematocrit ≥55%) or pulmonary hypertension 25870317.
ICS, inhaled corticosteroid; LABA, long-acting inhaled β_2-agonist; LAMA, long-acting inhaled muscarinic anticholinergic.
Data from: Global Strategy for the Diagnosis, Management and Prevention of COPD, Global Initiative for Chronic Obstructive Lung Disease (GOLD) 2016. Available from: http://goldcopd.org/. Accessed October 2016; Kew KM, Dias S, Cates CJ. Long-acting inhaled therapy (beta-agonists, anticholinergics and steroids) for COPD: a network meta-analysis. *Cochrane Database Syst Rev.* 2014;3:CD010844; Cranston JM, Crockett A, Moss J, et al. Domiciliary oxygen for chronic obstructive pulmonary disease. *Cochrane Database Syst Rev.* 2005;4:CD001744.

Other medications may have a role in treatment but their role is not clear. These are:

▶ Phosphodiesterase 4 (PDE4) inhibitors (roflumilast, cilomilast) reduce exacerbations but have little impact on quality of life and are expensive.[20]

▶ Oral theophylline improves exercise performance in patients with moderate to severe COPD.[21]

▶ Mucolytics (e.g., guaifenesin) reduce COPD exacerbations and disability days and may be useful, particularly in winter, for patients with more advanced COPD.[22]

Surgery. Lung volume reduction surgery is sometimes used for patients with severe diffuse emphysema. Although there is an increased 90-day mortality for patients undergoing surgery, in those who survive, quality of life and exercise capacity are improved.[23]

Treatment of Acute Exacerbation.[24–26] Treatment of COPD exacerbation depends on severity and usually includes antibiotics and systemic steroids. As shown in the CXR below, patients have hyperexpanded lungs and prominent substernal airspace.

Acute Exacerbation

• Symptom control: Short-acting inhaled bronchodilators

• Moderate–severe COPD: 5–7 days of oral or parenteral **systemic steroids** (SOR A)

• Purulent sputum and increased dyspnea or increased sputum production: **Empiric antibiotics** (macrolide, amoxicillin, amoxicillin/clavulanate, respiratory quinolone) (SOR B)

• Hypoxia: Oxygen

• Severe exacerbation/respiratory distress: Noninvasive positive pressure ventilation

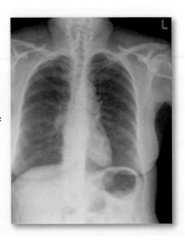

For inpatients, especially those admitted to the intensive care unit, antibiotics reduce treatment failure and mortality (number needed to treat = 14) but data are conflicting on benefit for outpatients, although treatment failure is reduced.[26] **Pulmonary rehabilitation** following an acute exacerbation of COPD is highly effective in improving quality of life and reducing subsequent hospital admissions and mortality.[27]

When to Hospitalize

▶ GOLD recommends hospital assessment or admission for patients with:

• Marked increase in intensity of symptoms
• Severe underlying COPD
• Onset of new physical signs (e.g., cyanosis, peripheral edema)
• Failure of an exacerbation to respond to initial medical management
• Presence of serious comorbidities (e.g., newly occurring arrhythmias)
• Frequent exacerbations
• Older age
• Insufficient home support

▶ Consider ICU admission for patients with severe dyspnea unresponsive to initial therapy; changes in mental status (e.g., confusion); persistent/worsening hypoxemia (PaO_2 <40 mm Hg) or severe/worsening respiratory acidosis (pH <7.25) despite supplemental oxygen and noninvasive ventilation, need for invasive mechanical ventilation, and hemodynamic instability.

Secondary Prevention

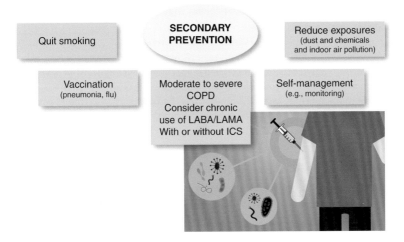

Monitoring

▶ Quantify and monitor dyspnea using the **MRC dyspnea scale** that ranges from Grade 1 (not troubled by dyspnea) to Grade 5 (too breathless to leave the house or breathless when dressing or undressing) (http://occmed.oxfordjournals.org/content/58/3/226.full).

▶ The **COPD Assessment Test** (CAT) is an eight-item questionnaire that assesses and quantifies the impact of COPD symptoms on health status (http://www.catestonline.org/). Higher baseline CAT scores are seen in those with frequent COPD exacerbations. CAT scores can also predict health status deterioration, depression, and mortality.[28]

▶ Encourage your patient to monitor their symptoms—looking for signs of acute exacerbation (increased dyspnea or increased purulent sputum production) or worsening symptoms such as inability to walk as far as usual—and to report these to their clinician.

▶ Ask about need for refills; if COPD is not controlled, proceed to step care and educate about new prescriptions.

▶ Because patients with severe COPD have a poor 5-year survival, consider conducting end-of-life care conversations and completion of a living will or similar document (Chapter 10). This includes preferences for intubation.

Eugenia is seen 1 week after hospital discharge. She is on home oxygen and has stopped smoking. She feels much better on her two long-acting inhalers and her medication for HF. You review her medications and refer her for pulmonary rehabilitation with the hope that she will be able to discontinue oxygen therapy in the future.

Coronary Artery Disease

Pathologic narrowing or occlusion of the coronary arteries is known as CAD or ischemic heart disease (IHD). CAD results from chronic deposition of lipid-rich atherosclerotic plaques beneath the arterial endothelium (intima). Over time, this deposition induces inflammatory and fibrotic blood vessel changes. As the occlusion expands, reduced blood flow (ischemia) may cause clinical symptoms such as **angina**. Rupture of the endothelial layer exposes the plaque to the bloodstream, triggering the coagulation cascade and thrombus formation; if sizeable enough, this process may lead to myocardial infarction (MI), resulting cardiac dysfunction or death.

> Your first patient of the day is Bill, a 76-year-old man with chest pain described as vague chest tightness with high levels of exertion, such as when shoveling snow or walking up more than two flights of stairs. The pain has been present for a few weeks. He had an episode of unprovoked pain this morning as well, accompanied by nausea. You decide to send him to the emergency room for work up and possible hospitalization.

How Common is CAD?

CAD accounts for one in four deaths in the United States, and is the leading cause of death for both men and women (>600,000 deaths/year).[29] Over 16 million adults in the United States have CAD and around 0.75 million people suffer MIs each year in the United States.[30]

How to Assess Severity/Control

In patients with known CAD, the presence, absence, or relative quality of a patient's chest pain, or *angina pectoris,* can give clues into the severity of their CAD (Table 12.7). Bill's description of pain which occurred initially with exertion and this morning accompanied by nausea is suspicious for angina.

Table 12.7 ▶ Types and Features of Different Types of Chest Pain

Type of Chest Pain	Characteristics	Diagnostic Clues	
Typical angina	• Substernal chest discomfort of pressure • Symptoms provoked by exertion or emotional stress • Symptoms relieved by rest or nitroglycerin	• Diaphoresis • Dizziness • Nausea	• Stable Angina: predictable pattern of symptoms (e.g., pain always occurs with certain degree of exertion, resolves with rest) • Unstable Angina: new, changing or unpredictable pattern (e.g., symptoms at rest)
Atypical angina	• Any two of the above characteristics of typical angina		
Noncardiac chest pain	• Any one of the above characteristics of typical angina	• Heartburn or acid indigestion symptoms • Pain reproducible with palpation of chest wall	

Table 12.8 ▶ Canadian Cardiovascular Society Classification System for Angina Pectoris

Class I Patient does not have limitations with ordinary physical activity, e.g.,
- Walking
- Climbing stairs
- Angina occurs with strenuous, rapid, or prolonged exertion

Class II Patient experiences *slight* limitations with ordinary physical activity, e.g.,
- Walking rapidly, climbing stairs rapidly, walking uphill
- Walking after meals, in the cold, in the wind, or under emotional stress
- Walking more than two level blocks or climbing more than one flight of ordinary stairs at normal pace

Class III Patient experiences *marked* limitations with ordinary physical activity, e.g.,
- Walking one to two level blocks, climbing more than one flight of stairs at a normal pace

Class IV Patient experiences *severe* limitations.
- Inability to carry out any physical activity without angina
- Symptoms may be present at rest

The Canadian Cardiovascular Society Classification System grades angina into functional classes based on patient limitations (Table 12.8).[31]

Diagnostics

Initial testing for patients with either known CAD or with symptoms of angina include:

▶ **History and physical examination,** with attention toward any signs of ischemic or chronic heart disease (HD) including diminished peripheral pulses, carotid/aortic/renal/femoral bruits, cardiac murmurs, third heart sound, pulmonary rales, jugular venous distension, or peripheral edema

▶ **Electrocardiogram**

Laboratory and imaging testing (e.g., hemoglobin, fasting glucose, creatinine, chest x-ray) can uncover underlying conditions or cardiovascular risk factors (diabetes, HF, anemia), but normal results do not rule out CAD. In the emergency room, Bill had abnormal EKG changes and elevated troponin, indicating myocardial injury.

Patients with unstable angina (chest pain with a new or changing pattern, particularly if at rest) should be risk-stratified to determine next steps for diagnosis as shown in Table 12.9.[32]

Once risk-stratified, cardiac stress testing is commonly used to diagnose new CAD or to determine progression of known CAD (Table 12.10).[32,33] Figure 12.3 illustrates a basic algorithm that may be used when selecting a stress test.

In patients with known CAD, consider coronary angiography (catheterization):

▶ Following survival of cardiac arrest or life-threatening ventricular arrhythmia

▶ With development of any signs of symptoms of HF

▶ High pretest probability of severe CAD

Table 12.9 ▶ Risk Stratification for Patients with Unstable Angina

High Risk	Intermediate Risk	Low Risk
At least one of the following: • Angina >20 minutes at rest • Angina with hypotension • Angina with new or worsening mitral regurgitation murmur • Angina at rest with ST segment changes ≥1 mm • Angina with S3 or new/worsening rales • Pulmonary edema, most likely related to ischemia	No high-risk features, but any of the following: • Angina at rest (>20 minutes or relieved by nitroglycerin) • Angina >20 minutes, resolved, with moderate or high likelihood of CAD • Angina with dynamic T-wave changes • New-onset CCSC Grade III or IV angina in past 2 weeks, with moderate or high likelihood of CAD • Nocturnal angina • Pathologic Q waves or resting ST-segment depression ≤1 mm in multiple lead groups • Age >65 years	No high- or intermediate-risk features, but any of the following: • Angina provoked at lower threshold • Increased angina frequency, severity, or duration • New-onset angina 2 weeks–2 months before presentation • Normal or unchanged ECG

CAD, coronary artery disease; CCSC, Canadian Cardiovascular Society Classification; ECG, electrocardiogram.

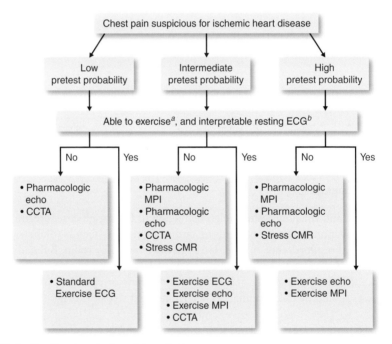

Figure 12.3 ▶ Algorithm for selection of stress tests.
[a]Must be able to achieve ≥85% of age-predicted target heart rate and ≥5 metabolic equivalents.
[b]Uninterpretable ECG findings include: left bundle branch block, ventricular pacing, ST segment elevation or depression ≥1 mm, left ventricular hypertrophy, pre-excitation (e.g., Wolf–Parkinson–White syndrome), digoxin effects. CCTA, coronary computed tomography angiography; CMR, cardiac magnetic resonance; ECG, electrocardiogram; echo, echocardiography; MPI, myocardial perfusion imaging. (Data from: Kirali K. Coronary artery disease—assessment, surgery, prevention. *InTech.* 2015. https://www.intechopen.com/books/coronary-artery-disease-assessment-surgery-prevention.)

Table 12.10 ▶ Types of Cardiac Stress Testing

Type of Test	Description
Standard exercise ECG	**Stress:** Exercise (treadmill or stationary bike) **Measurement:** heart rate, blood pressure, and ECG changes • Useful if low-intermediate risk of IHD
Exercise stress with radionuclide MPI	**Stress:** Exercise **Measurement:** myocardial perfusion is measured via single photon emission computed tomography (SPECT) or positron emission tomography (PET) following injection of radioactive tracer (typically technetium-99m or thallium-201)
Pharmacologic stress with radionuclide MPI	**Stress:** Vasodilator (adenosine, dipyridamole, regadenoson) or inotrope/chronotrope (dobutamine) **Measurement:** myocardial perfusion measured via SPECT or PET following injection of radioactive tracer;
Exercise stress with echo	**Stress:** Exercise **Measurement:** wall motion is measured via echocardiography
Pharmacologic stress with echo	**Stress:** Vasodilator or inotrope/chronotrope **Measurement:** wall motion measured via echocardiography
Cardiac MRI	**Stress:** usually vasodilator (adenosine) **Measurement:** myocardial perfusion is measured via magnetic resonance following injection of gadolinium • Useful if known stenosis of undetermined significance being considered for revascularization
Cardiac CT	**Stress:** None **Measurement:** coronary artery calcification and patency measured via computed tomography angiography, following injection of contrast media • Beta blockers and nitrates used to slow the heart and dilate vessels, respectively • Useful if indeterminate result from functional testing

CT, computed tomography; MRI, magnetic resonance imaging; ECG, electrocardiogram; echo, echocardiogram; IHD, ischemic heart disease; MPI, myocardial perfusion imaging.

Coronary angiography is **not appropriate** if:

▶ Patient would not want or could not tolerate revascularization (stenting or angioplasty)
▶ Low pretest probability of CAD and patient has not undergone noninvasive (stress) testing
▶ Patient is asymptomatic and has normal noninvasive testing

Bill falls into an intermediate risk category but with evidence of myocardial injury, he is sent for immediate cardiac catheterization which reveals near total occlusion of the left anterior descending (LAD) artery. He is treated with placement of a drug-eluting stent.

Treatment Goals and Options

Physicians treating patients with CAD should focus on the following treatment goals:

▶ Symptom monitoring:
  • Assess for changes in frequency, severity, patterns of angina
  • Treatment of angina

▶ Preventing progression of CAD
  • Cardiac risk factor modification

Following recovery from stenting, Bill was discharged home with follow-up to you as well as with cardiology. He has been feeling well but has not tested his exercise limits by walking any more than one block at a slow speed. He wonders whether exercise is safe for him after his procedure.

Methods to achieve treatment goals in patients with CAD are outlined in Tables 12.11 and 12.12.[34,35] Primary and secondary prevention efforts are key to reducing CAD global burden (economic cost, morbidity, mortality).

Table 12.11 ▶ Strategies for Management of Coronary Artery Disease Risk Factors

Risk Factor (SOR)	Office Strategies	Notes/Comments
Depression (B)	• Screen patients with PHQ-2 or PHQ-9	• Depression three times more common following MI • Treatment of patients with SSRI or CBT may give modest reduction in risk of symptoms[36]; evidence is inconclusive in terms of risk reduction for recurrent MI or death
Diabetes mellitus (C)	• Treatment per ADA guidelines	• RCTs have not shown reduction in CV events or mortality with intensive glycemic control
Hypertension (A)	• Limit dietary sodium • Increase intake of fresh fruits and vegetables; low fat dairy • Educate on DASH diet	• Target BP <140/90 mm Hg (JNC 8)[37]
Influenza vaccination (B)	• Annual vaccination for all patients with CAD	• Reduces risk of hospitalization for heart disease and all-cause mortality in elderly
Lipid Management (A)	• Increase physical activity • Advocate Mediterranean or plant-based diet	• Statin therapy should be considered if no contraindications or known side effects
Physical activity (A)	• Encourage walking during work breaks, gardening, increase household chores • Referral to medically supervised cardiac rehab for at-risk patients	• 30–60 minutes of moderate-intensity aerobic activity at least 5 days/week • Exercise-based cardiac rehabilitation programs may be started shortly after ACS or revascularization procedure
Smoking cessation (A)	• 5 As (Ask, Advise, Assess, Assist, Arrange) • Offer counseling and pharmacotherapy	• Reduces all-cause mortality in patients with CAD
Weight management (C)	• Assess weight and BMI at every visit	• Target BMI of 18.5–24.9 kg/m^2 • Reduce body weight by 5–10% from baseline

ACS, acute coronary syndrome; ADA, American Diabetes Association; BMI, body mass index; BP, blood pressure; CAD, coronary artery disease; CBT, cognitive behavioral therapy; CV, cardiovascular; DASH, dietary approaches to stopping hypertension; HDL, high-density lipoprotein; HF, heart failure; JNC, Joint National Committee on Prevention, Detection, Evaluation, and Treatment of High Blood Pressure; LDL, low-density lipoprotein; MI, myocardial infarction; PHQ, patient health questionnaire; RCT, randomized controlled trial; SOR, strength of recommendation; SSRI, selective serotonin reuptake inhibitor.

Table 12.12 ▶ Pharmacotherapy for Stable Coronary Artery Disease

Medications for Treatment of Stable Angina		
Medication Class	**Examples**	**Notes/Comments**
Nitrates	• Isosorbide mono or dinitrate • Nitroglycerin	• No reduction in mortality • Reduce frequency and severity of angina • Common side effects: hypotension, headache • Contraindicated with PDE5 inhibitors
Calcium channel blockers	• Amlodipine • Diltiazem • Nifedipine • Verapamil	• Dihydropyridines (nifedipine, amlodipine) plus a nitrate may cause hypotension • Nondihydropyridines (verapamil, diltiazem) plus a beta-blocker may cause bradycardia
Medications that Improve Risk Factor Control and Decrease CAD Mortality		
ACE Inhibitors	• Benazepril • Lisinopril • Ramipril	• Strong evidence for consistent CV protection, improved survival, and reduced morbidity/mortality
Antiplatelet/anticoagulant	• Aspirin • Clopidogrel	• Aspirin 81–162 mg/day in all with CAD, continue indefinitely (SOR A) • Clopidogrel effective alternative if patient cannot take aspirin. • Consider both ASA and clopidogrel for up to 12 months after acute MI or stent placement
Beta blockers	• Atenolol • Bisoprolol • Metoprolol • Propranolol	• Reduce recurrent MI, sudden cardiac death, mortality (SOR A) • Contraindicated in patients with asthma, cardiogenic shock, bradycardia, high-degree heart block, severe heart failure requiring inotropes or IV diuretics, hypotension
Lipid-lowering therapies	• Statins	• Statins reduce recurrent vascular events and all-cause mortality in patients following ACS (SOR A) • Reduce saturated fat intake to <7% of total calories, total cholesterol intake <200 mg, and trans-fatty acids <1% of total calories

ACE, angiotensin-converting enzyme; ACS, acute coronary syndrome; ASA, aspirin; CAD, coronary artery disease; CBT, cognitive behavioral therapy; CV, cardiovascular; IV, intravenous; MI, myocardial infarction; PDE5, phosphodiesterase-5; SOR, strength of recommendation.

Revascularization

In the acute setting of unstable angina, MI, ventricular arrhythmia, or development of HF symptoms, coronary artery revascularization may be necessary. As noted above, coronary angiography is a diagnostic procedure that can deliver therapeutic options of stenting, as in Bill's case, or angioplasty. For more severe coronary lesions or multi-vessel disease, coronary artery bypass graft surgery (CABG) may be required (Table 12.13).[38]

> Bill's symptoms are well controlled. You reassure him that exercise is safe following his procedure, but advise him to enroll in a medically-supervised cardiac rehabilitation program. You ensure that he is taking high-dose atorvastatin as well as aspirin, metoprolol, and lisinopril. You provide him with resources and information for the Mediterranean diet and order his annual influenza vaccine. You and your preceptor arrange for him to follow up at regular intervals for BP, weight checks, and depression screening.

Table 12.13 ▶ Indications and Contraindications for Coronary Artery Bypass Grafting

CABG Recommended

- Angina despite maximal medical therapy
- Proximal LAD stenosis >70%
- Substantial left main coronary artery stenosis
- 1- or 2-vessel CAD without proximal LAD stenosis but with large area of viable myocardium and high-risk criteria on noninvasive testing
- 2-vessel disease with proximal LAD stenosis and either EF <50% or ischemia on noninvasive testing
- 3-vessel disease

CABG May Be Considered

- Proximal LAD stenosis with 1-vessel disease
- 1- or 2-vessel disease without proximal LAD stenosis but with moderate area of viable myocardium and ischemia on noninvasive testing

CABG Not Recommended

- Coronary artery stenosis <60% in locations other than the left main coronary artery and no ischemia on noninvasive testing
- Coronary artery stenosis <50%
- 1- or 2-vessel disease w/o proximal LAD stenosis, mild symptoms, or inadequate trial of medical therapy and a small area of viable myocardium or no ischemia on noninvasive testing

CABG, coronary artery bypass graft; CAD, coronary artery disease; EF, ejection fraction; LAD, left anterior descending.

Diabetes Mellitus

DM is a metabolic disorder resulting from insulin deficiency, cellular resistance to insulin, or both; the body's inability to properly process food results in hyperglycemia.

Type 1 DM results from autoimmune-mediated destruction of pancreatic beta-cells resulting in absolute insulin deficiency. Glutamic acid decarboxylase (GAD65) is a major autoantigen in type 1 DM. Type 1 DM accounts for about 5% of cases of diabetes; most are young (<15 years), but type 1 DM can present at any age. These patients require exogenous insulin to maintain euglycemia.

Type 2 DM results from insulin resistance which places increasing demand on the pancreas to produce higher levels of insulin to maintain euglycemia. Those with type 2 DM are usually over 40 years of age, although younger age at presentation is increasing due to higher rates of obesity. These patients can often be treated with diet, exercise, and oral agents. This section will address type 2 DM.

Jamal is a 56-year-old obese man who presents for ongoing care for his diabetes of 4 years and HTN of 8 years. He reports that he has managed to lose 5 lb this month by going to weight watchers and feels well. He is a nonsmoker and drinks occasional beer on weekends. He needs refills his metformin, lisinopril, and statin, and requests his flu shot. His hemoglobin A1c from last week was 8%, LDL-C 96 mg/dL, and his creatinine was in the normal range. BP today is 150/84 mm Hg.

How Common is Diabetes Mellitus?

About 22 million people in the US have diagnosed DM, according to the Centers for Disease Control and Prevention (CDC). The age-adjusted rate is 6.4/100, unchanged since

2009. DM incidence increases with advancing age—from 1.9/100 for those <44 years to 19.2/100 for those >75 years (2014). Rates are slightly higher in men and in blacks versus whites or Asians.

How to Assess Severity/Control

There are two issues to consider when assessing severity: the continued exposure of the patient to elevated blood sugar which increases their risk of complications, and the comorbidities that increase the patient's risk of adverse outcomes when he/she has diabetes.

▶ *Hyperglycemia:* Exposure to elevated blood sugar places patients at higher risk of cardiovascular disease (CVD), stroke, renal disease, visual impairment from diabetic retinopathy, and sometimes death. Ask the patient about the duration of their diabetes, medication(s) used to control it, and any complications already experienced; these will provide some idea about severity (e.g., longer duration (over 10 years), more than monotherapy, and any complications).

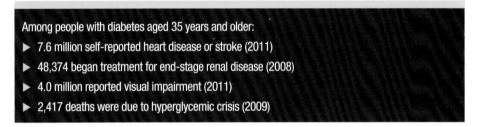

Among people with diabetes aged 35 years and older:

▶ 7.6 million self-reported heart disease or stroke (2011)

▶ 48,374 began treatment for end-stage renal disease (2008)

▶ 4.0 million reported visual impairment (2011)

▶ 2,417 deaths were due to hyperglycemic crisis (2009)

Control of blood sugar is usually assessed with serum hemoglobin A1c level. **The target level A1c is individualized based on life expectancy, disease duration, presence of complications,** CVD risk factors, comorbid conditions and risk for severe hypoglycemia. The acceptable range for control is between 6.5% (below this is normal) and 8%.[39,40]

▶ *Comorbidities:* Risk factors for the above complications include smoking, inactivity, HTN, CVD, and elevated lipids. Jamal has only had diabetes for 4 years, his kidney function is normal, and his LDL is acceptable. His A1c level, however, is at the upper range of acceptable and his BP is higher than recommended.

According to the CDC, 19.9% of US adults with diabetes smoked, 84.7% were overweight or obese, and 36.1% reported being physically inactive (2010). In 2009, 57.1% of US adults with diabetes reported having HTN and 58.4% reported elevated cholesterol. Controlling comorbidities will lower the risk of adverse outcomes such as stroke, MI, ESRD, and death.

Diagnostics

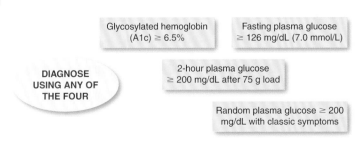

Glycosylated hemoglobin (A1c) ≥ 6.5%

Fasting plasma glucose ≥ 126 mg/dL (7.0 mmol/L)

DIAGNOSE USING ANY OF THE FOUR

2-hour plasma glucose ≥ 200 mg/dL after 75 g load

Random plasma glucose ≥ 200 mg/dL with classic symptoms

The American Diabetes Association (ADA) and the American Association of Clinical Endocrinologists (AACE) recommend repeating an abnormal fasting plasma glucose test for confirmation, particularly if the result is borderline.[39,40]

Risk factors for diabetes include obesity, family history of diabetes, CVD, previous impaired glucose tolerance, prior gestational diabetes, and polycystic ovary syndrome (for complete list see AACE guidelines).

Screening for type 2 diabetes:

▶ The United States Preventive Services Task Force recommends screening for abnormal blood glucose as part of cardiovascular risk assessment in adults aged 40 to 70 years who are overweight or obese.

▶ The ADA and AACE recommend screening other asymptomatic adults for type 2 diabetes if they have risk factors (noted above).

▶ Pregnant women are screened for gestational diabetes between 24 and 28 weeks gestation with a 2-hour oral glucose tolerance test (OGTT) using a 75-g glucose load.

Treatment Goals

The goals for treatment are to prevent episodes of hyper- and hypoglycemia (during treatment) and to reduce complications of DM primarily by controlling risk factors and comorbidities. **Risk factors for complications** of diabetes include CVD or major risk factors for CVD (smoking, HTN, family history of CVD, and HDL-C <35 mg/dL). AACE has constructed a number of algorithms to assist in identifying treatment options which intensify based on risk (https://www.aace.com/files/aace_algorithm.pdf).

In keeping with those goals, tests obtained for patients with type 2 DM include those listed in Table 12.14. Patients should be asked about smoking and advised to quit, if smokers; for individuals with diabetes, **smoking cessation** offers the greatest benefit for morbidity and mortality.

Table 12.14 ▶ Testing Recommended for Patients with Type 2 Diabetes Mellitus

Test (Normal)	Rationale	Initial Assessment	Subsequent Monitoring
BP (<140/80 mm Hg)[a]	Detect hypertension	2 BP measures at least 6 hours apart	Each visit
BMI (<25 kg/m²)	Identify obesity	Height and weight	Recheck weight if needed or yearly
Lipid panel (LDL <100 mg/dL; triglycerides <150 mg/dL)[b]	Detect hyperlipidemia	Nonfasted acceptable	Every 3 months until at goal, then yearly
Hemoglobin A1c	Establish diagnosis or average BS	Once at (or for) diagnosis	Every 3 months if not at goal, then every 6 months
Urinary albumin[c] or albumin-to-creatinine ratio and eGFR	Detect kidney disease	At diagnosis	Yearly

[a]Based on evidence of fewer cardiovascular events and lower mortality at this BP level.[43]
[b]<70 mg/dL recommended by AACE if high risk.
[c]An angiotensin-converting enzyme inhibitor or an angiotensin receptor blocker is recommended for nonpregnant patients with diabetes and elevated urinary albumin excretion (>300 mg/day) and/or estimated glomerular filtration rate, 60 mL/min/1.73 m²; however, there is no evidence that the treatment influences mortality or end-stage renal disease.
BMI, body mass index; BP, blood pressure; eGFR, estimated glomerular filtration rate; LDL, low density lipid.

Jamal's repeat BP is 148/84 mm Hg and his examination is significant only for obesity. His foot examination shows no lesions and normal sensation. You congratulate him on his weight loss and good lipid control and discuss his target BP of 140/80 mm Hg and A1c target of <7.5%. Jamal takes his medication regularly and is not opposed to changes. He is in touch with the nurse in the practice who is helping him with his weight loss program. He does not monitor his blood sugar as the test strips are expensive but he has a BP machine at home. He has not had an eye examination this year and you note that he never received his pneumonia vaccination.

Treatment Options

Prediabetes (impaired glucose tolerance) is identified through laboratory tests showing plasma glucose value of 140 to 199 mg/dL 2 hours after ingesting 75 g of glucose and/ or fasting glucose 100 to 125 mg/dL. Patients with prediabetes can be managed with lifestyle and risk factor modification and considered for low-risk medications (i.e., metformin, acarbose).

Diet modification is suggested to help patients reduce weight and regulate glucose by preventing large fluctuation in calories. Patients should eat regular meals with a largely plant-based diet with limited saturated fat. While low-glycemic index diets can help reduce HgbA1c and risk of hypoglycemia, no studies assessed morbidity or mortality benefits and there is insufficient evidence to recommend them.[41] The Mediterranean diet has been shown to reduce incidence of diabetes in those with prediabetes.

Exercise is encouraged at 150 minutes or more per week of moderate-intensity exercise such as brisk walking (15- to 20-minute mile) or its equivalent.

Risk factor modification is outlined in Table 12.15. Factors are listed in the order of importance with respect to decreasing morbidity and mortality.

The benefit of BP control in patients with diabetes was demonstrated in the United Kingdom Prospective Diabetes Study (UKPDS). In this study of 5,102 adults with type 2 diabetes, controlled BP (<150/85 mm Hg) decreased diabetes-related mortality, diabetes-related outcomes (NNT 61 to prevent one serious diabetes-related outcome), and overall mortality.[42] For Jamal, control of his BP to a systolic pressure of <140 mm Hg is a priority. Tight control of BP (<120 mm Hg), however, does not confer additional benefit.[43]

Oral agents can be used to control hyperglycemia. These act in various ways including decreasing hepatic glucose production, decreasing intestinal absorption of glucose,

Table 12.15 ▶ Risk Factor Modification for Patients with Diabetes Mellitus

Risk Factor	Goal	Options	Comment
Smoking	Cessation	Counseling, nicotine replacement, medication[a]	Encourage smokers to quit at each visit
Hypertension	BP 130–140/80 mm Hg	Diet (reduce salt or weight control), exercise, medication[b]	See hypertension section below. Check serum Cr and K^+ level after drug initiation and once or twice a year
Hyperlipidemia	LDL-C <100 mg/dL or <70 mg/dL if CVD	Diet (low cholesterol), exercise, statin	Yearly lipid profiles, more often if uncontrolled

[a]Bupropion hydrochloride or varenicline tartrate currently FDA-approved (Chapter 23).
[b]Thiazide or angiotensin-converting enzyme inhibitor classes may be the best first-line treatment.
Cr, creatinine; CVD, cardiovascular disease; K^+, potassium.

delaying gastric emptying, increasing peripheral uptake of glucose, increasing insulin secretion, decreasing glucagon secretion, and increasing insulin sensitivity in peripheral tissues.

Hypoglycemia is also dangerous, and care must be taken to avoid hypoglycemia when treating hyperglycemia. In an economic analysis, drug-induced hypoglycemia was highest for basal insulin and sulfonylureas; rates of hypoglycemia were 8.64 and 4.32 events per person-year in 65- to 79-year olds and 12.06 and 6.03 events per person-year for those 80 years and older.[44]

In addition, **tight glucose control** (A1c <6% to 7%) has not been shown to affect mortality and there is no compelling evidence that aggressive glycemic control reduces the risk of most macrovascular or microvascular complications such as cardiovascular events, stroke, or risk of dialysis or blindness.[45,46] The studies reporting these findings include the United Kingdom Prospective Diabetes Study (**UKPDS**),[47] Action to Control Cardiovascular Risk in Diabetes (**ACCORD**),[48] Action in Diabetes and Vascular Disease Preterax and Diamicron Modified Release Controlled Evaluation (**ADVANCE**),[49] and the Veterans Administration Diabetes Trial (**VADT**).[50]

To achieve optimal, individualized glycemic control, a tiered system is recommended by AACE as shown in Figure 12.4 (SOR C). When possible, **begin with metformin** for overweight patients with diabetes as it has been shown to prolong life regardless of its effect on hemoglobin A1c (NNT 141 to prevent one death).[51] Jamal is already taking metformin but the dose could be increased. A discussion of insulin use can be found in the AACE guidelines.

You and your attending discuss medication options with Jamal and decide to increase his metformin to the maximum daily dose and add hydrochlorothiazide 25 mg for BP control. You review potential medication side effects. His prescriptions for all his medications are sent electronically to the pharmacy.

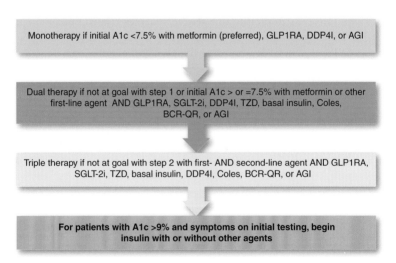

Monotherapy if initial A1c <7.5% with metformin (preferred), GLP1RA, DDP4I, or AGI

Dual therapy if not at goal with step 1 or initial A1c > or =7.5% with metformin or other first-line agent AND GLP1RA, SGLT-2i, DDP4I, TZD, basal insulin, Coles, BCR-QR, or AGI

Triple therapy if not at goal with step 2 with first- AND second-line agent AND GLP1RA, SGLT-2i, TZD, basal insulin, DDP4I, Coles, BCR-QR, or AGI

For patients with A1c >9% and symptoms on initial testing, begin insulin with or without other agents

Figure 12.4 ▶ Steps for assisting patients with glycemic control. AGI, α-glucosidase inhibitors; BCR-QR, bromocriptine quick release; Coles, colesevelam; DPP4I, dipeptidyl peptidase 4 inhibitors; GLP1RA, glucagon-like peptide 1 receptor agonists; SGLT2I, sodium glucose cotransporter 2 inhibitors; SU, sulfonylureas; TZD, thiazolidinediones.

Table 12.16 ▶ Prevention Efforts for Diabetic Complications

Complication	Recommendations from AACE	Monitoring
Nephropathy	Optimal glucose and blood pressure control (ACE or ARB may be most helpful), salt and protein restriction if progressive, supplement if iron or vitamin deficiencies	Per KDIGO; assess GFR and early morning albuminuria at least annually Nephrology referral if chronic kidney disease
Neuropathy, somatic[a]	Exercise to improve strength and balance; daily feet inspection, protective socks, appropriate footwear, and avoidance of injury	Check sensation of feet regularly, ask about symptoms of neuropathy, treat neuropathic pain[b]
Neuropathy, autonomic[c]	Bladder: bethanechol, intermittent cath Cardiac: graded exercise, medications GI: frequent small meals, prokinetic agents, fiber for constipation/diarrhea Sexual: counseling, lubricants, medication, or devices for erectile dysfunction	Monitor symptoms regularly
Retinopathy	Optimal glucose and blood pressure control (ACE or ARB may be most helpful), panretinal scatter laser photocoagulation if high-risk proliferative retinopathy	Annual dilated eye examination with ophthalmologist

[a]Includes focal involving single nerves or entrapment neuropathies (e.g., carpal tunnel syndrome), proximal lumbosacral, thoracic, and cervical radiculoplexus neuropathies, or distal neuropathies (characteristically symmetric, glove and stocking distribution).
[b]Medication options include tricyclic antidepressants, gabapentin or pregabalin, duloxetine, or the opioid tapentadol.
[c]Includes cardiac, gastrointestinal, sexual, bladder, sudomotor (e.g., anhidrosis, dry skin) pupillomotor, and visceral dysfunction.
AACE, American Association of Clinical Endocrinologists; ACE, angiotensin-converting enzyme inhibitor; ARB, angiotensin receptor blocker; GFR, glomerular filtration rate; GI, gastrointestinal; KDIGO, Kidney Disease: Improving Global Outcomes (http://kdigo.org/home/guidelines/ckd-evaluation-management/).

Secondary Prevention

Routine preventive care should be provided to patients with diabetes (Chapter 7); this aspect of care is often neglected when working on improved control of the disease and comorbidities, to the patient's detriment. Information about prevention of diabetic nephropathy, neuropathy, retinopathy is shown in Table 12.16.

Monitoring/Case Management

Monitoring of risk factors and complications are shown in Tables 12.15 and 12.16. At each visit, asking patients about results of self-monitoring efforts (blood sugar, BP, symptoms) and any new or persistent symptoms will help target avenues for intervention. Although the value of self-monitored blood glucose is limited in patients with type 2 DM on oral agents or diet alone,[52] a patient's self-monitoring can be used to adjust insulin therapy, identify hypoglycemic episodes, and adjust medications during attempts to improve control or illness.

Many practices have case managers for patients with chronic illness. These members of the care team can assist patients with monitoring, appointments, and education.

You ask the nurse to give Jamal both flu and pneumonia vaccinations today and he will meet next with the case manager to discuss monitoring his BP, continued work on his diet and exercise, and to arrange an ophthalmology examination. He will follow-up in 1 month.

Heart Failure

HF refers to any condition in which the heart's left ventricular function (either systolic or diastolic) is impaired. The resulting dysfunction in the filling and ejection of blood triggers maladaptive responses of the renal, endocrine, and sympathetic nervous systems. Common symptoms of HF include dyspnea, fatigue, and volume overload. HF is associated with high morbidity and mortality.

> Gerry, a 68-year-old man with history of coronary artery disease, chronic kidney disease stage 3, and systolic HF (left ventricular ejection fraction 35%) comes into the clinic for a routine medication review. He notes that he has been more short of breath recently. You observe that his weight has increased 7 pounds from 3 months ago. His medications include lisinopril (10 mg daily), carvedilol (25 mg twice daily), aspirin (81 mg daily), and atorvastatin (40 mg daily).

How Common is Heart Failure?

Given its interrelation with CAD (the leading cause of death in the United States),[53] HF is a highly prevalent condition. It is a contributing factor in approximately one in ten deaths in the United States, with a higher prevalence among the elderly and African Americans.[54,55]

HF has a variety of causes (Fig. 12.5).[56,57] Other risk factors for HF include DM (relative risk 1.9), cigarette smoking (RR 1.6), and obesity (RR 1.3).[58]

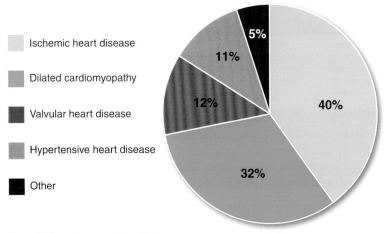

- Ischemic heart disease
- Dilated cardiomyopathy
- Valvular heart disease
- Hypertensive heart disease
- Other

Figure 12.5 ▶ Causes of heart failure.

How to Assess Severity/Control

Terminology, abbreviations, and severity classification systems related to HF have evolved in recent years. Table 12.17 provides clarification of nomenclature and definitions for HF.[59] The term "congestive heart failure" is less frequently used today, as patients may have HF without evidence of congestion or volume overload. As shown in Table 12.17, Gerry's left ventricular ejection fraction of 35% places him in the category of HF with reduced ejection fraction.

The American College of Cardiology Foundation (ACCF)/American Heart Association (AHA) Stages of Heart Failure and the New York Heart Association (NYHA) Functional Class system are the two most common methods of stratifying HF severity. Figure 12.6 illustrates the relationship between the two systems.

Table 12.17 ▶ Abbreviations and Definitions of Heart Failure Terms

Abbreviation	Full Name	Colloquial Term	Definition	Heart Failure Cases (%)	Comments
HF*r*EF	Heart failure with reduced ejection fraction	Systolic heart failure	LVEF <40%	~50–60	More common in younger men, with CAD
HF*p*EF	Heart failure with preserved ejection fraction	Diastolic Heart Failure	LVEF >50%	~40–50	More common in older women, with HTN, A-fib, and LVH

A-fib, atrial fibrillation; CAD, coronary artery disease; HTN, hypertension; LVEF, left ventricular ejection fraction; LVH, left ventricular hypertrophy.

Gerry's oxygen saturation is 96% on room air and his BP and heart rate are normal. On examination, he has rales in both lung bases, as well as jugular venous distension and pitting edema in both legs to his mid-shins. He states that he is comfortable at rest but tires with walking about 1 block. More recently, he cannot walk more than half a block without pausing for breath. Based on his symptoms and known ejection fraction (35%), you determine that he has at least Stage C/NYHA Class III HF.

Diagnostics

HF is a diagnosis in which the history and physical examination very strongly corroborate clinical suspicion. The Framingham criteria (Table 12.18) are used to help diagnose HF*r*EF.[60–62]

The most commonly assessed laboratory and imaging studies include B-type natriuretic peptide (BNP), chest radiography, electrocardiography, and echocardiography. **Echocardiography** is used both to confirm the diagnosis of HF and to distinguish whether it is systolic or diastolic in nature.

Other laboratory tests (e.g., complete blood count, electrolytes, creatinine, liver function tests, thyroid function studies, and urinalysis) can help identify underlying conditions which

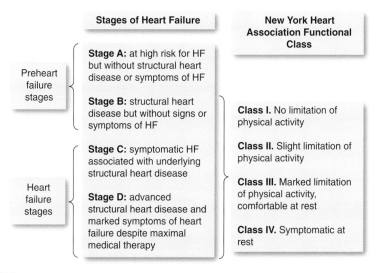

Figure 12.6 ▶ Interrelation between ACCF/AHA stages of heart failure and the NYHA functional classes.

Table 12.18 ▶ Framingham Criteria (Modified) for Diagnosis of Heart Failure

Major Criteria	Minor Criteria
• Acute pulmonary edema • Cardiomegaly • Central venous pressure >16 cm H_2O • Hepatojugular reflex • Neck vein distension • Paroxysmal nocturnal dyspnea or orthopnea • Pulmonary rales • Third heart sound (S3 gallop) • Weight loss ≥4.5 kg in 5 days in response to diuretic therapy	• Ankle edema • Dyspnea on exertion • Hepatomegaly • Nocturnal cough • Pleural effusion • Tachycardia (heart rate >120 bpm) • Weight loss ≥4.5 kg in 5 days

Diagnosis of heart failure requires two major or one major criterion and two minor criteria.
Sensitivity: 97%; Specificity: 79%.

may contribute to HF. Patients with HF who do not have a known history of IHD should be assessed for CAD, as it is the leading cause of HF. Presence of chest pain or angina warrants coronary angiography.[59] Figure 12.7 provides a framework for diagnosis of patients with HF.

Considering Gerry's weight gain and increased symptoms, you diagnose a HF exacerbation. His clinical appearance, normal BP and oxygen saturation suggest that Gerry can be managed as an outpatient. You order electrolytes and creatinine today and consider how you can best effect diuresis.

Treatment Goals

The goals of treatment for patients with HF are to improve quality of life and prevent disease progression. Mechanisms to achieve each of these goals are listed below, along with the SOR, when known.

Improve Quality of Life: Prevent Hospitalization for Acute Exacerbations, Reduce Morbidity

- Assess NYHA Functional Class routinely
- Evaluate for common symptoms of heart failure
- Assess blood pressure, signs of volume overload
- Encourage patients to monitor daily weights (SOR C)
- Encourage low-sodium diet, limited alcohol intake, diabetic control (SOR B)
- Encourage daily aerobic exercise as it improves functional capacity (SOR B)
- Avoid NSAIDs (SOR B)

Prevent Disease Progression: Prevent Long-term Hospitalization, Reduce Morbidity

- Hypertension: maintain blood pressure <140/80 mm Hg (SOR C)
- Hyperlipidemia: reduce lipid levels (SOR C)
- Diabetes: maintain HgA1c at target (SOR C)
- Coronary artery disease: control ischemia, consider revascularization (SOR C)
- Atrial fibrillation: rate control
- Tobacco use: encourage smoking cessation
- Enroll patient in multidisciplinary disease management program (SOR B)

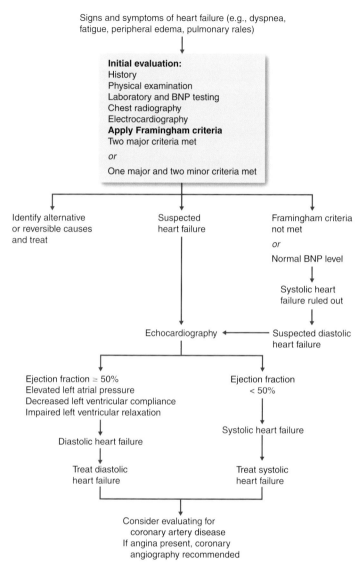

Figure 12.7 ▶ Algorithm for the evaluation and diagnosis of heart failure. BNP, B-type natriuretic peptide. (From: King M, Kingery J, Casey B. Diagnosis and evaluation of heart failure. *Am Fam Physician*. 2012;85(12):1161–1168. http://www.aafp.org/afp/2012/0615/p1161.html)

Treatment Options

In the setting of acute decompensation of HF (so-called "exacerbations"), diuretics (mainly loop diuretics) are used routinely for removal of excess fluid from the body's extracellular (interstitial) compartment. Diuresis improves symptoms of leg swelling and dyspnea due to pulmonary edema.

Pharmacologic therapy for chronic HF centers on reducing cardiac afterload, reducing systemic vascular resistance, and blocking activation of the renin–angiotensin–aldosterone neurohormonal system. Table 12.19 summarizes the major drugs used in treatment of HF*r*EF.[63] Gerry is already taking an angiotensin converting enzyme inhibitor and a beta-blocker for his HF. He is not on a diuretic, and furosemide would be an appropriate choice.

> You prescribe oral furosemide (40 mg daily for 3 days) to reduce his volume overload. You advise him to continue taking his lisinopril, carvedilol, aspirin, and atorvastatin, and to check daily weights. He is scheduled to return to clinic in 3 days to check his progress and ensure that your diuresis did not harm his renal function by reassessing electrolytes and creatinine.

Unlike HF*r*EF, there is little evidence to guide medication management for HF with preserved ejection fraction (HF*p*EF). Controlling patients' HTN, DM, obesity, tobacco use, hyperlipidemia, and IHD remain priorities. It is reasonable to consider angiotensin-converting enzyme inhibitors, beta blockers, angiotensin receptor blockers, and calcium channel blockers for these patients if HTN is present.[63]

Nonpharmacologic therapies for HF include:

▶ Exercise training: Exercise training reduces the risk of hospital admissions, improves health-related quality of life, and may reduce mortality in the long-term (SOR A).[64]

▶ Surgical therapy:
  - *Implantable defibrillators:* reduce mortality in patients with nonischemic cardiomyopathy, but not when implanted within 40 days following MI in ischemic cardiomyopathy[65]
  - *Coronary artery bypass grafting:* does not affect overall mortality but reduces cardiovascular death and death from any cause in patients with ischemic cardiomyopathy and LVEF<35%.[66]

▶ Complementary therapies: Hawthorn extract improves symptoms and exercise tolerance when used as adjunctive therapy for HF,[67] Tai Chi may be beneficial.[68]

▶ Salt-restricted diet: no evidence for reduction in morbidity or mortality.[69]

Figure 12.8 outlines the comprehensive ACCF/AHA strategy for linking treatments with stages of HF.

Secondary Prevention

Secondary prevention of HF is essentially the same as that of CAD (see CAD section in this chapter), and includes prevention and guideline-directed management of hyperlipidemia, DM, HTN, smoking, and administration of influenza and pneumococcal vaccines.[63]

Monitoring/Key Points in Patient Education and Self-Care

Family practitioners are ideally suited to take care of patients with HF, as there is great benefit in knowing a patient's story and managing this condition over time; ongoing patient education is key to preventing disease progression, hospitalizations, and ensuring maximal quality of life. Components of patient education include:

▶ Dietary guidance, including avoidance of triggers such as salt and alcohol

▶ Resources for management of tobacco use disorders

▶ Ensuring patients receive influenza and pneumococcal vaccines

▶ Encouraging patients to check daily weights

▶ Encouraging medication compliance[70]

Table 12.19 ▶ Pharmacotherapy for Heart Failure with Reduced Ejection Fraction (HF*r*EF)

Drug Class	Use	Evidence	Examples	Contra-indications	Adverse Effects	Monitoring
ACEIs	All NYHA Classes (SOR A)	Improve symptoms and QOL, **reduce mortality** and hospitalizations	Captopril, enalapril, lisinopril	Angioedema, bilateral RAS, hyperkalemia, hypotension, pregnancy, renal failure	Dry cough, hypotension, kidney injury	Blood pressure, BUN, creatinine, potassium
ARBs	Patient intolerant to ACEIs (SOR A)	Equivalent to ACEIs in **reducing mortality**	Candesartan, losartan, valsartan	Bilateral RAS, hyperkalemia, hypotension, pregnancy, renal failure	Hypotension, kidney injury	Blood pressure, BUN, creatinine, potassium
Aldosterone antagonists	NYHA Class III and IV; recent MI (SOR B)	**Reduce morbidity and mortality**	Eplerenone, spironolactone	Addison disease, hyperkalemia, renal failure	Electrolyte abnormalities, hypotension, hyperkalemia, kidney injury	Blood pressure, creatinine, weigh daily, potassium
β-blockers	NYHA Class II and III (SOR A)	Delay clinical progression of HF, **reduce mortality**	Bisoprolol, carvedilol, extended-release metoprolol	Asthma/COPD (relative), bradycardia, fluid retention, heart block, hypotension	Bradycardia, bronchospasm, hypotension	Blood pressure, heart rate
Digitalis	HF with refractory atrial fibrillation (SOR B)	May improve symptoms, but may increase mortality in women	Digoxin	Hypersensitivity, ventricular fibrillation	Arrhythmias, GI upset, neurologic complaints	Creatinine, digoxin level, electrolytes, ECG
Loop diuretics	Patients with volume overload (SOR B)	Improve symptoms	Bumetanide, furosemide, torsemide	Hypersensitivity, renal failure	Hypokalemia, hypotension, kidney injury	Blood pressure, creatinine, potassium
Vasodilator	Black patients with NYHA Class II-III (SOR B)	**Reduce mortality** when used with ACEIs and β-blockers	Isosorbide dinitrate, hydralazine	Hypersensitivity, concurrent use with PDE-5 inhibitors	Chest pain, dizziness, headache, hypotension, weakness	Blood pressure, heart rate

ACEIs, angiotensin-converting enzyme inhibitors; ARBs, angiotensin receptor blockers; BUN, blood urea nitrogen; COPD, chronic obstructive pulmonary disease; ECG, electrocardiogram; GI, gastrointestinal; HF, heart failure; HFrEF, heart failure with reduced ejection fraction; LOE, level of evidence; NYHA, New York Heart Association; PDE-5, phosphodiesterase-5; QOL, quality of life; RAS, renal artery stenosis.

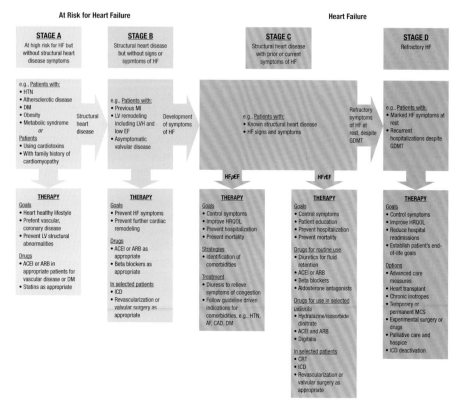

Figure 12.8 ▶ Stages in the development of heart failure and recommended therapy by stage. ACEI, angiotensin-converting enzyme inhibitor; AF, atrial fibrillation; ARB, angiotensin-receptor blocker; CAD, coronary artery disease; CRT, cardiac resynchronization therapy; DM, diabetes mellitus; EF, ejection fraction; GDMT, guideline-directed medical therapy; HF, heart failure; HPpEF, heart failure with preserved ejection fraction; HFrEF, heart failure with reduced ejection fraction; HRQOL, health-related quality of life; HTN, hypertension; ICD, implantable cardioverter-defibrillator; LV, left ventricular; LVH, left ventricular hypertrophy; MCS, mechanical circulatory support; MI, myocardial infarction. (From: Yancy CW, Jessup M, Bozkurt B, et al. 2013 ACCF/AHA guideline for the management of heart failure: executive summary: a report of the American College of Cardiology Foundation/American Heart Association Task Force on practice guidelines. *Circulation.* 2013;128(16):1810. http://circ.ahajournals.org/content/128/16/1810)

At 3-day follow-up, you are pleased to see that Gerry's symptoms have improved and his weight is down 5 pounds. You discuss with your attending that the addition of spironolactone may be beneficial for Gerry in the near future. You also ensure that Gerry is up to date on his influenza and pneumococcal vaccines and encourage him to consider enrolling in a free community aerobics class for seniors.

Hyperlipidemia

Ms. Maples is a 46-year-old healthy Caucasian woman who presents to talk to you about her cholesterol. She does not have either HTN or diabetes. She does not smoke. She had biometric screening at her workplace and was told that her cholesterol was too high. Her lipid panel results (mg/dL) are total cholesterol (TC) 264, low-density lipids (LDL) 181, high-density lipids (HDL) 46, and triglycerides (TG) 143. She asks if she should start a statin.

Table 12.20 ► Normal Lipid Levels

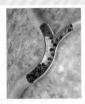

- Total cholesterol (TC) <200 mg/dL
- Low Density Lipids (LDL) <130 mg/dL
- High Density Lipids (HDL) >40 mg/dL
- Triglycerides (TG) <150 mg/dL

Most CVD is related to atherosclerosis which is described as buildup of plaque on the walls of the arteries. These plaques contain cholesterol, protein, calcium and inflammatory cells. Increased serum cholesterol is associated with elevated risk of plaque development. Normal lipid levels are displayed in Table 12.20.

How Common is Hyperlipidemia?

Heart disease (HD) is the leading cause of death in the United States and hyperlipidemia is an important risk factor for HD. Almost 33% of all adults in the US have high LDL levels and only one third of them have their LDL under control. People with high TC levels have twice the risk for HD compared to those with ideal levels.

Racial and Gender Variations in Prevalence of Hyperlipidemia		
Racial or Ethnic Group	Men (%)	Women (%)
Non-Hispanic Blacks	30.7	33.6
Mexican Americans	38.8	31.8
Non-Hispanic Whites	29.4	32.0
All	31.0	32.0

Source: *High Cholesterol Facts.* CDC, https://www.cdc.gov/cholesterol/facts.htm,

LDL levels have a continuous relationship with CVD risk. As LDL levels increase so too do CV risk levels in a dose-response relationship. This is true even in populations with normal TC levels.[71]

Diagnostics

Hyperlipidemia is diagnosed on laboratory testing of lipid levels. Based on the normal lipid levels shown in Table 12.20, Ms. Maples has hyperlipidemia with elevated TC and LDL levels. However, this diagnosis alone does not determine her need for medication.

Who Should be Screened? Since hyperlipidemia does not cause symptoms but is a risk factor for CVD, screening is the only way to find people with elevated lipid levels. Most guidelines recommend screening in the context of CVD risk reduction.

Screening recommendations from the USPSTF are shown in Table 12.21.

Risk Assessment. Most new guidelines recommend an assessment of each person's 10-year risk of developing complications from hyperlipidemia (e.g., CVA or MI) and basing pharmacologic treatment on that risk. The guidelines disagree as to the level of risk for initiating statin

Table 12.21 ▸ USPSTF Recommendations on Screening for Hyperlipidemia

Population	Grade of Recommendation[a]
Children age 1–20 years	Insufficient evidence
Men 35 years and older	A
Men 20–35 years at increased risk for CHD	B
Women 45 and older at increased risk for CHD	A
Women 20–45 at increased risk for CHD	B
Men 20–35 and women (any age) not at increased risk for CHD	C

[a]For additional information on grading see www.uspreventiveservicestaskforce.org. Information from: https://www.uspreventiveservicestaskforce.org/Page/Document/UpdateSummaryFinal/lipid-disorders-in-adults-cholesterol-dyslipidemia-screening; https://www.uspreventiveservicestaskforce.org/Page/Document/UpdateSummaryFinal/lipid-disorders-in-children-screening

treatment (see below).[72,74] Online risk calculators use data from the Framingham study that includes age, gender, race, lipid levels, BP, presence of diabetes, and smoking status to determine risk (http://www.cvriskcalculator.com/, www.healthdecision.org). Using an online calculator, you determine that Ms. Maples 10-year CVD risk is 1.7%.

> Nonfasting lipid levels are appropriate to use for screening. They have the benefit of being more convenient for patients and still are accurate in predicting future risk of ASCVD.[72]

Who Benefits from Statin Therapy?

The 2013 American College of Cardiology (ACC)/American Heart Association (AHA) guideline identifies four benefit groups, listed in Table 12.22, for whom ASCVD risk reduction outweighs the risk of medication (SOR A).[72] Ms. Maples does not meet criteria for medication treatment by either the ACC/AHA guideline or the guideline below.

The Veterans Administration/Department of Defense guidelines differ somewhat:[73]

▸ Individuals with 10-year risk under 6% do not qualify for treatment and should be rescreened in 5 years

▸ For individuals with 10-year risk between 6% and 12% conduct a shared decision-making conversation, with the option of lifestyle changes and/or statin therapy. They should be rescreened in 2 years if deciding against statin therapy

▸ Individuals with 10-year risk over 12% should be started on statin therapy

Table 12.22 ▸ AHA/ACC Benefit Groups for Statin Therapy[74]

Benefit Groups
• People with clinical evidence of ASCVD
• Individuals with DM between 40 and 75 years with LDL >70 mg/dL
• Individuals with LDL >190 mg/dL
• Individuals with LDL between 70 and 189 mg/dL and 10-year risk of ASCVD >7.5%[a]

[a]The 7.5% risk level is controversial as other guidelines have determined a risk level of 10% or 12% to be a cut off where benefits of statin therapy definitively outweigh risks.
ASCVD, atherosclerotic cardiovascular disease; LDL, low density lipids.

Table 12.23 ▸ Factors to Consider in Treatment Decisions for Statin Therapy

Additional Factors for Treatment

- LDL >160 mg/dL
- Evidence of genetic hyperlipidemia
- Family history of premature ASCVD (onset <55 years in a first-degree male relative and <65 years in a first-degree female relative)
- High sensitivity C-reactive protein >2 mg/L
- Coronary artery calcium score >300 Agatston units or >75th percentile
- Elevated lifetime risk of ASCVD

There is no evidence to order HS-CRP or do coronary artery calcium measurements in otherwise low-risk people

LDL, low density lipids; ASCVD, atherosclerotic cardiovascular disease.

For individuals who are not in one of the 4 statin benefit groups described in Table 12.22, the AHA suggests additional factors be considered to inform treatment decision making.[72] These factors are shown in Table 12.23.

Treatment Goal

Decrease CVD risk by reducing TC and LDL to ideal levels.

The new cholesterol guidelines recommend **AGAINST** adjusting pharmacologic therapy to achieve specific TC or LDL goals.[72,73] Instead, they recommend initiation of statin therapy, at different levels of intensity, based on lipid levels and 10-year CVD risk without repeating lipid levels.

Treatment Options

Lifestyle changes to reduce CVD risk that should be encouraged in all patients are listed in Table 12.24.

In addition to primary interventions noted above, medication therapy is usually initiated with statin therapy. There is good evidence that treatment with statins is effective for primary and secondary prevention of ASCVD.[72] Types of statins and recommendations for their use are shown in Table 12.25.

Other pharmacotherapy options are shown in Table 12.26.

Table 12.24 ▸ Primary Prevention to Reduce CVD Risk

Prevention Steps

- Exercise
- Dietary modification (low fat, high fiber, Mediterranean diet)
- Avoidance of smoking
- Limiting alcohol ingestion
- Weight loss if BMI >25

Table 12.25 ▶ Statins and Recommendations for Treatment

Level of Treatment	Medication	Recommendations
Low intensity (daily doses lower LDL on average less than 30%)	Simvastatin 10 mg Pravastatin 10–20 mg Lovastatin 20 mg	Shared-decision making based on 10-year risk of CVD
Moderate intensity (lowers LDL on average between 30% and 50%)	Atorvastatin 10–20 mg[a] Rosuvastatin 5–10 mg Simvastatin 20–40 mg Pravastatin 40–80 mg	10-year risk <6% (Veterans Administration guideline)
High intensity (lowers LDL levels by over 50%)	Atorvastatin 40–80 mg Rosuvastatin 20–40 mg[b]	Member of Benefit Group (Table 12.25)

[a]Effects of atorvastatin are greater in women than men.[74]
[b]Although both atorvastatin and rosuvastatin lower LDL in a dose-related manner, atorvastatin is three times less potent than rosuvastatin.[72,74]

Although Ms. Maples does not quality for statin therapy, you use this visit to talk about lifestyle factors to control her lipids including exercise, healthy diet, and weight loss. She is motivated to exercise more and eat more vegetables. Rescreening in 5 years is recommended.

Monitoring

These new lipid-lowering guidelines do not recommend following lipid profiles as treatment is not predicated on getting levels to a certain goal. So, the recommendation is to start appropriate candidates on moderate- or high-intensity statins and follow them clinically for any side effects or evidence of newly developing ASCVD.

Table 12.26 ▶ Nonstatin Pharmacologic Therapy

Agent	Supporting Evidence
Fibrates[75]	• Moderate evidence for benefit in secondary prevention • Many studies included clofibrate which is off the market; less strong evidence without this drug
Fish oil[72]	• Can reduce cholesterol • Works especially well in conjunction with medical therapy
Chinese herbal medicine[76]	• May have positive effects on risk of ASCVD • Many studies with bias • Lack of long-term patient outcomes.
Niacin[77]	• Does not affect all-cause mortality • Increases HDL by 15–35% • When combined with a statin improves disease-oriented outcomes

ASCVD, atherosclerotic cardiovascular disease; HDL, high density lipids.

Hypertension

Ms. Noble is a 47-year-old African American woman who presents after she was seen in the emergency department for a laceration and told that her BP was high. She has no history of HTN but has not been seen in your clinic for 10 years. She had gestational HTN with her last pregnancy 10 years ago and a family history of HTN in both her parents and a sister—risk factors for HTN. Her review of systems is negative for headaches, chest pain, shortness of breath or edema. You review her chart and see that her BP was 167/106 mm Hg in the ED; her BP today is 159/102 mm Hg.

What is hypertension?

A condition wherein the heart must pump blood against abnormally elevated vascular resistance. The high blood pressure needed to disseminate oxygen and other nutrients throughout the body can damage small and large blood vessels.

Blood pressure = Cardiac output × systemic vascular resistance

Blood Pressure Definitions

▶ Normal blood pressure: <120/80 mm Hg

▶ Prehypertension:120–139/80–89 mm Hg

▶ Hypertension:

  ▶ Stage 1: 140–159/90–99 mm Hg

  ▶ Stage 2: >160/100 mm Hg

Consequences of Hypertension

▶ Left ventricular hypertrophy (itself a risk factor for heart failure, myocardial infarction, sudden death, and stroke)

▶ Heart failure

▶ Ischemic stroke

▶ Intracerebral hemorrhage

▶ Ischemic heart disease, myocardial infarction

▶ Chronic kidney disease

How Common is Hypertension?

Hypertension is one of the most common reasons for primary care visits. The majority of the population over age 55 years will have HTN.

Over 70 million Americans over the age of 20 years have HTN, which is more common among blacks/African Americans than whites or Hispanics.[78]

Prevalence of Hypertension by Age and Gender

Age	Men (%)	Women (%)
20–34	11.1	6.8
35–44	25.1	19.0
45–54	37.1	35.2
55–64	54.0	53.3
65–74	64.0	69.3
75+	66.7	78.5
All	34.1	32.7

From National Center for Chronic Disease Prevention and Health Promotion, Division for Heart Disease and Stroke Prevention: *High Blood Pressure Facts*. November 30, 2016. https://www.cdc.gov/bloodpressure/facts.htm

Prevalence of Hypertension by Race and Ethnicity

Race of Ethnic Group	Men (%)	Women (%)
African American	43.0	45.7
Mexican Americans	27.8	28.9
Whites	33.9	31.3
All	34.1	32.7

From National Center for Chronic Disease Prevention and Health Promotion, Division for Heart Disease and Stroke Prevention: *High Blood Pressure Facts*. November 30, 2016. https://www.cdc.gov/bloodpressure/facts.htm

Table 12.27 ▸ Risk Factors for Hypertension

Risk Factors

- African American
- Depression
- Diabetes or gestational diabetes
- Family history of hypertension
- High alcohol intake

- High sodium diet
- Increasing age
- Obesity
- Physical inactivity
- Personality traits (hostile attitude, impatience)

Risk factors for HTN are shown in Table 12.27 and secondary causes of HTN are listed in Table 12.28.

Diagnostics

The **United States Preventive Services Task Force (USPSTF)** recommends screening for high BP in adults aged 18 years or older.[78] It also recommends obtaining measurements outside of the clinical setting for diagnostic confirmation before starting treatment (SOR A).

To diagnose HTN, measure BP using proper technique as noted below. An approach to patients with newly-diagnosed HTN is shown in Figure 12.9.

Proper Technique for Taking a Blood Pressure

▶ Use appropriate cuff size

▶ Take blood pressure in both arms

▶ Make sure you are in a calm environment

▶ Link to how to take a blood pressure:
   https://www.youtube.com/watch?v=tB8nISCEcs8

▶ For patients who you suspect may have white-coat hypertension, ambulatory outpatient blood pressure monitoring is an important adjunct diagnostic test

---

Table 12.28 ▸ Secondary Causes of Hypertension

Secondary Cause

- Medications (common include OCs, steroids, NSAIDs, antidepressants)
- Nonprescription medications (e.g., decongestants or weight-loss drugs)
- Illicit drugs (e.g., cocaine or methamphetamine)
- Primary renal disease (i.e., fibromuscular dysplasia, renal artery stenosis)
- Obstructive sleep apnea
- Primary aldosteronism (HTN, hypokalemia, and metabolic acidosis)
- Pheochromocytoma (rare, sometimes causes paroxysmal HTN)
- Endocrine disorders (Cushing syndrome, hypo or hyperthyroidism, hyperparathyroidism)
- Coarctation of the aorta (more often seen in young people)

HTN, hypertension; NSAID, nonsteroidal anti-inflammatory drug; OC, oral contraceptive.

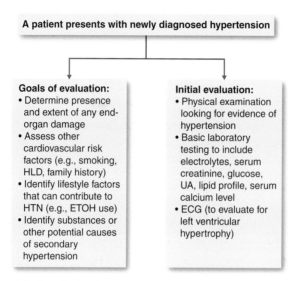

Figure 12.9 ▶ Approach to the patient with newly diagnosed hypertension. ECG, electrocardiogram; ETOH, ethanol; HLD, hypersensitivity lung disease; HTN, hypertension; UA, urinalysis.

You complete an initial evaluation of Ms. Noble, noting no evidence of end-organ damage, other cardiovascular risk factors, or secondary causes of HTN. You discuss the likelihood that she has HTN and order some basic tests and an ECG with a plan for follow-up in the next two weeks. You also talk to her about lifestyle modification, limiting salt, the DASH diet, and incorporating more exercise into her daily regimen.

Treatment Goals

▶ Prevent end organ damage, stroke or CVD by decreasing BP

▶ The Joint National Commission (JNC)-8 sets goals of BP under 140/90 mm Hg for people under 60 years and under 150/90 mm Hg for people over 60 years (somewhat controversial in that many cardiologists aim for goal BPs closer to 135/85 mm Hg and less than 120/80 mm Hg in people with known CAD or DM).[37]

> **Treatment of HTN can decrease the risk of heart failure by 50%, the risk of stroke by 30–40% and the risk of MI by 20–25%.[79]**

Treatment

For treatment options: http//www.nmhs.net/documents/27JNC8HTNGuidelinesBookBooklet. pdf. Nonpharmacologic options for treating HTN are displayed in Table 12.29.[80,81] Medication recommendations from the JNC 8 for treating HTN are shown in Table 12.30.[37]

At her return visit, Ms. Noble's BP continues to be elevated but her laboratory tests and ECG are normal. You discuss the medication options (shown below) and, given her race and lack of kidney disease, you start her on hydrochlorothiazide 25 mg daily. Your nurse instructs her in checking her BP at home, and she will follow up in 1 month.

Table 12.29 ▶ Nonpharmacologic Treatment Options for Hypertension

Nonpharmacologic Options (expected decrease in BP)

Can also prevent development of HTN and progression of prehypertension to HTN
- Weight loss (decrease in systolic BP by 5–20 mm Hg per 10 kg weight loss)
- DASH diet (8 mm Hg)
- Restrict dietary sodium intake (2–8 mm Hg)
- Exercise at least 30 minutes a day most days of the week (4–9 mm Hg)
- Decrease alcohol consumption (2–4 mm Hg)
- Stop smoking

 Table 12.30 ▶ Joint National Committee Medication Recommendations

JNC Recommendations

General Treatment
- Initial treatment of the non-black population should include a thiazide diuretic, CCB, ACEI, or ARB
- In the general black population (including those with diabetes), initial treatment should include a thiazide diuretic or CCB
- All patients with chronic kidney disease should be on an ACEI or ARB as an initial agent or add on to protect kidney function
- All patients should be re-evaluated in 1 month and if blood pressure is not controlled, the dose of their initial agent should be increased or another agent should be added
- If needed, a third medication may be added from other classes of agents (e.g., β blockers, α blockers, aldosterone antagonists)
- ACEIs and ARBs should not be used together in the same patient

Specific Recommendations[37,82]
- Thiazide diuretics are first-line therapy in JNC 7 and 8 due to their favorable side effect profile, low cost, and evidence of improved patient outcomes
- There is no evidence to favor chlorthalidone over hydrochlorothiazide and there is no evidence to use doses of hydrochlorothiazide over 25 mg daily
- Beta blockers are no longer recommended as first- or second-line treatments for the majority of patients due to lack of evidence on mortality benefits
- Beta blockers are considered in people after a MI, with heart failure, or with other conditions that can be treated with beta blockers (e.g., migraine headaches or tremor)

ACEI, angiotensin-converting enzyme inhibitor; ARB, angiotensin receptor blocker; BP, blood pressure; CCB, calcium channel blocker; MI, myocardial infarction.

Monitoring

After initial diagnosis, patients should follow up in 1 month to see if their BP is controlled. In addition, they can check BPs at home and follow up sooner if they are not well controlled. People with HTN are at increased risk of HD, so screening for other risk factors such as hyperlipidemia and diabetes is important.

Patient Education and Self-Care

Patients should be asked to check their BP at home on a regular basis (SOR C). They can also bring in their home BP cuffs periodically and test their accuracy against the office

BP cuffs. Patients should be encouraged to follow a healthy lifestyle. Good resources for patients include:

▶ CDC informational page on HTN, https://www.cdc.gov/bloodpressure/

▶ American Heart Association: www.heart.org.

> At her 1-month follow-up, Ms. Noble's BP is now 146/95 mm Hg in the office, so you add amlodipine 5 mg daily. She calls 2 weeks later and reports BPs in the 130s/80s at home which is confirmed at her next follow-up visit with you. She is able to lose a little weight and has started exercising. You discuss increasing dietary fruits and vegetables and long-term plans to prevent HD or stroke.

Obesity

How Common is Obesity?

Almost 35% of the US adult population is classified as obese (body mass index [BMI] = 30 mg/kg^2 or greater) and an additional 33.6% of adults is classified as overweight (BMI = 25 to 29.9 mg/kg^2).[83] Among children, one third of those aged 6–9 years are overweight or obese.

The United States Preventive Services Task Force recommends screening all adult patients for obesity (calculating BMI from height and weight) and offering intensive counseling and behavioral interventions to promote sustained weight loss for obese adults (SOR B).[84]

Associated Health Conditions Include

Coronary artery disease	Diabetes
Gallbladder disease	Hypertension
Liver disease	Osteoarthritis
Sleep apnea	Stroke

> Julian is a 58-year-old man with a BMI of 34. He presents for a routine health maintenance examination. He has a positive family history of HD in his father and diabetes in his mother. He is married and has one child. He is in a high-pressure job and has little time for exercise but would really like to lose weight.

How to Assess Severity

Waist circumference is a predictor of all-cause mortality,[85] and an important risk factor for CVD, and type-2 diabetes.[86] It is a particularly important measure when assessing obesity in older adults who may have reduced height from OP (falsely high BMI) or reduced weight from lower muscle mass (falsely low BMI). **Waist circumference over 88.9 cm (35 in) for women or 101 cm (40 in) for men is considered high risk** (see Chapter 13 and https://www.youtube.com/watch?v=Qc-4kwgzg4Y). Julian's weight circumference is 105 cm placing him at higher mortality risk.

Assessing severity is more about identifying and controlling medical conditions associated with obesity than with weight. A first step is to **review any medications,**

Table 12.31 ▶ Medications that can Promote Weight Gain and Alternatives

Drug Category	Alternatives: Weight Neutral or Weight Loss
Antidepressants	
• Tricyclics (amitriptyline, nortriptyline) • Mirtazapine	• Bupropion (weight loss) • Fluoxetine
Antidiabetic Agents	
• Insulin (all forms) • Sulfonylureas (e.g., glyburide) • Thiazolidinediones (e.g., pioglitazone)	• Metformin (weight loss) • Others including: acarbose, DPP-4 inhibitors, GLP-I receptor agonists (weight loss)
Antipsychotic Agents	
• Olanzapine • Quetiapine • Risperidone	• Ziprasidone
Anti-seizure Agents	
• Carbamazepine • Gabapentin	• Topiramate (weight loss) • Zonisamide (weight loss)
Hormones	
• Corticosteroids (prednisone, oral) • Depo Provera	• Intermittent use or other forms • Other forms of contraception

Data from: Domecq JP, Prutsky G, Leppin A, et al. Clinical review: Drugs commonly associated with weight change: a systematic review and meta-analysis. *J Clin Endocrinol Metab.* 2015;100(2):363–370.

including nonprescription drugs, that the patient may be taking that promote weight gain (Table 12.31). Most of these drugs only increase weight by an average of 1 to 3 kg, but can sometimes be substituted for drugs that are weight-neutral or promote weight loss, if a drug is needed. Julian is not on medications associated with weight gain. While it is uncommon to have an endocrine condition that is responsible for obesity, thyroid disease, Cushing's syndrome, or polycystic ovarian syndrome can promote weight gain.

Screen patients with obesity for the health conditions listed above. Julian's BP is mildly elevated at 145/90 mm Hg. Adults with a BMI >40 kg/m² have higher rates of cancer of the breast, endometrium, colon, and prostate in addition to a reduced life expectancy; obese women may have difficulty with abnormal menses and infertility. In the case presented, Julian could be questioned about chest pain and sleep apnea, his BP measured, and laboratory testing considered for blood sugar and lipids. He could also be recommended for colorectal cancer screening (Chapter 7).

An approach to patients with obesity is shown in Figure 12.10.

Julian agrees to obtain laboratory tests, park farther from work to get in more walking and join Weight Watchers. You help him identify foods that he might eliminate from his diet. He will follow-up in 1 month.

Treatment Goals

Treatment goals for BP, glucose, and lipids, if elevated, are discussed in other sections within this chapter. Treatment goals for obesity should be individualized, but even a 3% to 5% weight loss can decrease risk of CVD and diabetes.[87]

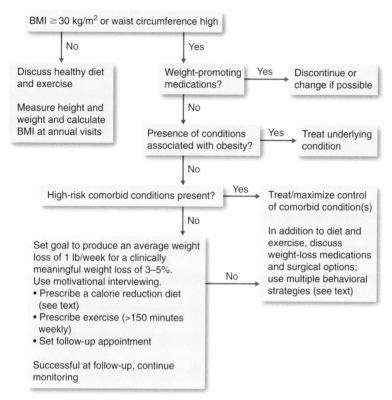

Figure 12.10 ▶ Approach to the patient with obesity.

Evidence-based recommendations from the 2013 Obesity Guideline include:[87]

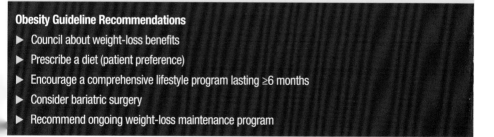

Obesity Guideline Recommendations
▶ Council about weight-loss benefits
▶ Prescribe a diet (patient preference)
▶ Encourage a comprehensive lifestyle program lasting ≥6 months
▶ Consider bariatric surgery
▶ Recommend ongoing weight-loss maintenance program

To assist patients with lifestyle change, use the specific behavioral and cognitive-behavioral strategies discussed in Chapter 5. Effective behavioral strategies include support such as goal-setting and encouraging self-monitoring, motivational interviewing and simple tasks such as reducing sitting and TV screen time.

Treatment Options

Diet. Even when combined with lifestyle modification, dieting results in only modest weight loss (<5 kg weight loss over 2 to 4 years) (SOR A).[88] There is no single diet that is better than any other—any diet that creates a **deficit of about 500 kcal/day** below what is needed to maintain weight can be successful. This can be accomplished in many ways such as:

▸ Following a specific diet

▸ Eliminating specific high-calorie foods

▸ Substituting low-calorie drinks for meals

Commercial weight-reduction programs like Weight Watchers or Slimming World appear to be more effective in helping patients achieve weight loss than primary care-directed weight loss efforts.

Exercise. Adding exercise to diet may result in modest weight loss or additional weight loss of about 1 to 3 kg. However, exercise improves metabolic profiles, and exercise at levels of 60 to 90 minutes per day can help maintain weight loss. Many kinds of exercise can be suggested including walking and water aerobics.

> Julian returns to the office. His weight is down 3 lb and his BP is unchanged. His laboratory test results indicate mildly elevated LDL but are otherwise normal. He has not had a chance to join Weight Watchers yet but plans to do so. He has eliminated fast food lunches and feels better. You congratulate him on this good start and encourage continued diet and exercise, noting that he can likely avoid the need for medication for his BP and cholesterol if weight loss continues. Telephone follow-up is planned for one month and an office visit in 3 months.

Medication. Offer pharmacologic therapy to patients with obesity (or with a BMI of 27 kg/m^2 or 30 kg/m^2 or more with concomitant obesity-related risk factors or diseases) who fail to achieve their weight loss goals through diet and exercise alone.[89,90] Medication remains an option for Julian, but there is no need to begin medication at this time given his lack of comorbid obesity-related diseases.

Medication options include lorcaserin, orlistat, phentermine/topiramate, and sympathomimetics (Table 12.32). No drug appears to be better than another, although orlistat is often considered a first-line agent based on long-term safety.

Average weight loss with medication varies from 2 to 10 kg. Other drugs with weight loss as a side effect have also been used including fluoxetine and bupropion. Most weight loss occurs in the first 6 months of treatment.[91] If weight loss is less than 3% in three months, re-evaluate.

Bariatric Surgery. Bariatric surgery (i.e., gastric banding and gastric bypass) creates restriction of stomach size and inability to absorb consumed calories due to bypassing sections of bowel. Offer referral to an experienced bariatric surgeon to patients with a BMI ≥40 kg/m^2 or BMI ≥35 kg/m^2 with obesity-related comorbid conditions who are motivated to lose weight but have failed to achieve their weight loss goals through diet and exercise with or without pharmacotherapy.[87]

Surgery provides a range of 25 to 75 kg of weight loss after 2 to 4 years (higher loss following bypass),[92] and has been shown to reduce all-cause mortality[93] as well as rates of diabetes, sleep apnea and symptoms of dyspnea and chest pain.[94] Diagrams of gastric banding and gastric bypass procedures are shown in Figure 12.11. Bariatric surgery is also an option for Julian if his efforts to reduce his weight prove unsuccessful.

Table 12.32 ▶ Medication Options for Obesity

Medication	How It Works	Side Effects	Cautions
Lorcaserin (10 mg daily)	Anorectic with serotonergic properties	Nausea, dry mouth, constipation, priapism	Multiple drug interactions Avoid with other serotonergic agents or heart disease; caution with diabetes
Orlistat (120 mg three times daily)	Lipase inhibitor—prevents fat absorption	Diarrhea, gas, bloating abdominal pain, dyspepsia	Inhibits pancreatic lipase
Phentermine–topiramate (multiple formulations, once daily)	(see below) plus anticonvulsant with weight loss side effect	Nausea, dry mouth, constipation, altered taste	Multiple drug interactions, Avoid if heart disease, uncontrolled hypertension, glaucoma, or hyperthyroidism
Naltrexone/bupropion (8 mg/90 mg daily to 16/180 twice daily)	Opioid receptor antagonist plus dopamine/norepinephrine reuptake inhibitor	Nausea, constipation, headache, dizziness	Not for children or adolescence Can raise blood pressure
Sympathomimetics • Phentermine (15–37.5 mg in am) • Diethylpropion (25 mg 3 times daily or 75 mg ER daily)	Appetite suppressants (psychostimulants)	Palpitations, tachycardia, hypertension, nausea	Major drug interactions Addiction potential Avoid if heart disease or uncontrolled hypertension

ER, extended release.
Data from: Li Z, Maglione M, Tu W, et al. Meta-analysis: pharmacologic treatment of obesity. *Ann Internal Med.* 2005;142(7):532–546; Bray GA, Ryan DH. Medical therapy for the patient with obesity. *Circulation.* 2012;125(13):1695–1703; Bray GA, Ryan DH. Update on obesity pharmacotherapy. *Ann N Y Acad Sci.* 2014;1311(1):1–13; http://www.arenapharm.com/belviq (Accessed May 2014); Early J, Whitten JS. Naltrexone/bupropion (Contrave) for weight loss. *Am Fam Physician.* 2015; 91(8):554–556.

Operative mortality is about 1% for gastric bypass and 0.4% for gastric banding with similar rates of other postoperative adverse events.[95] **Potential side effects** include vitamin B_{12} deficiency, incisional hernia, possible need for reoperation, gastritis, gallbladder disease, dumping syndrome, and malabsorption.[87]

To prevent nutritional deficiencies, bariatric patients should take[96]:

▶ 1–2 adult multivitamins plus minerals containing iron, folic acid, and thiamine

▶ 1,200–1,500 mg elemental calcium from dietary sources and/or supplements

▶ 3,000 IU of vitamin D (titrated to therapeutic 25-D levels >30 ng/mL)

▶ Vitamin B_{12}

Devices. Several devices are available to assist with weight loss. These fall into the categories of space-occupying devices (ReShape, Orbera Gastric Balloon, Transpyloric Shuttle, Sati-Sphere), aspiration therapy (AspireAssist), gastric volume reduction (Transoral Endoscopic

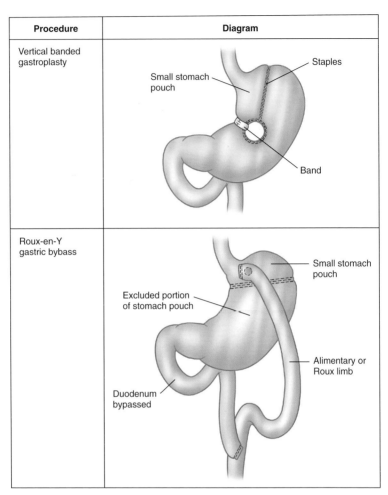

Procedure	Diagram
Vertical banded gastroplasty	
Roux-en-Y gastric bybass	

Figure 12.11 ▶ Gastric banding and bypass procedures. (Images from National Heart, Lung, and Blood Institute: Managing overweight and obesity in adults: systematic evidence review from the obesity expert panel. 2013:97. US Department of Health and Human Services. https://www.nhlbi.nih.gov/health-topics/managing-overweight-obesity-in-adults)

Restrictive Implant System), and vagal-blocking therapy (Maestro Rechargeable System). Initial (3-month) weight loss ranges from about 7 to 17 kg.[97] There is limited data on longer-term effectiveness and safety. ReShape and Orbera, have been FDA-approved for use up to 6 months in patients with a BMI of 30 to 40 mg/kg^2. Images of the FDA-approved devices can be found at https://www.fda.gov/medicaldevices/productsandmedicalprocedures/obesitydevices/default.htm.

Adverse effects of balloon-type devices include abdominal pain or distention, gastric ulceration, gastritis, and nausea/vomiting. Other devices are awaiting FDA approval.

Secondary Prevention

Preventive health screening should occur based on age and risk factors (Chapter 7). However, obese women appear to be less likely to obtain Pap smears and mammograms and may need additional encouragement.[98]

Monitoring

Weight loss efforts can be frustrating and ongoing support and monitoring can be help-ful. Work with the patient to determine appropriate follow-up intervals. If the patient is on anti-obesity drugs or recently following bariatric surgery, intervals of every 3 months may be appropriate for follow-up assessing for successful weight loss and side effects as noted above.

Your office nurse continues to provide monthly telephone follow-up via text messages to Julian and at his 3-month follow-up, his steady weight-loss has continued.

Resources

Weight control like any attempt at a healthier lifestyle is an ongoing issue. Reliable Inter-net resources for patients (and for you) include: https://medlineplus.gov/obesity.html and https://www.cdc.gov/obesity/index.html.

Osteoporosis

Ms. Cho is a 63-year-old woman who presents to follow up after a recent hospitalization for back pain. Her work up revealed vertebral compression fractures at T4 to T6. She presents to talk about pain control and OP. She has never had a bone density test and does not have any other risk factors for secondary OP. You talk to Ms. Cho about OP and counsel her on the importance of weight-bearing exercise and a diet rich in calcium and vitamin D. You also do a fall evaluation which is negative. You order a dual energy x-ray absorptiometry (DEXA) scan and advise her to continue her calcitonin nasal spray that was started in the hospital and has helped with her pain.

OP is a bone disease that is characterized by low bone mass, microarchitectural distortion of the bone matrix, and an increased fracture risk (Fig. 12.12). Osteopenia is low bone

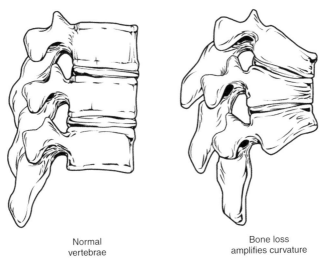

Normal
vertebrae

Bone loss
amplifies curvature

Figure 12.12 ▶ Normal and osteoporotic vertebrae. (From Openstax. The vertebral column. *Anatomy & Physiology.* Houston: Rice University; 2017;8:103. Download for free at http://cnx.org.)

Table 12.33 ► Risk Factors for Osteoporosis

Risk Factors	
• Age	• Low body weight (<127 lb)
• Excess alcohol use	• Personal history of fracture
• Smoking	• Family history of osteoporotic fracture
• Immobilization and inadequate activity	• Low calcium or vitamin D intake

density but not at the same level as OP. The **main consequences** of osteopenia and OP are **hip fracture** and consequent loss of independence and **vertebral compression fractures** which lead to chronic pain. After a hip fracture, only 40% to 60% of people regain their prefracture level of mobility.[99,100] In addition, 10% to 20% of people are institutionalized after a hip fracture.

Peak bone density occurs around age 30 years for both men and women. Men experience a gradual decline in bone density with age, while women experience an accelerated period of bone loss right after menopause in addition to bone loss with age. Risk factors for OP are shown in Table 12.33 and secondary causes of OP are shown in Table 12.34.[101–103]

How Common is Osteoporosis

► 16% of women over age 50 years and 24.8% of women over age 65 years have OP?[99,100]

► 4% of men over age 50 years and 5.6% of men over age 65 years have OP (Fig. 12.13)

► Over 10 million people in the United States have OP

► 1 in 2 women and 1 in 4 men will have an osteoporotic-related fracture during their lives

Diagnostics

DEXA is an x-ray able to measure bone density (Fig. 12.14). The examination calculates the actual bone density at the lumbar spine and hip and compares it to the bone density

Table 12.34 ► Common Causes of Secondary Osteoporosis

Causes	
Autoimmune disorders: rheumatoid arthritis, systemic lupus	**Medications:**
Chronic obstructive pulmonary disease	• Anticonvulsants
Endocrine disorders: adrenal insufficiency, female athlete triad, hypothyroidism, hyperthyroidism, type 1 diabetes mellitus, primary ovarian insufficiency, hyperprolactinemia	• Chemotherapy agents
	• Glucocorticoids
	• Heparin
GI disorders: celiac disease, gastric bypass, inflammatory bowel disease, malabsorption, pancreatic insufficiency	• Lithium
	• Methotrexate
Liver disease	• Proton pump inhibitors
Nutritional disorders: heavy alcohol use, eating disorders, vitamin D deficiency	• Thyroid hormone excess
Renal insufficiency or failure	

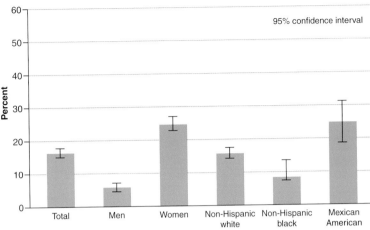

Figure 12.13 ► Age-adjusted percentage of adults aged 65 years old and over with osteoporosis. (From CDC Osteoporosis fast facts, available at: http://www.cdc.gov/nchs/data/hestat/osteoporsis/osteoporosis2005_2010.htm.)

standard of a 35-year-old white woman. Two numbers are calculated. The T-score is the relationship of the patient's bone density to the standard and is scored as:

▶ **Normal** bone density is within 1 standard deviation from the standard

▶ **Osteopenia** (or low bone density) is defined as −1 to −2.5 SD below the standard

▶ **Osteoporosis** is defined as ≥−2.5 SD below the standard

The Z-score compares bone density to age and gender averages. This score is helpful to signal the possible presence of secondary OP (i.e., if the person's bone density is significantly below expected for their age and gender). On DEXA scan, Ms. Cho a T-score of −2.2, placing her in the range of osteopenia.

FRAX or fracture risk assessment tool (https://www.shef.ac.uk/FRAX/) is based on large population-based cohorts around the world. The calculator uses DEXA results, along with clinical risk factors, to calculate the 10-year risk of a hip or other major osteoporotic

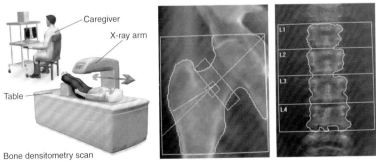

Figure 12.14 ► Bone density measurement with DEXA. (**Left:** From https://en.wikipedia.org/wiki/Dual-energy_ X-ray_absorptiometry. Images from Blausen.com staff, 2014. Medical gallery of Blausen Medical 2014. *WikiJournal of Medicine* 1 (2). DOI:10.15347/wjm/2014.010.) (**Right:** From Germain DP. Fabry disease. *Orphanet J Rare Dis.* 2010;5:30.)

fracture. Calculating Ms, Cho's FRAX score, her 10-year probability of major osteoporotic fracture is 11% and for hip fracture is 2%.

Screen for Osteoporosis (US Preventive Services Task Force Recommendation)

▶ In women 65 years and older and in younger women whose fracture risk is that of a 65-year-old woman with no other risk factors **(SOR B)**

▶ Evidence is insufficient to recommend for or against screening men for OP

Treatment decisions are based on FRAX results and T scores.

Consider treatment if:

▶ FRAX score is ≥3% 10-year risk for hip fracture or ≥20% risk of other major osteoporotic fractures

▶ T score is ≤−2.5 at the femoral neck

▶ T score is between −1 and −2.5 and the patient has an elevated 10-year risk of fracture

▶ The patient has a history of a previous osteoporotic-related fracture

---

Treatment Goals

▶ Maximize peak bone density in all young men and women by counseling about avoidance of risks for secondary OP, ingesting adequate amounts of calcium and vitamin D-rich foods, getting adequate exercise.

▶ Identify women with osteopenia or OP before fracture occurs through screening.

▶ Counsel all community-dwelling adults over 65 years about exercise, physical therapy, and vitamin D supplementation to prevent falls (SOR B).[104]

▶ Treat all adults who are diagnosed with OP, who have had a previous osteoporotic fracture, or who have osteopenia and other risk factors for fracture with one of the FDA-approved medications.

Treatment Options

▶ Exercise, eat a diet rich in calcium and vitamin D, avoid causes of secondary OP.

▶ USPSTF—insufficient evidence to recommend supplementation with calcium and vitamin D.

▶ For OP, choose a medication listed in Table 12.35.

At follow-up, you discuss her test result and FRAX score. Although you would normally not start her on medications based on her scores, since she has already had an OP-related fracture, you talk to her about the benefits and risks of starting a bisphosphonate to prevent future vertebral compression fractures. She elects to start alendronate.

Monitoring

▶ ***When should we repeat a DEXA scan?*** There is no clear answer to that question. In people who are started on medications to prevent fractures, repeat BMD assessment may be considered in 1 to 2 years after initiation of medication.[104]

Table 12.35 ▶ Medications for Treating Osteoporosis to Prevent Fractures

Medications	Mechanism of Action	Comments
Bisphosphonates • Alendronate (Fosamax) • Ibandronate (Boniva) • Risedronate (Actonel) • Zoledronic acid (Reclast)	Inhibit osteoclastic activity and works as antiresorptive agents	Reduces hip and vertebral fractures in RCTs Oral bisphosphonates can lead to esophagitis and long-term use has been linked to osteonecrosis of the jaw and atypical femur fractures
SERM • Raloxifene (Evista)	Systemic estrogen reuptake modulator that decreases bone resorption and bone turnover	Can cause hot flashes and increase risk of VTE Reduces vertebral fractures in RCTs, but not hip fractures.
Calcitonin nasal spray	Antiresorptive agent.	Used commonly for treating pain related to vertebral compression fractures
Teriparatide (Forteo)	Synthetic parathyroid hormone that has bone anabolic activity and stimulates bone growth	Frequent side effects include leg cramps, dizziness, and nausea Increased the risk of osteosarcoma in rats
Denosumab (Prolia)	Inhibits the formation and activity of osteoclasts	Often used second line in people who do not improve with bisphosphonates

RCT, randomized clinical trial; SERM, selective estrogen receptor modulator; VTE, venous thromboembolism.

▶ *What should you do if your patient is taking prednisone?* Because the risk of developing OP is so high in patients on chronic steroids, the American College of Rheumatology recommends prophylactic treatment with a bisphosphonate for postmenopausal women or men over age 50 years who are going to be on >7.5 mg of prednisone for more than 3 months.[105]

Patient Education and Self-Care

People with osteopenia or OP should be encouraged to focus on exercise and dietary changes to prevent fractures. There are many specific exercises that will help prevent fractures.

▶ https://www.youtube.com/watch?v=DAv1oLk_XGM

▶ https://www.youtube.com/watch?v=LTS7R3Zsu2Q

▶ http://www.webmd.com/osteoporosis/video/prevent-fractures-osteoporosis

Exercise to prevent fractures focuses on weight bearing exercise to maintain bone density in the legs and hips and weight lifting to maintain strong bones in the upper body.

You refer Ms. Cho to physical therapy to work on core strengthening and arrange to follow up in 6 months.

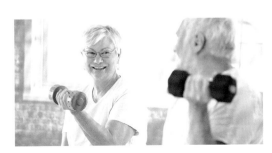

QUESTIONS

1. Which one of the following is an aspect of successful chronic disease management in addition to community resources, healthcare organizations, clinical information systems, decision support, and self-management support?
   A. Telemedicine
   B. Provision of medical equipment
   C. Delivery system redesign
   D. Access to advanced imaging

2. You receive a call from a parent of an 8-year-old child with worsening asthma. Which one of the following is the first step in the home management of an acute asthma exacerbation?
   A. Assess severity
   B. Prescribe antibiotics
   C. Prescribe a trial of a treatment of an inhaled short-acting beta agonist
   D. Prescribe a trial of an inhaled corticosteroid
   E. Advise the parent to bring the child to the office for assessment

3. Which one of the following should be done to confirm a diagnosis of chronic obstructive pulmonary disease?
   A. Assess clinical features
   B. Perform spirometry
   C. Obtain a chest x-ray
   D. Perform an arterial blood gas
   E. Obtain an echocardiogram

4. You are working with a 70-year-old man who has stable coronary artery disease to prevent progression of his heart disease. He is a nonsmoker. Which one of the following, done as part of risk factor modification, will likely reduce his risk of dying?
   A. Screen for and treat depression, if present
   B. Attempt to normalize his blood sugar, if diabetic
   C. Provide influenza vaccination
   D. Increase his physical activity
   E. Help him reduce his weight to a target BMI <25 kg/m^2

5. Blood pressure control in patients with diabetes to $<150/85$ mm Hg decreases diabetes-related mortality, diabetes-related outcomes and overall mortality?
   A. True
   B. False

6. Which one of the following is true of heart failure with preserved ejection fraction?
   A. It is more common in young men.
   B. Left ventricular ejection fraction is $>80\%$.
   C. It is considered preheart failure.
   D. Echocardiogram can be used to establish the diagnosis.
   E. There is strong evidence to guide medication management.

7. Which one of the following is one of the American College of Cardiology/American Heart Association benefit groups for statin therapy (atherosclerotic cardiovascular disease [ASCVD] risk reduction outweighs the risk of medication)?

A. People with clinical evidence of ASCVD
B. People with hypertension
C. Men who are over age 50 years
D. Women who are postmenopausal
E. Individuals with a low density lipid level of >100 mg/dL and 10-year ASCVD risk >5%

8. Which one of the following is recommended by the Joint National Committee 8 for treatment of hypertension?
   A. Initial treatment of the non-black population should include a beta blocker.
   B. Initial treatment of the black population should include a thiazide diuretic.
   C. Patients with chronic kidney disease should be treated with a calcium channel blocker.
   D. If blood pressure is not controlled in 6 months, another agent should be added.
   E. If blood pressure is not controlled on an angiotensin converting enzyme inhibitor, and angiotensin receptor blocker should be added.

9. You are seeing an obese patient who asks about strategies for weight loss, having failed to achieve weight loss with diet and exercise. Which one of the following is true of managing obesity in this patient?
   A. He should try a different type of diet as certain diets are better for weight loss.
   B. He should increase his exercise as it can reduce weight by about 7 kg.
   C. Medication should be tried before considering surgery.
   D. He should be offered surgery if his BMI is ≥40 kg/m².

10. Which one of the following is true of diagnosis and management of osteoporosis (OP)?
    A. Half of women over age 50 years have OP.
    B. Women should be screened for OP at age 50 years or older.
    C. Treatment decisions are based on fracture risk assessment tool (FRAX) results.
    D. Treatment of OP is calcium and vitamin D.
    E. Women with OP should be monitored annually with dual energy x-ray absorptiometry.

ANSWERS

Question 1: The correct answer is C.
The 6 different aspects of successful chronic disease care, shown in Table 12.1, are community resources, healthcare organizations, decision support, delivery system redesign, clinical information systems, and self-management support.

Question 2: The correct answer is A.
For acute asthma-induced wheezing, the initial step is to determine severity based on peak expiratory flow.

Question 3: The correct answer is B.
Diagnose COPD with spirometry showing persistent airflow limitation.

Question 4: The correct answer is C.
As shown in Table 12.11, providing annual influenza vaccination for all patients with coronary artery disease reduces risk of hospitalization for heart disease and all-cause mortality in the elderly.

Question 5: The correct answer is A.

The benefit of blood pressure control in patients with diabetes was demonstrated in the United Kingdom Prospective Diabetes Study (UKPDS). In this study of 5,102 adults with type 2 diabetes, controlled blood pressure (<150/85 mm Hg) decreased diabetes-related mortality, diabetes-related outcomes (NNT 61 to prevent one serious diabetes-related outcome), and overall mortality.

Question 6: The correct answer is D.

Echocardiography is used both to confirm the diagnosis of HF and to distinguish whether it is systolic or diastolic in nature. Features of heart failure with reduced or preserved ejection fraction are shown in Table 12.17.

Question 7: The correct answer is A.

The 2013 American College of Cardiology (ACC)/American Heart Association (AHA) guideline identifies four benefit groups, listed in Table 12.22, for whom atherosclerotic cardiovascular disease (ASCVD) risk reduction outweighs the risk of medication (SOR A). The four groups are: people with clinical evidence of ASCVD, individuals with DM between 40 and 75 years with LDL >70 mg/dL, individuals with LDL >190 mg/dL, and individuals with LDL between 70 and 189 mg/dL and 10-year risk of ASCVD >7.5%.

Question 8: The correct answer is B.

Table 12.3: In the general black population (including those with diabetes), initial treatment should include a thiazide diuretic or calcium channel blocker.

Question 9: The correct answer is D.

Offer referral to an experienced bariatric surgeon to patients with a BMI ≥40 kg/m² or BMI ≥35 kg/m² with obesity-related comorbid conditions who are motivated to lose weight but have failed to achieve their weight loss goals through diet and exercise with or without pharmacotherapy.

Question 10: The correct answer is C.

FRAX or fracture risk assessment tool is based on large population-based cohorts around the world. The calculator uses DEXA results, along with clinical risk factors, to calculate the 10-year risk of a hip or other major osteoporotic fracture. Treatment decisions are based on these scores...

REFERENCES

1. Bodenheimer T, Wagner EH, Grumbach K. Improving primary care for patients with chronic illness, part 1. *JAMA.* 2002;288(14):1775–1779.
2. Chronic disease prevention and health promotion, facts about chronic diseases. Available from: http://www.cdc.gov/chronicdisease/overview/index.htm. Accessed October 2016.
3. National Asthma Education and Prevention Program: *Expert panel report III: Guidelines for the Diagnosis and Management of Asthma.* Bethesda, MD: National Heart, Lung, and Blood Institute, 2007. (NIH publication no. 08–4051). Available from: www.nhlbi.nih.gov/guidelines/asthma/asthgdln.htm
4. Fahy JV, O'Byrne PM. "Reactive airways disease." A lazy term of uncertain meaning that should be abandoned. *Am J Respir Crit Care Med.* 2001;163(4):822.
5. 2014 National Health Interview Survey (NHIS) Data. Available from: https://www.cdc.gov/asthma/most_recent_data.htm. Accessed September 25, 2016.
6. Liu AH, Zeiger R, Sorkness C, et al. Development and cross-sectional validation of the childhood asthma control test. *J Allergy Clin Immunol.* 2007;119:817.
7. Nathan RA, Sorkness CA, Kosinski M, et al. Development of the asthma control test: a survey for assessing asthma control. *J Allergy Clin Immunol.* 2004;113(1):59–65.

8. National Asthma Education and Prevention Program. *Expert Panel Report III: Guidelines for the Diagnosis and Management of Asthma.* Bethesda, MD: National Heart, Lung, and Blood Institute, 2007. (NIH publication no. 08–4051). Available from: www.nhlbi.nih.gov/guidelines/asthma/asthgdln.htm. Accessed October 2016.

9. Pellegrino R, Viegi G, Brusasco V, et al. Interpretative strategies for lung function tests. *Eur Respir J.* 2005;26:948–968.

10. Eldeirawi K, Persky VW. History of ear infections and prevalence of asthma in a national sample of children aged 2 to 11 years: the Third National Health and Nutrition Examination Survey, 1988 to 1994. *Chest.* 2004;125(5):1685–1692.

11. Arif AA, Delclos GL, Lee ES, et al. Prevalence and risk factors of asthma and wheezing among US adults: an analysis of the NHANES III data. *Eur Respir J.* 2003;21(5):827–833.

12. Miller KE. Metered-dose inhalers vs. nebulizers in treating asthma. *Am Fam Physician.* 2002;66(7):1311.

13. Platts-Mills T, Leung DY, Schatz M. The role of allergens in asthma. *Am Fam Physician.* 2007;76(5):675–680.

14. Williams SG, Schmidt DK, Redd SC, et al. Key clinical activities for quality asthma care. Recommendations of the national asthma education and prevention program. *MMWR Recomm Rep.* 2003;52(RR-6):1–8.

15. Global Strategy for the Diagnosis, Management and Prevention of COPD, Global Initiative for Chronic Obstructive Lung Disease (GOLD) 2016. Available from: http://goldcopd.org/. Accessed October 2016.

16. Centers for Disease Control and Prevention, COPD. Available from: http://www.cdc.gov/copd/index.html. Accessed October 2016.

17. National Heart Lung and Blood Institute. Available from: http://www.nhlbi.nih.gov/health/health-topics/topics/aat. Accessed October 2016.

18. Centers for Disease Control and Prevention. Available from: http://www.cdc.gov/nchs/fastats/leading-causes-of-death.htm. Accessed October 2016.

19. Anthonisen NR, Skeans MA, Wise RA, et al. Lung Health Study Research Group. The effects of a smoking cessation intervention on 14.5-year mortality: a randomized clinical trial. *Ann Intern Med.* 2005;142(4):233–239.

20. Chong J, Leung B, Poole P. Phosphodiesterase 4 inhibitors for chronic obstructive pulmonary disease. *Cochrane Database Syst Rev.* 2013;(11):CD002309.

21. Ram FS, Jones PW, Castro AA. Oral theophylline for chronic obstructive pulmonary disease. *Cochrane Database Syst Rev.* 2002;(4):CD003902.

22. Poole P, Chong J, Cates CJ. Mucolytic agents versus placebo for chronic bronchitis or chronic obstructive pulmonary disease. *Cochrane Database Syst Rev.* 2015;(7):CD001287.

23. van Agteren JE, Carson KV, Tiong LU, et al. Lung volume reduction surgery for diffuse emphysema. *Cochrane Database Syst Rev.* 2016;(10):CD001001.

24. Walters JA, Tan DJ, White CJ, et al. Systemic corticosteroids for acute exacerbations of chronic obstructive pulmonary disease. *Cochrane Database Syst Rev.* 2014;(9):CD001288.

25. Walters JA, Tan DJ, White CJ, et al. Different durations of corticosteroid therapy for exacerbations of chronic obstructive pulmonary disease. *Cochrane Database Syst Rev.* 2014;(12):CD006897.

26. Vollenweider DJ, Jarrett H, Steurer-Stey CA, et al. Antibiotics for exacerbations of chronic obstructive pulmonary disease. *Cochrane Database Syst Rev.* 2012;(12):CD010257.

27. Gimeno-Santos E, Scharplatz M, Troosters T, et al. Pulmonary rehabilitation following exacerbations of chronic obstructive pulmonary disease.*Cochrane Database Syst Rev.* 2011;(5):CD005305.

28. Karloh M, Fleig Mayer A, Maurici R, et al. The COPD assessment test: What do we know so far? A systematic review and meta-analysis about clinical outcomes prediction and classification of patients into GOLD stages. *Chest.* 2016;149(2):413–425.

29. Heart Disease Facts. Centers for Disease Control and Prevention. Available from: http://www.cdc.gov/heartdisease/facts.htm. Accessed October 2016.

30. Rodney KZ. Coronary heart disease. *Essential Evidence Plus.* Updated 1/3/2016, Accessed October 25, 2016.

31. Campeau L. Grading of angina pectoris. *Circulation.* 1976;54(3):522–523.

32. Qaseem A, Fihn SD, Williams S, et al. Diagnosis of stable ischemic heart disease: Summary of a clinical practice guideline from the American college of physicians/American college of cardiology foundation/American heart association/American association for thoracic surgery/preventive cardiovascular nurses Association/society of thoracic surgeons. *Ann Intern Med.* 2012;157(10):729–734.

33. Wells Askew J, et al. Selecting the optimal cardiac stress test. UpToDate. Dec 16, 2015. Available from: https://www.uptodate.com/contents/selecting-the-optimal-cardiac-stress-test?source=search_result&search=exercise%20mpi&selectedTitle=1~14#H458218820. Accessed December 2016.

34. Practice Guidelines. Management of stable ischemic heart disease: Recommendations from the ACP. *Am Fam Physician.* 2013;88(9):612–616.

35. Hall SL, Lorenc T. Secondary prevention of coronary artery disease. *Am Fam Physician.* 2010;81(3):289–296.
36. Thombs BD, de Jonge P, Coyne JC, et al. Depression screening and patient outcomes in cardiovascular care: a systematic review. *JAMA.* 2008;300(18):2161–2171.
37. James PA, Oparil S, Carter BL, et al. 2014 evidence-based guideline for the management of high blood pressure in adults: Report from the panel members appointed to the Eighth Joint National Committee (JNC 8). *JAMA.* 2014;311:507–520.
38. Eagle KA, Guyton RA, Davidoff R, et al. for the American college of cardiology, American heart association task force on practice guidelines, American society for thoracic surgery and the society of thoracic surgeons. ACC/AHA 2004 guideline update for coronary artery graft surgery: summary article: a report of the American college of cardiology/American heart association task force on practice guidelines (Committee to Update the 1999 Guidelines for Coronary Artery Bypass Graft Surgery). *Circulation.* 2004;110(9):1168–1176.
39. Handelsman Y, Bloomgarden ZT, Grunberger G, et al. American Association of Clinical Endocrinologists medical guidelines for a diabetes mellitus comprehensive care plan – 2015. *Endocr Pract.* 2015;21(Suppl 1):1–87.
40. American Diabetes Association. Standards of medical care in diabetes – 2016. *Diabetes Care.* 2016;39(1): S1–S112.
41. Thomas D, Elliott EJ. Low glycaemic index, or low glycaemic load, diets for diabetes mellitus. *Cochrane Database Syst Rev.* 2009;(1):CD006296.
42. Tight blood pressure control and risk of macrovascular and microvascular complications in type 2 diabetes: UKPDS 38. UK Prospective Diabetes Study Group. *BMJ.* 1998;317(7160):703–713.
43. ACCORD Study Group. Cushman WC, Evans GW, Byington RP, et al. Effects of intensive blood-pressure control in type 2 diabetes mellitus. *N Engl J Med.* 2010;362(17):1575–1585.
44. Boulin M, Diaby V, Tannenbaum C. Preventing unnecessary costs of drug-induced hypoglycemia in older adults with type 2 diabetes in the United States and Canada. *PLoS One.* 2016;11(9):e0162951.
45. Tandon N, Ali MK, Narayan KM. Pharmacologic prevention of microvascular and macrovascular complications in diabetes mellitus: implications of the results of recent clinical trials in type 2 diabetes. *Am J Cardiovasc Drugs.* 2012;12(1):7–22.
46. Rodríguez-Gutiérrez R, Montori VM. Glycemic control for patients with type 2 diabetes mellitus: our evolving faith in the face of evidence. *Circ Cardiovasc Qual Outcomes.* 2016;9(5):504–512.
47. UK Prospective Diabetes Study Group. Intensive blood-glucose control with sulphonylureas or insulin compared with conventional treatment and risk of complications in patients with type 2 diabetes (UKPDS 33). *Lancet.* 1998;352:837–853.
48. The Action to Control Cardiovascular Risk in Diabetes Study Group. Effects of intensive glucose lowering in type 2 diabetes. *N Engl J Med.* 2008;358:2545–2559.
49. The ADVANCE Collaborative Group. Intensive blood glucose control and vascular outcomes in patients with type 2 diabetes. *N Engl J Med.* 2008;358:2560–2572.
50. Duckworth W, Abraira C, Moritz T, et al. Glucose control and vascular complications in veterans with type 2 diabetes. *N Engl J Med.* 2009;360:129–139.
51. Effect of intensive blood-glucose control with metformin on complications in overweight patients with type 2 diabetes (UKPDS 34). UK Prospective Diabetes Study (UKPDS) Group. *Lancet.* 1998;352(9131):854–865.
52. O'Kane MJ, Bunting B, Copeland M, et al. Efficacy of self monitoring of blood glucose in patients with newly diagnosed type 2 diabetes (ESMON study): randomised controlled trial. *BMJ.* 2008;336(7654):1174–1177.
53. CDC, NCHS. Underlying cause of death 1999–2013 on CDC WONDER online database, released 2015. Data are from the multiple cause of death Files, 1999–2013, as compiled from data provided by the 57 vital statistics jurisdictions through the Vital Statistics Cooperative Program. Accessed February 3, 2015.
54. Mozzafarian D, Benjamin EJ, Go AS, et al. on behalf of the American Heart association statistics committee and stroke statistics subcommittee. Heart disease and stroke statistics—2016 update: a report from the American heart association. *Circulation.* 2016;133:e38–e360.
55. Kalogeropoulos A, Georgiopoulou V, Kritchevsky SB, et al. Epidemiology of incident heart failure in a contemporary elderly cohort: the health, aging, and body composition study. *Arch Intern Med.* 2009;169(7):708–715.
56. Felker GM, Thompson RE, Hare JM, et al. Underlying causes and long-term survival in patients with initially unexplained cardiomyopathy. *N Engl J Med.* 2000;342(15):1077–1084.
57. Baldasseroni S, Opasich C, Gorini M, et al. Italian network on congestive heart failure investigators. Left bundle-branch block is associated with increased 1-year sudden and total mortality rate in 5517 outpatients with congestive heart failure: a report from the Italian network on congestive heart failure. *Am Heart J.* 2002;143(3):398–405.
58. He J, Ogden LG, Bazzano LA, et al. Risk factors for congestive heart failure in US men and women: NHANES I epidemiologic follow-up study. *Arch Intern Med.* 2001;161(7):996–1002.

59. King M, Kingery J, Casey B. Diagnosis and evaluation of heart failure. *Am Fam Physician*. 2012;85(12):1161–1168.
60. Maestre A, Gil V, Gallego J, et al. Diagnostic accuracy of clinical criteria for identifying systolic and diastolic heart failure: cross-sectional study. *J Eval Clin Pract*. 2009;15(1):55–61.
61. McKee PA, Castelli WP, McNamara PM, et al. The natural history of congestive heart failure: the Framingham study. *N Engl J Med*. 1971;285:1441–1446.
62. Senni M, Tribouilloy CM, Rodeheffer RJ, et al. Congestive heart failure in the community: a study of all incident cases in Olmsted County, Minnesota, in 1991. *Circulation*. 1998;98(21):2282–2289.
63. Yancy CW, Jessup M, Bozkurt B, et al. 2013 ACCF/AHA guideline for the management of heart failure: executive summary: a report of the American College of Cardiology Foundation/American Heart Association Task Force on practice guidelines. *Circulation*. 2013;128(16):1810–1852.
64. Taylor RS, Sagar VA, Davies EJ, et al. Exercise based rehabilitation for heart failure. *Cochrane Database Syst Rev*. 2014;(4):CD003331.
65. Desai AS, Fang JC, Maisel WH, et al. Implantable defibrillators for the prevention of mortality in patients with nonischemic cardiomyopathy: a meta-analysis of randomized controlled trials. *JAMA*. 2004;292:2874–2879.
66. Velazquez EJ, Lee KL, Deja MA, et al.; STICH Investigators. Coronary-artery bypass surgery in patients with left ventricular dysfunction. *N Engl J Med*. 2011;364:1607–1616.
67. Pittler MH, Guo R, Ernst E, et al. Hawthorn extract for treating chronic heart failure. *Cochrane Database Syst Rev*. 2008;(1):CD005312.
68. Yeh GY, Wang C, Wayne PM, et al. Tai chi exercise for patients with cardiovascular conditions and risk factors: a systematic review. *Cardiopulm Rehabil Prev*. 2009;29:152–160.
69. Taylor RS, Ashton KE, Moxham T, et al. Reduced dietary salt for the prevention of cardiovascular disease: a meta-analysis of randomized controlled trials (Cochrane review). *Am J Hypertens*. 2011;24:843–853.
70. Doust JA. Heart failure (systolic). Essential Evidence Plus. Updated 1/3/2016. Available from: http://www.essentialevidenceplus.com.ezproxy.library.wisc.edu/content/eee/33. Accessed October 5, 2016.
71. Mannu GS, Zaman MJ, Gupta A, et al. Evidence of lifestyle modifications in the management of hypercholesterolemia. *Current Cardiology Rev*. 2013;9:2–14.
72. Stone NJ, Robinson JG, Lichtenstein AH, et al. 2013 ACC/AHA guidelines on the treatment of blood cholesterol to reduce atherosclerotic cardiovascular risk in adults: a report of the American College of Cardiology/American Heart Association task force on practice guidelines. *Circulation*. 2014;129(25 Suppl 2):S1–S45.
73. VA DOD Guideline: Diagnosis and management of dyslipidemia for cardiovascular risk reduction. Available from: http://www.healthquality.va.gov/guidelines/CD/lipids/LipidSumOptSinglePg31Aug15.pdf. Accessed October 2016.
74. Adams SP, Sekhon SS, Wright JM. Lipid-lowering efficacy of rosuvastatin. *Cochrane Database Syst Rev*. 2014;(11):CD010254.
75. Wang D, Liu B, Tao W, et al. Fibrates for secondary prevention of cardiovascular disease and stroke. *Cochrane Database Syst Rev*. 2015;(10):CD009580.
76. Liu ZL, Li GQ, Bensoussan A, et al. Chinese herbal medicines for hypertriglyceridemia. *Cochrane Database Syst Rev*. 2013;(6):CD009560.
77. Last A, Ference JD, Falleroni J. Pharmacologic treatment of hyperlipidemia. *Am Fam Physician*. 2011;84(5):551–558.
78. United States Preventive Services Task Force. Availabla from: https://www.uspreventiveservicestaskforce.org/Page/Document/RecommendationStatementFinal/high-blood-pressure-in-adults-screening. Accessed November 2016.
79. Turnbull F, Beal B, Ninomiya T, et al. Effects of different regimens to lower blood pressure on major cardiovascular events in older and younger adults: meta-analysis of randomized trials. *BMJ*. 2008;336(7653):1121–1124.
80. Oza R, Garcellano. Nonpharmacologic management of hypertension: what works? *Am Fam Physician*. 2015;91(11):772–776.
81. Basile J, Bloch MJ. Overview of hypertension in adults. *Up to Date* 2016. Available from: www.uptodate.com. Accessed October 2016.
82. Langan R, Jones K. Common questions about the initial management of hypertension. *Am Fam Physician*. 2015;91(3):172–177.
83. Ogden CL, Carroll MD, Kit BK, et al. Prevalence of childhood and adult obesity in the United States, 2011–2012. *JAMA*. 2014;311(8):806–814.
84. US Preventive Services Task Force. Screening for Obesity in Adults. Available from: http://www.uspreventiveservicestaskforce.org/uspstf/uspsobes.htm. Accessed September 2016.

85. Cerhan JR, Moore SC, Jacobs EJ, et al. A pooled analysis of waist circumference and mortality in 650,000 adults. *Mayo Clin Proc*. 2014;89(3):334–345.
86. National Institutes of Health. The Practical Guide: Identification, Evaluation and Treatment of Over-weight and Obesity in Adults. Bethesda, MD: National Institutes of Health, National Heart, Lung, and Blood Institute, and North American Association for the Study of Obesity; 2000 NIH publication 00–4084. Available from: http://www.nhlbi.nih.gov/health-pro/guidelines/archive/clinical-guidelines-obesity-adults-evidence-report. Accessed September 2016.
87. Jensen MD, Ryan DH, Apovian CM, et al. 2013 AHA/ACC/TOS Guideline for the Management of Overweight and Obesity in Adults. Circulation. Published online 2013 Nov 12. Available from: https://www.guideline.gov/summaries/summary/48339/2013-ahaacctos-guideline-for-the-management-of-overweight-and-obesity-in-adults-a-report-of-the-american-college-of-cardiologyamerican-heart-association-task-force-on-practice-guidelines-and-the-obesity-society. Accessed September 2016.
88. Douketis JD, Macie C, Thabane L, et al. Systematic review of long-term weight loss studies in obese adults: clinical significance and applicability to clinical practice. *Int J Obes (Lond)*. 2005;29(10):1153–1167.
89. Snow V, Barry P, Fitterman N, et al. Pharmacologic and surgical management of obesity in primary care: a clinical practice guideline from the American college of physicians. *Ann Intern Med*. 2005;142(7):525–531.
90. Endocrinology Society. Available from: https://www.guideline.gov/summaries/summary/49254/pharmacological-management-of-obesity-an-endocrine-society-clinical-practice-guideline. Accessed September 2016.
91. Greenway FL, Caruso MK. Safety of obesity drugs. *Expert Opin Drug Saf*. 2005;4(6):1083–1095.
92. Douketis JD, Macie C, Thabane L, et al. Systematic review of long-term weight loss studies in obese adults: clinical significance and applicability to clinical practice. *Int J Obes (Lond)*. 2005;29(10):1153–1167.
93. Pontiroli AE, Morabito A. Long-term prevention of mortality in morbid obesity through bariatric surgery. A systematic review and meta-analysis of trials performed with gastric banding and gastric bypass. *Ann Surg*. 2011;253(3):484–487.
94. Karason K, Lindroos AK, Stenlof K, et al. Relief of cardiorespiratory symptoms and increased physical activity after surgically induced weight loss: results from the Swedish Obese Subjects study. *Arch Intern Med*. 2000;160(12):1797–1802.
95. Maggard MA, Shugarman LR, Suttorp M, et al. Meta-analysis: surgical treatment of obesity. *Ann Intern Med*. 2005;142(7):547–559.
96. Mechanick JI, Youdim A, Jones DB, et al. Clinical practice guidelines for the perioperative nutritional, metabolic, and nonsurgical support of the bariatric surgery patient—2013 update: cosponsored by American Association of Clinical Endocrinologists, The Obesity Society, and American Society for Metabolic & Bariatric Surgery. *Surg Obes Relat Dis*. 2013;9(2):159–191.
97. Kumar N. Endoscopic therapy for weight loss: gastroplasty, duodenal sleeves, intragastric balloons, and aspiration. *World J Gastrointest Endosc*. 2015;7(9):847–859.
98. Ferrante JM, Chen PH, Crabtree BF, et al. Cancer screening in women: body mass index and adherence to physician recommendations. *Am J Prev Med*. 2007;32(6):525–531.
99. CDC Health statistics on osteoporosis. Available from: http://www.cdc.gov/nchs/data/hestat/osteoporsis/osteoporosis2005_2010.htm. Accessed 10/13/16.
100. Dyer SM, Crotty M, Fairhall N, et al.; Fragility fracture network (FFN) rehabilitation research special interest group. A critical review of the long-term disability outcomes following hip fracture. *BMC Geriatrics*. 2016;16:158.
101. Cosman F, deBeur SJ, LeBoff MS, et al. Clinician's guide to prevention and treatment of osteoporosis. *Osteoporos Int*. 2014;25:2359–2381.
102. *Bone Health and Osteoporosis: a Report of the Surgeon General*. Rockville, MD: US Dept. of Health and Human Services, Public Health Service, Office of the Surgeon General; Washington, D.C.: For sale by the Supt. of Docs., US G.P.O; 2004.
103. Jeremiah MP, Unwin BK, Greenawald MH, et al. Diagnosis and management of osteoporosis. *Am Fam Physician*. 2015;92(4):261–268.
104. Final update summary: osteoporosis screening US Preventive Services Task Force, July 2015. Available from: https://www.uspreventiveservicestaskforce.org/Page/Document/UpdateSummaryFinal/osteoporosis-screening. Accessed October 2016.
105. Grossman JM, Gordon R, Ranganath VK, et al. American College of Rheumatology 2010 recommendations for the prevention and treatment of glucocorticoid-induced osteoporosis. *Arthritis Care Res*. 2010;62(11):1515–1526.

Weight Management and Nutrition

KEY POINTS

1 ▶ Nutritional assessment is important in any patient with abnormal weight or unusual weight gain or weight loss; overweight patients may suffer from undernutrition.

2 ▶ Mediterranean and DASH diets are two dietary patterns that have strong supporting evidence for improving health and lowering disease risk.

3 ▶ Physicians should use shared decision making with patients who need to lose weight.

4 ▶ Weight loss of even 5% of body weight can significantly reduce morbidity in obese individuals.

5 ▶ Prevention and management of obesity in children is important and should emphasize positive behaviors (e.g., eating meals with family) while avoiding diet restriction, bullying and shaming.

Sally is a 45-year-old woman who presents to the office with bilateral knee pain which has been getting worse over the past 2 months. She denies swelling in either knee and has no other joint pain. She played basketball and softball in high school. She has a long history of being overweight or obese, and would like to try to lose weight, but is limited in exercising because of knee pain. She frequently tries diets that she finds in magazines or on the Internet, and will lose up to 30 lb in a few months, but always regains the weight.

On physical exam, Sally appears obese, with no signs of distress. Her height is 65 in (1.65 M), and weight is 223 lb (101 kg). Her body mass index (BMI) is 37. Her blood pressure is 142/89 mm Hg. Her knee exam shows no sign of erythema or effusion. She has full range of motion and mild joint-line tenderness laterally in both knees. Her gait and other joints appear normal.

You determine that she has mild knee degenerative joint disease, with the ongoing stress of her body mass contributing to her joint pain. No imaging studies are warranted at this time.

NUTRITION ASSESSMENT

The fact that an individual is overweight or obese does not guarantee that his or her nutrition is adequate. In any patient with abnormal weight, it is essential to perform a nutrition assessment to determine whether that person is consuming adequate nutrients to maintain health. Table 13.1 outlines an approach to office-based assessment of nutritional status.

Dietary History

The dietary history is a key component of nutritional assessment and in evaluating overweight and obesity. Ask about specific dietary patterns such as vegan, vegetarian, gluten-free, or other patterns. Sally has tried many different diets and it is important to get information about what she is currently eating to provide further counseling. You notice that she is carrying a smartphone.

Table 13.1 ▶ Approach to Office-Based Assessment of Nutritional Status

Characteristic	Elements	Hints
History	• Weight loss or gain • Dietary history • Nutritional supplements • Medications current and past use • Access to nutritionally dense food • Ability to prepare, eat, absorb, and digest food • Cultural norms • Activity level • Alcohol use • Family history • Social and emotional history	• Obtain usual weight • General or restricted diet (e.g., gluten-free, Atkins) • Are medications necessary (some medications cause weight gain, suppress appetite, alter metabolism) • Poverty, age issues • Frailty, disability, dental or GI issues
Physical exam	• Weight/height/BMI • Waist circumference[a] • Temporal/intermetacarpal wasting • Hair loss • Specific nutrient deficiencies • Thyroid exam	• BMI not always a good indicator of body composition (e.g., elderly and athletes) • Lanugo-type hair consistent with anorexia nervosa • Enlarged thyroid may indicate hypothyroidism
Laboratory tests	• Complete blood count • Transferrin[b] • Albumin[c] • Pre-albumin (transthyretin)[c] • Electrolytes • Thyroid-stimulating hormone	• Anemias, iron deficiency • Electrolytes may be abnormal with acute deficiency, vomiting, diarrhea

[a]See Figure 13.1 for correct measurement of waist circumference.
[b]Negative acute phase reactant but short half-life, changes more rapidly in cases of acute disease.
[c]Albumin is a negative acute phase reactant that has a long serum half-life and decreases during acute inflammation; pre-albumin is an acute phase reactant with a short half-life.

Dietary recall is an important tool that can be performed either prospectively or retrospectively. There are several dietary diary software applications available for smartphones and other devices, which may make prospective dietary history easier (Table 13.2). This type of prospective food diary, which is entered at the time of eating, has more validity than retrospective recall-based food diaries.[1] The major weakness of food diaries is that patients tend to underreport foods consumed; the heavier a person is, the more underreporting that occurs.[2] In addition, most do not implement customized behavioral interventions or motivational interviewing benefits. Prescribing these apps alone is unlikely to result in long-term weight loss.[3]

A Food Frequency Questionnaire (FFQ; http://epi.grants.cancer.gov/diet/usualintakes/ffq.html?&url=/diet/usualintakes/ffq.html) consists of a list of foods and beverages. The patient marks foods consumed and how many times each was consumed over a defined time period, usually during the last year. These questionnaires are used frequently in epidemiologic studies, but are not as valid as food diaries for patients.

> You tell Sally that it would be helpful to have her keep a food diary and suggest using an app such as LoseIt or MyFitnessPal. You also ask her to document her meals and snacks immediately after consumption to help with accuracy and return for a follow-up appointment.

Table 13.2 ▶ Nutrition and Weight Loss Applications

Application and Link	Description
Lose It! (https://www.loseit.com)	Free app for computer, Android, or iOS that helps with calorie budgeting. Tracks common foods, exercise; some links to health tips
MyFitnessPal (https://www.myfitnesspal.com/)	Free app for computer, Android, or iOS; calorie counter, diet and exercise journal
Healthy Out (https://healthyout.com/)	Free app for Android or iOS, helps locate restaurants in the area and identifies menu items by type of diet (e.g., vegan, low calorie, gluten free)
Weight Watchers (www.weightwatchers.com)	Part of a comprehensive system that uses social support, education, and a points (not calories) system for tracking intake and activity. Free with Weight Watchers membership
Sparkpeople (www.sparkpeople.com)	Free app for computer, Android, or iOS; tracks calories, creates personalized fitness program, some community support components
Cronometer (www.cronometer.com)	Free app for computer, paid for Android or iOS that allows tracking of calories as well as exercise, biometrics, vitamins, minerals, and a breakdown of macronutrients. No specific coaching or community

Physical Exam

Most electronic medical records (EMRs) will automatically calculate the body mass index (BMI) from height and weight, using the formula BMI = weight in kilograms/height in meters^2. A BMI calculator is available at https://www.nhlbi.nih.gov/. Table 13.3 lists BMI categories for adults.

In children and adolescents, the BMI is compared with norms on a standard growth chart, using the BMI-for-age percentile, which shows how the patient's BMI compares with that of others of the same age. The Centers for Disease Control and Prevention have a BMI-for-age calculator, found at https://nccd.cdc.gov/dnpabmi/calculator.aspx. Table 13.4 lists the BMI-for-age percentiles.

Waist circumference can give an indication of abdominal fat. The waist circumference should be measured just above the iliac crests. Waist circumference greater than 40 in in men, and greater than 35 in in nonpregnant women, may indicate an increased risk of heart disease and type 2 diabetes. It is important to actually measure waist circumference in a standardized manner, as shown in Figure 13.1.[4]

Table 13.3 ▶ Adult Body Mass Index Definitions

BMI	Category
18.5–24.9	Normal weight
25.0–29.9	Overweight
30.0–39.9	Obese
40 and above	Extreme obesity

Table 13.4 ▶ BMI Categories for Children and Adolescents

BMI-for-Age Percentile	Category
Less than 5th percentile	Underweight
5th percentile to less than the 85th percentile	Healthy weight
85th percentile to less than the 95th percentile	Risk of overweight
95th percentile or greater	Overweight

Waist circumference appears to be a better predictor of risk for cardiovascular disease and diabetes than does the waist–hip ratio. Increased waist circumference, and not BMI, is a criterion for metabolic syndrome.

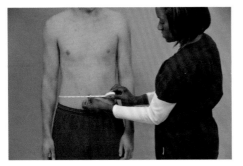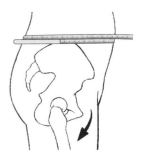

Figure 13.1 ▶ Measuring waist circumference. (From The Centers for Disease Control and Prevention: Healthy Weight: Assessing Your Weight. May 15, 2015. Available at: https://www.cdc.gov/healthyweight/assessing/)

Skin fold thickness can also help indicate body composition, but standardizing how this is measured can be difficult. Neither BMI, waist circumference, nor skin fold thickness is a perfect measure of body fat content. While the only true gold standard of this measurement would be cadaver analysis, other somewhat more accurate measures include dual-energy x-ray absorptiometry (DEXA) and underwater weighing, neither of which is practical in an office setting.[5] However, BMI and waist circumference appear to be adequate proxies in terms of predicting potential for weight-related diseases.

PHYSICAL SIGNS OF SPECIFIC NUTRIENT DEFICIENCIES

Deficiencies in particular macronutrients (carbohydrate, fat, and protein) or micronutrients can cause specific physical signs, as outlined in Tables 13.5 and 13.6. Classic findings are noted in bold. Note that individuals rarely display signs of a single nutritional deficiency, since so many are related to intake. Any patient with a deficiency in one nutrient is likely deficient in multiple nutritional components. Sally's diet summary that she sends to you through the patient portal, shows no evidence of nutrient deficiency, but like most patients in primary care, she consumes too many calories.

Table 13.5 ▶ Specific Nutrient Deficiencies

Nutrient	Signs of Deficiency	Causes of Deficiency
Biotin	**Dermatitis,** decreased appetite, neuritis, **glossitis**	Decreased intake
Calcium	Symptoms occur late; poor growth, bone loss, **osteomalacia, osteoporosis, tetany, muscle cramps, heart dysrhythmias**	Poor intake, poor vitamin D consumption, postmenopausal status or other low estrogen state in women, lactose intolerance, vegetarianism
Carbohydrate	Weight loss, poor growth	Decreased intake, malabsorption, genetic diseases related to carbohydrate metabolism
Fat	Poor growth, flaky skin, impaired immune response, impaired wound healing, hair loss	Decreased intake, malabsorption
Folate	**Megaloblastic anemia,** weakness, **fatigue,** poor concentration, mucosal ulcers, **neural tube defects in infants born to mothers with deficiency**	Alcoholism, malabsorption
Iron	**Microcytic, hypochromic anemia; fatigue;** poor immune response	Blood loss, poor intake
Magnesium	Behavioral disturbances, tremor, **neuromuscular irritability,** anorexia, **heart dysrhythmias,** coronary spasm	Alcoholism, gastrointestinal disease (diarrhea, malabsorption), ileal resection, type 2 diabetes, elderly
Niacin	Pellagra—**confusion,** delusions, diarrhea, nausea, **mucositis, scaly skin**	Decreased intake, malabsorption, dialysis
Pantothenic acid	Fatigue, malaise, insomnia, paresthesias, depression	Decreased intake, malabsorption
Phosphorus	Poor growth, anorexia, anxiety, weakness, paresthesias in hands and feet	Alcoholism, diabetes, starvation, excessive use of antacids or diuretics
Potassium	Muscle weakness, **arrhythmias,** paralysis	Medications such as diuretics
Protein	Poor growth and development, impaired immune response, edema, muscular weakness (*Kwashiorkor* is mainly a protein deficiency; *marasmus* is protein and calorie deficiency)	Decreased intake, increased wasting (kidney disease), malabsorption, inborn errors of metabolism
Selenium	Cardiac myopathy, muscle pain, male infertility	Rare; some parts of China are low-selenium regions (soil) with decreased plant and animal content of selenium; dialysis, HIV infection
Zinc	**Poor growth, impaired wound healing,** anorexia, poor immune function, hypogonadism in males, hair loss, diarrhea	Impaired absorption (GI surgery, inflammatory bowel disease), chronic liver or kidney disease, sickle cell disease, diabetes, cancer, chronic diarrhea. Vegetarians may be at risk

Table 13.6 ▶ Specific Vitamin Deficiencies

Vitamin	Sign of Deficiency	Cause of Deficiency
Vitamin B$_1$ (thiamine)	*Beriberi*—**neuropathy,** confusion, pain, numbness in hands and feet	Decreased intake, malabsorption, dialysis
Vitamin B$_2$ (riboflavin)	Anemia, **cheilitis, oral lesions,** poor growth, gingivitis	Decreased intake, malabsorption
Vitamin B$_6$ (pyridoxal compounds)	Anemia, **rash,** depression, confusion, infantile seizures	Decreased intake, malabsorption, medication induced
Vitamin B$_{12}$ (cobalamin)	**Macrocytic anemia,** fatigue, **neuropathy,** unsteadiness, confusion, **glossitis**	Decreased stomach hydrochloric acid, decreased intake (strict vegetarians at risk), post-gastrectomy, ileal disease (e.g., Crohn disease)
Vitamin A	**Xerophthalmia and night blindness** (women and children), can have low iron stores	Prematurity (infants), decreased intake (poor access to animal food sources), pancreatic insufficiency (poor fat absorption)
Vitamin C (ascorbic acid)	Scurvy (acute deficiency)—fatigue, **gingivitis, petechiae, ecchymoses,** joint pain, poor collagen production leading to weakened connective tissue and hyperkeratosis. Iron deficiency may result long-term bone disease in children	Decreased intake (poor food variety with lack of fruits and vegetables), alcohol abuse, malabsorption, severe kidney disease
Vitamin D	**Rickets, osteomalacia, bone pain**	Breastfed infants at risk (require supplement), poor sunlight exposure, decreased intake
Vitamin E	**Newborns—hemolytic anemia;** peripheral neuropathy, ataxia, myopathy, retinopathy, **impaired immune response**	Poor fat absorption, low–birth-weight infants
Vitamin K	**Bleeding, poor clotting,** ecchymosis can contribute to osteoporosis	Poor fat absorption, liver disease

Table 13.7 contains photographs of physical findings related to nutritional deficiencies. A good resource for information on the individual micronutrients is the Office of Dietary Supplements at the National Institutes of Health (https://ods.od.nih.gov/factsheets/list-all/).

It is important to emphasize to patients that the best way to consume all nutrients is through **food sources rather than supplements.** While many patients may have a preference for fresh fruits and vegetables, the most important message is that they consume those foods in one form or another. Commercial canning and freezing take place close to the food sources, and fruits and vegetables to be frozen or canned are typically grown for that purpose, maximizing the nutrient value at the time of preservation. Suggesting to patients that they try to consume fresh over preserved products may be counterproductive, as many may not have access to, or be able to afford, fresh vegetables.

Table 13.7 ▶ Photographs of Physical Manifestations of Nutrient Deficiencies

Kwashiorkor—severe protein deficiency; protuberant abdomen, edema in hands and feet[a]

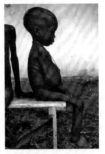

Marasmus—protein and calorie deficiency; loose, saggy skin, edema, protuberant ribs[b]

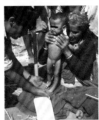

Vitamin B₂ deficiency—angular cheilitis; dry swollen lips, lesions at corners of the mouth. Gingiva are inflamed.[c]

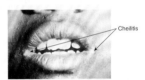

Vitamin B₆ (niacin) and vitamin C deficiency (pellagra and scurvy)—hyperkeratosis, mottled pigment[c]

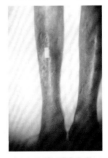

Vitamin D deficiency (nutritional rickets)—bowed legs, joint enlargement at wrist[c]

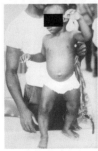

[a]CDC and Dr. Lyle Conrad. Centers for Disease Control and Prevention, Public Health Image Library (PHIL), https://phil.cdc.gov/phil/home.asp
[b]CDC and Dr. Edward Brink. Centers for Disease Control and Prevention, Public Health Image Library (PHIL), https://phil.cdc.gov/phil/home.asp
[c]CDC. Centers for Disease Control and Prevention, Public Health Image Library (PHIL), https://phil.cdc.gov/phil/home.asp

The Office of Dietary Supplements also has a range of tables providing information about recommended intakes and sources for macronutrients, water, vitamins, and minerals: https://ods.od.nih.gov/Health_Information/Dietary_Reference_Intakes.aspx.

What Is a Healthy Diet?

When discussing eating patterns with patients, the use of the word "diet" may connote a temporary change, such as "going on a diet." Patients should work toward establishing an overall healthy eating pattern that is permanent. It is important to give patients information on specifics of what makes up a healthy diet, rather than simply counseling them to "eat more healthy foods." In Sally's case, you identify specific areas to improve based on her food diary such as reducing portion sizes and elimination of fast food lunches and late-night snacking.

People have individual preferences for foods, and dietary patterns that are based on their own cultural, religious, and health beliefs, so using shared decision making in helping to maximize healthy food intake is essential.

The United States government periodically publishes consumer information on healthy eating. The most recent iteration of these recommendations, Dietary Guidelines for Americans 2015 to 2020, can be found at http://health.gov/dietaryguidelines/2015/guidelines/. This publication is based on making changes to align with healthy eating patterns. A summary of the healthy eating pattern includes eating a variety of vegetables, whole fruits, grains (at least half should be whole grains), low or nonfat dairy products, a variety of protein-containing foods, and limiting the amount of saturated and trans fats. The appendices for the online document contain useful tables about physical activity, caloric requirements, and sources of particular nutrients.

In general, the Mediterranean diet and the DASH (Dietary Approaches to Stop Hypertension) dietary patterns have the strongest supporting evidence in terms of preventing chronic disease in decreasing mortality.[6,7] There are variations of the **Mediterranean diet**, but in general, it consists of a relatively high intake of olive oil, fruit, nuts, vegetables, and whole grains, with a much lower intake of red meat, whole fat dairy products, processed meats, and sugars, and includes wine (in moderation), as well as moderate amounts of fish and poultry.

The **DASH diet** is very similar to the Mediterranean diet, and emphasizes whole grains, vegetables, fruits, low-fat dairy products, fish, poultry, legumes, and vegetable oils. The DASH diet calls for limiting foods high in saturated fat, as well as sugar-sweetened beverages and sweets. More about the DASH diet may be found at http://www.nhlbi.nih. gov/health/health-topics/topics/dash/followdash. Tables recommending food servings in a variety of dietary patterns, including the Mediterranean diet, may be found at https:// health.gov/dietaryguidelines/2015/guidelines/#subnav-4.

Patients may present with questions about diets to which they adhere or would like to try. Table 13.8 summarizes some of the popular diets. Note that many of these diets are considered "fads" and patients have difficulty adhering to them long term.

Sally returns for follow-up and after discussing areas in her diet for improvement, she states that she does best when following a specific diet. You provide her with the link to the Dietary Guidelines website along with printouts of the DASH and Mediterranean diets. You discuss the pros and cons of the different diets which she is tempted to try. Sally notes her preferences with respect to changing her eating pattern and activity level as part of shared decision making (see Chapter 5).

Table 13.8 ▶ Popular Dietary Plans

Diet	Description	Positive/Negative Attributes
Anti-inflammatory diet	Proposed by Dr. Andrew Weil; based on variety, fresh foods, and fruits and vegetables	+Rich in optimal foods −Complicated, with different requirements for each nutrient
Atkins diet[a]	Focuses on controlling insulin through diet; restricting carbohydrates	+Some lose weight on diet −Ketosis and vitamin and mineral deficiencies possible; side effects of headaches, dizziness, weakness/fatigue
DASH diet (dietary approaches to stop hypertension)	Nonstarchy vegetables and fruits, low fat dairy, whole grains, lean meat and poultry, fish, nuts and seeds, healthy fats (like olive oil); more dairy foods and meat than Mediterranean diet	+Healthy range of foods −Much higher in fruits and vegetables than most Americans usually eat
Gluten-free diet[b]	Diet omits all forms of cereal grains of wheat, rye, barley, triticale (combination of wheat and rye) originally used for those who are gluten intolerant	+Helps individuals who are gluten intolerant −Can be higher in calories; nutrient deficiencies prevalent (calcium, fiber, iron, B vitamins)
Juice cleanses	3–10-day periods of a diet of fruit and vegetable juices, intended to reduce weight and flush toxins	−Case reports of oxalate nephropathy as oxalate concentrations are high in many vegetables and nuts
Mediterranean diet	Emphasis on plant foods as well as moderate amounts of fish and poultry (including eggs) and small amounts of meat; cheese and yogurt main dairy products; olive oil is main fat source	+Strong research on health benefits including decreased mortality, CVD, cancer, and neurodegenerative diseases −Different from what most Americans follow
Raw food diet	Foods are not processed or cooked (at least 3/4 not cooked); completely plant based and ideally organic	+Weight loss; high fiber −Deficiencies if practiced too restrictively, high fiber can cause bloating and GI discomfort, certain raw foods have higher toxins or contaminates[c]
South Beach Diet	Focuses on control of insulin levels and benefits of unrefined carbohydrates; emphasis is on low saturated fats with fish and olive oil; moderately low carbohydrate diet	+Low in refined carbohydrate −Higher in fats and proteins than usually thought healthy
Vegan diet	Focus is a way of life as much as a particular diet, more for environmental and ethical reasons than health; eats nothing that is animal based including eggs, dairy, and honey	+Contains lots of plant-based fiber −Vitamin and mineral (especially calcium, B$_{12}$) deficiencies are probable if strict adherence

(continued)

Table 13.8 ▶ Popular Dietary Plans *(Continued)*

Diet	Description	Positive/Negative Attributes
Vegetarian diet	Excludes animal-based foods from the diet. Types include Lacto (allows dairy products), Fruitarian (fruit only), Lacto-ovo (allows dairy and eggs), Ovo (allows eggs), Pesco (allows fish), Semi (seems to determine what will be excluded/included)	+Lower weight, longer life expectancy than meat eaters, fewer diseases −Vitamin B_{12} deficiency as well as other vitamin and mineral deficiencies depending on how restrictive the diet
Weight Watchers Plan	Focuses on losing weight through diet, exercise, and social support	+Effective for weight loss −Must maintain as lifestyle change
Zone Diet	Aims for nutritional balance at each meal/time eating; includes at least two snacks daily with protein at each snack and meal; emphasizes good quality carbohydrate and fats such as olive oil, avocado and nuts; diet does not prescribe number of calories	+Often used in athletic clubs to regiment eating −Can be difficult to follow exactly and person needs to be attentive continuously to what they are eating

[a]Those who have high blood pressure, diabetes, heart disease, or high blood cholesterol need to check with a health provider before starting.
[b]About 18 million Americans are thought to be gluten intolerant; originally for celiac disease but expanded to those who are gluten sensitive (some symptoms as celiac but without stomach damage) and gluten intolerant (symptoms of cramping, bloating, nausea, and diarrhea with or without celiac disease).
[c]Potential toxicities: alfalfa sprouts (toxin canavanine), kale (a thyrotoxin in large raw amounts), kidney beans (toxin phytohemagglutinin), raw eggs (salmonella), apricot kernels (cyanide), parsnips (furanocoumarin), raw meat (bacteria, parasites, viruses), raw milk (mycobacteria bovis). CVD, cardiovascular disease; GI, gastrointestinal.

Dietary Patterns for Children

A Healthy Eating Calculator for children may be found at https://www.bcm.edu/cnrc-apps/healthyeatingcalculator/eatingCal.html.

EATING DISORDERS

As part of a nutritional assessment, physicians need to be aware of the potential for eating disorders. Table 13.9 summarizes types of disordered eating, including signs, symptoms, and risk factors. Note that while laboratory findings cannot be used to diagnose eating disorders, both anorexia nervosa and bulimia may result in significant metabolic derangements.[8,9]

OVERWEIGHT AND OBESITY

According to the National Health and Nutrition Examination Survey (NHANES), about 40% of men and 30% of women were overweight, and 35% of men and 37% of women were obese.[10] The prevalence of overweight and obesity in children and adolescents has not increased as dramatically in the same time period; in 2009 to 2010, about % of infants and toddlers had a high weight-for-recumbent length and about 17% of children and adolescents aged 2 to 19 years were obese.[11] Patients who are overweight or obese are at increased risk

Table 13.9 ▶ Eating Disorders and Complications

Type of Eating Disorder	Description	Complications	Potential Causes	Risk Factors	Common Treatments
Anorexia nervosa (1 in 20 people will be affected in lifetime; prevalence 9/1,000 women, 3/1,000 men)	Person becomes too thin because the person thinks she/he is too fat; relentless pursuit of thinness and severe food restriction. More common in women; usually starts in teenage years but can be in elderly; often occurs with depression, anxiety disorders, and substance abuse; commonly associated with perfectionism	OP; brittle hair/nails; dry, yellow skin; lanugo; anemia; muscle wasting and weakness; amenorrhea; severe constipation; low BP; temperature, and pulse; arrhythmias, heart and brain damage; multi-organ failure; edema; acrocyanosis; tiredness; infertility; heavy physical and emotional toll; potentially fatal Labs: hypokalemia, hyponatremia, hypoglycemia, hypercortisolism; low TSH, normal T3 and T4, hypomagnesemia	• Genetics • Environment (cultural pressures to be thin) • Peer pressure (teasing, bullying, ridicule) • Potentially history of physical/sexual abuse • Perfectionism, impulsive behavior, difficulty with relationships that contribute to low self-esteem	• Age (early teens and 20s more common) • Gender (female, though males are less likely to seek help [1 out of every 10 diagnoses are males]) • Family history (parent or sibling with eating disorder increases risk) • Dieting • Life changes (e.g., starting a new school, new job, divorce) • Certain activities (gymnasts, runners, wrestlers, dancers)	• Early diagnosis has the best recovery outcome; mental health professional for psychological evaluation • Monitoring food intake and medical care for medical problems as listed • Psychotherapy—individual, group, or family • Nutrition counseling • Sometimes medications (particularly for depression and anxiety, can also act as an appetite stimulant)
Bulimia nervosa (prevalence 15/1,000 women, 5/1,000 men)	Person has periods of overeating followed by self-induced vomiting or use of laxatives (several times weekly to multiple times daily); recurrent with frequent episodes that cause a feeling of lack of control; usually at normal weight, possibly overweight. More common in women; usually starts in teenage years; associated with depression, anxiety, and substance abuse	Chronically inflamed sore throat; swollen salivary glands in neck and jaw; worn tooth enamel with sensitive and decaying teeth; acid reflux and GI problems; intestinal irritation from laxative abuse; severe dehydration; electrolyte imbalance; low self-esteem; electrolyte and hydration problems can cause cardiac arrhythmias, heart failure, and death Labs: hypokalemic, hypochloremic metabolic alkalosis; possibly low sodium	Potentially same as anorexia nervosa	Potentially same as anorexia nervosa	• Similar to anorexia nervosa • CBT and/or interpersonal therapy effective • Antidepressants can be offered as primary therapy

(continued)

301

Table 13.9 ▶ Eating Disorders and Complications *(Continued)*

Type of Eating Disorder	Description	Complications	Potential Causes	Risk Factors	Common Treatments
Binge-eating disorder (35/1,000 women, 2/1,000 men)	Out-of-control eating without compensatory purging, excessive exercise or fasting. More common in women; usually starts in teenage years; person may be normal weight, over-weight or obese	Obesity with more risk for CVD and high BP; mental stressors of guilt, shame and distress about binge eating which leads to more binge eating	Potentially same as anorexia nervosa	Potentially same as anorexia nervosa	Potentially same as bulimia nervosa
Disordered eating	Often used in clinical practice for dieters who are unhappy with their body and constantly dieting ineffectively; usually have low self-esteem and life satisfaction	Life dissatisfaction; low nutrient intakes; potentially could lead to a labeled eating disorder	Causes are usually attributed to culture that glorifies the inordinately thin images in the media that are unrealistic for most	US media with reinforce-ment from peers and others	Discouragement of dieting for the sake of appearances and encour-aging healthy eating

BP, blood pressure; CBT, cognitive behavioral therapy; OP, osteoporosis.
Data from Williams PM, Goodie JL. Anorexia, bulimia, and eating disorders (amended 2016 June 13; cited 2016 November 10). In: *Essential Evidence Plus*, Hoboken, NJ: John Wiley & Sons, Inc. ©2012]. Available from http://www.essentialevidenceplus.com/content/eee/620; and from Mehler PS. Bulimia nervosa. *N Engl J Med*. 2003;349:875–881.

for developing cardiovascular disease, and obese patients have an elevated risk of all-cause mortality.[12] Notably, when patients are able to lose even 3% to 5% of their body weight, morbidity declines.[12] This is often a motivator for patients who sometimes set unreachable goals.

During your visit with Sally, you emphasize that if she could achieve even moderate weight loss, she could improve her overall health and decrease her risk of chronic diseases, which include cardiovascular disease (she already has a family history of hypertension, and her blood pressure is high today), cancer (she has a family history of breast cancer), and osteoarthritis. Sally appears to be ready to take action. You encourage her to choose one or two small changes from the areas of improvement that you identified, and to make gradual changes. In addition, you also provide information about ways to increase her activity. You plan regular follow-up appointments.

A discussion of obesity in adults can be found in Chapter 12. Management options include diet, exercise, medication, bariatric surgery, and medical devices.

Obesity in Children

Current thinking is that obesity in children is multifactorial in origin. Influences such as maternal nutrition, stress, and physical activity, as well as environmental toxic stress, family stress, genetics, and epigenetics, all play a role, and are out of the child's control.[13]

Management of overweight and obesity in children is becoming increasingly necessary. Evidence shows that encouraging a healthy diet in a positive way and avoiding the suggestion of any type of food restriction is important. Additionally, parents can play a role in encouraging a healthy lifestyle without emphasizing appearance or weight status. Table 13.10 outlines current recommendations regarding weight management in children

 Table 13.10 ▶ Management of Overweight and Obesity in Children and Adolescents

Strategies for Preventing Weight-Related Problems

Encourage and support
- Healthy eating
- Physical activity
- Healthy lifestyle
- Healthy habits
- Positive body image
- Frequent family meals

Discourage
- Dieting
- Skipping meals
- Use of diet pills
- Body dissatisfaction
- Talking about weight
- More than 2 hours of screen time daily

Inquire about
- Bullying
- Mistreatment

Monitor carefully
- Weight loss to prevent medical complications of semistarvation

and adolescents. Note that medications are not safe or efficacious for inducing weight loss in children. Orlistat may be useful in children aged 12 years or older.[14]

COMMON MYTHS AND TRENDS

Colonic Cleanse

The notion of colonic cleansing has been around for decades, maybe even centuries. "Spring cleaning" is an idea that seemed to hold true for our bodies as well as our homes in some people's minds. The idea of taking a strong laxative in the springtime to cleanse our bodies was held strongly throughout the United States through the 1950s and fell out of vogue in most communities at that time, with few practicing this regularly.

With increasing interest in healthy lifestyles, there seems to be a resurgence of this idea that cleansing the body regularly helps it flush wastes that "stick to the walls of the colon." Individuals use products such as nutritional supplements, laxatives, enemas, herbal teas, or colon hydrotherapy (at a doctor's visit) to attempt to wash out the colon.

Practitioners of this exercise claim that it may help maladies such as arthritis, asthma, irritable bowel disease, and other chronic problems. Potential side effects of cleansing regimens include vomiting, nausea, and cramps; dizziness; dehydration; bowel perforation; infection; depletion of probiotics, sodium and potassium; and kidney damage. Colon cleansing changes the microflora in the intestinal tract, which may, in fact, be detrimental to health. There is no strong evidence that colonic cleansing is beneficial for any chronic disease.[15]

Overweight Means Overnutrition

Many times, physicians neglect to assess nutritional status in patients who are overweight. In fact, especially in the elderly, overweight patients may suffer from malnourishment and even sarcopenia (decreased muscle, or lean body mass). Sarcopenia is a significant problem in the elderly, who grow progressively weaker; and, lack of skeletal muscle strength and mass puts them at risk for falls and inability to meet activities of daily living (see Chapter 10). It is important that even overweight individuals obtain adequate protein calories in the diet to maintain muscle mass. Protein supplements in the absence of some form of resistance exercise are not helpful for building lean body mass.

Overweight is Always Unhealthy

It is important to avoid judging an individual's health status solely on BMI. While overweight and obesity predispose people to multiple chronic diseases, many overweight individuals are otherwise healthy and not at great risk for other diseases. In fact, research has shown that as people grow older, being mildly overweight may in fact improve longevity.[16]

FUTURE DIRECTIONS IN OBESITY AND WEIGHT MANAGEMENT

Nutritional Ecology

Nutrition scientists are beginning to take an in-depth look at the many factors that influence nutrition and obesity. Nutritional ecology is the study of how evolution (and change in gene frequencies) and ecology influence nutrition, or how the human organism interacts with its environment. Nutrition ecologists are studying how the combination of nutrients, rather than the sum of individual nutrients, interacts with body systems. Dietary patterns, rather than quantities of individual nutrients, may have more influence over body weight and health.[17]

Gut Microbiome and Influence on Weight

Related to nutritional ecology is the current study of how the intestinal microbiome influences nutritional status and weight. Studies have demonstrated that in obese individuals, the type of microflora in the intestine is able to cause the intestinal tract to efficiently absorb energy from the diet. Altered composition of the gut microflora can result in disruption of the mucus barrier lining the intestinal tract, along with changes in immune and metabolic function in the intestinal tissues. Current theories hold that these disruptions may contribute to the development of obesity. In turn, factors that influence the gut microbiome include age, diet, exercise, use of antibiotics, and in children, breast versus bottle feeding and exposures during birth. Diet plays a major role in regulating intestinal flora; breast-fed infants are less likely to become obese than those who are not breastfed.[18] Part of the negative influence of a diet high in refined sugars is that the concentration of metabolic products of these sugars results in a change in the bacterial composition of the intestine, which may increase the propensity to weight gain. The mechanisms by which a change in the microbiome affects weight gain are not entirely elucidated, but may include changes in absorption and/or metabolism of nutrients, as well in neurohormonal modulation affecting appetite and satiety.[19]

Role of Fat Type in Energy Balance

A third recent area of study is how different types of fat tissue relate to energy metabolism. Recent studies in animals show that brown adipose tissue is highly efficient in changing chemical energy into heat. Researchers hypothesize that by inducing greater amounts of this so-called "beige fat," we may be able to find treatments for obesity and related metabolic diseases.[20]

Nutrigenomics

Researchers are demonstrating that how individuals metabolize and use nutrients may be influenced by genetic factors. There may also be genetic influence in how individuals select a dietary pattern. Some companies are currently marketing tests for genes that may predispose a person to different nutritionally related diseases or deficiencies, and thus can allow for customized advice. At this time, there is not enough evidence to recommend routine genetic testing for nutrition management, but this is a rapidly growing field of knowledge.

QUESTIONS

1. Obese patients often must lose over 20% of their body weight to see significant health effects.
   A. True
   B. False

2. Which diet is associated with decreased mortality in patients with cardiovascular disease?
   A. Mediterranean diet
   B. Low fat diet
   C. The Atkins diet
   D. Low calorie diet

3. Which one of the following is a predictor of diabetes and a criterion for metabolic syndrome?
   A. Family history
   B. BMI
   C. Actual weight
   D. Age
   E. Waist circumference

4. Kwashiorkor is characterized by which one of the following?
   A. Protein deficiency
   B. B_{12} deficiency
   C. Vitamin C deficiency
   D. Vitamin D deficiency

5. Which one of the following is true of most people with bulimia nervosa?
   A. They are underweight
   B. They are teenaged
   C. They are taking oral contraceptives
   D. They are normal or overweight

ANSWERS

Question 1: The correct answer is B.
Notably, when patients are able to lose even 3% to 5% of their body weight, morbidity declines.

Question 2: The correct answer is A.
In general, the Mediterranean diet and the DASH (Dietary Approaches to Stop Hypertension) dietary patterns have the strongest supporting evidence in terms of preventing chronic disease in decreasing mortality.

Question 3: The correct answer is E.
Waist circumference appears to be a better predictor of risk for cardiovascular disease and diabetes than does the waist–hip ratio. Increased waist circumference, and not BMI, is a criterion for metabolic syndrome.

Question 4: The correct answer is A.
Table 13.7. Kwashiorkor is due to severe protein deficiency; children typically have a protuberant abdomen and edema in their hands and feet.

Question 5: The correct answer is D.
Table 13.9. A person with bulimia nervosa has periods of overeating followed by self-induced vomiting or use of laxatives (several times weekly to multiple times daily); recurrent with frequent episodes that cause a feeling of lack of control; and is usually at normal weight, possibly overweight.

REFERENCES

1. Hammond KA. Dietary and clinical assessment. In: Mahan LK, Escott-Stump S, eds. *Krause's Food, Nutrition, and Diet Therapy.* Philadelphia, PA: Saunders-Elsevier; 2004:403–435.
2. Lichtman SW, Pisarska K, Berman ER, et al. Discrepancy between self-reported and actual caloric intake and exercise in obese subjects. *N Engl J Med.* 1992;327:1893–1898.
3. Laing BY, Mangione CM, Tsent C, et al. Effectiveness of a smartphone application for weight loss compared with usual care in overweight primary care patients: a randomized, controlled trial. *Ann Intern Med.* 2014;161(10 Suppl):S5–S12.
4. Centers for Disease Control and Prevention. Available at: https://www.cdc.gov/healthyweight/assessing./ Also, Impact of obesity at: https://www.youtube.com/watch?v=9Y1MAN23FSQ. Accessed November 10, 2016.
5. Talma H, Chinapaw JM, Bakker B, et al. Bioelectrical impedance analysis to estimate body composition in children and adolescents: a systematic review and evidence appraisal of validity, responsiveness, reliability and measurement error. *Obesity Rev.* 2013;14:895–905.
6. Sofi F, Abbate R, Gensini GF, et al. Accruing evidence on benefits of adherence to the Mediterranean diet on health: an updated systematic review and meta-analysis. *Am J Clin Nutr.* 2010;92:1189–1196.
7. Sotos-Prieto M, Bhupathiraju SN, Mattei J, et al. Changes in three diet quality scores and total and cause-specific mortality. *Circulation.* 2016;133(Suppl 1), Available at: http://circ.ahajournals.org/content/133/Suppl_1/A29.short. Accessed August 31, 2016.
8. Williams PM, Goodie JL. Anorexia, bulimia, and eating disorders (amended 2016 June 13). In: *Essential Evidence Plus.* Hoboken, NJ: John Wiley & Sons, Inc.; 2012. Available from http://www.essentialevidenceplus.com/content/eee/620. Accessed November 2016.
9. Mehler PS. Bulimia nervosa. *N Engl J Med.* 2003;349:875–881.
10. Yang L, Colditz GA. Prevalence of overweight and obesity in the United States, 2007–2012. *JAMA Intern Med.* 2015;175(8):1412–1413.
11. Ogden CL, Carroll MD, Kit BK, et al. Prevalence of obesity and trends in body mass index among US children and adolescents, 1999–2010. *JAMA.* 2012;307(5):483–490.
12. National Heart, Lung, and Blood Institute, Managing overweight and obesity in adults: systematic evidence review from the obesity expert panel, 2013. U.S. Department of Health and Human Services. Available at: https://www.nhlbi.nih.gov/health/educational/lose_wt/guidelines.htm. Accessed December 2017.
13. McGuire S. Examining a developmental approach to childhood obesity: the fetal and early childhood years: workshop in brief. *Adv Nutr.* 2015;6:487–488.
14. McDuffie JR, Callis KA, Uwaifo GI, et al. Three-month tolerability of orlistat in adolescents with obesity-related comorbid conditions. *Obes Res.* 2002;10(7):642–650.
15. Mishori R, Otubu A, Jones AA. The dangers of colon cleansing. *J Fam Practice.* 2010;60:454.
16. Chapman IM. Obesity paradox during aging. *Interdiscip Top Gerontol.* 2010;37:20–36.
17. Raubenheimer D, Simpson D. Nutritional ecology and human health. *Ann Rev Nutrition.* 2016;36:603–626.
18. Nahera VV. Gut microbiota: modulation of host physiology in obesity. *Physiology.* 2016;31(5):327–335.
19. Boroni Moreira AP, Fiche Salles Teixeira T, do C Gouveia Peluzio M, et al. Gut microbiota and the development of obesity. *Nutr Hosp.* 2012;27:1408–1414.
20. Wu J, Cohen P, Spiegelman B. Adaptive thermogenesis in adipocytes: is beige the new brown? *Genes Dev.* 2013;27:234–250.

14

Contraception

KEY POINTS

1 ▶ Using shared decision making, the clinician has responsibility of evaluating medical contraindications and the women need to be heard about her contraceptive method preferences.

2 ▶ Many myths are still taught, past abuses forgotten, and much distrust exists around contraceptive methods.

3 ▶ Screening for pregnancy intendedness in a culturally sensitive way is part of any office visit for women of reproductive age. If she is already on a method, check for method satisfaction.

4 ▶ Excellent resources exist for both clinicians and patients: phone apps, educational web sites, and instructional videos are all available.

5 ▶ Although there is a hierarchy of contraceptive efficacy among various methods, efficacy may not be the most important attribute for an individual woman and that outlook must be respected.

6 ▶ Best practices are an important goal and include refills for 1 year, same day start, provision of emergency contraception pills with all user-dependent methods, and overlap when switching methods to avoid gaps.

7 ▶ Abortion has very high efficacy and rare complications and should be presented as an option when an unwanted pregnancy has occurred.

8 ▶ For patients who feel that they are finished with childbearing, permanent contraceptive options are available. Of these, vasectomy can be safely performed as an outpatient procedure without the risks associated with surgical sterilization of women.

Maria is an 18-year-old new patient who presents to your office requesting contraception. She's about to go to college and is afraid that she would forget to take a pill every day. She's worried about getting pregnant and wants something that works very well.

You take a history and determine that Maria is healthy without medical problems and takes no medications.

CONTRACEPTIVE OPTIONS FOR MARIA AND HOW WE TALK TO HER ABOUT THEM

▶ Presentation of contraceptive options includes information on and/or a discussion of all options.

▶ Handouts that present options and the pros and cons of each method can be a very effective tool; see http://www.reproductiveaccess.org/resource/birth-control-choices-fact-sheet/

▶ Take a history that elicits not only medical history, but also a patient's contraceptive needs and beliefs and need for protection against sexually transmitted infections (STIs).

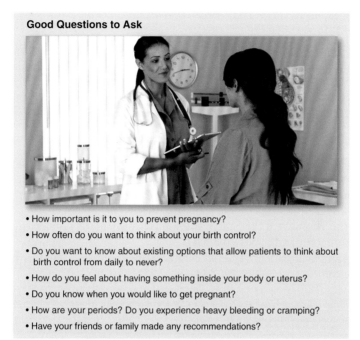

Good Questions to Ask

• How important is it to you to prevent pregnancy?
• How often do you want to think about your birth control?
• Do you want to know about existing options that allow patients to think about birth control from daily to never?
• How do you feel about having something inside your body or uterus?
• Do you know when you would like to get pregnant?
• How are your periods? Do you experience heavy bleeding or cramping?
• Have your friends or family made any recommendations?

▶ Maria has stated that effectiveness is very important to her, but other patients may have different priorities including the following:

• Side effects, especially bleeding profile and weight gain
• Being able to stop/start on own (control)
• Return to fertility
• Need for protection against STIs and human immunodeficiency virus (e.g., condoms)

Shared decision making is the counseling model that best fits contraception counseling, as there is not one method that is always better for everyone (see Chapter 5). A good resource for counseling is https://bedsider.org/. This is a great interactive website, especially for teens/young people.

Clinicians should also know about the **history of contraceptive abuses** in our country may affect how patients may feel about contraception and clinicians who provide contraception. These include:

▶ Involuntary sterilization of people of color

• In the late 1960s to early 1970s, a small but significant number of Mexican immigrants were coerced into tubal ligation at the time of emergency C-sections. Many of these women describe signing papers in English during labor and did not know that they were sterilized until much later (see PBS documentary *No Mas Bebes*).
• As recently as the 1970s women were sterilized in the California prisons without explanations or consent.

▶ Contraceptive coercion

- In the 1980s, the contraceptive method, Norplant, was pushed on women as a condition for keeping their welfare benefits. For further reading about this see Roberts, Dorothy. *Killing the Black Body: Race, Reproduction, and the Meaning of Liberty.* Vintage, 2014.
- Monetary incentives have been offered to poor women for use of contraception

▶ Conducting contraceptive trials in non-white populations without informed consent (see original oral contraceptive trials in Puerto Rico).

- Current studies have demonstrated provider biases in counseling toward pushing long-acting reversible contraceptives (LARCs, e.g., intrauterine device [IUD] or implant) on women of color.

Being sensitive to these issues and using patient-centered counseling approaches can help overcome distrust. For example, if a patient is interested in switching from a more effective form of contraception such as an IUD to a less effective form of contraception such as condoms, it is the physician's responsibility to discuss the potential effect of this choice with the patient. However, if the patient still wants to switch, the provider needs to honor the patient's autonomy and remove the IUD.

For an example of patient-centered contraceptive counseling, see this video: https://www.youtube.com/watch?v=OP9klE0JLLU

After counseling, Maria decides that she doesn't want anything in her uterus and opts for the contraceptive implant (Brand name Nexplanon).

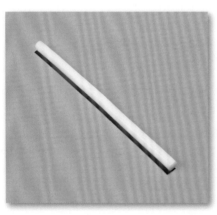

- The contraceptive implant is a small plastic rod inserted in the upper arm after administration of local anesthesia. It is FDA-approved for 3 years. No women in the contraceptive trials got pregnant!
- Link to video of Nexplanon placement/pop out (these links may change with time, it is possible to google alternative videos)
  - https://youtu.be/ug7q_1RUMio insertion
  - https://vimeo.com/182511752 pop out

WHEN CAN MARIA HAVE HER IMPLANT PLACED?

Best Practice: Same day start of contraceptives whenever possible.

The Centers for Disease Control and Prevention (CDC) Selected Practice Recommendations are immediate start of all methods after pregnancy is reliably ruled out: within 7 days of LMP or an abortion, no history of unprotected sex, within 4 weeks postpartum,

Table 14.1 ▶ When to Start Using Specific Contraceptive Methods

Contraceptive Method	When to Start (if the provider is reasonably certain that the woman is not pregnant)	Additional Contraception (i.e., back-up) Needed	Examinations or Tests Needed Before Initiation[a]
Copper-containing IUD	Anytime	Not needed	Bimanual examination and cervical inspection[b]
Levonorgestrel-releasing IUD	Anytime	If >7 days after menses started, use back-up method or abstain for 7 days	Bimanual examination and cervical inspection[b]
Implant	Anytime	If >5 days after menses started, use back-up method or abstain for 7 days	None
Injectable	Anytime	If >7 days after menses started, use back-up method or abstain for 7 days	None
Combined hormonal contraceptive	Anytime	If >5 days after menses started, use back-up method or abstain for 7 days	Blood pressure measurement
Progestin-only pill	Anytime	If >5 days after menses started, use back-up method or abstain for 2 days	None

[a]Weight (BMI) measurement is not needed to determine medical eligibility for any methods of contraception because all methods can be used (U.S. MEC 1) or generally can be used (U.S. MEC 2) among obese women. However, measuring weight and calculating BMI (weight [kg]/height [m^2] at baseline might be helpful for monitoring any changes and counseling women who might be concerned about weight change perceived to be associated with their contraceptive method.
[b]Most women do not require additional STD screening at the time of IUD insertion. If a woman with risk factors for STDs has not been screened for gonorrhea and chlamydia according to CDC's STD Treatment Guidelines (http://www.cdc.gov/std/treatment), screening can be performed at the time of IUD insertion, and insertion should not be delayed. Women with current purulent cervicitis or chlamydial infection or gonococcal infection should not undergo IUD insertion (U.S. MEC 4).
BMI, body mass index; IUD, intrauterine device; STD, sexually transmitted disease; U.S. MEC, U.S. Medical Eligibility Criteria for Contraceptive Use.
From CDC. US Selected Practice Recommendations (US SPR) for contraceptive use, 2016: When to start contraceptive methods and routine followup. Available at: http://www.cdc.gov/reproductivehealth/contraception/pdf/when-to-start_508tagged.pdf

currently on a reliable method, fully or nearly fully breastfeeding and <6 months postpartum. Additional information is shown in Table 14.1 (http://www.cdc.gov/reproductive-health/contraception/usspr.htm)

▶ If pregnancy status is unsure, the CDC recommends quick start anyway for OCs and depot medroxyprogesterone with a follow-up pregnancy test in 2 weeks.

• http://www.reproductiveaccess.org/resource/quick-start-algorithm/

- Hormonal contraception (combined oral contraceptives, progestin-only pills, patch, ring, implant and progesterone IUD) requires 7-day use of back-up contraception

▶ Maria **does not** need a pelvic exam before getting her implant.

- Pap smears do not start until age 21. Gonorrhea and chlamydia testing can be done from urine. There is no indication for routine pelvic exams prior to contraceptive initiation.

Best Practice: De-link Pap smears and pelvic exams from contraceptive prescriptions to improve access.

Maria was so happy after her visit with you, that she referred her friend Joy to see you. Joy is 17 years old and has never been pregnant. She is upset because her neurologist told her to stop her birth control pills after her new diagnosis of migraines with aura. She wonders if there is something else she can take.

The CDC categorizes medical eligibility for contraceptive use with four levels:

WHO Medical Eligibility Criteria: Categories

1	A condition for which there is no restriction for the use of the contraceptive method
2	A condition where the advantages of using the method generally outweigh the theoretical or proven risks
3	A condition where the theoretical or proven risks usually outweigh the advantages of using the method
4	A condition which represents an unacceptable health risk if the contraceptive method is used

▶ As a general rule, it is safe to routinely provide contraceptive methods that are a level 1 or 2. Methods that are a level 4 should never be prescribed. Methods that are a level 3 are generally not prescribed, but, in specific cases, the benefits may outweigh the risks.

▶ Migraines with aura are a "4" for initiation or continuation of estrogen-containing methods due to the increased risk of stroke.

WHAT CONTRACEPTION CAN JOY TAKE?

▶ Joy can use any method that does not contain estrogen such as IUD, contraceptive implant, medroxyprogesterone (Depo-Provera), progestin-only pills, and barrier methods.

- WHO MEC criteria
  - http://www.reproductiveaccess.org/resource/medical-eligibility-initiating-contraception/
  - CDC app for iPhone and Android http://www.cdc.gov/mobile/mobileapp.html
  - http://www.cdc.gov/mmwr/volumes/65/rr/rr6503a1.htm?s_cid=rr6503a1_w

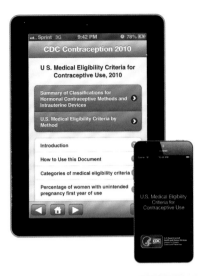

After counseling, Joy is interested in an IUD. However, she thought she couldn't have an IUD because she's never had children. She also heard from her mother that IUDs (Table 14.2) increase your risk of infections.

▶ IUDs are divided into two main categories:
- Hormonal progestin-only IUDs (left-hand picture)
  - Mirena, FDA approved for 5 years (studies support 7 years)
  - Skyla, FDA approved for 3 years
  - Liletta, FDA approved for 3 years (but has the same hormone concentration as Mirena so likely lasts 5 to 7 years)
  - Kyleena, FDA approved for 5 years
- Nonhormonal or Copper IUD (right-hand picture)
  - Paragard, FDA approved for 10 years (good data, i.e., lasts 12 years)

▶ Video for IUD insertion can be seen at https://youtube/hlfV8tKgw6E (video links may change over time. Additional videos can be found on YouTube)

IUD Myth vs. IUD Fact	
IUDs cannot be used in patients who have not given birth	IUDs can be first-line contraception in teens and nulliparous woman[1]
IUDs cause pelvic infections	This myth is based on the now defunct Dalkon Shield of the 1980s. There is new evidence that modern IUDs may protect against pelvic infections once placed[2]
IUDs cause ectopic pregnancy	IUDs overall decrease risk of ectopic pregnancy. However, if a woman becomes pregnant with an IUD in place, one-third to one-half of the time it is ectopic
You need to have testing for gonorrhea and chlamydia before having an IUD placed	Advanced testing for gonorrhea and chlamydia before having the IUD placed is not recommended. Same day testing and treating if positive does decrease PID[3]

Table 14.2 ▶ Switching Between Contraceptive Methods

Switching FROM	Switching TO						
	Pill	Patch	Ring	Progestin Shot ("Depo")	Progestin Implant	Hormone IUD	Copper IUD (Nonhormone)
Pill	No gap: take first pill of new pack the day after taking any pill in old pack	Start patch 1 day before stopping pill	No gap: insert ring the day after taking any pill in pack	First shot 7 days before stopping pill	Insert implant 4 days before stopping pill	Insert hormone IUD 7 days before stopping pill	Can insert copper IUD up to 5 days after stopping pill
Patch	Start pill 1 day before stopping patch		No gap: insert ring and remove patch on the same day	First shot 7 days before stopping patch	Insert implant 4 days before stopping patch	Insert hormone IUD 7 days before stopping patch	Can insert copper IUD up to 5 days after stopping patch
Ring	Start pill 1 day before stopping ring	Start patch 2 days before stopping ring		First shot 7 days before stopping ring	Insert implant 4 days before stopping ring	Insert hormone IUD 7 days before stopping ring	Can insert copper IUD up to 5 days after stopping ring
Progestin shot ("Depo")	Can take first pill up to 15 weeks after the last shot	Can start patch up to 15 weeks after the last shot	Can insert ring up to 15 weeks after the last shot		Can insert implant up to 15 weeks after the last shot	Can insert hormone IUD up to 15 weeks after the last shot	Can insert copper IUD up to 16 weeks after the last shot
Progestin implant	Start pill 7 days before implant is removed	Start patch 7 days before implant is removed	Start ring 7 days before implant is removed	First shot 7 days before implant is removed		Insert hormone IUD 7 days before implant is removed	Can insert copper IUD up to 5 days after implant is removed
Hormone IUD	Start pill 7 days before IUD is removed	Start patch 7 days before IUD is removed	Start ring 7 days before IUD is removed	First shot 7 days before IUD is removed	Insert implant 4 days before IUD is removed		Can insert copper IUD right after hormone IUD is removed
Copper IUD	Start pill 7 days before IUD is removed	Start patch 7 days before IUD is removed	Start ring 7 days before IUD is removed	First shot 7 days before IUD is removed	Insert implant 4 days before IUD is removed	Insert hormone IUD right after copper IUD is removed. Use back-up method for 7 days	

From Reproductive Health Access Project: How to switch birth control methods, June, 2015. Available at: http://www.reproductiveaccess.org/resource/switch-birth-control-methods/

Joy is nervous about having an IUD placed since she's never had a pelvic exam. You suggest using ibuprofen 600 mg prior to insertion, having a support person in the room, using a heat pack during insertion, playing music, and provide verbal preparation—all of which can help any patient (especially a teen) to be more comfortable during LARC insertion (see http://www.reproductiveaccess.org/resource/contraceptive-pearl-non-pharmacologic-pain-management/).

Best Practice: Perform same day insertion of LARC methods including IUDs if pregnancy can be reliably ruled out.

Six years later, Maria returns to see you again. She was so happy with her implant that she had it removed 3 years ago and had another one placed. When you ask her what she would like to do now, she remarks that she would like to get pregnant within the next year. However, she is still concerned that she may forget to take pills every day.

HOW DO YOU COUNSEL MARIA?

Options for women considering pregnancy soon, but who want good protection include the following:

▶ Depot medroxyprogesterone acetate (Depo, Depo-Provera), however, there is evidence of delayed return to fertility.

▶ IUD and implants have quick return to fertility after removal, but are high cost if only used for short term.

▶ Methods like diaphragm or condoms and foam, that patients can start and stop on their own.

▶ The contraceptive ring (NuvaRing) (keep in place for 3 weeks then remove for 1 week) and contraceptive patch (shown below) (change weekly for 3 weeks then 1 week without) can be good options for patients who do not want LARC, but do not want to think about contraception daily.

▶ There is also some evidence that the implant is effective for 4 years.[4] Maria could choose to keep the implant and delay removal until she is ready to attempt conception.

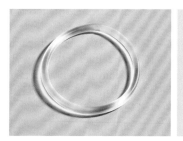 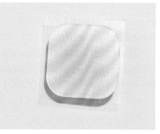

After counseling, Maria opts for the contraceptive ring since she is still concerned that she would forget to take pills daily.

A link to a video of how to use a vaginal ring (NuvaRing). This link may change with time, so it is possible to google alternative videos. https://www.youtube.com/watch?v=nF1IshIHjBE

What's the Best Timing?

▶ Information about optimal timing for switching birth control methods is shown in Table 14.2. For Maria, she should start the contraceptive ring 1 week before implant removal to prevent gaps.

Best Practice: When possible, overlap methods to prevent gaps in contraception.

> You write Maria a prescription for the contraceptive ring. She plans to start this tomorrow and return in 1 week to have her implant removed.

How Many Refills Should You Give?

Best Practice is to provide 1 year of contraception such as a 90-day supply plus 1 year of refills.

> A few months later, Maria walks in to see you for an urgent visit. She is feeling very anxious because she forgot to put her NuvaRing back in after her period last week and had unprotected sex with her husband last night.

WHAT OPTIONS ARE THERE FOR UNPROTECTED INTERCOURSE?

▶ Emergency contraception (EC): http://www.reproductiveaccess.org/wp-content/uploads/2014/12/emergency-contraception.pdf
- Levonorgestrel EC (brand name "Plan B")
  - Effective up to 72 hours from unprotected intercourse.
  - Effectiveness sharply drops at weight of 155 lb and/or BMI >25.
  - No medical contraindications.
  - Delays ovulation. More fertile in week after taking!
  - Does NOT require a prescription.
- Ulipristal acetate (UPA), brand name Ella, a selective progesterone receptor modulator (mimics progesterone and binds to receptors)
  - Effective up to 120 hours (5 days) from unprotected intercourse.
  - Effectiveness start to drop at BMI >35. Delays ovulation. More fertile in week after taking!
  - The progestin in many methods may interact with UPA, rendering it less effective. The CDC Selected Practice Recommendation guidelines (http://www.cdc.gov/reproductivehealth/contraception/usspr.htm) recommend not to start progestin-containing methods for 5 days after taking UPA. This must be weighed against the likelihood of another episode of unprotected sex.
  - REQUIRES a prescription.
- Copper IUD
  - The most effective type of EC (99%).
  - Effective up to 120 hours from unprotected intercourse (maybe more).
  - No BMI/weight restrictions.
  - Can continue as routine contraception.

Best Practice: Provide an EC prescription at time of prescription of any user-dependent contraceptive method (e.g., condoms, patch, pill, ring).[5]

Maria's weight today is 135 lb. You give her levonorgestrel EC (brand Plan B) which you have available in your clinic, and counsel her to take a pregnancy test at home or in the office in 2 weeks.

▶ **When should she restart her NuvaRing?** With levonorgestrel EC, restart contraception on the same day as taking EC. With UPA EC, the 2016 CDC Selected Practice Recommendations say to wait 5 days before restarting a progestin-containing method (http://www.cdc.gov/mmwr/volumes/65/rr/pdfs/rr6504.pdf).

- She asks you what her options would be if the EC doesn't work (levonorgestrel EC prevents pregnancy around 85% of the time)[5]
- Options for unplanned pregnancy include abortion, continued pregnancy, and adoption.
- Explain that no contraceptive method is perfect! Unplanned pregnancy can occur even in women who are doing everything they can to prevent it.
- Conversely, a woman may choose a less effective form of contraception due to medical problems, past side effects or other personal factors and use abortion as a back-up or continue the pregnancy if it is just mistimed but not unwanted.

Maria has just been laid off from work. Although she and her husband want to have a child soon, now is just not the right time!

Unplanned pregnancy makes up about half of the pregnancies in the United States each year. Of these, approximately half end in abortion and half are continued.[6]

▶ First-trimester abortion options include surgical abortion and medical abortion which is effective up to 70 days from last menstrual period.

▶ Both types of abortion are safe (safer than continuing the pregnancy).

▶ No effect on future fertility, no increased risk of breast cancer. Good quality evidence also shows that there are no long-term psychological sequelae to having an abortion.[7]

▶ All physicians should be able to counsel a woman who presents with an unplanned pregnancy regardless of their own beliefs and refer for the treatment the patient requests.

Maria returns to see you in 2 weeks for her follow-up pregnancy test. She is very relieved when the test is negative. She thanks you for being so knowledgeable about contraception! You mention that she should begin folic acid prior to attempting pregnancy.

Two months later, Maria comes back with an upper respiratory infection. You check in with her about her birth control method and pregnancy plans. It turns out she stopped her ring and is now trying to get pregnant. She did start the folic acid. You are glad you checked on this so that you can discuss her overall health in preparation for pregnancy (see Chapter 8).

Best Practice: Screen for pregnancy intendedness and method satisfaction at every opportunity (http://www.onekeyquestion.org/).

Fast forward, 3 years. Maria is now pregnant with her second child and is seeing you for her prenatal care. She is 30 weeks' gestation and you are discussing her contraceptive plans for after delivery. Maria states that she and her husband are done having children after this pregnancy.

Table 14.3 ▸ Options for Postpartum Contraception

Method	Timing
Combined hormonal contraception (combined oral contraceptive pills, patch, ring)	For women without risk factors for venous thromboembolism. Can be started at 30 days' postpartum. May interfere with milk supply in breastfeeding women
Contraceptive injection (Depo-Provera)	Can be started any time in the postpartum period Ideally prior to hospital discharge
Implant	Can be placed any time in the postpartum period
IUD: hormonal and nonhormonal	Ideally placed 10 minutes post-delivery of placenta or at 4–6 weeks post-partum Can be placed any time in the postpartum period
Progestin only pills (POP)	Can be started any time in the postpartum period Ideally at the time of hospital discharge
Tubal ligation	Can be done at the time of a C-section or prior to hospital discharge after a vaginal delivery

PERMANENT CONTRACEPTION

▶ Patients who feel that they are done childbearing may ask for permanent contraceptive options.

▶ Appropriate counseling and allowing for time to decide is important. Although the procedures can sometimes be reversed, success of successful reversal is low.

What Are Maria's Options for Permanent Sterilization?

Options for female sterilization include surgical sterilization (tubal ligation) and hystero-scopically placed tubal implants (Essure). Of note is that Essure is currently undergoing post-market surveillance for reported adverse events including abdominal pain, vaginal bleeding, and uterine perforation.

Options for male sterilization include vasectomy, which can be performed as an outpatient procedure with minimal recovery. Options for postpartum contraception are shown in Table 14.3.

Maria thanks you for the information. She will consider her options, but thinks her partner may be interested in vasectomy. You set up a consult for her husband with a colleague in your office who performs vasectomies for them to find out more about the procedure (https://www.plannedparenthood.org/learn/birth-control/vasectomy).

QUESTIONS

1. Sexually active women should be counseled to start on the most effective method of contraception.
   A. True
   B. False

2. Which of the following is true of IUDs?
   A. They shouldn't be placed in women who have never had a baby.
   B. They shouldn't be placed in women who are under age 20 years.
   C. Once placed, IUDs may protect against pelvic infection.
   D. Advanced testing for STIs should be performed before IUD placement.

3. The Centers for Disease Control and Prevention medical eligibility criteria for contraceptive use grades contraceptive methods based on safety. A "1" classification means which one of the following?
   A. The method should not be used in any situation.
   B. The method can be used if benefits outweigh risks.
   C. There is no restriction for using the method.
   D. The method can be used if the patient wants it regardless of risk.

4. Which one of the following is appropriate management for a woman who presents with an unplanned pregnancy?
   A. The physician should advise her based on his/her beliefs.
   B. The physician should tell her that abortion is more dangerous than carrying the baby to term.
   C. The physicians should counsel her about her options (continuation of the pregnancy, abortion, or adoption) nonjudgmentally regardless of their personal beliefs.
   D. The physician should congratulate her.

5. Which of the following is the most effective method of emergency contraception 3 days after unprotected intercourse?
   A. Insertion of a copper IUD
   B. Insertion of a progestin IUD
   C. Plan B (levonorgestrel)
   D. Ella (ulipristal)
   E. High-dose combined oral contraceptive pills

ANSWERS

Question 1: The correct answer is B.
Presentation of contraceptive options includes information on and/or a discussion of all options.

Question 2: The correct answer is C.
IUD myth versus IUD fact text box: There is new evidence that modern IUDs may protect against pelvic infections once placed.

Question 3: The correct answer is C.
The CDC categorizes medical eligibility for contraceptive use with four levels: 1—a condition for which there is no restriction for the use of a contraceptive method.

Question 4: The correct answer is C.
All physicians should be able to counsel a woman who presents with an unplanned pregnancy regardless of their own beliefs and refer for the treatment the patient requests.

Question 5: The correct answer is A.
The copper IUD is the most effective type of EC (99%) and is effective up to 120 hours from unprotected intercourse (maybe more).

REFERENCES

1. Committee on Adolescent Health Care Long-Acting Reversible Contraception Working Group, The American College of Obstetricians and Gynecologists. Committee opinion no. 539: adolescents and long-acting reversible contraception: implants and intrauterine devices. *Obstet Gynecol.* 2012;120(4):983–988.
2. Jatlaoui TC, Simmons KB, Curtis KM. The safety of intrauterine contraception initiation among women with current asymptomatic cervical infections or at increased risk of sexually transmitted infections. *Contraception.* 2016;94(6):701–712.
3. Sufrin CB, Postlethwaite D, Armstrong MA, et al. Neisseria gonorrhea and Chlamydia trachomatis screening at intrauterine device insertion and pelvic inflammatory disease. *Obstet Gynecol.* 2012;120(6):1314–1321.
4. Ali M, Akin A, Bahamondes L, et al. Extended use up to 5 years of the etonogestrel-releasing subdermal contraceptive implant: comparison to levonorgestrel-releasing subdermal implant. *Hum Reprod.* 2016;31(11):2491–2498.
5. Practice bulletin no. 152: emergency contraception. *Obstet Gynecol.* 2015;126(3):e1–e11.
6. Guttmacher Institute. Available at: https://www.guttmacher.org/fact-sheet/unintended-pregnancy-united-states. Accessed November 2016.
7. Biggs MA, Neuhaus JN, Foster DG. Mental health diagnoses 3 years after receiving or being denied an abortion in the United States. *Am J Pub Health.* 2015;105(12):2557–2563.

Women's Health Care

1 ▶ Caring for women across the lifecycle requires an understanding of the unique hormonal, social, and physical changes at each stage of life.

2 ▶ Menstrual and breast complaints are common in a primary care office.

3 ▶ Taking a sexual history and doing a pelvic examination are important skills in becoming proficient in the care of women.

Tanya is a 46-year-old woman who presents as a new patient to your office for a health maintenance exam. She has never had a mammogram and reports that her last pap and pelvic exam were at least 5 years ago. She has always had irregular menstrual cycles, but reports 4 to 5 days of vaginal bleeding occurring every 14 to 21 days over the last few months with heavy bleeding and clotting for the first 1 to 2 days. Menarche was at age 12 years, with irregular cycles and typically heavy bleeding throughout her reproductive life. She has been told, from prior ultrasound, that she had some "cysts" on her ovaries, but has not had any evaluation recently. She also reports some vaginal itching with whitish discharge in between menses. She is sexually active with a male partner for the past 3 months, but has had 2 other male partners in the past year. She has never had testing for sexually transmitted infections (STIs), but considers herself low risk. She routinely uses condoms for contraception.

Caring for women across their lifespan requires an understanding of the unique health care needs at various stages of development. An understanding of the various hormonal changes at each stage allows providers to address appropriate screening and prevention, and to provide appropriate counseling and education. Family physicians are uniquely positioned to provide care for women across their lifespan. By counseling women about expectations of normal transitions from menarche to the reproductive years to menopause and beyond, providers can address specific reproductive and other concerns, and therefore mitigate their influence on a woman's overall health.

Figure 15.1 outlines various hormonal changes, immunizations, counseling, screening, and educational topics that should be addressed across the lifecycle when caring for women of various ages.

MENSTRUAL CYCLE

An understanding of hormonal changes during a normal, ovulatory menstrual cycle (Fig. 15.2) is important, as any deviation from these can result in hormonal changes and, ultimately, abnormalities in menstrual flow (see Table 15.1 for common terminology describing abnormal menstrual flow).

Concerns about menstruation are common in the primary care provider's office, such as those outlined in Figure 15.1 (hormonal changes). Although Tanya's menstrual pattern

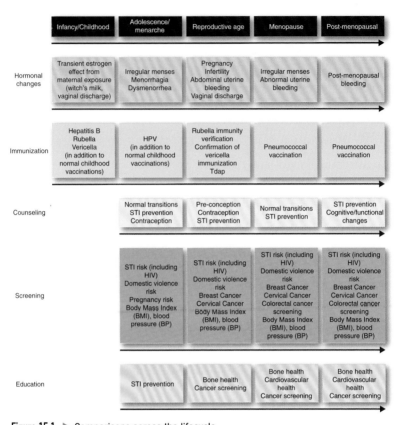

Figure 15.1 ▶ Comparisons across the lifecycle.

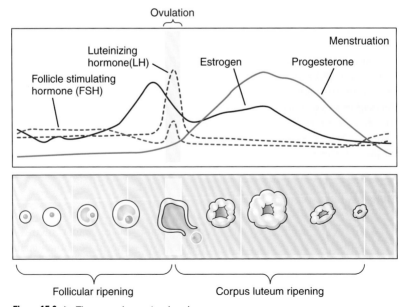

Figure 15.2 ▶ The normal menstrual cycle.

Table 15.1 ▶ Terms Describing Abnormal Menstrual Flow	
Term	**Definition**
Polymenorrhea	Abnormally frequent menses (<21 days between cycles)
Oligomenorrhea	Abnormally infrequent menses (>35 days between cycles)
Menorrhagia/hypermenorrhea	Abnormally heavy flow
Hypomenorrhea	Abnormally light menstrual flow
Metrorrhagia	Menstrual bleeding at irregular intervals (typically between expected menstrual periods
Dysmenorrhea	Painful menstrual bleeding
Menometrorrhagia	Abnormally heavy or prolonged bleeding occurring at irregular and more frequent intervals than normal

is irregular, it is normal for her. You might discuss anticipated perimenopausal changes with her. For example, excessive, unopposed estrogen production can result in failure of the normal luteinizing hormone surge, resulting in an anovulatory cycle and failure of normal menstruation. This is a typical hormonal finding in women with polycystic ovarian syndrome, in which unopposed estrogen is a common finding. Figure 15.2 demonstrates the normal rise and fall of progesterone levels required in order to trigger normal menstruation. A deficiency in this "luteal phase" progesterone surge can be a factor in impaired fertility, as well as in shortened or irregular menstrual cycles.

Familiarity with the PALM-COEIN categorization system, proposed by the Menstrual Disorders Working Group of the International Federation of Gynecology and Obstetrics, will help in classifying the likely cause of abnormal uterine bleeding (AUB) and ultimately help guide management (Fig. 15.3).[1]

TAKING A SEXUAL HISTORY

In order to appropriately address common concerns and diagnoses, it is important to feel comfortable in taking a complete sexual history. Familiarity with "The 5 P's" can guide

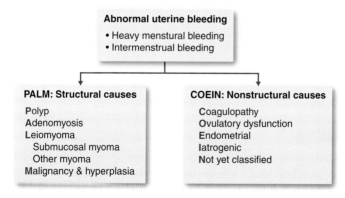

Figure 15.3 ▶ PALM-COEIN categorization system for abnormal uterine bleeding.

The 5 P's:
▶ Partners
▶ Practices
▶ Protection from STIs
▶ Past history of STIs
▶ Pregnancy

providers to address the important elements or sexual history (see Chapter 18). Tanya has had three partners in the past year and, although she considers herself low risk for sexually transmitted infections, she should be offered testing. In addition, as condom is not the most effective contraceptive choice, a discussion of contraception would be appropriate.

The Centers for Disease Control and Prevention and the American Academy of Family Physicians (AAFP) provide guides to taking a sexual history (http://www.cdc.gov/STD/treatment/SexualHistory.pdf, http://www.aafp.org/afp/2002/1101/p1705.html). Addressing a patient's sexual concerns is a vital part of caring for the entire person and is also an important screening tool, since organic disease, psychiatric disease, and medication side effects can all manifest as sexual dysfunction, which may go unrecognized if an adequate history is not elicited (see https://www.youtube.com/watch?v=1NjCUKJ04dg).

SCREENING FOR INTIMATE PARTNER VIOLENCE

Ask patients about intimate partner violence (IPV). Approximately, 1 in 7 women is victim to physical, sexual, or psychological harm by a current or former partner or spouse.[2] Several screening questionnaires have been devised to guide history-taking, including the "HITS" screening tool (How often does your partner: physically hurt you, insult you, threaten you with harm, scream, or curse at you?). More information about IPV can be found at http://www.ncbi.nlm.nih.gov/pmc/articles/PMC2688958/table/T1/ and in Chapter 21.

Although women may be reluctant to disclose IPV (https://www.youtube.com/watch?v=qdJFDUj0ErE), discussing the topic openly gives the patient permission to discuss concerns, either during the current visit, or future ones. When asked, Tanya denies any threats or abuse in her current relationship, but does admit that a former partner would threaten her "and sometimes put his hands on me" when they were arguing. She reports feeling safe in her current relationship.

Becoming comfortable with screening and offering help for IPV is an important skill to develop. Additional resources discussing state laws (https://www.youtube.com/watch?v=3GuDnKf0iPU) and other resources available for patients (https://www.youtube.com/watch?v=E6y3qCx4-V4) can be accessed online.

BREAST EXAMINATION

During your examination, Tanya mentions that she has noticed a "lump" in her breast, and would like you to examine it. You notice a firm, 2-cm, poorly mobile mass in the upper, outer quadrant of her right breast. There is no dimpling, erythema, or pain over the area, and you cannot elicit any nipple discharge. You also cannot appreciate any axillary or supraclavicular adenopathy. You recommend that TS undergo a diagnostic mammogram of the right breast with an ultrasound, and a screening study of the left breast. Both of these return with normal results. You recommend referral for a diagnostic biopsy of the palpable lesion.

According to the U.S. Preventive Services Task Force (USPSTF), as well as the American Cancer Society, routine clinical breast exam does not improve outcomes in women of any age. The AAFP agrees with these groups, recommending that providers discuss the risks and benefits of clinical breast exam with patients and defer exam unless significant concern is expressed by the patient, or the benefit of exam is felt to outweigh the risk. Table 15.2

Table 15.2 ▶ Breast Cancer Screening Recommendations From Various Organizations

Organization	Self-Breast Exam	Clinical Breast Exam	Mammogram	MRI or DBT	BRCA Testing
United States Preventive Services Task Force (USPSTF)	Against screening (D)	Insufficient evidence to recommend for or against (I)	Most beneficial for women 50–74 years (B) (biennial screening) but especially ages 60–69 years	Insufficient evidence, even in individuals with dense breast tissue (I)	Insufficient evidence to recommend for all women (I) Discuss screening if family history in first-degree relative; counsel on results
American Academy of Family Physicians	Discuss risks/ benefits, but against screening	Discuss risks/ benefits with patient, but against routine screening	Agrees with USPSTF	Agrees with USPSTF	Agrees with USPSTF
American Cancer Society	Against screening	Against screening	Annually if age 45–54 years and every 2 years for 55 years and older if life expectancy is at least 10 years. Offer if aged 40–44 years	Perform in addition to mammogram if high risk and in good health beginning at age 30 years	No opinion offered
American Congress of Obstetricians and Gynecologists	"Breast self-awareness" for all women, which may include self-exam	Screen every 1–3 years for women 20–39 years and annually for those 40 years and older	Offer screening annually beginning at age 40 years	Not for women of average risk; discuss with those at increased risk	Appropriate for women with >20–25% chance of an inherited predisposition to breast or ovarian cancer

Guidelines can be accessed at the following sites: http://www.uspreventiveservicestaskforce.org/Page/Document/UpdateSummaryFinal/
breast-cancer-screening; http://www.aafp.org/patient-care/clinical-recommendations/all/breast-cancer.html; http://www.cancer.org/
healthy/findcancerearly/cancerscreeningguidelines/american-cancer-society-guidelines-for-the-early-detection-of-cancer;
http://www.acog.org/Resources-And-Publications/Committee-Opinions/Committee-on-Gynecologic-Practice/Well-Woman-Visit
DBT, digital breast tomosynthesis; MRI, magnetic resonance imaging.

presents a comparison of the recommendations from various organizations. Additional health screening information can be found in Chapter 7.

In the event that a clinical breast exam reveals an abnormality which is not detected by mammography, further exploration should be undertaken with radiologic studies (ultrasound, MRI, or digital breast tomosynthesis), as well as surgical referral for diagnostic biopsy. It is important to take a systematic approach to the patient presenting with breast mass (http://www.aafp.org/afp/2012/0815/afp20120815p343-f1.gif).

When a patient reports a breast mass, it is important to be aware of concerning symptoms for increased risk of breast cancer, such as those listed below. Tanya has none of these features, except perhaps poor mobility, but, given her age and a palpable mass, a biopsy of the mass is warranted.

 Clues or "red flags" for breast cancer:

▶ Unilateral noncyclic pain

▶ Watery or bloody nipple discharge

▶ Unilateral, hard, immobile mass

▶ Skin retraction/dimpling, or edema (orange peel)

▶ Previous history of breast cancer

▶ Family history of premenopausal breast cancer or ovarian cancer

Clinicians should also be familiar with other commonly presenting breast complaints including pain, nipple discharge (galactorrhea), or bleeding. Pain presenting in a cyclical manner is most often bilateral and related to normal hormonal changes; cyclic pain accounts for approximately 2/3 of such complaints. Noncyclical pain is more often unilateral and should raise concern about infection, trauma, or fibrocystic disease.

Although breast pain is a rare presentation of breast neoplasm, this should certainly be considered in the differential diagnosis. An approach to the patient presenting with breast pain can be found at http://www.aafp.org/afp/2000/0415/afp20000415p2371-f1.gif.

Patients presenting with nipple discharge should be evaluated for hormonal etiologies including recent cessation of breast feeding, supplemental hormone therapy (HT) (such as for contraception), thyroid disorders, and excess prolactin production (such as with prolactin-producing pituitary tumors), as well as infections, such as mastitis or abscess (http://www.aafp.org/afp/2012/0815/afp20120815p343-f3.gif). Bloody nipple discharge is a more ominous symptom and should be completely evaluated to rule out neoplasm, particularly ductal carcinoma in situ or intraductal papilloma. See Table 15.3 for medications that can cause galactorrhea.

PELVIC EXAMINATION

Since Tanya has not had a Pap test or pelvic exam in at least 5 years, you recommend that she undergo pelvic examination, with Pap test and cultures that she has agreed to have you obtain. You elect to do co-testing with liquid-based Pap test and HPV testing. You discuss that if both of these tests are normal, she will not need another screen for 5 years. She agrees. During your exam, you note a small amount of yellowish discharge with some mild vaginal irritation, but no cervical lesions.

Table 15.3 ▶ Pharmacologic Agents Causing Galactorrhea

Psychotropic medications	*Antianxiety drugs*: benzodiazepines, buspirone *Antidepressants*: MAOIs, SSRIs, tricyclic agents *Antipsychotics* (first or second generation): haloperidol, loxitane, mellaril, moban, navane, prolixin, risperidone, stelazine, thioxanthenes, thorazine, trilafon
Neurologic medications	Dihydroergotamine, sumatriptan, valproic acid
Antihypertensives	Atenolol, methyldopa, reserpine, verapamil
Gastrointestinal agents	Histamine 2 blockers (cimetidine, famotidine, ranitidine), metoclopramide
Hormonal preparations	Danazol, estrogen, medroxyprogesterone acetate, oral contraceptives
Controlled substances/illicit drugs	Amphetamines, cannabis, cocaine, opiates

MAOI, monoamine oxidase inhibitor; SSRI, selective serotonin receptor inhibitor.

Performing a pelvic examination is a vital skill in caring for women across the lifespan (https://www.apgo.org/educational-resources/basic-clinical-skills/pelvic-exam-2017/), and an important element of the well-woman visit.[3] The exam often elicits patient anxiety, and can elicit anxiety for the inexperienced provider as well. Communication during the exam, which involves visual inspection of the external genitalia, speculum examination, as typically bimanual examination, is of great importance and can relieve the apprehension, allowing for a more comfortable exam for both patient and provider (https://www.youtube.com/watch?v=3vwh-YCCQvo). Recommendations for cervical cancer screening are discussed in Chapter 7.[4] Management of abnormal Pap tests is outlined by ASCCP (www.asccp.org).

For women under age 21 years, examination of the external genitalia may be adequate in the absence of complaints which would require further investigation. Table 15.4 outlines some common pitfalls, as well as some "do's and don'ts," for inexperienced providers when performing a pelvic exam on a patient of any age. Offering a chaperone is recommended for all providers, but mandatory for male providers.

VAGINAL DISCHARGE AND LESIONS

While some testing will require a few days for results to return, a vaginal wet prep can be performed in the provider's office, and offer some information to the patient during the visit. Table 15.5 lists the steps in performing a wet prep in the office and Table 15.6 lists characteristic findings of several types of vaginal infections which may help the provider arrive at a diagnosis even prior to laboratory results becoming available. As Tanya's discharge appeared normal and she did not have typical signs or symptoms of a vaginal infection, you do not perform a wet prep.

Other STIs may present with genital lesions, such as herpes simplex virus, which typically presents with vesicular lesions with an erythematous base, and syphilis, which may initially present as a single, painless chancre. Genital warts, a manifestation of human papilloma virus infection, may also present as painless lesions, but typically are numerous at presentation. Treatment of various causes of vaginitis STIs is presented in Table 15.7.

Table 15.4 ▶ Common Pitfalls in Conducting a Pelvic Examination

Common Pitfalls	Do	Don't
Lack of comfort with equipment or availability	Ensure that all equipment is working and available including speculum, light source, lubricant, culture tubes, sample cups, and gloves	Assume that all of the needed equipment is in the room, and begin the exam without verifying that you have everything you will need
Forgetting to communicate prior to the exam	Explain to the patient your plans for the exam	Assume that the patient knows what will be done
Forgetting to communicate during the exam	Communicate with the patient during the exam	Forget to communicate during the exam
Forgetting to pay attention to the patient's discomfort	Be sensitive to the patient's discomfort during the exam and ask about discomfort	Rush through the exam, thinking that this will decrease discomfort
Using words that may make the patient uncomfortable	Use words such as "examine" or "check" during the exam	Use words such as "feel" or "touch" during the exam
Failing to appropriately locate the cervix during the speculum exam	Exert pressure posteriorly as you insert the speculum rotated at a 45-degree angle, then rotate flat at full insertion angling anteriorly until the cervix is visualized	Insert the speculum without 45-degree rotation or exert pressure anteriorly (toward the urethra) during insertion
Forgetting to close the speculum prior to removal	Be sure to close the speculum completely prior to removal	
Forgetting to communicate your findings after the exam	Inform the patient of any normal and abnormal findings as well as expected follow-up	Avoid re-entering the room after the exam to save time or avoid further interaction

Table 15.5 ▶ Steps to Performing a Wet Pep[a]

Steps

1. Proceed as for vaginal culture collection and obtain (self or patient) a sample of vaginal fluid
2. On a single glass slide, place a drop of NaCl and a drop of KOH
3. Mix a small amount of vaginal fluid with each solution and apply coverslip
4. Immediately after preparation, take the prepared slide to the microscope and use low magnification (10×) to focus
5. Look for clue cells, white cells and trichomonads on the NaCl field and for budding hypha on the KOH field
6. Perform a whiff test and, if available, check pH
7. Discuss findings and treatment with patient

[a]https://www.youtube.com/watch?v=Vl5y1mZ4iZk&feature=youtube
KOH, potassium hydroxide; NaCl, sodium chloride.

Table 15.6 ▶ Common Vaginal Infections

Type of Infection	Bacterial Vaginosis	Candidiasis	Trichomoniasis	Gonorrhea or Chlamydia	Normal Physiologic	Atrophic Vaginitis
Symptoms	Odor Mild discharge Mild itch	Itch (severe) Thick discharge	Itch Discharge **Many asymptomatic**	Itch Discharge **Many asymptomatic**	Discharge	Itching, burning, discomfort
Discharge	Thin, white	White, curdy	Gray/yellow, thin, frothy	Clear, mucoid	Clear to white, variable	Yellowish, foul smelling (at times)
Exam	Fishy odor	Edema, erythema of vaginal epithelium	Malodorous, cervical petechiae (strawberry cervix)		No lesions or irritation	Thin, inflamed mucosa; vaginal dryness
pH	4.5–7.0	<4.5	>5.0–7.0	<4.5	3.8–4.2	>5
Laboratory	Clue Cells[a] on microscopy (NaCl)	Pseudohyphae and budding yeast[b] on microscopy (KOH)	Flagellated protozoa[c] on microscopy (NaCl); culture	Culture, PCR	Lactobacilli on microscopy (NaCl)	Atrophic cytologic changes; increase in parabasal cells

[a]http://images.slideplayer.com/25/7840100/slides/slide_63.jpg
[b]https://www.tcd.ie/Biology_Teaching_Centre/assets/pdf/by2205/by2205-webgalleries2011/by2205-gallery1/candida.pdf
[c]http://images.slideplayer.com/16/5002629/slides/slide_51.jpg

Table 15.7 ▶ Treatment of Vaginitis and Sexually Transmitted Infections

Infection	Treatment[a]
Vaginal Candidiasis	Clotrimazole 1% vaginal cream 5 g intravaginally daily for 7–14 days OR Fluconazole 150 mg orally one time
Bacterial Vaginosis/Gardnerella	Metronidazole 500 mg orally twice daily for 7 days (alternative: 2 g orally one time) OR Clindamycin 300 mg orally twice daily for 7 days
Trichomoniasis	Metronidazole 2 g orally one time PR Metronidazole 500 mg orally twice daily for 7 days
Gonorrhea	Ceftriaxone 250 mg IM one time PLUS Azithromycin 1 g orally one time
Chlamydia trachomatis	Azithromycin 1 g orally one time OR Doxycycline 100 mg PO BID for 7 days
Herpes simplex virus (HSV)[b]	Acyclovir 400 mg orally 3 times daily for 7–10 days OR valacyclovir 1 g orally twice for 7–10 days
Syphilis	Benzathine penicillin G 2.4 million units IM one time
Human papilloma virus (HPV)	Not necessary for external lesions; screen for cervical cancer

[a]For additional information, see https://www.cdc.gov/std/tg2015/2015-wall-chart.pdf
[b]See http://www.cdc.gov/std/tg2015/herpes.htm

You inform Tanya of all of these findings, including findings on exam, and discuss appropriate follow-up once the results of her Pap test and cultures are complete. You discuss appropriate anticipatory guidance and screening, including screening for osteoporosis and cardiovascular disease. Since she has no significant risk factors for osteoporosis, you recommend that she consider formal screening at age 65 years, and until that time, you recommend preventive measures, including routine weight-bearing exercise and appropriate calcium and vitamin D intake (http://www.washingtonarthritisrheumors.com/wp-content/uploads/2016/06/Osteoporosis-prevention.jpg).[5] Because her BMI is normal at 22.5 and her blood pressure is 110/72, you recommend continued annual screening. You also discuss colorectal cancer screening to begin at age 50 years. She also agrees to HIV screening, since she has never had this performed before.

ABNORMAL UTERINE BLEEDING

When you call TS to inform her that her cultures and Pap test all returned with normal results and that her breast biopsy revealed a fibroadenoma, she informs you that she has been having vaginal bleeding for the past 10 days since she saw you in the office. The bleeding has become heavier over the past 3 to 4 days and she is noticing some clotting and cramping. You ask her to return to the office for reevaluation of this abnormal bleeding.

AUB is a commonly presenting condition in primary care. Terms used to describe AUB were previously presented in Table 15.1. Differentiation of whether menstrual bleeding is ovulatory or anovulatory can assist in workup and management. Inquiring about signs or symptoms of ovulation, such as mittelschmerz (ovulatory pelvic pain), typical changes in cervical mucus throughout the cycle, and premenstrual symptoms, suggest ovulatory cycle. In addition to the PALM-COEIN classification (Fig. 15.3), AUB can be divided into ovulatory and anovulatory causes as shown in Table 15.8. Tanya had been having normal cycles and reports no signs of infection, so her heavier bleeding would represent ovulatory bleeding likely related to menopause, a structural problem like a fibroid or polyp, or possibly a complication of pregnancy or cancer.

Understanding the hormonal levels involved in a normal, ovulatory menstrual cycle (Fig. 15.1), as well as factors that can alter risk of serious cause (such as age) can help the provider decide on further workup, treatment, and adjustment of therapy (http://www.aafp.org/afp/1999/1001/afp19991001p1371-f3.gif). Ultimately, management of AUB depends primarily on the clinical presentation, including results of history and physical exam (Table 15.8). In addition, a pregnancy test should be obtained on women of reproductive age to rule out complications of pregnancy, and a thyroid-stimulating hormone (thyroid disorder) and serum prolactin levels (pituitary adenoma) should be obtained in women with anovulation.

When TS returns to your office, you obtain a pregnancy test which is negative, and order a pelvic ultrasound. Her ultrasound demonstrates a thickened endometrium and the radiologist recommends a saline infused ultrasound (sonohysterogram—https://www.bocafertility.com/images/figg_3.png). The sonohysterogram reveals an endometrial polyp (http://www.advancedwomensimaging.com.au/files/imagecache/page-image-enlarged/img/page/ConfirmedEndometrialPolyp.jpg) with a 5-mm endometrial stripe, and no ovarian abnormalities noted. You send her for surgical evaluation and she undergoes hysteroscopy and D&C with removal of the polyp. She returns for follow-up 3 months later, and is feeling much better with no further menstrual bleeding. She reports increasing symptoms of night sweats, however, as well as some hot flushing during the day.

Table 15.8 ▶ Causes and Management of Abnormal Uterine Bleeding by Ovulatory Status

Ovulatory Causes of AUB		Anovulatory Causes of AUB	
Cause	**Management**	**Cause**	**Management**
Shortened luteal phase	LNG-IUD (most effective for heavy menstrual bleeding), hormonal treatment (e.g., combined OCs, cyclic progestin)	Hypothalamic/pituitary/ovarian dysregulation (especially at extremes of reproductive age)	Hormonal treatment (e.g., combined OCs, cyclic or continuous progestin); surgical options if uncontrolled
Structural lesions (cervical or endometrial polyps, leiomyomata, or adenomyosis)	Removal	Thyroid dysfunction	Thyroid replacement for hypothyroidism or medication, surgery or RAI for hyperthyroidism
Infections (PID or cervicitis)	Antibiotics	Estrogen excess states (PCOS)	Metformin, OCs
Coagulopathies	Treat underlying disorder	Insulin excess states (impaired glucose metabolism)	Metformin; treat underlying disorder
Neoplasms (cervical, uterine, endometrial)	Surgical management	Contraceptive-related bleeding	Adjust hormone content (OC), NSAID

AUB, abnormal uterine bleeding; IUD, intrauterine device; LNG, levonorgestrel; OC, oral contraceptive; PID, pelvic inflammatory disease; PCOS, polycystic ovarian syndrome.
Data from Keehbaugh J, Burns E, Smith MA. Abnormal uterine bleeding (amended 2016 May 7; cited 2016 Dec 09). In: *Essential Evidence Plus [Internet]*. Hoboken (NJ): John Wiley & Sons, Inc.; 2012. Available from: http://www.essentialevidenceplus.com/content/eee/225; Paladine HL, Shah PA. Abnormal vaginal bleeding. In: Smith MA, Shimp LA, Schrager S, eds. *Lange: Family Medicine Ambulatory Care and Prevention*. 6th ed. New York: McGraw-Hill; 2014.

MENOPAUSE AND MENOPAUSAL SYMPTOMS

The mean age for natural menopause among US women is about 52 years, with a range of 45 to 55 years.[6] Early menopause occurs at 40 to 45 years of age and an age earlier than 40 years is called primary ovarian insufficiency, usually due to an autoimmune condition. Ablation procedures also can lead to permanent cessation of menses.

Menopause is diagnosed based on traditional criterion of no menses for 1 year, a retrospective diagnosis. Serum markers of menopause are not always easy to interpret. FSH can be quite variable in the years leading up to menopause and levels above 30 mIU/mL can occur prior to menopause. For women who wish to know if they can stop OCs and not be worried about pregnancy, a cut-off of 40 to 60 mIU/mL is fairly reliable—the hormone level should be drawn at least 10 days after stopping OCs.

Symptoms

The majority of women in the United States have menopausal symptoms during the menopausal transition and beyond. The most common is vasomotor (hot flashes) like those reported by Tanya. The majority of peri- and postmenopausal women have bothersome hot flashes which peak in the year following the last menstrual period and, for about 10%

of women, are lifelong. Other common symptoms are mood and sleep disturbances and decreased libido. Over time, the vaginal mucosa atrophies which can cause symptoms such as dyspareunia and vaginal irritation. The conglomeration of GU symptoms attributable to menopause is now called genitourinary syndrome of menopause.

Management With Hormone Therapy

Estrogen supplementation to treat menopausal symptoms was introduced in the 1960s. For women with a uterus, it became clear that there was an increased risk of endometrial cancer with unopposed estrogen. By the 1980s it was common practice to add a progestin for uterine protection. By the 1990s, prescribing menopausal HT was routine practice with the expectation of health benefits based on a large body of observational data. That practice ended in 2002 when the results of the Women's Health Initiative (WHI) study of combined HT was published. In that study, oral conjugated equine estrogens plus medroxyprogesterone (MP) (Prempro) was compared with placebo on multiple outcomes.[7] On balance there were 19 adverse events per 10,000 women per year in the treated group or about 1% over a 5-year period (Table 15.9). **Since then, governmental and professional organizations recommend HT only for treatment of menopausal symptoms at the lowest dose for the shortest duration feasible.[8]**

There are at least two important considerations for prescribing HT to symptomatic women. The first is the route of administration of estrogen. Several studies have demonstrated that the prothrombotic effects of estrogen can be nearly eliminated by using a transdermal formulation, which avoids the first liver pass. The second consideration is the choice of progestin. There was a large French cohort study over more than 20 years that showed very different breast cancer risk according to the progestin used.[9] The risk of breast cancer was highest with MP (similar to the WHI results) and not increased at all with oral micronized progesterone, intermediate with others. So, for symptomatic women who request treatment, the safest choice appears to be a **transdermal estrogen and micronized progesterone**. The latter only has FDA approval for cyclic use, for example, 200 mg 10 to

Table 15.9 ▶ Main Outcomes of the Women's Health Initiative Study

Beneficial Outcomes	NNT for 1 Year	NNT for 5 Years
Hip fracture	2,000	400
Vertebral fracture	2,000	400
Colorectal cancer	1,667	333
Harmful Outcomes	**NNH for 1 Year**	**NNH for 5 Years**
Venous thromboembolism	555	111
Myocardial infarction	1,429	286
Stroke	1,250	250
Breast cancer[a]	1,250	250

[a]No increase in breast cancer seen with estrogen only.
Data from Writing Group for the Women's Health Initiative. Risks and benefits of estrogen plus progestin in healthy postmenopausal women: Principle results from the Women's Health Initiative randomized controlled trial. *JAMA*. 2002;288:321–333; Shumaker SA, Legault C, Rapp SR, et al. Estrogen plus progestin and the incidence of dementia and mild cognitive impairment in postmenopausal women: the Women's Health Initiative Memory Study: a randomized controlled trial. *JAMA*. 2003;289:2651–2662;[14] The Women's Health Initiative Steering Committee. Effects of conjugated equine estrogen in postmenopausal women with hysterectomy: the Women's Health Initiative randomized controlled trial. *JAMA*. 2004;291:1701–1712.[15]

15 days per month. If Tanya's symptoms become more severe, a discussion of HT or other options for vasomotor symptoms, as discussed below, would be appropriate.

Vaginal dryness can be managed with low-dose topical estrogen preparations without risk of endometrial stimulation. Alternatively, or additionally, vaginal lubricants may be helpful.

Other Management Options

For women with troublesome hot flashes who are not candidates for HT or who do not want to use HT, there are other alternatives.[10] Gabapentin (300 mg three times daily), for example, reduces hot flashes by 20% to 30% compared with placebo.[11]

Venlafaxine is also somewhat effective as are some SSRIs, although study results are conflicting. Low-dose paroxetine (brand name Brisdelle) is the only FDA-approved non-hormonal treatment of menopause.

With respect to complementary therapies, a well-designed study of black cohosh showed no difference from placebo. Studies of phytoestrogens have been conflicting. Limited evidence suggests that relaxation techniques may be effective,[12] but not exercise.[13]

QUESTIONS

1. ACOG's PALM-COEIN mnemonic describes etiologies of which one of the following?
   A. Miscarriage
   B. Menopause
   C. Abnormal vaginal bleeding
   D. Contraception

2. The US Preventive Services Task Force, American Academy of Family Physicians, and the American Cancer Society recommend that women do self-breast examinations regularly.
   A. True
   B. False

3. When a woman presents with a breast mass, which one of the following are "red flags" for breast cancer?
   A. Bilateral pain
   B. A mass that comes and goes with the menstrual cycle
   C. Unilateral bloody nipple discharge
   D. A grandmother with breast cancer at age 76 years

4. Which of the following is a characteristic of bacterial vaginosis?
   A. Low pH
   B. Petechiae on the cervix ("strawberry cervix")
   C. Erythema of the vaginal epithelium
   D. Clue cells
   E. Thick, white discharge

ANSWERS

Question 1: The correct answer is C.
Familiarity with the PALM-COEIN categorization system, proposed by the Menstrual Disorders Working Group of the International Federation of Gynecology and Obstetrics, will help in classifying the likely cause of abnormal uterine bleeding and ultimately help guide management.

Question 2: The correct answer is B.

Table 15.2, The US Preventive Services Task Force and American Cancer Society recommend against self-breast examination; the American Academy of Family Physicians recommends against this practice as well, but suggest a discussion of risks and benefits.

Question 3: The correct answer is C.

When a patient reports a breast mass, it is important to be aware of concerning symptoms for increased risk of breast cancer, such as those listed below: (Text Box) Unilateral noncyclic pain, watery or bloody nipple discharge.

Question 4: The correct answer is D.

(Table 15.6): Bacterial vaginosis is associated with mild discharge and itching, thin white discharge, fishy odor, high pH, fishy odor, and clue cells on microscopy.

REFERENCES

1. ACOG practice bulletin 136: management of abnormal uterine bleeding associated with ovulatory dysfunction. *Obstet Gynecol.* 2014;122:176–185.
2. Centers for Disease Control and Prevention. Available at: http://www.cdc.gov/violenceprevention/pdf/intimatepartnerviolence.pdf. Accessed November 2016.
3. American Congress of Obstetricians and Gynecologists. Available at: http://www.acog.org/Resources-And-Publications/Committee-Opinions/Committee-on-Gynecologic-Practice/Well-Woman-Visit. Accessed November 2016.
4. United States Preventive Services Task Force. Available at: https://www.uspreventiveservicestaskforce.org/Page/Name/us-preventive-services-task-force-issues-new-cervical-cancer-screening-recommendations. Accessed November 2016.
5. National Academies. Available at: http://www.nationalacademies.org/hmd/~/media/Files/Report%20Files/2010/Dietary-Reference-Intakes-for-Calcium-and-Vitamin-D/Vitamin%20D%20and%20Calcium%202010%20Report%20Brief.pdf. Accessed December 2016.
6. Cramer DW, Xu H. Predicting age at menopause. *Maturitas.* 1996;23:319–326.
7. Writing Group for the Women's Health Initiative. Risks and benefits of estrogen plus progestin in healthy postmenopausal women: Principle results from the Women's Health Initiative randomized controlled trial. *JAMA.* 2002;288:321–333.
8. North American Menopause Society clinical recommendations. Available at: https://www.menopause.org/publications/clinical-care-recommendations/chapter-8-prescription-therapies. Accessed December 2016.
9. Fournier A, Berrino F, Riboli E, et al. Breast cancer risk in relation to different types of hormone replacement therapy in the E3N-EPIC cohort. *Int J Cancer.* 2005;114:448–454.
10. Hill DA, Crider M, Hill SR. Hormone therapy and other treatments for symptoms of menopause. *Am Fam Physician.* 2016;94(11):884–889.
11. Toulis KA, Tzellos T, Kouvelas D, et al. Gabapentin for the treatment of hot flashes in women with natural or tamoxifen-induced menopause: a systematic review and meta-analysis. *Clin Ther.* 2009;31(2):221–235.
12. Freedman RR, Woodward S. Behavioral treatment of menopausal hot flushes: evaluation by ambulatory monitoring. *Am J Obstet Gynecol.* 1992;167:436–439.
13. Aiello EJ, Yasui Y, Toworger SS, et al. Effect of a yearlong, moderate-intensity exercise intervention on the occurrence and severity of menopause symptoms in postmenopausal women. *Menopause.* 2004;11:382–388.
14. Shumaker SA, Legault C, Rapp SR, et al. Estrogen plus progestin and the incidence of dementia and mild cognitive impairment in postmenopausal women: the Women's Health Initiative Memory Study: a randomized controlled trial. *JAMA.* 2003;289:2651–2662.
15. The Women's Health Initiative Steering Committee. Effects of conjugated equine estrogen in postmenopausal women with hysterectomy: the Women's Health Initiative randomized controlled trial. *JAMA.* 2004;291:1701–1712.

Men's Health Care

1 ▶ The leading causes of death in men of all ages include cardiovascular disease, cancer, unintentional injuries, and suicide.

2 ▶ Men, particularly those under 45 years, are significantly less likely to have a regular or primary source of health care. Consider each episode of care as an opportunity to review screening, prevention, risk assessment.

3 ▶ Prostate cancer screening and treatment of age-related hypogonadism are topics best approached with shared decision-making strategies.

CARE OF THE YOUNG ADULT MAN

Cole is a 20-year-old man who presents to your office for a "check-up." He is a full-time college student and works part-time waiting tables. He says he is feeling well but was hoping to be tested for sexually transmitted infections (STIs) because a childhood friend of his was recently diagnosed with human immunodeficiency virus (HIV), which scared him. He denies having any chronic medical problems and does not take any medications.

Prioritizing Care for Young Adult Men

Young adult men seek preventive care significantly less often than women.[1] In the United States, nearly 25% of men aged 18 to 64 years have no true source of primary care and tend to visit emergency departments or urgent care facilities for acute health care needs.[2] This equates to missed opportunities to identify potentially harmful behaviors and to provide education on safety, healthy lifestyles and sexual health. Evidence-based clinical decision-making tools, such as the United States Preventive Services Task Force (USPSTF) AHRQ's Electronic Preventive Services Selector (https://epss.ahrq.gov/PDA/index.jsp) are easy to access and help provide efficient comprehensive care.

Mortality in Young Adult Men

While Cole's primary concern is screening for STIs, you should also discuss other preventive health items (Tables 16.1; Fig. 16.1).

Unintentional injuries and suicide rank first and second among the top five leading cause of death among US men aged 15 to 44 years. Homicide ranks fourth.[12] While there is a paucity of evidence to routinely recommend screening and intervention for these issues, one should consider prioritizing time for education in injury and death prevention. Building rapport and establishing trust can encourage your patient to share this and other sensitive information.

Table 16.1 ▶ Screening for High Risk Behaviors in Young Adult Men			
Behavior	USPSTF or Other Recommendations	Screening Tools	Counseling and Intervention Tools
Alcohol misuse[3]	USPSTF: Grade B for adults age 18 years and older	AUDIT-C[4] (3-item questionnaire)	Brief counseling (>5 minutes) on 1 or more occasions is most effective (e.g., NIAAA pocket guide[5])
Illicit drug use[6]	USPSTF: Insufficient evidence for adult screening	CAGE-AID[4] (5-item questionnaire)	Limited data for use in screening populations with low-prevalence
Tobacco use[7]	USPSTF: Grade A for screening, counseling, and interventions to promote cessation	5-As framework[8] • **A**sk (with vital signs) • **A**dvise to quit • **A**ssess willingness • **A**ssist with quitting • **A**rrange follow-up (see Chapter 23)	Behavioral therapy (in-person, telephone, online) Example: I Want to Quit: American Lung Association (ALA Pharmacotherapy) • Nicotine replacement (gum, lozenges, patches, nasal spray, etc.) • Bupropion SR Varenicline combination therapy
Driver safety	No evidence-based or consensus guidelines. Consider education (motor vehicle crashes are the leading cause of injury-related death in teens and young adults)[9]	None available	Various websites promoting driver safety: http://youth.gov/ https://www.cdc.gov/
Weapon use	No evidence-based or consensus guidelines. Consider asking about gun ownership or recreational use.[a]	None available	Encourage firearm safety training and safe storage. Consider discouraging personal ownership of weapons that fire >10 rounds.[10]

[a]Some states have legislation prohibiting physician inquiry into gun ownerships ("gag" laws).[11]

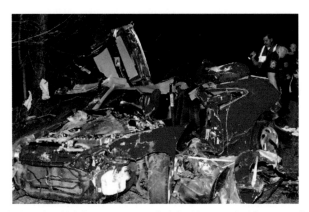

Figure 16.1 ▶ Wrecked car in which three teenagers died. Accident resulted from use of alcohol. All three had been drinking. (From CDC and Gwinnett County Police Department 1999. Centers for Disease Control and Prevention, Public Health Image Library (PHIL). https://phil.cdc.gov/phil/home.asp.)

Further conversation with Cole reveals that he drinks four to five beers on weekends usually at social functions. He uses marijuana occasionally but denies use of tobacco products, illicit drugs or controlled substances, including prescription medications. He enjoys rock-climbing and playing basketball on a college intramural team. He is doing well in school, studying political science, and has not had any academic struggles. His father has hypertension and takes cholesterol medication. His mother has migraine headaches. He is not aware of any early cardiovascular disease or other cancers in his family.

Screening and Prevention of High-Risk Behaviors in the Young Adult Men

Screening for Alcohol and Substance Use

An estimated 30% of men age 18 years and older have consumed moderate to high amounts of alcohol (defined by the CDC as having five or more drinks in 1 day) at least once in the preceding year. Alcohol misuse may account for over 85,000 deaths in the United States each year and is a leading cause of preventable death.[3] Evidence suggests that screening and brief interventions in the primary care setting can effectively reduce risky drinking in adults (see Chapter 23). The most effective interventions targeting alcohol misuse were at least 6 to 15 minutes in duration and included various formats such as face-to-face counseling or provision of written or online materials.[3]

There is limited evidence supporting screening for illicit drug use in primary care. However, in the United States, the rate of illicit drug use is highest among adults age 18 to 20,[6] thus a simple yes or no question about illicit substance use may signal the need for further attention. Since Cole admits to occasional marijuana use, he may be at risk for use of other substances. In addition to illegal substances, providers should inquire about misuse of prescription drugs, which accounts for an increasing percentage of misuse and overdose in the United States.

Sexually Transmitted Infection Screening for Men

Cole reports that he has been sexually active for 4 years. He has had four female partners, one which was long-term, and the others single encounters. He has practiced oral sex and vaginal-insertive intercourse. He uses condoms most of the time. He denies ever having anal sex. He has never been tested for STIs and is not aware of any known exposures. He has no genitourinary symptoms. He drives, wears seat belts 100% of the time, and states he does not own a firearm.

Though asymptomatic and without any known exposures, Cole is at increased risk for STIs based on his age, multiple partners, and inconsistent condom use. Chapter 18 provides further information on obtaining an appropriate sexual history, a key in determining what screening to offer. The AHRQ preventive services selector tools referenced earlier can help you determine what tests he might need. Be sure to check the Risk Info and Details sections for each recommendation. In viewing these sections, you will find that the levels of evidence to support these choices are mixed. There is also no clear recommendation for frequency of STI screening in heterosexual HIV-negative men; assessment of risk factors including type and number of sexual partners and types of sexual behaviors should be taken into consideration.

There is insufficient evidence for screening for **chlamydia and gonorrhea** in sexually active men who are exclusively heterosexual,[13] however it may be reasonable to offer him screening with nucleic-acid amplification testing of urine or urethral samples for gonorrhea and chlamydia due to multiple partners and inconsistent use of condoms. The urine sample is preferentially a first-catch specimen to increase the sensitivity. Treatment without any symptoms or without a confirmed exposure to chlamydia or gonorrhea is not warranted. The primary benefit of testing is to reduce transmission to female partners, who are at much higher risk of complications from chlamydia and gonorrhea.[14]

Regardless of gender (self or partner), **high-risk sexual behaviors** confer greater risk. Men who have sex with men (MSM) are at significantly higher risk of STIs compared to men who exclusively have sex with women, likely due to higher frequencies of insertive and receptive anal sex. MSM are at higher risk of STIs including hepatitis B and C. For all patients, it is important to inquire about sexual behaviors that include oral, anal, and vaginal receptive and insertive intercourse, appropriate for the sex of the patient, numbers of partners and condom use. Screening should be offered for HIV, syphilis, hepatitis B and C, and gonorrhea and chlamydia (at both genital and nongenital sites such as rectal and pharyngeal sampling) for those at higher risk. STI screening for MSM should be done annually and potentially more frequently for those with HIV or higher-risk sexual behaviors.[14]

Sexual Health Counseling

The USPSTF recommends intensive behavioral counseling for sexually active adults at increased risk for STI.[15] This is based on evidence primarily in adolescent women that demonstrated decreased STI rates after exposure to frequent and lengthy group counseling programs. Intensive intervention is generally not possible for young adults busy with work and/or school. Prioritizing this topic during a clinic visit is often the best option.

Preventive measures against STIs include sexual abstinence and condom use. Condoms do not protect against STIs spread through skin contact including herpes, syphilis, and human papilloma virus.

Pregnancy and contraception should be discussed during sexual education for men who have sex with women. Condom use or sexual abstinence are the only current forms of easily reversible contraception for men.

Physical Examination

Per the USPSTF, periodic screening for high blood pressure (BP) and obesity would warrant obtaining vital signs and height and weight at this visit.[16,17] In the absence of symptoms, there is no other mandatory physical examination for a young adult man.

Many providers might choose to briefly examine the head and neck, auscultate heart and lungs, and possibly examine the genitalia if requested by the patient as part of an STI screening. While the individual benefits are uncertain, the physical exam can promote connection between provider and patient and may foster rapport-building and patient education.

Cancer Screening

Testicular cancer is the most frequent cancer affecting men ages 15 to 34 years, but remains a very rare cancer (0.4% lifetime risk for all men). As of 2013, there were 5.7 new cases of testicular cancer per 100,000 men, with a 95% 5-year survival rate.[18] The USPSTF gives screening for testicular cancer a D recommendation based on its rare incidence, overall good prognosis, and risk of harm from screening.[19,20] See Chapter 7 for other prevention recommendations.

You conclude the visit with Cole today having performed a brief exam that includes vital signs and heart/lung exam. You administer the PHQ-2 and AUDIT-C which are both negative, or low risk. You review screening guidelines for STIs; test him for HIV, syphilis, and gonorrhea and chlamydia; and encourage him to use condoms regularly. You educate him that unintentional injuries are the major cause of mortality in his age group and encourage him to drive responsibly and use appropriate safety precautions for recreational sports.

CARE OF THE MIDDLE-AGED MAN

Tom, a 47-year-old man, presents for a wellness exam. He has not been to a doctor's office in about 10 years, and agreed to come because he was getting tired of his wife's nagging. His tone of voice portrays annoyance and he makes limited eye contact. He is married to his second wife for 10 years and they have two school-aged children. He works full-time in a desk job, but notes his company will be downsizing in the next year and he worries about losing his job, including his and his family's health benefits. He does not exercise regularly but considers himself active with maintaining his home and coaching his son's soccer team. His family history is significant for his father having died from a heart attack at age 52. He does not smoke. He drinks two to three beers on the weekends. He is overweight.

Prioritizing Care of Middle-Aged Men

Nearly 12% of adult men rate their health status as "fair" or "poor"; this figure increases to 17% among men aged 45 to 64 years and continues to increase with age.[21] Tom's lack of regular medical care over the prior decade presents a challenge for providing comprehensive care in what is likely to be a clinic visit with only 20 to 30 minutes of time allotted. Effectively establishing rapport and setting a shared agenda with the expectation of follow-up visits may help promote continued high-quality comprehensive care.[22]

While Tom is changing for his exam, you use the AHRQ EPSS website to search for **recommended screening and preventive services** (https://epss.ahrq.gov/ePSS/search.jsp). As men age, cardiovascular disease (CVD) risk increases and becomes a more prominent cause of morbidity and mortality. Many of the recommended preventive health items in this age group are centered around prevention and/or detection of CVD. These include screening for obesity, hypertension, hyperlipidemia, diabetes, and assessing lifestyle behaviors such as substance use, dietary habits, and physical activity. See Chapter 7 for other prevention recommendations.

In addition to preventive care, men may seek primary care for a variety of issues.[23] Standardized male wellness visit forms may help to screen efficiently for common conditions. An example form is here: http://www.aafp.org/fpm/2003/0700/fpm20030700p35-rt1.pdf.

After spending a few minutes getting to know Tom, you review the standardized wellness form he has filled out and notice he identified concerns about his marriage and erectile dysfunction (ED). Further discussion reveals that he and his wife have been arguing frequently at home, usually about finances. He says they have not been sexually active in about 3 months and he has been

BOX 16.1 SAMPLE PLAN FOR INITIAL AND FOLLOW-UP VISITS FOR TOM

1. Address Tom's main concerns (decreased libido and erectile dysfunction [ED])
2. Cardiovascular Disease Screening and Risk Stratification
    a. Measure blood pressure, height/weight (calculate BMI), abdominal circumference
    b. Physical examination (nondilated funduscopic exam [if blood pressure elevated], heart and lung auscultation, palpate abdomen for pulsatile mass and organomegaly, genital exam because of ED concerns, palpate/observe extremities for edema, hair loss)
    c. Order labs: lipid panel, hemoglobin A1C; once available, calculate 10-year cardiovascular disease risk (e.g., ASCVD Risk Estimator at http://tools.acc.org/ASCVD-Risk-estimator/)
    d. Brief Health Counseling, if applicable on healthy diet and exercise (>150 min/week of moderate intensity cardiovascular exercise; consider strength training 2–3 times weekly)
3. Other Screening
    a. Depression: PHQ-2 or PHQ-9

unable to maintain an erection for more than a few minutes. His libido is poor. He jokes that this is probably the real reason his wife wanted him to come see you. You assure him that you are glad he is here to discuss his health and offer to focus today's visit on his marital strain and sexual concerns, which seem most important. You propose to address these issues, then order some screening labs to be reviewed at a follow-up visit. Tom agrees with this plan, noted in Box 16.1.

Erectile Dysfunction

Tom has briefly mentioned his concern about erectile dysfunction (ED), but, like many men, it is likely a much greater concern that he will admit. ED is probably more common than statistics demonstrate, and is known to increase with age. ED has a variety of causes including heart disease, hypertension, hyperlipidemia, diabetes, overweight/obesity, tobacco use, anxiety, relationship strain, life stressors, history of abuse, sedentary lifestyle, hypogonadism, thyroid disorders, genital pain, and many medications including opiates, antidepressants, antihistamines, antihypertensives, diuretics, and anxiolytics.[24] Tom's situation presents a valuable opportunity for shared agenda setting, and, in the process of more thoroughly evaluating Tom for ED, you will gain the opportunity to screen for CVD and potentially help the patient initiate preventive measures that may improve both ED and his CVD risk.

Men may be embarrassed or reluctant to describe their struggles with ED, making evaluation difficult. Several validated clinical tools are available to help both provider and patient. One such tool is the five-item International Index of Erectile Function (IIEF-5) which can be used for both diagnosis and monitoring treatment efficacy (Table 16.2).[24]

Attention to medication use is important, as many common medications have the adverse effect of ED. Both a cardiovascular and genital examination (noting testicular size and presence of any masses), as well as assessment of secondary male characteristics (body hair) should be performed. Testing for testosterone deficiency should be considered if, in addition to decreased libido and ED, the patient notes loss of spontaneous erections, decreased physical stamina and strength, depressed mood, fatigue, increased visceral adiposity, sleep disturbance, and/or poor concentration and memory.[25] Testosterone deficiency is defined by experts as a serum concentration <300 ng/dL on a first-morning test

Table 16.2 ▶ Five-Item Version of the International Index of Erectile Function Questionnaire

Questions	Scores				
	1	**2**	**3**	**4**	**5**
How do you rate your confidence that you could get and keep an erection?	Very low	Low	Moderate	High	Very high
When you had erections with sexual stimulation, how often were your erections hard enough for penetration?	Almost never or never	A few times[a]	Sometimes[b]	Most times[c]	Almost always or always
During sexual intercourse, how often were you able to maintain your erection after you had penetrated (entered) your partner?	Almost never or never	A few times[a]	Sometimes[b]	Most times[c]	Almost always or always
During sexual intercourse, how difficult was it to maintain your erection to completion of intercourse?	Extremely difficult	Very difficult	Difficult	Slightly difficult	Not difficult
When you attempted sexual intercourse, how often was it satisfactory for you?	Almost never or never	A few times[a]	Sometimes[b]	Most times[c]	Almost always or always

Note: The score is the sum of the above five questions responses. Erectile dysfunction is classified based on these scores: 17–21 = mild; 12–16 = mild to moderate; 8–11 = moderate; 5–7 severe.
[a]Much less than one-half the time.
[b]About one-half the time.
[c]Much more than one-half the time.

via radioimmunoassay coupled with symptoms (see Care of the Elderly Man).[25] Laboratory testing may otherwise be limited to routine cardiovascular screening, though additional lab tests may be ordered if clinically warranted.

Treatment of ED depends on the cause and may require several modalities including relationship or mental health counseling, lifestyle modification, and targeted medical therapies shown in Table 16.3.[24]

Table 16.3 ▶ Treatment for Erectile Dysfunction

First Line

- Manage chronic conditions—diabetes, HTN, etc.
- Lifestyle modification—weight loss, regular exercise
- Smoking cessation
- Individual or couples counseling and/or treatment for mood disorder or anxiety
- Oral PDE-5 inhibitors

Second Line

- Vacuum device
- Alprostadil—intracavernous or intraurethral

Third Line

- Urology referral
- Penile prostheses

Cardiovascular Disease Screening Middle-Aged Men

Hypertension

While there is no evidence to suggest an optimal interval for hypertension screening, the USPSTF recommends annual BP screening for adults aged 40 years or older and for those at increased risk for high BP (e.g., those who have high-normal BP [130 to 139/85 to 89 mm Hg], those who are overweight or obese, and African Americans).[26] BPs that are elevated should be confirmed with additional measurements either at home, or during a repeat office visit. The USPSTF found evidence that ambulatory BP monitoring (ABPM) is the best method for diagnosing hypertension.[26]

Overweight/Obesity

In the United States, 34.5% of men age 20 years and older are considered obese and only 50% of men over 18 years meet the federal guidelines for adequate physical activity shown in Table 16.4.[27] All adults should be screened for obesity with BMI calculation and potentially abdominal/waist circumference to detect metabolic syndrome.[28]

The USPSTF recommends (grade B) dietary and physical activity counseling for adults who are obese and have cardiovascular risk factors. There is moderate evidence supporting the effectiveness of counseling interventions consisting of 5 to 16 contacts over a 9- to 12-month period. Obese adults should be offered referral to intensive interventions targeting obesity. Such interventions are most effective if comprehensive, including at least 12 to 26 sessions annually.[29]

Lipid Measurement

The lipid panel can be utilized as one of several parameters in determining a calculated 10-year risk for CVD. The American College of Cardiology and American Heart Association ASCVD risk estimator (http://tools.acc.org/ascvd-risk-estimator/) is one such example. The USPSTF, in line with ACC/AHA and other organizations, recommends offering a statin for primary prevention of CVD in adults age 40 to 75 with an estimated 10-year CVD event risk of 10% or greater.[30]

Suicide in Middle-Aged Men

Suicide remains a leading cause of death in men ages 35 to 65 years. Death rates from suicide have increased in recent decades and account for the largest proportion of suicides

Table 16.4 ▶ CDC Guidelines for Physical Activity in Adults

Aerobic Activity
- 150 min/week of moderate-intensity exercise (e.g., brisk walking), or
- 75 min/week of vigorous-intensity exercise (e.g., running/jogging), or
- Equal mix of moderate and vigorous-intensity activities

Muscle-Strengthening Exercise
- 2 or more days a week
- Works all major muscle groups

Data from https://www.cdc.gov/physicalactivity/basics/adults/index.htm

in the United States,[31] yet efforts at prevention have not generally been focused on this age group. Men who die by suicide are more likely to have more severe feelings of hopelessness and resolve to die; are more likely to be intoxicated at the time of death; and are more likely to act quickly once suicidal ideation occurs.[32] Risk factors for suicide in men include stressors in family and work environments, as well as coexistent substance abuse. While recommendations for screening and prevention of suicide are unclear, screening for depression is recommended (USPSTF grade B). As men are less likely to seek mental health care, primary care providers may be the sole point of contact in the health care system for men at risk of suicide.

> Tom scores moderate on the IIEF-5 tool for ED. He also screens positive for depression on the PHQ-9 but answers no to question #9 for suicidal ideation. He accepts a referral to a behavioral health counselor and plans to discuss marital counseling with his wife. He declines medications for depression and ED today, and wants to try counseling and lifestyle modifications first. You perform a physical exam including genitalia which is normal. You order a lipid panel, HbA1c, and schedule a follow-up visit in 2 weeks to review the results. You recommend initiation of a regular exercise routine with the goal of 150 minutes of moderate intensity cardiovascular exercise each week.

CARE OF THE ELDERLY MAN

> Jack is a 68-year-old man with hypertension, hyperlipidemia, hypothyroidism, and benign prostatic hyperplasia who presents requesting refills of his chronic medications. He sees his physician twice annually. He is retired and spends his days with his wife gardening or working around their home, collecting and selling antiques, and helping care for his mother who lives in a long-term care facility. He checks his BP twice weekly at the gym, with typical readings of 135/80 mm Hg. He walks 2 miles about three times weekly and lifts weights twice weekly. He is concerned about chronic bilateral knee pain. He also asks about his testosterone level, as he has several friends who have started using testosterone patches and feel stronger and healthier on it.

Prioritizing Care of the Elderly Man

For the elderly man, providers may encounter multiple chronic medical conditions, an increasing number of age-appropriate screening items and immunizations required, and often acute or new concerns brought by the patient. For patients receiving Medicare, providers are tasked with balancing the needs or desires of the patient with limitations set on covered services. Prioritizing goals, setting a shared agenda, and maintaining transparency will help ensure appropriate and cost-effective care.

When chronic conditions appear to be stable and well-controlled, more time can be dedicated to the patient's acute concerns and prevention. A pre-visit chart review by medical assistants can quickly establish which screening items are due, if any. Use the AHRQ EPSS tool (https://epss.ahrq.gov/ePSS/search.jsp) to review appropriate screening and preventive recommendations for Jack now.

Issues common to elderly men may include lower urinary tract symptoms (LUTS) related to benign prostatic hyperplasia, ED, concerns about testosterone levels and prostate cancer.

Jack has nocturia about three times each night, but says this is not bothersome to him. He has no difficulty with his urine stream. He and his wife are sexually active several times monthly and he does not report any problems with libido or ED. Jack's medications include lisinopril, amlodipine, levothyroxine, lovastatin, and low-dose aspirin once daily. He takes acetaminophen as needed for knee pain. His past surgeries include a total knee replacement, an arthroscopic shoulder surgery, and cholecystectomy. He has no allergies. He is a former smoker but stopped over 30 years ago. He receives dental care twice yearly; his last vision screen was 6 months ago and he received a new eyeglasses prescription. He and his wife live in a single family two-story home. They are completely independent and both still drive. Jack and his wife are planning a cross-country trip in an RV in about 1 month, and he would like to make sure his prescriptions will last him until he returns in about 5 months.

Lower Urinary Tract Symptoms

Symptoms of urinary frequency, nocturia, and weak urine stream, collectively known as LUTS, are common in elderly men but often not reported directly by the patient. These may only be recognized through a review of symptoms on a standardized screening form or indirectly during a patient's report of insomnia or after an acute presentation for bladder obstruction. Benign prostatic hypertrophy (BPH) is a very common cause of LUTS and increases with age, but other etiologies should be considered (Box 16.2).[33]

For patients with LUTS due to BPH, providers may administer the American Urological Association Symptom Score Index Questionnaire to grade severity and assess efficacy of treatment (Table 16.5).[34]

BOX 16.2 CAUSES OF LUTS OTHER THAN BPH

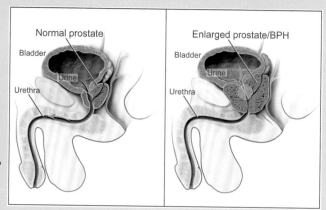

▶ Infection of bladder or prostate

▶ Diabetes mellitus

▶ Bladder calculus

▶ Cancer of bladder or prostate

▶ Urethral stricture

▶ Medications including diuretics, antihistamines, anticholinergics, opioids, sympathomimetics

▶ Caffeine (bladder irritant)

▶ Neurogenic bladder

▶ Overactive bladder

Image from National Cancer Institute. Benign prostatic hyperplasia. 2005. https://visualsonline.cancer.gov/details.cfm?imageid=7137.

Table 16.5 ▶ American Urological Association BPH Symptom Score Index Questionnaire

Over the Past Month or So	Not at All	Less than 1 in 5 Times	Less than One-Half of the Time	About One-Half of the Time	More than One-Half of the Time	Almost Always
How often have you had the sensation of not completely emptying your bladder after you finished urinating?	0	1	2	3	4	5
How often have you had to urinate again less than 2 hours after you finished urinating?	0	1	2	3	4	5
How often have you found that you stopped and started again when urinating?	0	1	2	3	4	5
How often have you found it difficult to postpone urinating?	0	1	2	3	4	5
How often have you had a weak urinary stream?	0	1	2	3	4	5
How often have you had to push or strain to begin urinating?	0	1	2	3	4	5

	None	1 time	2 times	3 times	4 times	5 times
How many times do you typically get up to urinate from the time you go to bed at night until the time you get up on the morning?	0	1	2	3	4	5

Evaluation and Management of LUTS

A digital rectal examination, though limited and subject to provider skill, should be performed in the evaluation of LUTS to help assess prostate size, tenderness, and irregular contour or masses.[33] A urinalysis and serum prostate-specific antigen (PSA) should be ordered and may suggest alternative causes of LUTS; however, the PSA is often mildly or moderately elevated in BPH and is not specific for prostate cancer.

Many men with mild symptoms due to BPH may simply choose to monitor the condition while others may desire treatment; current evidence suggests that in the absence of acute urinary obstruction or other complications, either approach is reasonable. Those who prefer to monitor symptoms may benefit from lifestyle modifications including reducing evening fluid intake, weight loss, avoidance of bladder irritants, or discontinuing medications that worsen symptoms. Patients desiring treatment can be offered either medications (Table 16.6) or surgical management. Current surgical options include various transurethral ablative or excisional techniques.[33]

Table 16.6 ▶ Medications for Benign Prostatic Hypertrophy

Medication	Formulations/Drugs	Side Effects/Caution	Comments
α 1 receptor blockers (cause smooth muscle relaxation of prostatic urethra)	• Uroselective preferred due to low risk of hypotension (e.g., alfuzosin 10 mg daily) • Nonselective (e.g., doxazosin 1–8 mg daily)	Can cause retrograde or decreased ejaculation (uroselective), orthostatic hypotension (nonselective)	Symptom improvement in 2–4 weeks Uroselective drugs are costly; nonselective agents more prone to side effects
5-α reductase inhibitors (reduce prostate size)	• Example: finasteride 5 mg daily	Erectile dysfunction, decreased libido, ejaculation disorders	Symptom improvement in several months; can be initiated with alpha blockers PSA levels will decrease on these drugs
Anticholinergics (decrease bladder contractions; second line agent)	• Example: tolterodine extended release 4 mg daily	Urinary retention, dry mouth, constipation	Used to reduce irritative symptoms Often used in combination with first-line medications

Data from Pearson R, Williams PM. Common questions about the diagnosis and management of benign prostatic hyperplasia. *Am Fam Physician*. 2014;90(11):769–774.

Prostate Cancer Screening

In May, 2012, the USPSTF recommended against prostate cancer screening with PSA. In 2017 this was under review with draft changes suggesting grade C for men at average risk ages 55 to 69 years and grade D for men 70 years and older. Screening guidelines differ and screening for prostate cancer with PSA remains an evolving and highly controversial both within and outside of the medical community. This, coupled with media attention, understandably creates confusion among patients, particular those who may have been routinely screened in the past or who may be considered at greater risk (Table 16.7). Providers should be aware of the major screening guidelines shown in Table 16.7 and promote shared-decision making.[35]

For men who are considering prostate cancer screening, it is difficult to have an adequate discussion within the confines of a comprehensive wellness visit. It may be best to provide educational materials and have the patient return to the office if screening is still desired. The ChoosingWisely campaign provides an excellent patient resource on prostate screening available here: http://www.choosingwisely.org/patient-resources/psa-test-for-prostate-cancer/.

Testosterone and Andropause

Age-related hypogonadism, sometimes labeled "andropause," is a poorly understood condition involving low serum testosterone levels in association with a constellation of symptoms including but not limited to decreased libido, fatigue or perceived muscle weakness, and ED.[36] In middle-aged and elderly men without known hypogonadism related to testicular, pituitary or hypothalamic disorders or to adverse effects of specific antiandrogen

Table 16.7 ▶ Comparison of Prostate Cancer Screening Guidelines

USPSTF: Grade C for ages 55–69, Grade D for ages 70 and older r.e. PSA screening for men at average risk—(Draft recommendation as of July, 2017)

• Men ages 55–69—Shared decision-making

American Urological Association (AUA)

• Age <40 years: recommends against PSA screening

• Age 40–54 years
  • Does not recommend routine screening for average risk
  • Higher risk (e.g., positive family history or African-American race), decisions regarding prostate cancer screening should be individualized

• Age 55–69 years
  • Weigh benefit of preventing prostate cancer mortality in one man for every 1,000 men screened over a decade against the known potential harms
  • Use shared decision-making for men who are considering PSA screening, and proceed based on men's values and preferences
  • Screening interval: routine screening interval of 2 years or more may be preferred over annual screening

• Age 70+ years or men with <10–15-year life expectancy: Not recommended

American College of Physicians (ACP)

• Age 50–69 years: inform men about limited potential benefits and substantial harms

• Harms of screening at many levels:
  • PSA screening test: anxiety, high false-positive and negative rates
  • Biopsy: infections, pain, overdiagnosis, and overtreatment
  • Treatment of prostate cancer: urinary/gastrointestinal dysfunction, sexual problems, other risks inherent to major surgery

• Base decision to screen on a man's risk for prostate cancer, his health status and life expectancy, and his preferences. Do NOT screen when it is not desired.

• Not recommended for <50 years, >69 years; or life expectancy <10–15 years

Data from AHRQ National Guidelines Clearinghouse. Guideline synthesis "screening for prostate cancer". Available at: https://www.guideline.gov/syntheses/synthesis/49682/screening-for-prostate-cancer?q=prostate±cancer±screening. Accessed March 2017.

treatments, testosterone replacement therapy (TST) for andropause remains controversial.[37,38] Patients seeking evaluation and treatment for andropause should be made aware that evidence surrounding the benefits and risks of TST are conflicting at best (Table 16.8).

There are no widely accepted definitions for low serum total testosterone; commonly used levels include <200 or <300 ng/dL.[36] Serum testosterone levels also vary throughout the day, although to a lesser degree in middle-aged and elderly men. At least two tests should be performed to confirm low levels before treatment is offered. Traditionally, tests have been done in the early morning. In patients with persistently low testosterone levels, follicle stimulating hormone and luteinizing hormone should be performed to evaluate for primary or secondary hypogonadism.[25]

Men who choose to start testosterone therapy should be appropriately monitored for complications (Table 16.8).[25] The testosterone dose should be adjusted to achieve serum levels in the mid-normal range, rather than levels above the accepted normal ranges.

Table 16.8 ▶ Potential Benefits, Risks and Contraindications for Testosterone Replacement

Potential Benefits	Risks	Contraindications
• Improved sexual desire and erectile function	• Prostate cancer	• Prostate or breast cancer
• Improved mood	• Benign prostatic hyperplasia	• Prostate nodule
• Improved physical strength and performance	• Decreased urine stream flow • Cardiovascular disease • Sleep apnea • Erythrocytosis	• Elevated PSA >4 ng/mL • PSA>3 in African American men or those with a family history of prostate cancer • Severe untreated obstructive sleep apnea • Poorly controlled congestive heart failure • Baseline hematocrit >50% • Severe lower urinary tract symptoms (IPSS score >19)

Record review confirms that Jack was screened for diabetes 2 years ago with a hemoglobin A1C of 6.3%. His last lipid panel was also obtained 2 years ago. A TSH level last year was within normal limits, and prior TSH levels have also been normal for the past decade. He underwent a colonoscopy 5 years ago; two biopsies returned as tubular adenomas, each less than 10 mm in size and he was told to repeat the test in 5 to 10 years. He has received an annual influenza vaccine this year. His other vaccinations are up to date and include a tetanus/pertussis booster 4 years ago, both PCV13 and PPSV23 within the last 3 years and the zoster vaccine 5 years ago.

Preventive Services for Medicare-Covered Men

Men age 65 years and over may choose to use Medicare for all or most of their health care coverage. Medicare covers an initial preventive health visit at the age of 65 years, and then annual wellness visits thereafter. The focus of these visits includes thorough reviews of medical and social history, ordering or planning preventive services such as screenings and immunizations, end-of-life planning and screening for cognitive and other functional decline. A wide range of preventive services are covered and generally align with USPSTF services grades A and B recommendation.[39] Patients and providers should be aware that a head-to-toe physical examination is not covered as part of an annual wellness visit.[40] Medicare provides an interactive and user-friendly website to guide patients and their physicians. https://www.cms.gov/Medicare/Prevention/PrevntionGenInfo/medicare-preventive-services/MPS-QuickReferenceChart-1.html.

Jack had previously established care and had an initial wellness visit at the age of 65 years using his Medicare coverage. He is hoping today's visit will be covered as an annual wellness visit through Medicare. You obtain vital signs, height/weight, and calculate BMI. You examine his knees and determine that his chronic knee pain is likely osteoarthritis; since it does not seem to limit his activities you advise that he remain active and continue taking acetaminophen as needed. Since his current chronic medical conditions appear well-controlled, you refill his medications without any changes to his therapy.

BOX 16.3 SAMPLE PLAN FOR INITIAL AND FOLLOW-UP VISITS FOR JACK

1. Address Jack's main concern of bilateral knee pain
2. Refill his medications
3. Discuss his questions about his testosterone level
4. Evaluate control of chronic problems
   a. Hypertension—controlled to target BP
   b. Hyperlipidemia—appears controlled but last test 2 years ago
   c. Hypothyroidism—controlled
   d. Benign prostatic hypertrophy—evaluate LUTS with AUA questionnaire
5. Screening
   a. Colon cancer (recommended for adults age 50–75)[41]: had colonoscopy 5 years ago showing small tubular adenomas. Consider repeat screening within next 5 years.
   b. Abdominal aortic aneurysm (one-time screening for men ages 65–75 who have ever smoked)[42]: offer abdominal ultrasonography
   c. Hepatitis C (one-time screening for adults born between 1945–1965)[43]: done
   d. Fall prevention—Jack is active and does not appear at risk currently[44]

On the AUA SI questionnaire he scores 2, in the mild range for LUTS. As he is not bothered by his symptoms, you discuss continued observation for worsening symptoms. You educate Jack on the indications for checking testosterone levels and on the potential risks and benefits of testosterone replacement. Since he does not have any clear symptoms of age-related hypogonadism, you recommend no testing and he agrees. You discuss the risks and benefits of screening for prostate cancer using PSA. He had a friend die of prostate cancer but Jack had previously reviewed the risks and benefits of prostate cancer testing and he has decided he does not want this.

You order a lipid panel and refer Jack for a follow-up screening colonoscopy after discussing appropriate timing since he is interested in testing now. You offer ultrasonography for aortic aneurysm screening which he declines. All other preventive items are up to date. You ask him to return in 1 year for his next wellness visit, or sooner if any problems arise (Box 16.3).

QUESTIONS

1. A 21-year-old man comes to your office to establish care. He has no particular concerns but wants testing done for "whatever I'm supposed to get." He is sexually active with multiple male partners, drinks alcohol, and smokes cigarettes. Which one of the following screening exams, tests, or behavior tools has level A United States Preventive Services Task Force evidence for someone like this patient?
   A. Screening lipid panel
   B. Tobacco use
   C. Careful cardiovascular exam
   D. Alcohol misuse
   E. Testicular exam

2. Which one of the following physical exam components is recommended for well middle-aged nonsmoking men?
   A. Screening for obesity
   B. Assessment for carotid bruits
   C. Thyroid palpation
   D. Inguinal hernia assessment
   E. Rectal examination

3. Which one of the following is considered a first-line intervention in a man with erectile dysfunction without obvious cause?
   A. Limiting alcohol
   B. Individual or couples counseling
   C. Intracavernous alprostadil
   D. Vacuum device
   E. Urology referral

4. Ronald, a 75-year-old Taiwanese man, returns to see you to discuss longstanding symptoms he has had with benign prostatic hypertrophy (BPH) and lower urinary tract symptoms. His American Urological Association BPH Symptom Score at his last visit 4 months ago was 8. At today's visit, his score is 10. He uses an alpha blocker at maximal doses without side effects and finasteride once daily. He does not have symptoms of urinary retention and a creatinine, checked as part of the management of concurrent hypertension, was normal. Which one of the following should he do now?
   A. No change in management. While his symptoms have exacerbated some he is not concerned, and there is no evidence of end-organ damage.
   B. Refer him to a urologist for further nonsurgical management.
   C. Refer him to a urologist for surgical management.
   D. Stop the alpha blockers since symptoms worsened with their use.

ANSWERS

Question 1: The correct answer is B.
(Table 16.1): The USPSTF gives an A rating to screening for tobacco use in young adult men. The section on Screening and Prevention of High-Risk Behaviors in Young Adult Men as well as the USPSTF screening tool, found at https://epss.ahrq.gov/ePSS/search.jsp speak to this.

Question 2: The correct answer is A.
Many of the recommended preventive health items in this age group are centered around prevention and/or detection of CVD. These include screening for obesity, hypertension, hyperlipidemia, diabetes, and assessing lifestyle behaviors such as substance use, dietary habits, and physical activity.

Question 3: The correct answer is B.
Table 16.3. First-line treatment for erective dysfunction includes management of chronic conditions, lifestyle modification (weight loss, exercise), smoking cessation, individual or couples counseling, and oral PDE-5 inhibitors.

Question 4: The correct answer is A.
Many men with mild symptoms due to BPH may simply choose to monitor the condition while others may desire treatment; current evidence suggests that in the absence of acute urinary obstruction or other complications, either approach is reasonable.

REFERENCES

1. Marcell AV, Klein JD, Fischer I, et al. Male adolescent use of health care services: where are the boys? *J Adolesc Health*. 2002;30(1):35–43.
2. Centers for Disease Control and Prevention (CDC)/National Center for Health Statistics(NCHS). Table 62. No usual source of health care among adults aged 18–64, by selected characteristics: United States, average annual, selected years 1993–1994 through 2013–2014. In Health, United States, 2015 – Utilization of Health Resources, Ambulatory Care Trend Tables. Available at: https://www.cdc.gov/nchs/data/hus/2015/062.pdf. Accessed January 2017.
3. U.S. Preventive Services Task Force. Final Recommendation Statement: Alcohol misuse: screening and behavioral counseling interventions in primary care. 2013. Available at: https://www.uspreventiveservicestaskforce.org/Page/Document/UpdateSummaryFinal/alcohol-misuse-screening-and-behavioral-counseling-interventions-in-primary-care. Accessed March 2017.
4. Substance Abuse and Mental Health Services Administration (SAMHSA) – Health Resources and Services Administration (HRSA) Center for Integrated Health Solutions website. Screening Tools. Available at: http://www.integration.samhsa.gov/clinical-practice/screening-tools. Accessed March 2017.
5. National Institute on Alcohol Abuse and Alcoholism (NIAAA). A Pocket Guide for Screening and Brief Intervention. 2005 edition. Available at: https://pubs.niaaa.nih.gov/publications/practitioner/PocketGuide/pocket.pdf. Accessed March 2017.
6. U.S. Preventive Services Task Force. Final Recommendation Statement: Drug use, illicit: screening. 2014. Available at: https://www.uspreventiveservicestaskforce.org/Page/Document/RecommendationStatementFinal/drug-use-illicit-screening. Accessed March 2017.
7. U.S. Preventive Services Task Force. Final Recommendation Statement: Tobacco smoking cessation in adults, including pregnant women: behavioral and pharmacotherapy interventions. 2016. Available at: https://www.uspreventiveservicestaskforce.org/Page/Document/RecommendationStatementFinal/tobacco-use-in-adults-and-pregnant-women-counseling-and-interventions1. Accessed March 2017.
8. Agency for Healthcare Research and Quality, Rockville, MD. Five major steps to intervention (The "5 A's"). 2012. Available at: http://www.ahrq.gov/professionals/clinicians-providers/guidelines-recommendations/tobacco/5steps.html. Accessed March 2017.
9. CDC, National Center for Injury Prevention and Control, Division of Unintentional Injury Prevention. Teen drivers: get the facts. 2016. Available at: https://www.cdc.gov/motorvehiclesafety/teen_drivers/teendrivers_factsheet.html. Accessed March 2017.
10. AAFP policy statement. Firearms and safety issues. Available at: http://www.aafp.org/about/policies/all/weapons-laws.html. Accessed March 2017.
11. Weinberger SE, Hoyt DB, Lawrence HC, et al. Firearm-related injury and death in the united states: a call to action from 8 health professional organizations and the American Bar Association. *Ann Intern Med*. 2015;162:513–516.
12. CDC/NCHS. Table 19. Leading causes of death and numbers of deaths, by sex, race, and Hispanic origin: United States, 1980 and 2014. In *Health, United States, 2015 – Health Status and Determinants, Mortality Trend Tables*. Available at: https://www.cdc.gov/nchs/data/hus/2015/019.pdf. Accessed January 2017.
13. U.S. Preventive Services Task Force. Final Update Summary: Chlamydia and Gonorrhea: screening. 2016. Available at: https://www.uspreventiveservicestaskforce.org/Page/Document/UpdateSummaryFinal/chlamydia-and-gonorrhea-screening?ds=1&s=gonorrhea. Accessed February 2017.
14. Ghanem KG, Tuddenham S. Screening for sexually transmitted infections. *UpToDate*. 2016. Accessed online 24 February 2017.
15. U.S. Preventive Services Task Force. Final Update Summary: Sexually Transmitted Infections: behavioral counseling. 2016. Available at: https://www.uspreventiveservicestaskforce.org/Page/Document/UpdateSummaryFinal/sexually-transmitted-infections-behavioral-counseling1. Accessed February 2017.
16. U.S. Preventive Services Task Force. Final Update Summary: High blood pressure in adults: screening. 2016. Available at: https://www.uspreventiveservicestaskforce.org/Page/Document/UpdateSummaryFinal/high-blood-pressure-in-adults-screening?ds=1&s=hypertension. Accessed April 2017.
17. U.S. Preventive Services Task Force. Final Update Summary: Obesity in adults: screening and management. 2016. Available at: https://www.uspreventiveservicestaskforce.org/Page/Document/UpdateSummaryFinal/obesity-in-adults-screening-and-management. Accessed April 2017.
18. National Cancer Institute Surveillance, Epidemiology and End Results Program. Cancer stat facts: testis cancer. Available at: https://seer.cancer.gov/statfacts/html/testis.html. Accessed April 2017.

19. U.S. Preventive Services Task Force. Final Evidence Review: Testicular cancer: screening. 2014. Available at: https://www.uspreventiveservicestaskforce.org/Page/Document/EvidenceReportFinal/testicular-cancer-screening-february-2004. Accessed February 2017.

20. U.S. Preventive Services Task Force. Final Recommendation Statement: Testicular cancer: screening. 2016. Available at: https://www.uspreventiveservicestaskforce.org/Page/Document/RecommendationStatementFinal/testicular-cancer-screening. Accessed February 2017.

21. CDC/NCHS National Health Interview Survey. Table A-11a. Age-adjusted percent distribution (with standard errors) of respondent-assessed health status among adults aged 18 and over, by selected characteristics: United States, 2014. Available at: https://ftp.cdc.gov/pub/Health_Statistics/NCHS/NHIS/SHS/2014_SHS_Table_A-11.pdf. Accessed March 2017.

22. Mauksch LB, Dugdale DC, Dodson S, et al. Relationship, communication and efficiency in the medical encounter. *Arch Intern Med.* 2008;168(13):1387–1395.

23. CDC/NCHS National Ambulatory Medical Care Survey. Table 11. Twenty leading principal reasons for office visits, by patient sex: United States, 2013. Available at: https://www.cdc.gov/nchs/data/ahcd/namcs_summary/2013_namcs_web_tables.pdf. Accessed March 2017.

24. Rew KT, Heidelbaugh JJ. Erectile dysfunction. *Am Fam Physician.* 2016;94(10):820–827.

25. Bhasin S, Cunningham GR, Hayes FJ, et al. Testosterone therapy in men with androgen deficiency syndromes: an Endocrine Society clinical practice guideline. *J Clin Endocrinol Metab.* 2010;95(6): 2536–2559.

26. U.S. Preventive Services Task Force. Final Recommendation Statement: High blood pressure in adults: screening. 2016. https://www.uspreventiveservicestaskforce.org/Page/Document/RecommendationStatementFinal/high-blood-pressure-in-adults-screening. Accessed 2 April 2017.

27. CDC Fast Stats. Men's health. http://www.cdc.gov/nchs/fastats/mens-health.htm. Accessed 8 Mar 2017.

28. U.S. Preventive Services Task Force. Final Recommendation Statement: Obesity in adults: screening and management. 2016. https://www.uspreventiveservicestaskforce.org/Page/Document/RecommendationStatementFinal/obesity-in-adults-screening-and-management. Accessed 2 April 2017.

29. U.S. Preventive Services Task Force. Final Recommendation Statement: Healthful diet and physical activity for cardiovascular disease prevention in adults with cardiovascular risk factors: behavioral counseling. 2016. Available at: https://www.uspreventiveservicestaskforce.org/Page/Document/UpdateSummaryFinal/healthy-diet-and-physical-activity-counseling-adults-with-high-risk-of-cvd. Accessed April 2017.

30. U.S. Preventive Services Task Force. Final Recommendation Statement: Statin use for the primary prevention of cardiovascular disease in adults: preventive medication. 2016. Available at: https://www.uspreventiveservicestaskforce.org/Page/Document/UpdateSummaryFinal/statin-use-in-adults-preventive-medication1. Accessed April 2, 2017.

31. CDC National Center for Injury Prevention and Control. Suicide facts at a glance 2015. Available at: https://www.cdc.gov/violenceprevention/pdf/suicide-datasheet-a.pdf. Accessed April 2, 2017.

32. Bilsker D, White J. The silent epidemic of male suicide. *BCMJ.* 2011;53(10):529–534.

33. Pearson R, Williams PM. Common questions about the diagnosis and management of benign prostatic hyperplasia. *Am Fam Physician.* 2014;90(11):769–774.

34. American Urological Association. Benign prostatic hypertrophy. https://www.auanet.org/education/benign-prostatic-hypertrophy.cfm. Accessed April 2, 2017.

35. AHRQ National Guidelines Clearinghouse. Guideline synthesis "screening for prostate cancer". https://www.guideline.gov/syntheses/synthesis/49682/screening-for-prostate-cancer?q=prostate±cancer±screening. Accessed April 2, 2017.

36. Snyder PJ. Overview of testosterone deficiency in older men. *UptoDate.* 2016. Accessed March 17, 2017.

37. Fugh-Berman A. Editorials: Should family physicians screen for testosterone deficiency in men? No: screening may be harmful, and benefits are unproven. *Am Fam Physician.* 2015;91(4):226–228.

38. Heidelbaugh JJ. Editorials: Should family physicians screen for testosterone deficiency in men? Yes: screening for testosterone deficiency is worthwhile for most older men. *Am Fam Physician.* 2015;91(4):220–221.

39. Medicare Learning Network. Medicare preventive services. Available at: https://www.cms.gov/Medicare/Prevention/PrevntionGenInfo/medicare-preventive-services/MPS-QuickReferenceChart-1.html. Accessed April 2, 2017.

40. Medicare.gov website. https://www.medicare.gov/coverage/preventive-visit-and-yearly-wellness-exams.html. Accessed March 17, 2017.

41. U.S. Preventive Services Task Force. Final Recommendation Statement: Colorectal cancer: screening. 2016. https://www.uspreventiveservicestaskforce.org/Page/Document/RecommendationStatementFinal/ colorectal-cancer-screening2. Accessed April 2, 2017.

42. U.S. Preventive Services Task Force. Final Recommendation Statement: Abdominal aortic aneurysm: screening. 2014. https://www.uspreventiveservicestaskforce.org/Page/Document/ RecommendationStatementFinal/abdominal-aortic-aneurysm-screening. Accessed April 2, 2017.

43. U.S. Preventive Services Task Force. Final Recommendation Statement: Hepatitis C: screening. 2016. Available at: https://www.uspreventiveservicestaskforce.org/Page/Document/ RecommendationStatementFinal/hepatitis-c-screening. Accessed April 2, 2017.

44. U.S. Preventive Services Task Force. Final Recommendation Statement: Falls prevention in older adults: counseling and preventive medication. 2016. Available at: https://www.uspreventiveservicestaskforce. org/Page/Document/UpdateSummaryFinal/falls-prevention-in-older-adults-counseling-and-preventive-medication. Accessed April 2, 2017.

Musculoskeletal Problems

KEY POINTS

1 ▸ Use the Ottawa ankle rules when deciding about imaging an acute ankle sprain

2 ▸ Use specific testing to help diagnose and determine treatment for shoulder injuries

3 ▸ Age, onset, and duration of symptoms can help in the diagnosis of knee pain

4 ▸ Imaging in cases of acute nonspecific back pain should be reserved for cases with red flag symptoms and signs

In this chapter on musculoskeletal problems, we will cover ankle pain, knee pain, shoulder pain, and low back pain (LBP). As you evaluate patients with these problems, it is helpful to organize your history as shown below, using the mnemonic **OPQRST** to characterize their pain. Take care to focus on occupation and hobbies, as this usually contributes to both mechanisms of injury and rehabilitation plan.

▸ **O**nset (acute vs. chronic and traumatic vs. overuse), **P**rovocation and palliation (what makes pain worse or better), **Q**uality (sharp, cramping, dull, aching), **R**adiation (to other body part), **S**everity (on pain scale 1–10), **T**iming (constant vs. intermittent) and therapies trialed (medication, ice, physical therapy)

▸ Age (different diagnoses are more or less likely depending on age)

▸ Occupation or sport

▸ Dominant hand (can help determine cause and prognosis)

▸ Previous injury

▸ Comorbidities (e.g., adhesive capsulitis is more common in diabetes; inflammatory arthritis is common with autoimmune disease)

Standard components of a joint physical exam usually include inspection, palpation, range of motion (ROM; passive and active), strength/pain with resisted motion, sensation, reflexes, and special tests.

ANKLE PAIN

Sasha is a 15-year-old girl who presents to your office with ankle pain. She has had intermittent pain since an ankle sprain 2 years ago, but the pain has gotten worse over the last month. Sasha takes ballet, jazz, and tap, and dances approximately 15 hours weekly.

Ankle pain is a common problem in the primary care office, accounting for 750,000 outpatient visits each year.[1] Ankle injuries can be acute or chronic. They can involve trauma to the bones, ligaments, and tendons but can also be degenerative, inflammatory, or infectious in nature. Most acute ankle injuries heal quite nicely. However, a subset of people who experience ankle sprains develop permanent laxity and are predisposed to further sprains and a feeling of ankle instability. It is likely that Sasha is continually reinjuring her ankle due to permanent ligament laxity.

Functional Anatomy

The ankle joint is a hinge joint with some extra features. The ankle is composed of the distal fibula, talus, and distal tibia. The mortise of the ankle joint allows dorsiflexion, plantarflexion, internal rotation, and external rotation (Fig. 17.1). The subtalar joint, formed by the calcaneus and talus, allows inversion, eversion, and internal and external rotation.

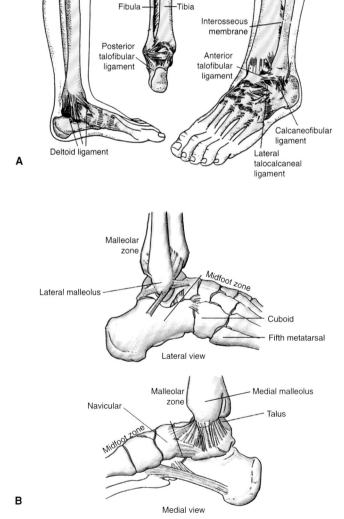

Figure 17.1 ► Anatomy of the ankle joint. **A:** Ligamentous structure; **(B)** bony structures; *(continued)*

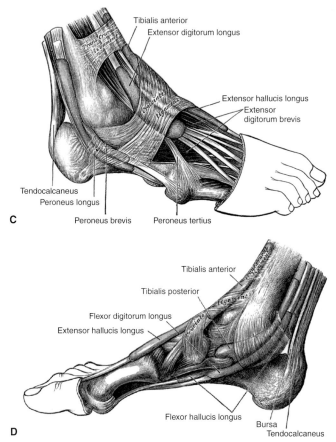

Figure 17.1 ▶ *(Continued)* **(C)** ankle tendons, lateral; and **(D)** ankle tendons, medial. (**C**, **D** from Gray H. Anatomy of the Human Body. Philadelphia, PA: Lea & Febiger; 1918; Bartleby.com, 2000. www.bartleby.com/107/)

The lateral stabilizers of the ankle are the anterior talofibular, the calcaneal fibular, and the posterior talofibular ligaments (ATFL, CLF, PTFL) plus peroneus longus and brevis tendons. The medial stabilizers are the deltoid ligament and the tibialis anterior and posterior tendons. The ankle mortise is stabilized by a number of ligaments, including the ATFL, CLF, PTFL, and peroneus longus and brevis tendons. The syndesmosis is an interosseous membrane between the tibia and fibula (for anatomy, see https://www.youtube.com/watch?v=4hCS1O2LP_c). Injury to the syndesmosis is called a high ankle sprain.

Initial Evaluation

In the initial evaluation of ankle pain, be sure to first determine whether the condition is a result of a traumatic or overuse injury. Use the mnemonic **OPQRST** and the points shown at the beginning of this chapter to help organize your history.

Components of the ankle exam are outlined in Table 17.1.

Once you have completed your history and physical examination, formulate a differential diagnosis as shown in Table 17.2. On exam, Sasha had tenderness over her ATFL and some mild laxity with anterior drawer testing.

Table 17.1 ▶ Examination of the Ankle

Inspection	Note any ecchymoses or edema. Evaluate stance and gait. Note foot supination or pronation[a]
Palpate bony structures, ligaments and tendons	Look for pain over the distal fibula/lateral malleolus; distal tibia/medial malleolus; metatarsals (with attention to base of the 5th metatarsal and navicular [Fig. 17.1B]); ligaments (Fig. 17.1A); and tendons (Fig. 17.1C,D). Other: Palpate the retrocalcaneal bursa, located directly anteriorly to the distal Achilles tendon
Range of motion (ROM)	Test active and passive dorsiflexion, plantarflexion, inversion, and eversion noting any limitation or pain
Strength	Test-resisted dorsiflexion, plantarflexion, inversion, eversion[b]
Sensation	Dermatomes for sciatic or common peroneal nerve or polyneuropathy[c]
Reflexes	Test Achilles reflex, taking note of differences in the reflex with respect to the other side. Asymmetry between sides can indicate a neurologic deficit, specifically the S1 nerve root

Special Testing[b]	Meaning of Positive Test
Anterior drawer test: Slightly plantarflex and externally rotate the ankle, grasp the calcaneus and try to slide the heel forward	Greater movement than on the contralateral side indicates injury to the ATFL ligament
Talar tilt test: Stabilize the distal lower leg. Using other hand, grasp the foot at the talus and apply varus stress	Greater laxity on affected side may indicate CFL injury
Hop test: Have the patient hop several times on one foot	Pain with an overuse injury may indicate a stress fracture
Squeeze test: Compress the gastrocnemius and soleus by squeezing the calf	Pain over the area of the syndesmosis indicates a high ankle sprain
Thompson test: With patient prone, squeeze the calf	No plantarflexion of the foot indicates Achilles rupture

[a]In flatfoot deformity, look for "too many toes sign"—looking at the foot with the patient facing away from you, all the toes will be visible laterally (see http://orthoinfo.aaos.org/topic.cfm?topic=a00166).
[b]For a good review of the special signs, see: https://www.youtube.com/watch?v=QiSm8rz2cmo.
[c]For dermatomes, see http://www.backpain-guide.com/Chapter_Fig_folders/Ch06_Path_Folder/4Radiculopathy.html.
ATFL, anterior talofibular ligament; CLF, calcaneal fibular ligament; PTFL, posterior talofibular ligament.

When to Order Imaging

To help determine whether imaging is needed, use the **Ottawa ankle rules**.[2] Order x-rays of the ankle or foot (AP, lateral, and mortise view) if the patient has **pain in the malleolar area** OR **midfoot** AND **one of the following**:

▶ Bony tenderness at the posterior edge or tip of lateral or medial malleolus
▶ Bony tenderness over the navicular

Table 17.2 ▶ Differential Diagnosis of Ankle Pain

Diagnosis Suggested[a]	Key History	Key Physical Exam Findings
Traumatic Injury		
Lateral ankle sprain	Inversion mechanism, lateral ankle pain, history of ankle sprain	ATFL (most common), CLF, or PTFL tenderness. Positive (+) anterior drawer test
Fifth metatarsal fracture	Inversion injury, direct force to lateral midfoot, lateral foot pain	Tenderness over 5th metatarsal
Medial ankle sprain	Eversion injury, medial ankle pain, history of ankle sprain	Tenderness over deltoid ligament, + talar tilt test
Distal fibular/lateral malleolar fracture	Inversion injury, direct force to lateral ankle	Tenderness over fibula/lateral malleolus, distortion of lateral malleolus
Medial malleolar fracture	Eversion injury, direct force to medial ankle	Tenderness over tibia/medial malleolus, distortion of medial malleolus
Syndesmosis injury/ high ankle sprain	External rotation mechanism	Anterolateral ankle pain, syndesmosis tenderness, + squeeze test
Overuse		
Achilles tendonitis	Running or high impact maneuvers	Pain over Achilles tendon or calcaneus, thickening of the tendon
Posterior tibial tendonitis	Running or high impact maneuvers	Tenderness over posterior tibial tendon, pain with resisted inversion and plantarflexion
Peroneal tendonitis	Running, high impact maneuvers or dancing, especially ballet	Tenderness over peroneal tendons, pain with resisted eversion and plantarflexion
Tibial or fibular stress fracture	Running	Pinpoint tenderness over bone. + Hop test. Axial loading produces pain
Chronic ankle instability	Chronic ankle pain after multiple or poorly rehabilitated ankle sprain(s)	Nonspecific pain, can be localized to lateral ligaments. + anterior drawer test

[a]Listed in order of most common to least common.

▶ Bony tenderness at the base of the 5th metatarsal

▶ Inability to bear weight (defined as four steps) during your evaluation

A mortise view helps evaluate the integrity of the syndesmosis and the deltoid ligament. A widened space between the talus and the medial malleolus may indicate an injury to these ligaments. These would not apply to Sasha as she does not have an acute injury.

You discuss with Sasha and her father who is here with her today that she had chronic instability of the ankle due to her previous ankle sprain.

Ankle Injury Management

▶ Ankle sprain

- SOR C: Acetaminophen or nonsteroidal anti-inflammatory drugs (NSAIDs) for pain[3]; short-term bracing or taping; physical therapy to increase ankle ROM, to strengthen stabilizing muscles, and to improve balance.[4]

▶ Syndesmosis injury: Refer to orthopedics (SOR C).

▶ Tendonitis (SOR C):

- Physical therapy to strengthen the tendons and muscles of the ankle, steroid injection to decrease inflammation, consider platelet-rich plasma injection or percutaneous tenotomy to promote healing.[5]

▶ Chronic ankle instability, as in Sasha's case (SOR C):

- Physical therapy to strengthen the tendons and muscles of the ankle.[6]
- Tape or brace for stability.
- Refer refractory cases for surgical consultation.[7]

Management of fractures is presented in Table 17.3.

Table 17.3 ▶ Management of Ankle Fractures

Fracture	Initial Management	Follow-up or if Complicated
Stress fracture: Nondisplaced/high risk[a]	Non–weight bearing and immobilization for 6–8 weeks	Referral to orthopedics for surgical evaluation
Stress fracture: Nondisplaced/low risk	Walking boot for 2–8 weeks, activity modification	MRI and/or referral if no improvement after 8 weeks
Fifth metatarsal: Avulsion	If nondisplaced: Short leg walking boot for 2 weeks; activity as tolerated	If displaced, refer for surgical consultation
Fifth metatarsal: Diaphysis stress fracture or metaphyseal–diaphyseal junction	Refer to orthopedics for surgical consultation	
Distal fibula: Isolated, nondisplaced	Ice and compression for swelling. Short leg cast or boot for 4–8 weeks	X-ray every 2 weeks until callous formation to assess displacement and healing; consider orthopedics referral
Distal fibula: Displaced fracture, bimalleolar fracture, or widened mortise	Refer to orthopedics for surgical consultation	

[a]High risk for nonunion includes navicular, 5th metatarsal, medial malleolus.
ND, nondisplaced.
Data from Patel DS, Roth M, Kapil N. Stress fractures: diagnosis, treatment and prevention. *Am Fam Physician*. 2011;83(1):39–46; Hatch RL, Alsobrook JA, Clugston JR. Diagnosis and management of metatarsal fractures. *Am Fam Physician*. 2007;76(6):817–826; Herscovici D, Scaduto JM, Infante A. Conservative treatment of isolated fractures of the medial malleolus. *J Bone Joint Surg*. 2007;89(1):89–99.

Sasha was referred to physical therapy. There, she worked on ankle mobility and strengthening. After therapy, she slowly weaned out of her brace. At her follow-up appointment, she reported being back to dance and had full resolution of her ankle pain. She was instructed to continue the daily exercise program that she learned in therapy.

KNEE PAIN

Jose is a 45-year-old man with lateral knee pain which started 2 months ago when training for a half marathon. He is running 3 to 8 miles per day, 5 days per week. He denies any swelling or trauma. Denies any catching but states when standing up sometimes he feels like it is locking. He has worked in construction daily for the last 20 years and reports difficulty going up and down stairs due to the pain most days.

Knee pain accounts for 2 million visits to family physicians annually.[1] The incidence of osteoarthritis is 240 cases per 100,000-person years and is one of the leading causes of disability in the United States. Women are two to eight times as likely to sustain an ACL injury as men.

Risk factors for knee pain include obesity; malalignment; poor flexibility; poor training equipment or poor technique; sudden increase in training intensity; and activities involving cutting, jumping, pivoting, and sudden deceleration.

Functional Anatomy

The knee is a hinge joint that allows forward translation, internal rotation of the knee during flexion, and posterior translation and external rotation during extension. The bony articulations that make the knee joint consist of femur, tibia, fibula, and patella. The stabilizers of the knee are anterior cruciate ligament (ACL), posterior cruciate ligament (PCL), medial collateral ligament (MCL), lateral collateral ligament (LCL), menisci, and joint capsule. Secondary stabilizers are made up of the iliotibial band; quadriceps, hamstrings, and popliteus muscles (Fig. 17.2).

The ACL prevents anterior movement. PCL resists posterior movement. MCL stabilizes during lateral stress and the LCL stabilizes during medial stress. As Jose did not report

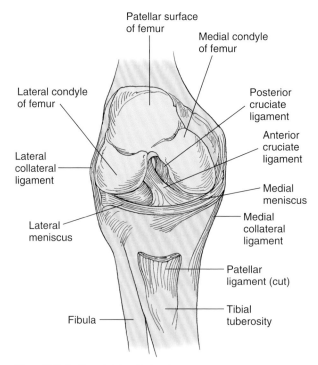

Figure 17.2 ▶ Knee joint, anterior view.

an injury and does not experience instability, it is unlikely that he has a torn ligament. Menisci are shock absorbers. The popliteus has multiple jobs including stopping the lateral meniscus from becoming stuck between the tibia and femur during flexion and helps lock the knee in extension and unlock during start of flexion. Locking is often reported in a meniscus injury when a torn piece of cartilage catches in the knee joint.

Initial Evaluation

The approach to knee pain can be broken down based on chronicity of pain with an under-standing of anatomy and mechanism of injury. Use the mnemonic **OPQRST** and the points shown at the beginning of this chapter to help organize your history. The patient may have heard an audible "pop" when the knee pain was felt. Table 17.4 lists components of the knee examination and, based on the examination and special tests (Table 17.5), a differen-tial diagnosis of knee pain can be formulated (Table 17.6). As injury to ligaments and the meniscus are common, you would include Lachman's, McMurray's, and posterior drawer tests during your examination of Jose.

Table 17.4 ▶ Examination of Painful Knee

Inspection	Erythema, effusion (milk fluid into suprapatellar pouch and test for fluid wave)
Palpation	Medial and lateral joint lines and patellar facets; insertions of MCL, LCL, pes anserine bursa, biceps femoris, semimembranosus, iliotibial band
Range of motion (ROM)	Flexion (normal 135 degrees), extension (normal −5 to −10), straight leg raising (hamstring)
Strength	Flexion/extension of knee, hip flexion, hip extension, abduction, adduction
Sensation	Follow dermatome
Reflexes	Patellar

LCL, lateral collateral ligament; MCL, medial collateral ligament.

Jose has no swelling, effusions, or deformities on exam. He has pain at the lateral joint line. He has decreased ROM to straight leg raise to 60 degrees and has pain with knee flexion past 90 degrees but full ROM to 135 degrees. Negative Lachman's, varus and valgus stress testing. He has pain and clicking with flexion and external rotation while rotating the foot (positive McMurray test).

When to Order Imaging

Use the Ottawa knee rules to help determine when to order plain films of the knee:[8] Order if one or more of the following applies:

▶ Age 55 years or older

▶ Tenderness at the head of the fibula

▶ Isolated patellar tenderness

▶ Inability to flex to 90 degrees

▶ Inability to bear weight both immediately and in the emergency department (four weight transfers onto each leg, regardless of limping)

Table 17.5 ▶ Specialized Tests in the Evaluation of a Painful Knee[a]

Specialized Tests (Focus of Test)	Method	Meaning of Positive Test
Lachman's (ACL)	Flex leg to 30 degrees, stabilize femur and shift tibia anteriorly	No end point indicates an ACL tear
McMurray's (meniscus)	With fingers on joint line, flex and internally rotate while bringing knee into extension; then repeat while externally rotating	Clicking of lateral meniscus and/or pain (with internal rotation) or clicking of medial meniscus and/or pain (with external rotation)
Ober test (ITB)	Side-lying patient with unaffected leg under bent at 90 degrees. Examiner stabilizes pelvis and abducts and extends the affected leg. While keeping abduction, attempt to lower knee into adduction	Tenderness or tightness in ITB will cause leg to remain in abducted position OR pain in lateral knee
Patellar compression test (OA, PFS)	With leg extended, apply force to superior aspect of patella inferiorly and distally. Ask patient to contract quadriceps muscle	Pain with maneuver indicates patellofemoral pain. Age <25 years: PFS. Age >25 years: Chondromalacia of patella or OA
Posterior drawer (PCL)	Flex knees to 90 degrees, sit on foot and translate tibia posterior	No end point indicates a PCL tear
Posterior sag test	While supine, flex hip and knee to 90 degrees, supporting calf	Posterior sag of the tibia caused by gravitational pull indicates PCL deficiency
Varus (LCL)	With leg flexed to 30 degrees, apply varus stress	Joint opens more if laxity. If laxity persists with leg extended to 0 degrees, this indicates a full tear of the LCL
Valgus (MCL)	With leg flexed to 30 degrees, apply valgus stress	Joint opens more if laxity. Full tear, laxity persists with leg extended to 0 degrees

[a]For an excellent overview of the knee exam, see the series "Dr. Mark Hutchinson's knee exam" on YouTube.
ACL, anterior cruciate ligament; LCL, lateral collateral ligament; MCL, medial collateral ligament; OA, osteoarthritis; PCL, posterior cruciate ligament; PFS, patellofemoral syndrome.

Order an MRI:

▶ If acute injury with effusion, laxity on examination

▶ If no improvement in pain or ROM after 6 to 8 weeks of physical therapy

Jose also does not have an acute injury, so these rules would not apply.

Knee Pain Management

In the acute phase of most knee injuries, rest, ice, compression, and elevation (RICE) are the mainstays of treatment.

▶ Posterior cruciate ligament tear (SOR C): Acute: RICE

▶ Medial collateral ligament tear (SOR C):

- Acute: RICE; weight bearing as tolerated, early ROM and strength; hinge bracing to decrease valgus deformity
- Partial tears can be treated nonoperatively.[9]

Table 17.6 ▶ Differential Diagnosis, Mechanism of Injury, and Key Physical Exam Findings in Knee Pain

Diagnosis	Mechanism of Injury	Key Physical Exam Findings
Traumatic		
ACL tear	Hyperextension, deceleration, cutting	Effusion (bloody aspiration), positive (+) Lachman's, + anterior drawer test
PCL tear	Hyperextension or falling on to flexed knee	+ Posterior drawer test +/– Posterior sag test
MCL tear	Lateral force	+ Valgus stress test[a]
LCL tear	Medial force	+ Varus stress test[a]
Meniscus tear	Twisting on planted foot	+/– Effusion, + McMurray test, joint line tenderness
Overuse		
PFS	Sudden increase in activity, pain with prolonged sitting	+ Patellar compression, age <25 years
Chondromalacia of patella	Sudden increase in activity, pain with prolonged sitting	+ Patellar compression, age >25 years
OA	Pain with going up and down stairs or weight bearing, stiffness improves with activity. May have a feeling of instability and functional limitations	+/– Effusion, +/– joint line tenderness. + patellar compression if patellofemoral joint OA. Age >45 years
ITB	Sudden increase in activity; pain running, biking, climbing hills, or at heel strike during gait	+ Ober testing. Pain over greater trochanter and lateral femoral condyle

[a]Grade I: <5-mm open but solid end point, grade II: 5- to 8-mm open but solid end point, grade III: 8- to 11-mm open and no or soft end point, and grade IV: >11-mm open and no or soft end point.
ACL, anterior cruciate ligament; ITB, iliotibial band; LCL, lateral collateral ligament; MCL, medial collateral ligament; OA, osteoarthritis; PCL, posterior cruciate ligament; PFS, patellofemoral syndrome.

▶ Lateral collateral ligament tear (SOR C):
- Acute: RICE; weight bearing as tolerated.
- Return to work, play. Grade 1 average 4 weeks, grade 2 average 10 weeks, and grade 3 average 10 to 14 weeks.

▶ Anterior cruciate ligament tear (SOR C): Acute: RICE
- Nonoperative: SOR C: More sedentary lifestyles; modify sports to swimming, running, and cycling.
- Operative: Young adults 18 to 35 years with ACL tear (moderate recommendation from AAOS; SOR B); return to sports at 6 months following reconstruction

▶ Mensicus tear, as in Jose's case (SOR C):
- Conservative treatment: Ice; NSAIDs; physical therapy to reduce pain, swelling, and improve ROM and strength. Conservative management appears to be as effective as arthroscopic partial meniscectomy for improving symptoms and function at 12 to 24 months in patients with degenerative meniscal tears.[10]
  - Used for degenerative tears, nondisplaced/nonsymptomatic tears, root tears in poor candidates (multiple comorbidities, advanced OA)

- Surgical treatment
  - Repair—reducible in red–red zone (vascular periphery) age <60 years or red–white zone, age <40 years
  - Meniscectomy—white–white zone (vascular central portion)
  - Repair associated with better long-term activity levels than meniscectomy (SOR B)
▸ Patellofemoral pain syndrome/chondromalacia patella

- Ice, compression, NSAIDs in acute painful stage
- Six weeks of physical therapy focusing on medial quadriceps, hip, core strength, and increased proprioception/functional training.[11] (SOR B)
- Patellar taping, foot orthoses may be used an adjunct to help immediately reduce pain.[12] (SOR B)
- Surgery (rare); if not improving, look for alternative diagnosis. Does not improve pain at 5 years.[13] (SOR B)

▸ OA

- Strength/resistance training reduces pain and improves physical function.[14] (SOR B)
  - Aerobic exercise and aquatic versus land based are equally effective in improving pain and function.[15] (SOR A)
- NSAIDs may be less effective but have fewer side effects.[16] (SOR B)
- If not improving, may benefit from intra-articular corticosteroids.[17] (SOR C)
- Viscosupplementation has conflicting evidences on efficacy; used if no effect with exercise or corticosteroid injection (SOR C).
- Surgery for patients with continued pain with treatment and x-rays showing OA, if conservative measures fail.

▸ ITB

- Initially avoid repetitive knee flexion. Physical therapy for foam rolling and breakup of soft tissue adhesions; strengthen hip abductor (gluteus medius), and core stabilize pelvis. Neuromuscular gait retraining.
- Use NSAID and physical therapy during acute phase.[18] (SOR C)
- Corticosteroid injection to decrease pain during running in first 2 weeks after treatment.[19] (SOR C)
- Surgical intervention (SOR C)

> Jose was diagnosed with a lateral meniscus tear. He iced his knee and took a week off from running after a steroid injection. He started formal physical therapy and increased his hip and core strength. He gradually returned to running without pain.

SHOULDER PAIN

> You are seeing Kim, a 50-year-old female postal worker, who has delivered packages over the past 20 years. She comes in for worsening anterior-lateral shoulder pain exacerbated by lifting packages above her head. She denies any acute injury or trauma. She states that the pain has worsened and now she can't sleep at night. Ice makes it better, and she is able to complete her job while taking ibuprofen (Motrin).

Shoulder pain has a yearly incidence of 15 episodes per 1,000 patients seen in primary care.[20] The differential diagnosis in the primary care setting can be narrowed to the four most common reasons for pain: rotator cuff disorder (tendinopathy, partial tear, and complete tear), adhesive capsulitis, osteoarthritis (glenohumeral and acromioclavicular), and shoulder instability (subluxation, dislocation).

Functional Anatomy

It is important for diagnosis to understand shoulder anatomy and its four articulations: sternoclavicular, acromioclavicular, glenohumeral, and scapulothoracic joints. Shoulder stability is maintained by static and dynamic stabilizers. The static stabilizers are the body support, joint capsule, glenohumeral ligaments, and glenoid labrum. The dynamic stabilizers are the rotator cuff muscles (supraspinatus, infraspinatus, teres minor, and subscapularis) and the long head of biceps tendon (Fig. 17.3) (see also https://www.youtube.com/watch?v=D3GVKjeY1FM).

After obtaining the initial history using the OPQRST (call out box at the beginning of the chapter), complete a physical exam paying attention to deficits in active and passive ROM and strength. Specialized tests can also help you make the diagnosis (Table 17.7).

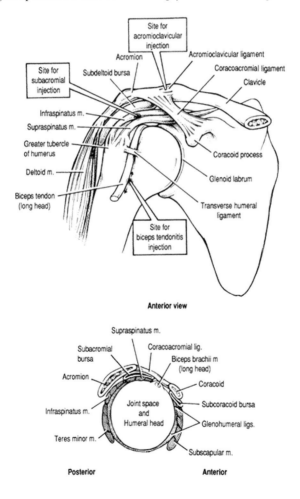

Figure 17.3 ▶ Anatomy of the shoulder joint.

Table 17.7 ▶ Examination of the Shoulder

Inspection	Symmetry, effusions
Palpation	Sternoclavicular joint, clavicle, AC joint, biceps tendon, subacromial bursa. Assessing for pain.
Range of motion (ROM)	Passive and active. Forward flexion (180 degrees), abduction (180 degrees), adduction, internal and external rotation; pain between 60–120 degrees is a painful arc associated with rotator cuff
Strength	Forward flexion, abduction (supraspinatus), internal rotation (subscapularis), external rotation (infraspinatus, teres minor)
Sensation	Dermatomes looking for brachial plexus injuries or cervical radiculopathy[a]
Reflexes	Biceps, triceps, brachioradialis; absence indicates injury at brachial plexus or cervical radiculopathy

Special Testing[b]	Meaning of Positive Test
Apprehension test (anterior stability): Patient supine and relaxed. Arm brought to 90 degrees with elbow flexed to 90 degrees. Apply gentle external rotation	Positive if the patient becomes apprehensive indicating glenohumeral instability
Drop arm (rotator cuff): Passively abduct arm to 160 degrees, then ask patient to lower arm	Arm drops uncontrolled indicates large rotator cuff tear
Empty can testing (supraspinatus): Patient abducts to 90 degrees, then forward flexes to 30 degrees. Pronate hands like emptying a can. Examiner applies downward force that patient resists	Pain or weakness indicates supraspinatus pathology (either tendonitis or tear)
Hawkins (rotator cuff): Passively forward flex arm to 90 degrees with elbow flexed to 90 degrees, then passively internally rotate arm to end point (~90)	Pain indicates impingement of the rotator cuff, usually the supraspinatus tendon.
Lift off (subscapularis): Patient places dorsum of hand against low back while sitting and manually lifts hand away while examiner resists	Pain or weakness indicates subscapularis pathology (either tendonitis or tear)
Neer's (rotator cuff): Internally rotate the patient's arm and forcefully move arm through forward flexion	Pain in anterior-lateral aspect of shoulder indicates impingement of the rotator cuff, usually the supraspinatus tendon
O'Brien's (superior labrum): Passively flex to 90 degrees, then move to 10 degrees of adduction. Patient points thumb down. Examiner applies downward force and patient resists. Repeat with thumb up	Pain only while thumb down described as "deep" indicates labral lesion. If pain localized to AC joint, test is positive for AC pathology (sprain, OA)
Sulcus (multidirectional instability): Patients arm at side, examiner exerts force inferiorly by pulling arm down	Positive if sulcus or indentation is seen indicating instability

[a]For dermatomes: http://www.backpain-guide.com/Chapter_Fig_folders/Ch06_Path_Folder/4Radiculopathy.html
[b]See https://www.youtube.com/watch?v=r7xyq_I_Kcw. Accessed November 2016.

Table 17.8 ▶ Differential Diagnosis, Mechanism of Injury, and Key Physical Exam Findings in Shoulder Pain

Diagnosis Suggested	Mechanism	Key Physical Exam Findings
Traumatic		
Shoulder dislocation	Arm in abducted and externally rotated position. Feeling of pop or shift	Positive (+) Apprehension test, +/– sulcus (if multidirectional instability)
AC joint sprain	Fall onto abducted internally rotated arm	+ Cross-body adduction
Rotator cuff full-thickness tear	Grabbing onto something while falling	+ Drop arm test, + Hawkins, + Neer's, weakness with external rotation and empty can test, age >60 years
Overuse		
Rotator cuff disorders (tendinopathy, partial tears)	Repetitive overhead movements. Worse at night. Dull achy pain	Pain localized to deltoid. Pain when testing strength of rotator cuff (empty can; internal, external rotation). + Hawkins, + Neer's, age >40 years
Adhesive capsulitis	Pain with progressive loss of active and passive ROM. Associated with diabetes, female	Age 40–60 years. Pain and loss of ROM to passive and active motion
AC joint arthritis	Repetitive overhead lifting or heavy weight training. Pain at superior aspect of shoulder	Tenderness to palpation of AC joint. + cross-body adduction, + O'Brien test with pain localized to AC joint
Glenohumeral joint arthritis	History of fall/trauma. Deep diffuse pain	Loss of passive ROM. Decreased external rotation and abduction

AC, acromioclavicular; ROM, range of motion.

Following completion of your examination and special tests, a differential diagnosis of shoulder pain can be formulated as shown in Table 17.8. Based on Kim's history, you are suspecting an overuse injury, likely a rotator cuff tendinosis.

Figure 17.4 shows an algorithm for a patient presenting with acute shoulder pain, including when to order early advanced imaging. Figure 17.5 presents similar information for a patient with chronic shoulder pain.

On exam, Kim has no atrophy or scapular winging. There is tenderness to palpation over the greater tuberosity. She denies tenderness at the biceps tendon. She has decreased active compared to passive ROM due to pain. There is weakness to empty can testing (supraspinatus) but a negative drop arm test (no large rotator cuff tear). She has normal (5/5) strength to internal and external rotation. She has a positive Neer's, positive Hawkins tests (supraspinatus impingement), and negative O'Brien test (no labral or AC lesion).

Management of Shoulder Pain

▶ Anterior shoulder dislocation

- Reduction
    - Kocher external rotation technique: Flex patient's elbow to 90 degrees and externally rotate to 70 to 80 degrees. Slide patients elbow to midline chest and rotate

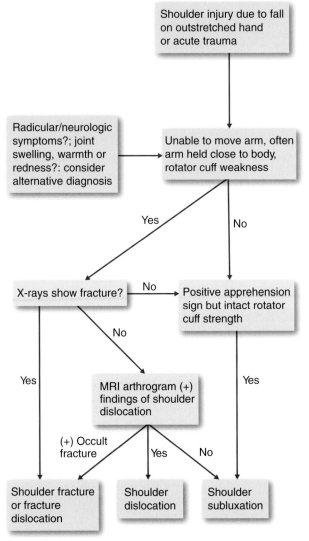

Figure 17.4 ▸ Approach to a patient with acute shoulder pain.

the elbow internally across the chest so palm touches opposite shoulder
(see: https://www.youtube.com/watch?v=2wiIlT6_YLM).

- Upright technique: Patient sitting, apply pressure to scapula moving it medially
  and then apply downward traction by holding the patient's flexed elbow in your
  arm and pushing down at the elbow, holding the wrist in place (see: https://www.
  youtube.com/watch?v=MkdCGV_MOCM).
- Immobilization with sling <1 week is as effective as >3 weeks.[21] (SOR C) Avoid
  excessive immobilization, as elbow will lose ROM. Patient should perform ROM and
  strengthening exercises.
- Surgical repair if >2 dislocations and age <25 years or associated fracture or
  instability.

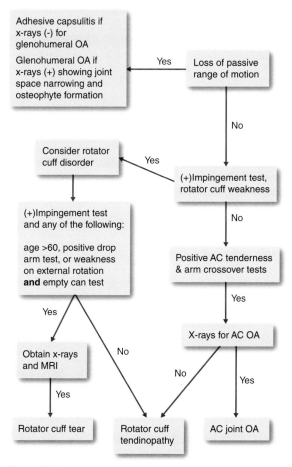

Figure 17.5 ▶ Approach to a patient with chronic shoulder pain.

▶ Posterior shoulder dislocation

- Posterior shoulder flattening anteriorly with prominent coracoid process and unable to externally rotate. Commonly associated with humeral fractures at neck and tuberosity and requires surgical treatment.

Information on management of sprains and tears is presented in Table 17.9. As therapy may differ based on whether Kim has an associated full-thickness rotator cuff tear, imaging is needed. Tendinosis generally improves with temporary avoidance of activities that worsen pain and physical therapy; in Kim's case, because her sleep is affected, she will need something for pain.

X-rays of Kim's shoulder are normal. Given her tenderness to palpation of the subacromial bursa and nighttime pain, you give her a steroid injection and refer her for physical therapy. Over the next month, she increases her periscapular strength and rotator cuff strength and her pain improves.

Table 17.9 ▶ Management of Shoulder Sprains, Tears, Arthritis, and Adhesive Capsulitis

Injury	Management[a]
AC Sprain	
Normal x-ray or lateral end of clavicle slightly elevated (grade I or II)	Sling 1–2 weeks, ice, NSAIDs; ROM and strength exercise after immobilization for 3–7 days
Twenty-five percent increase in coracoclavicular distance (III)	Controversial, but nonoperative trend; sling 2–4 weeks, ice, NSAIDs, ROM, and strength exercises
Posterior displaced clavicle, >100% clavicle to acromion distance or distal clavicle, subacromial, or subcoracoid (IV–VI)	Surgical: Primary repair versus augmentation versus ligament reconstruction
Rotator Cuff	
Partial-thickness tears	Ice, PT; single subacromial injection of steroid and lidocaine may be beneficial[22]; subacromial hyaluronate injection can help with symptoms in rotator cuff partial-thickness tears[23]
Full-thickness rotator cuff tear	Single intra-articular injection may reduce pain for up to 3 months,[24] surgery may be more effective than PT at 1 year with full-thickness tears >1–3 cm[25]
Tendonitis	Rest from activities that worsen it, perform activities at shoulder level, ice 2–3 times daily for 24–48 hours; topical (SOR A) or oral (SOR B) NSAID; progressive resistance training program/exercise (SOR B); subacromial injection may help for up to 12 weeks if not improving (SOR B)
Arthritis	
AC joint	Activity modification, ice, PT exercises to improve scapular retraction; AC joint injection with corticosteroid works for short-term relief for 6–12 months. Surgical: Distal clavicle resection
Glenohumeral joint	Activity modification (avoid excessive ROM), joint rest, intermittent ice, PT and strength training; intra-articular joint injection Surgical: Total shoulder arthroplasty
Adhesive Capsulitis	
Conservative: NSAIDs for pain, progressive ROM exercises; shoulder countertraction to physiotherapy improves shoulder function and pain (SOR A); single intraarticular injection may speed recovery (SOR B)	
Surgical: Manipulation under anesthesia if continued disability after 6 months (not more effective than home exercises, SOR B)	

[a]SOR C unless otherwise specified.

LOWER BACK PAIN

Sam is a 30-year-old man who presents with lower back pain. The onset of pain was gradual and began approximately 1 year ago. Location is in the central and left side of the lower back. He does not have any leg symptoms. Sam works at a desk job. He plays rugby on a club team.

LBP is extremely common with a population prevalence of 60% to 70%.[26] It is one of the top reasons for a visit to the family physician. LBP can be classified as acute or chronic (>3 months). Sam's pain has become chronic.

The differential diagnosis for both acute and chronic back pain is long. Mechanical back pain, including muscular dysfunction, degenerative disease, and disk disease, accounts for 97% of back pain diagnoses. Among adolescents, spondylolysis is a common cause of mechanical back pain. Despite a thorough evaluation, a significant percentage of mechanical LBP is idiopathic.

Usually, it is appropriate to be conservative in both evaluation and treatment of LBP. In general, LBP has a favorable prognosis with 30% of patients getting better in 1 week and 60% better by 6 to 7 weeks.[27] However, the condition can be relapsing and remitting, and 24% to 33% can have another episode of back pain within 6 months.[28]

Functional Anatomy

The spine is made up of vertebral bodies that articulate with each other via posterior facet joints and intervertebral disks. The vertebral column and ligaments house and protect the spinal cord (Fig. 17.6A). At each level of the cord, nerves exit the column via the neural foramina (Fig. 17.6B). Lateral to the spine are the paraspinal muscles, which are often the culprit of back pain.

Initial Evaluation

In the initial evaluation of back pain, be sure to take a thorough history using the **OPQRST** and additional questions detailed in the call box at the beginning of this chapter. Recognize that the majority of cases of back pain are not due to a serious underlying condition and are self-limited in nature, so take a conservative approach in the diagnostic strategy. Be sure to look for red flags and reasons to accelerate plain films and advanced imaging. Acknowledge that many cases of back pain are multifactorial and it may be impossible to pinpoint a diagnosis.

 Clues or "red flags" for early or emergent imaging in patients with LBP

▶ Urinary retention, overflow incontinence, fecal incontinence or decreased anal sphincter tone, saddle anesthesia, bilateral lower leg weakness or numbness, progressive neurologic deficit, major motor or sensory deficit (cauda equina syndrome)

▶ History of cancer, weight loss, night pain (cancer)

▶ History of prolonged corticosteroid use or significant trauma (fracture)

▶ Fever, history of intravenous drug abuse, recent or current bacterial infection, rest pain, immunocompromised (infection)

Table 17.10 lists components of the back exam and two special tests that help to establish a diagnosis. The neurologic exam is particularly important in localizing the level of a disk herniation (Table 17.11). Using your clinical evaluation, a differential diagnosis of LBP can be formulated as shown in Table 17.12.

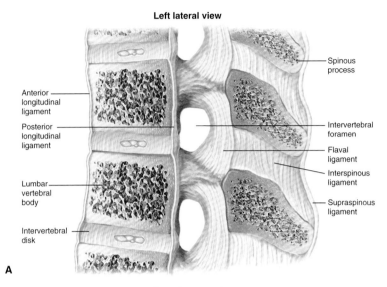

Left lateral view

Spinous process
Anterior longitudinal ligament
Posterior longitudinal ligament
Intervertebral foramen
Flaval ligament
Interspinous ligament
Lumbar vertebral body
Supraspinous ligament
Intervertebral disk

A

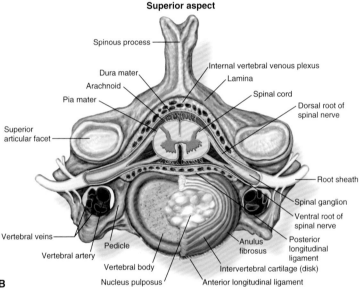

Superior aspect

Spinous process
Internal vertebral venous plexus
Dura mater
Lamina
Arachnoid
Pia mater
Spinal cord
Dorsal root of spinal nerve
Superior articular facet
Root sheath
Spinal ganglion
Ventral root of spinal nerve
Vertebral veins
Anulus fibrosus
Posterior longitudinal ligament
Pedicle
Vertebral artery
Intervertebral cartilage (disk)
Vertebral body
Nucleus pulposus
Anterior longitudinal ligament

B

Figure 17.6 ▶ **A:** Lateral view of spine ligaments. **B:** Cross-section, lumbar intervertebral disk unit.

Non-Spine Diagnoses to Consider

It is important to consider other causes of back pain, particularly if the history or physical exam findings are suggestive of these diagnoses:

▶ Pelvic
  • Nephrolithiasis: History of stones, flank pain, hematuria
  • Pyelonephritis: Fever, flank pain, pyuria
  • Pelvic inflammatory disease: History of sexually transmitted infection, purulent vaginal discharge, cervical motion tenderness

Table 17.10 ▶ Examination of the Back

Inspection	Evaluate posture and gait. Compare hip height to assess for asymmetry. Mild asymmetry is normal and common. However, a discrepancy in hip height could indicate a leg length discrepancy, lumbar spasm, or scoliosis
Palpation	Palpate spinous and transverse processes looking for pain. Palpate SI joints bilaterally looking for pain. Palpate paraspinal muscles to feel for increased tone or spasm. Palpate the piriformis in the buttock to evaluate for tenderness
Range of motion	Test forward flexion, extension, side-to-side flexion, and rotation to assess limited movement. Perform a hip exam to assess for hip ROM as well, as often back pain is either referred from the hip or caused by a primary hip issue
Strength	Test-resisted hip extension, knee extension and flexion, ankle dorsiflexion and plantarflexion, and great toe dorsiflexion to assess nerve function (see Table 17.11)
Sensation	Evaluate each dermatome[a] (see Table 17.11)
Reflexes	Test patellar and Achilles reflexes, noting asymmetry (see Table 17.11)
Special Testing[b]	**Meaning of Positive Test**
Straight leg raise: With patient supine, passively flex the patient's hip with knee in extension	Radicular pain reproduced that extend past the knee (caution in differentiating radicular symptoms from tight hamstrings)
Stork test (single-leg hyperextension test): Patients stands on one leg and extends backward	Pain at affected vertebral level

[a]For dermatomes: http://www.backpain-guide.com/Chapter_Fig_folders/Ch06_Path_Folder/4Radiculopathy.html
[b]See https://www.youtube.com/watch?v=4ik29RwqA3s; https://www.youtube.com/watch?v=9cb3iLlmTEA

▶ Gastrointestinal

- Pancreatitis: Epigastric pain radiating to the back, anorexia, fever, nausea
- Cholecystitis: RUQ abdominal pain, nausea, anorexia, fever, history of biliary colic
- Peptic ulcer: Colicky epigastric pain correlating with meals, bloating

▶ Shingles (*Herpes zoster*): Pain or rash confined to one dermatome

▶ Aortic aneurysm: "Tearing" pain in the upper back

Figure 17.7 presents a guide to the management of patients with LBP.

Table 17.11 ▶ Neurologic findings on Back Physical Exam

Level of Disk Herniation	Nerve Root Affected	Sensory Loss	Motor Weakness	Exam Maneuver	Reflex Affected
L3–L4 disk	L4	Medial foot	Knee extension	Squat and rise	Patellar
L4–L5 disk	L5	Dorsal foot	Dorsiflexion ankle/great toe	Heel walking	None
L5–S1	S1	Lateral foot	Plantarflexion ankle/toes	Walking on toes	Achilles

Table 17.12 ▶ Differential Diagnosis of Low Back Pain Using History and Physical Exam

Diagnosis Suggested[a]	Key History	Key Physical Exam Findings
Mechanical		
Spondylolysis (defect or fracture of the pars interarticularis, a section of the vertebral bone)	Adolescent, male gender, athletes involved in sports with repetitive flexion, extension, rotation. Pain with lumbar extension	Tenderness to deep palpation over affected area/spinous process. Single-leg hyperextension test causes pain on the weight-bearing side
Spondylolisthesis (forward displacement of a vertebral bone in relation to adjacent vertebra)	Adolescent or older adult (degenerative). Pain with lumbar extension. May experience radicular symptoms or rest pain	Tenderness to deep palpation of affected vertebrae. Step-off (an out-of-line vertebrae) may be present. Single-leg hyperextension test causes pain on weight-bearing side
Myofascial LBP/lumbar strain	Acute injury or insidious onset, lateral pain	May have increased muscle tone or spasm, tenderness over paraspinous muscles
Herniated disk[b] (extrusion of nucleus pulposus from intervertebral disk; can impinge spinal nerve root)	Age 30–55 years. Pain radiates into buttocks and legs, particularly below knee. Pain worse with flexion, cough, Valsalva. May have weakness or numbness of LE	Positive straight leg raise. May have weakness or numbness on LE strength and sensory exam in dermatomal distribution. May also have asymmetric reflexes
Degenerative facet joint/osteoarthritis (degeneration of articulation of the vertebral bones)	Age >40 years. Localized pain. May radiate to groin, buttock, thighs, but not below the knee. Sx worse in AM. Extension, rotation, standing, sitting can worsen Sx. No change with cough or Valsalva	Unable to palpate facet joints on exam. Pain with hyperextension and rotation
Degenerative disk (degradation of intervertebral disks in the vertebral column)	Age >40 years. Stiffness, pain that decreases after 20–30 minutes of activity. Worse with sitting, lumbar flexion and rotation, and Valsalva. Improved with lying on side with hips/knee bent	May have multiple levels of tender vertebrae or difficulty with ROM
Spinal stenosis (degenerative changes that facet joint and ligamentum flavum hypertrophy)	Age >60 years. Neurogenic claudication (LE pain, weakness or numbness with increased activity). Pain improved with sitting, flexion; worse with extension	Forward flexed posture. Lumbar extension may provoke symptoms. +/– LE weakness or sensation changes, but if present, may affect multiple dermatomes
Fracture (e.g., compression, traumatic)	Age >50 years. Female gender. Hx of osteoporosis or trauma	May be point tender over vertebrae

Diagnosis Suggested[a]	Key History	Key Physical Exam Findings
Nonmechanical		
Inflammatory Arthritis	Age <40 years. Gradual onset. Stiffness, pain that decreases after several hours of activity. Multiple joints involved	Limited spinal mobility
Infection	Fever, immunocompromised. Acute onset. Recent infectious source	May have vertebral point tenderness
Neoplasia	Night pain, weight loss, rest pain	

[a]Diagnoses in each section ordered from those that are most likely to appear in youngest to oldest ages.
[b]Red flag symptoms: urinary retention, fecal incontinence, saddle anesthesia, major motor or sensory deficit.
Hx, history; LE, lower extremity; Sx, symptoms.

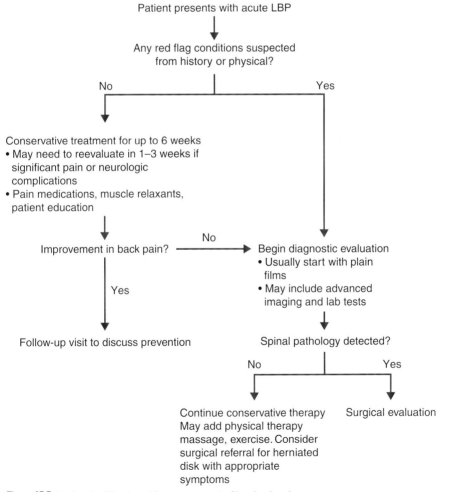

Patient presents with acute LBP

Any red flag conditions suspected from history or physical?

No — Yes

Conservative treatment for up to 6 weeks
• May need to reevaluate in 1–3 weeks if significant pain or neurologic complications
• Pain medications, muscle relaxants, patient education

Improvement in back pain? —No→ Begin diagnostic evaluation
• Usually start with plain films
• May include advanced imaging and lab tests

Yes

Follow-up visit to discuss prevention

Spinal pathology detected?

No — Yes

Continue conservative therapy May add physical therapy massage, exercise. Consider surgical referral for herniated disk with appropriate symptoms

Surgical evaluation

Figure 17.7 ▶ An algorithm to guide management of low back pain.

Table 17.13 ▶ Indications for Back Imaging

Modality	Indication	Possible Findings
Plain films (standing anteroposterior and lateral views of the lumbosacral spine)	• Consider if no improvement in 6 weeks • Image earlier if history of trauma, osteoporosis, chronic steroid use, or elderly patient	May identify degenerative changes, compression fractures, spondylolysis, spondylolisthesis
CT scan (without contrast)	• Consider if suspected fracture that is not identified on plain films	May identify occult fracture
Tc99m bone scan with SPECT spine	• Consider if suspected spondylolysis in a child or adolescent and plain films are negative	May identify occult spondylolysis (gold standard)
MRI	• Consider for suspected ligamentous injury, disk disease, spinal stenosis, neoplasm, or infection	May identify discogenic disease, acute spondylolysis, spinal stenosis, neoplasm, or infection

Data from Davis PC, Wippold FJ 2nd, Brunberg JA., et al ACR Appropriateness Criteria on low back pain. *J Am Coll Radiol.* 2009;6(6):401–407.

On exam, Sam has tenderness over his lumbar paraspinal muscles. He has full strength and sensation. His single-leg hyperextension test and straight leg test are negative. You discuss with Sam that he likely has chronic myofascial pain.

Imaging

Although imaging is usually unnecessary, consider use of these tests in situations listed in Table 17.13. It is important to recognize that many asymptomatic adults have pathology on back imaging, so positive findings may not be the cause of back symptoms. Sam had expected to get x-rays today, but given that his pain did not appear to be bony or radicular, a decision is made using shared decision making to obtain imaging at the next appointment if he does not improve.

Back Pain Management

Acute LBP without warning symptoms, including suspected myofascial pain, osteoarthritis, disk disease, and spinal stenosis, is often self-limited and usually improves in 6 to 8 weeks. Advise patients to do the following:

▶ Stay active and use pain relievers such as acetaminophen, although there is little supporting evidence.[29,30] (SOR C)

- NSAIDs and muscle relaxers have some short-term benefit but significant side effects.[31,32] (SOR B)
- Athletes with spondylolysis should rest from their sport for >3 months and then gradually return to their sport wearing a spinal brace for 3 to 6 months.[33] (SOR C)

For **chronic LBP**, conservative options can be continued or more invasive interventions explored (SOR C).

▶ Exercise therapy, spinal manipulation, and acupuncture may improve pain and function in patients with chronic LBP.[34] As Sam is a relatively young and active man, exercise therapy would be an appropriate choice. Options should be presented.

▶ Duloxetine may improve chronic LBP; however, selective serotonin reuptake inhibitors and tricyclic antidepressants have not been shown effective.[35,36]

▶ Patients with degenerative disk disease may gain short-term relief from epidural steroid injections.[37]

▶ For patients with degenerative facet joint/osteoarthritis, facet joint injections may not be better than placebo.[38]

Sam was referred to physical therapy. There, he worked on abdominal and gluteal muscle strengthening. After therapy, Sam worked the exercises he learned into his daily exercise routine. At his follow-up appointment, he reported he had eased back into rugby, and his pain was 80% improved. He was instructed to continue his daily exercise program.

Indications for Referral

Patients who have objective findings of **radiculopathy and spinal stenosis** on MRI with no improvement with conservative treatment or injections can be referred for surgical evaluation.

▶ Patients with spinal fractures should be managed on an individual basis. This may warrant consultation with an orthopedist.

▶ Patients with inflammatory arthritis of the spine should be referred to a rheumatologist.

▶ Patients with neoplasia should be referred to an oncologist.

QUESTIONS

1. You are evaluating a high-school athlete for a sprained ankle that occurred during football practice. He reports pain in the lateral malleolar area. Which one of the following is true of ankle imaging in this patient?
   A. Special ankle tests like the talar tilt test determine need for ankle x-rays.
   B. Provided there is no foot deformity, ankle x-rays are unnecessary.
   C. Order ankle x-rays because of his reported pain location.
   D. Use the Ottawa ankle rules to determine the need for ankle x-rays.
   E. X-rays should be obtained any time an injury occurs at school.

2. Which one of the following is true of surgical management of common knee problems in primary care practice?
   A. Surgery is recommended for lateral collateral ligament tears.
   B. Surgery is recommended for adults 18 to 35 years with ACL tears.
   C. Surgery for a partial meniscus tear is more effective than conservative management.
   D. Surgery for patellofemoral pain syndrome improves symptoms at 5 years.

3. In evaluation of a patient with shoulder pain, which one of the following points to the likely etiology?
   A. A positive apprehension test suggests glenohumeral instability/shoulder dislocation.
   B. Falling onto an abducted internally rotated arm suggests rotator cuff tear.

C. Loss of shoulder ROM in a teenager suggests adhesive capsulitis.

D. Heavy weight training suggests glenohumeral joint arthritis.

E. A positive cross-body test suggests a rotator cuff disorder.

4. Which one of the following is true of LBP?

A. Mechanical back pain accounts for less than half of the diagnoses.

B. Spondylolysis is a common cause of LBP in elderly patients.

C. It is usually appropriate to be conservative in both evaluation and treatment.

D. Most patients with LBP are better in 1 week.

E. Another episode of back pain within 6 months occurs in over half of patients.

5. Which one of the following is appropriate management for patients with LBP?

A. Bed rest for the first 2 days for acute LBP.

B. Opioids for short-term use in acute LBP.

C. Selective serotonin reuptake inhibitors for chronic LBP.

D. Exercise therapy, spinal manipulation, and acupuncture for chronic LBP.

E. Facet joint injections for back osteoarthritis.

ANSWERS

Question 1: The correct answer is D.

To help determine whether imaging is needed, use the Ottawa ankle rules. Order x-rays of the ankle or foot (AP, lateral, and mortise view) if the patient has pain in the malleolar area OR midfoot AND one of the following: bony tenderness at the posterior edge or tip of lateral or medial malleolus, bony tenderness over the navicular, bony tenderness at the base of the 5th metatarsal, or inability to bear weight (defined as 4 steps) during your evaluation.

Question 2: The correct answer is B.

For anterior cruciate ligament tears, operative management is suggested for young adults 18 to 35 years with ACL tear (moderate recommendation from AAOS; SOR B); return to sports at 6 months following reconstruction.

Question 3: The correct answer is A.

Table 17.7: The apprehension test is positive if the patient becomes apprehensive and indicates glenohumeral instability.

Question 4: The correct answer is C.

Usually, it is appropriate to be conservative in both evaluation and treatment of LBP. In general, LBP has a favorable prognosis with 30% of patients getting better in 1 week and 60% better by 6 to 7 weeks.

Question 5: The correct answer is D.

For chronic LBP, conservative options can be continued or more invasive interventions explored (SOR C). Exercise therapy, spinal manipulation, and acupuncture may improve pain and function in patients with chronic LBP.

REFERENCES

1. Centers for Disease Control and Prevention, National Center for Health Statistics. *National Ambulatory Medical Care Survey.* Hyattsville, MD: National Center for Health Statistics; 2000.

2. Stiell IG, McKnight RD, Greenberg GH., et al Implementation of the Ottawa ankle rules. *JAMA*. 1994;271(11): 827–832.
3. Jones P, Dalziel SR, Lamdin R., et al Oral non-steroidal anti-inflammatory drugs versus other oral analgesic agents for acute soft tissue injury. *Cochrane Database Syst Rev*. 2015;(7):CD007789.
4. van Rijn RM, van Ochten J, Luijsterburg PA., et al Effectiveness of additional supervised exercises compared with conventional treatment alone in patients with acute lateral ankle sprains: systematic review. *BMJ*. 2010;341:c5688.
5. Moraes VY, Lenza M, Tamaoki MJ., et al Platelet-rich therapies for musculoskeletal soft tissue injuries. *Cochrane Database Syst Rev*. 2014;(4):CD010071.
6. Sefton JM, Yarar C, Hicks-Little CA., et al Six weeks of balance training improves sensorimotor function in individuals with chronic ankle instability. *J Orthop Sports Phys Ther*. 2011;41(2):81–89.
7. de Vries JS, Krips R, Sierevelt IN., et al Interventions for treating chronic ankle instability. *Cochrane Database Syst Rev*. 2011;(8):CD004124.
8. Stiell IG, Greenberg GH, Wells GA., et al Derivation of a decision rule for the use of radiography in acute knee injuries. *Ann Emerg Med*. 1995;26:405–413.
9. Lundberg M, Messner K. Long-term prognosis of isolated partial medial collateral ligament ruptures. A ten-year clinical and radiographic evaluation of a prospectively observed group of patients. *Am J Sports Med*. 1996;24(2):160–163.
10. Swart NM, van Oudenaarde K, Reijnierse MJ., et al Effectiveness of exercise therapy for meniscal lesions in adults: a systematic review and meta-analysis. *J Sci Med Sport*. 2016;19(12):990–998.
11. van der Heijden RA, Lankhorst NE, van Linschoten R, et al. Exercise for treating patellofemoral pain syndrome. *Cochrane Database Syst Rev*. 2015;1:CD010387.
12. Callaghan MJ, Selfe J. Patellar taping for patellofemoral pain syndrome in adults. *Cochrane Database Syst Rev*. 2012;(4):CD006717.
13. Kettunen JA, Harilainen A, Sandelin J., et al Knee arthroscopy and exercise versus exercise only for chronic patellofemoral pain syndrome: 5-year follow-up. *Br J Sports Med*. 2012;46(4):243–246.
14. Lange AK, Vanwanseele B, Fiatarone Singh MA. Strength training for treatment of osteoarthritis of the knee: a systematic review. *Arthritis Rheum*. 2008;59(10):1488–1494.
15. Fransen M, McConnell S, Harmer AR., et al Exercise for osteoarthritis of the knee. *Cochrane Database Syst Rev*. 2015;(1):CD004376.
16. Towheed TE, Maxwell L, Judd MG., et al Acetaminophen for osteoarthritis. *Cochrane Database Syst Rev*. 2006;(1):CD004257.
17. Bannuru RR, Schmid CH, Kent DM., et al Comparative effectiveness of pharmacologic interventions for knee osteoarthritis: a systematic review and network meta-analysis. *Ann Intern Med*. 2015;162(1):46–54.
18. Schwellnus MP, Theunissen L, Noakes TD., et al Anti-inflammatory and combined anti-inflammatory/ analgesic medication in the early management of iliotibial band friction syndrome. A clinical trial. *S Afr Med J*. 1991;79(10):602–606.
19. Gunter P, Schwellnus MP. Local corticosteroid injection in iliotibial band friction syndrome in runners: a randomised controlled trial. *Br J Sports Med*. 2004;38(3):269–272.
20. Van der Windt DA, Koes BW, de Jong BA., et al Shoulder disorders in general practice: incidence, patient characteristics, and management. *Ann Rheum Dis*. 1995;54(12):959–964.
21. Hanchard NC, Goodchild LM, Kottam L. Conservative management following closed reduction of traumatic anterior dislocation of the shoulder. *Cochrane Database Syst Rev*. 2014;(4):CD004962.
22. Alvarez CM, Litchfield R, Jackowski D., et al A prospective, double-blind, randomized clinical trial comparing subacromial injection of betamethasone and xylocaine to xylocaine alone in chronic rotator cuff tendinosis. *Am J Sports Med*. 2005;33(2):255–262.
23. Chou WY, Ko JY, Wang FS., et al Effect of sodium hyaluronate treatment on rotator cuff lesions without complete tears: a randomized, double-blind, placebo-controlled study. *J Shoulder Elbow Surg*. 2010;19(4):557–563.
24. Gialanella B, Prometti P. Effects of corticosteroids injection in rotator cuff tears. *Pain Med*. 2011;12(10): 1559–1565.
25. Moosmayer S, Lund G, Seljom US., et al Tendon repair compared with physiotherapy in the treatment of rotator cuff tears: a randomized controlled study in 103 cases with a five-year follow-up. *J Bone Joint Surg Am*. 2014;96(18):1504–1514.
26. Deyo RA, Mirza SK, Martin BI. Back pain prevalence and visit rates: estimates from US national surveys, 2002. *Spine*. 2006;31:2724–2727.

27. Wolsko PM, Eisenberg DM, Davis RB., et al Patterns and perceptions of care for treatment of back and neck pain: results of a national survey. *Spine.* 2003;28(3):292–297; discussion 298.
28. Stanton TR, Henschke N, Maher CG., et al After an episode of acute back pain, recurrence is unpredictable and not as common as previously thought. *Spine.* 2008;33(26):2923–2928.
29. Dahm KT, Brurberg KG, Jamtvedt G., et al Advice to rest in bed versus advice to stay active for acute low-back pain and sciatica. *Cochrane Database Syst Rev.* 2009;(6):CD007612.
30. Williams CM, Maher CG, Latimer J., et al Efficacy of paracetamol for acute low-back pain: a double-blind, randomised controlled trial. *Lancet.* 2014;384(9954):1586–1596.
31. Roelofs PD, Deyo RA, Koes BW., et al Non-steroidal anti-inflammatory drugs for low back pain. *Cochrane Database Syst Rev.* 2008;(1):CD000396.
32. van Tulder MW, Touray T, Furlan AD., et al Muscle relaxants for non-specific low-back pain. *Cochrane Database Syst Rev.* 2003;(2):CD004252.
33. El Rassi G, Takemitsu M, Glutting J., et al Effect of sports modification on clinical outcome in children and adolescent athletes with symptomatic lumbar spondylolysis. *Am J Phys Med Rehabil.* 2013;92(12):1070–1074.
34. Chou R, Atlas SJ, Stanos SP., et al Nonsurgical interventional therapies for low back pain: a review of the evidence for an American Pain Society clinical practice guideline. *Spine.* 2009;34(10):1078–1093.
35. Skljarevski V, Zhang S, Desaiah D., et al Duloxetine versus placebo in patients with chronic low back pain: a 12-week, fixed-dose, randomized, double-blind trial. *J Pain.* 2010;11(12):1282–1290.
36. Urquhart DM, Hoving JL, Assendelft WW., et al Antidepressants for non-specific low back pain. *Cochrane Database Syst Rev.* 2008;(1):CD001703.
37. Bono CM, Ghiselli G, Gilbert TJ., et al An evidence-based clinical guideline for the diagnosis and treatment of cervical radiculopathy from degenerative disorders. *Spine J.* 2011;11(1):64–72.
38. Ribeiro LH, Furtado RN, Konai MS., et al Effect of facet joint injection versus systemic steroids in low back pain: a randomized controlled trial. *Spine.* 2013;38(23):1995–2002.

Sexuality and Relationship Issues

KEY POINTS

1 ▶ Taking a sexual history should be done in a private setting using open-ended, nonjudgmental language.

2 ▶ Specific questions about gender and sexuality are important in knowing how to take care of patients.

3 ▶ Sexuality in adolescents and older adults is unique from other adults.

4 ▶ The family physician is often called upon to counsel patients who are experiencing significant relationship issues such as sexual abuse, divorce, or death of a spouse.

TAKING A SEXUAL/RELATIONSHIP HISTORY

Your next patient of the day is Michaela, a 23-year-old woman who made an appointment to discuss starting the contraceptive injection. When you enter the room, you notice that Michaela has a very masculine appearance—short hair, slacks, button-down shirt, and a bowtie. You introduce yourself and ask, "what name do you go by?" The patient asks you to use the name "Mick." You say, "I see that you're here today to get the shot for birth control, is that right?" Mick answers, "Well, I guess so, but I also really just hate my period and want it to stop. I hear the shot is good for that." You begin to take a sexual history.

Definitions and Terminology

Before taking a sexual history, it is helpful to understand the terminology around sex, gender, and sexuality. Some basic definitions can be found in Table 18.1. Each of us has a distinct biologic sex, a gender identity, and a sexual orientation that may change and evolve over time.

General Structure of the Sexual/Relationship History

Before obtaining a sexual history, start with an opening statement that normalizes the questions you are about to ask.

You say to Mick, "I want to ask you some questions about your sexual health. I know these questions are personal, but they touch on issues that are very important for overall health. Just so you know, I ask all my patients these same questions regardless of age, gender, or marital status, and I take your privacy seriously. Do you have any questions before we begin?"

Keep in mind that the one of the main goals when taking a sexual history is to determine what, if any, screening is appropriate for this particular patient. To that end, the clinician needs to determine whether someone is sexually active, who are their partners, and the number of prior partners (Fig. 18.1). After obtaining this basic information, follow-up questions can be tailored.

Table 18.1 ▶ Gender and Sexuality Terminology

Sex	Biologic or anatomical characteristics used to assign sex at birth (e.g., chromosomes, hormones, and internal and external genitalia)
Gender	The socially constructed characteristics of men and women (e.g., roles, relationships, norms, behaviors); defined by culture and historical period
Gender Identity	One's innermost sense of self as male, female, both, or neither
Transgender or Gender Expansive	Sometimes used as umbrella terms to describe anyone whose identity or behavior falls outside of stereotypical gender norms. Refers to a person whose gender identity does not match their assigned birth sex
Sexual Orientation	Refers to being emotionally, romantically, or sexually attracted to people of a specific gender

The CDC recommends the "5 Ps" approach (Box 18.1) to gathering a more in-depth sexual history (http://www.cdc.gov/STD/treatment/SexualHistory.pdf).

Figure 18.1 summarizes how to approach taking a sexual history. Though not included in the algorithm, an important aspect of setting the stage and ensuring confidentiality is asking friends or family to step out of the exam room before taking a sexuality history.

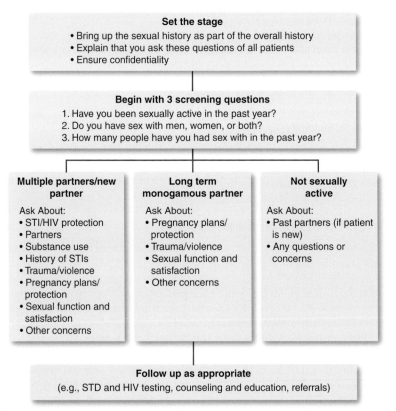

Figure 18.1 ▶ Conducting a sexual history. (Data from Taking routine histories of sexual health: a system-wide approach for health centers, by the National LGBT Health Education Center, November 2015. Available at: http://www.lgbthealtheducation.org/wp-content/uploads/COM-827-sexual-history_toolkit_2015.pdf)

BOX 18.1 THE 5 PS

Partners

▶ "Are your sex partners men, women, transgender people, or some combination?"

Practices

▶ "Do you have any questions or concerns about your sex life?"

▶ "Tell me about your sex practices."

Protection from STDs

▶ "How often do you use condoms when you have vaginal (or oral or anal) sex?"

▶ "Tell me about the reasons you do or don't use condoms."

▶ "Have you or any of your partners traded sex for things like rent, housing, drugs, or money?"

Past history of STDs

▶ "Have you ever had a sexually transmitted infection (STI)?"

▶ "Are you having any symptoms now that make you concerned you may have an infection?"

Protection from pregnancy

▶ "What are your plans for pregnancy and/or parenting?"

▶ "Do you want information about birth control?"

Tips and Special Considerations for Transgender Patients

▶ **DO** use the appropriate name and pronouns when taking a transgender patient's medical history. (Female pronouns are she, her, hers; male pronouns are he, him, his; examples of gender neutral pronouns are they, them, their, zie, and hir). You should use these terms of address even if they differ from what appears on the medical record. Mick shares with you that he identifies as a transgender male and uses male pronouns, so you should do the same.

▶ **DO** remember that a transgender person may identify as straight, gay, lesbian, queer, or some other sexual orientation, and this may evolve and change over time.

▶ **DO** use open-ended questions (e.g., "Can you tell me a bit about your sexual practices?") instead of asking questions about specific body parts, which may be hard for patients who are gender dysphoric.

▶ **DO** apologize if you make a mistake in regards to pronouns or gender identity.

▶ **DON'T** assume you know their sexual orientation.

You're doing WHAT in the bedroom?

Health care provider education is available at the Alternative Sexualities Health Research Alliance (http://www.tashra.org/provider-education), which is a community-based nonprofit dedicated to improving health and health care experiences for individuals with nontraditional sexual practices. There is also an excellent presentation at http://media.wix.com/ugd/3cd6ea_5ba09760d6c846bbbda846d793969419.pdf, which is geared specifically to medical students who would like to learn more about this area.

Mick describes his sexual orientation as "queer," and explains that he has one primary partner who is female, but they have an open relationship and his partner regularly has sex with both men and women. He gets tested regularly for HIV, and his last test was negative about 6 months ago. He has never had a pelvic exam because the thought of having an exam "down there" is frightening and because he assumed he didn't need one since all his sexual partners have been female.

GENITAL PHYSICAL EXAM

A video demonstrating how to do a complete female genital exam can be found at https://www.youtube.com/watch?v=lZnQ70WFsoQ. A series of videos on the complete male genital exam can be found at https://www.auanet.org/education/medical-student/gu-exam/index.cfm?video=opening. In addition, a focused exam is appropriate for patients coming in with a specific health concern.

Special Considerations When Examining Transgender Patients

UCSF's Center of Excellence for Transgender Health provides wonderful guidance on conducting a thoughtful physical exam with a transgender patient (http://transhealth.ucsf.edu/trans?page=guidelines-physical-examination). There is also excellent advice in this pamphlet called *Tips For Providing Paps to Trans Men* (http://checkitoutguys.ca/sites/default/files/Tips_Paps_TransMen_0.pdf).

SCREENING AND PREVENTION

Screening tests and examinations should be tailored to each patient's risk factors (see Chapter 7). Although Mick is a transgender man, he should be advised to undergo preventive tests appropriate for his age, sex, and sexual behaviors.

> **There's an App for That!**
>
> The US Preventive Services Task Force has a website (https://www.uspreventiveservicestaskforce.org/BrowseRec/Index) and a free app (http://epss.ahrq.gov/PDA/index.jsp) that can quickly help you determine which screening tests are recommended.

Pre-exposure prophylaxis is a powerful prevention tool for patients who are at high risk for becoming infected with HIV. This is a daily pill (emtricitabine/tenofovir) which, when used correctly, can lower the risk of HIV infection by as much as 92%.[1,2] For more detailed information, check out the CDC's website at https://www.cdc.gov/hiv/risk/prep/.

> **Resources for Further Self-Directed Learning**
>
> Video from University of California at Berkeley (https://www.youtube.com/watch?v=Dbtwj33N5pQ)
>
> ▸ Excellent lecture by a nurse practitioner from the City Clinic (free STD clinic) on taking a sexual history
>
> Video from the AMA on taking a sexual health history
>
> ▸ http://www.bigshouldersdubs.com/clients/AMA/23-AMA-HealthHistory.htm

Mick denies having receptive vaginal intercourse in the past 2 weeks. His urine pregnancy test is negative, so you offer the contraceptive injection today. You tell him that, based on his history, you recommend testing for HIV, chlamydia, and gonorrhea. You offer urine testing for chlamydia and gonorrhea, and recommend that he return for a Pap test at another visit when he can bring a support person.

CARING FOR UNMARRIED PEOPLE

Those who are not legally married (single people, unmarried LGBT couples, cohabiting couples, polyamorous people) should be counseled to take steps to make sure that their decision making is protected. Having an advance directive for health care (also called living will) and a health care power of attorney are important documents for people of all ages to have in place.

ADOLESCENT SEXUALITY: SPECIAL CONSIDERATIONS

Jessi, a 15-year-old female, has an appointment to discuss abdominal pain. Her mother is with her for the appointment, and describes pain that has been ongoing for about a month, severe enough that Jessi has been missing school for a day or two each week. Jessi says the pain is around her belly button, and does not radiate. No associated fevers, vomiting, diarrhea, blood in stool. After explaining about clinic and state policies about confidential health services for teens, you ask Jessi's mom to step out of the room, and you continue your history. When you start taking a social history and ask her about her relationship, Jessi starts to cry and says that she tried to break up with her boyfriend a few weeks ago because he was pressuring her to have sex and preventing her from hanging out with her friends. He shoved her, called her a bitch and threatened to post naked pictures of her to social media. She doesn't know what to do.

Tips for taking an adolescent's sexual history:

▸ **DO** familiarize yourself with your state's minor consent laws. The Guttmacher Institute is a good place to start (https://www.guttmacher.org/state-policy/explore/overview-minors-consent-law).

▸ **DO** explain in clear terms to adolescents and their parents/guardians about confidentiality and its limits.

▸ **DO** discuss healthy relationships with adolescents. This will be particularly important in working with Jessi who needs to know that it is not OK to be physically or emotionally bullied and will need support to end the relationship.

▸ **DO** use gender neutral terms (e.g., "do you have a crush on anyone?") until the patient established a sexual preference.

▸ **DO** avoid jargon (e.g., say "are you having sex?" instead of "do you have intercourse?")

▸ **DO** make every effort to spend some of the visit with the adolescent alone without parents, siblings, or partners in the room. As shown in the above case, Jessi only reported her situation to you once her mother was out of the room; this is often the case.

▶ **DON'T** ask questions in a judgmental way ("You don't have unprotected sex, do you?") or use body language that can be perceived as negative (shaking head "no," wrinkling up your nose) when asking questions.

▶ **DON'T** assume that adolescents with disabilities are not sexually active.

Talking About Consent

Consent is a topic that is important to everyone, regardless of age, but explicitly discussing consent is an important part of counseling adolescents on healthy relationships. One way to define consent is:

▶ **Consent is the presence of "yes," not the absence of "no," and it needs continued agreement.**

Resources for Further Self-Directed Learning

UCSF's Adolescent Health Toolkit (http://nahic.ucsf.edu/resource_center/toolkit-youth-centered-care/)

▶ Geared toward primary care providers

▶ Includes screening, assessment, and referral tools

▶ Handouts for teens and their parents/caregivers

Adolescent Health Working Group's Provider Toolkit Series (https://www.ahwg.net)

▶ Topics covered: Trauma and Resilience, Consent and Confidentiality, Sexual Health, Behavioral Health, Body Basics, Adolescent Health Care 101.

Physicians for Reproductive Health: Online Curriculum Adolescent Reproductive and Sexual Health Education Project (https://prh.org/)

▶ Standardized case videos on LARC, taking a sexual history with a gender-expansive patient, coming out, STIs, and more

Futures Without Violence (https://futureswithoutviolence.org)

▶ Guidelines for preventing, identifying, and addressing adolescent relationship abuse

▶ Free downloads: safety card for adolescents, poster to display in clinic

---

SEXUALITY IN OLDER ADULTS

In one large US survey, 39.5% of women and 67% of men aged 65 to 74 years reported sexual activity in the preceding 12 months. Approximately half of all of the survey respondents reported at least one bothersome sexual problem but only 38% of men and 22% of women reported having discussed sex with a physician since the age of 50 years.[3]

Some Questions to Help You Talk About Sex With Your Elderly Patients[4]

"I have a few sexual health questions I'd like to ask you; would that be OK?"

▶ "Are you comfortable with where things are at this point in your life with respect to your sexual activity?"

▶ Do you have any questions or concerns about your sexual health that you'd like to review?"

▶ "Are you sexually active?"

▶ "Have you had more than one partner in the last year?"

▶ "Have you been tested for sexually transmitted infections? They can still occur if either you or your partner are not entirely monogamous with each other."

▶ "Are there health or other concerns that limit the ability for you to be as sexually active as you would like to be?"

Health Conditions That Negatively Affect Sexual Functioning

Special consideration should be given to **health conditions** such as hypertension, diabetes, and arthritis, and **medications** such as antidepressants, antipsychotics, anticonvulsants, cholinesterase inhibitors, hormonal agents, and beta blockers that can negatively affect sexual functioning.[5] Additionally, the history should include questions about problems such as erectile dysfunction, vaginal dryness, pain during sexual intercourse, premature ejaculation, inability to climax, lack of pleasure during sex, anxiety about sexual performance, and problematic lack of interest in sex.

In discussing the sexual history with elderly patients, it is also important to note cognitive status. Patients may be reluctant or unable to discuss cognitive decline as it relates to sexuality. Dementia does not necessarily preclude consensual sexual activity. However, moderate to severe dementia can impair decisional capacity or lead to inappropriate sexual behavior including unwanted verbal or physical sexual advances, sexual aggression, public exposure of breasts and/or genitals, and public masturbation. If you suspect sexual abuse and/or exploitation, this must be reported to the appropriate authority. Inappropriate sexual behavior often requires a multimodal approach including behavioral management strategies and education of family and caregivers.[6]

RELATIONSHIPS

Navigating difficult relationships is another frequent concern that patients bring to their family physicians. While there are many situations that benefit from discussion and counseling, three that can be particularly devastating are separation and divorce, sexual assault, and bereavement.

Separation and Divorce

Almost half of all first marriages end in separation or divorce within 20 years.[7] Roughly one-third of first cohabitations end in separation within 5 years.[8] Divorce is second only to death of a spouse on the scale of stressful events.[9]

In helping patients navigate the complicated emotional landscape of separation and divorce, health care providers should listen without judgment and offer emotional support; reassure the patient that grief is a natural response to the loss of the partnership; encourage healthy eating, exercise, and adequate sleep; encourage engagement in healthy social interactions; screen for substance abuse and intervene where necessary; help patients recognize the signs and symptoms of depression; and refer to mental health services as appropriate.[10]

Supporting Children Through Separation and Divorce

Children of separating or divorcing parents require special attention and support at all stages of the process. The stress of divorce can affect children differently depending on developmental stage. At all ages, children frequently have psychosomatic symptoms as a response to anger, loss, grief, feeling unloved, and other stressors. However, feelings of guilt and responsibility for the family disruption are also common, and some children will feel that they should try to repair their parents' partnership.[11]

Health care providers should offer support and age-appropriate advice to the child and parents regarding reactions to divorce, especially guilt, anger, sadness, and perceived loss of love. Providers should refrain from choosing sides and try to maintain positive relationships with both parents. Parents should be advised not to argue in front of children, not to encourage children to take sides, and not to speak negatively about the other parent in front of children.[11] As much as possible, children's routines should be maintained. Any disruption of normal routines should be communicated by both parents in advance (http://www.helpguide.org/articles/family-divorce/children-and-divorce.htm).

Sexual Assault

The CDC defines sexual violence as "a sexual act committed against someone without that person's freely-given consent."[12] In a 2012 survey of US adults, nearly **1 in 5** (18.3%) women and **1 in 71** men (1.4%) reported experiencing rape at some time in their lives.[13] Additionally, 1 in 11 women have been raped by an intimate partner.[13] See Chapter 21.

Patients reporting sexual assault should be offered the option of sexual assault forensic examination by a Sexual Assault Nurse Examiner (SANE) or health care provider with similar certification (Fig. 18.2). This allows for prompt collection of DNA and other evidence which can be used in legal proceedings, and provision of appropriate health care services such as STI prophylaxis and referral for management of injuries. Health care providers should contact the National Sexual Assault Hotline 1-800-656-HOPE or the local health department to identify resources in their practice locations.

Long-term consequences for survivors of sexual violence are manifold and include anxiety, depression, posttraumatic stress disorder, strained interpersonal relationships, substance abuse, risky sexual behavior, chronic pain, gastrointestinal disorders, migraines, and other chronic headache conditions.[14]

BEREAVEMENT AND GRIEF

Jim is a 71-year-old man with hypertension and diabetes being seen in your clinic 13 months after the death of his wife of 40 years. He used to be a fun-loving guy and he and his wife had an active social life but he rarely gets out of the house now. He avoids places they used

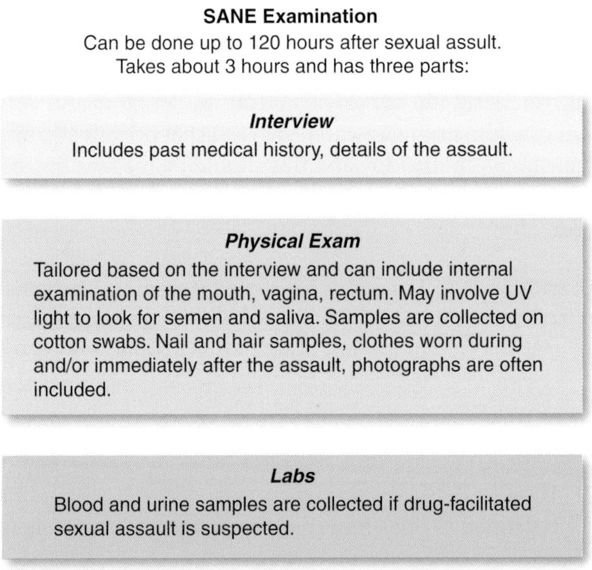

SANE Examination
Can be done up to 120 hours after sexual assult.
Takes about 3 hours and has three parts:

Interview
Includes past medical history, details of the assault.

Physical Exam
Tailored based on the interview and can include internal examination of the mouth, vagina, rectum. May involve UV light to look for semen and saliva. Samples are collected on cotton swabs. Nail and hair samples, clothes worn during and/or immediately after the assault, photographs are often included.

Labs
Blood and urine samples are collected if drug-facilitated sexual assault is suspected.

Figure 18.2 ▶ Sexual assault nurse examiner examination format. (Data from Washington University in St. Louis. What to expect from a SANE/forensic exam. 2012. Available at: https://shs.wustl.edu/SexualViolence/What-to-do-if-you-have-been-sexually-assaulted/Pages/What-to-expect-from-A-SANE-forensic-exam.aspx. Accessed November 21, 2016.)

to frequent as well as family functions because he doesn't want to be reminded of his wife. He sees no point to his life as it is now, and wishes for death so that he and his wife may be reunited, though he denies a suicidal plan. He thinks of her constantly and can't accept that she's gone. Jim reports feeling angry and bitter, and he is tearful on describing his life since his wife's death.

Death of a loved one is one of the most common adverse life events of older age. Bereavement is the state of having suffered a loss. Grief is a natural response to bereavement and is characterized by profound sadness that may be accompanied by yearning and longing, decreased interest in ongoing activities, and frequent thoughts of the deceased.[15] Usually acute grief becomes integrated into daily living and symptoms will not interfere with normal functioning.[16]

However, in a significant minority of cases, grief becomes **prolonged and symptoms remain severe and impairing**; this condition is called persistent complex bereavement disorder or complicated grief. This is shown with Jim whose emotional difficulty has gone beyond the usual grieving process and will require additional attention. Complicated grief is characterized by a prolonged course of intense yearning for the deceased, profound sorrow and emotional pain, preoccupation with the deceased and/or circumstances of the loved one's death, excessive avoidance of people, places, and situations that remind the patient of the loss, difficulty accepting the loss, self-blame for the loss, anger and bitterness surrounding the loss, feeling cut off from others, and/or feeling devoid of meaning and purpose in the absence of the loved one. Suicidal thoughts based on a wish to rejoin the deceased may be present.[15,17]

Patients suffering bereavement, grief, and persistent complex bereavement disorder may suffer adverse effects on their physical health and are at increased risk of death from heart disease and suicide.[15] Elderly patients should be asked directly about bereavement, and health care providers should consider referral to mental health services for patients suffering significant grief. Emerging research suggests that persistent complex bereavement disorder is amenable to psychotherapy and this should be the first line of treatment.[18] The role of antidepressant medication in the treatment of persistent complex bereavement disorder is not yet clear.[15,18]

> You diagnose Jim with persistent complex bereavement disorder. You refer him for mental health evaluation and counseling. Additionally, you encourage him to pursue social outlets such as civic organizations or volunteering as well as reengaging with family and friends as he is able.

QUESTIONS

1. Gender identity is defined as one's innermost sense of self as male, female, both, or neither.
   A. True.
   B. False.
2. Talking to adolescents about sexuality can be difficult. Which one of the following tips is recommended?
   A. Tell the patient that you don't think teenagers should be having sex.
   B. Hand them a pamphlet to avoid embarrassment and ask if they have any questions.
   C. Use gender neutral terms (e.g., "do you have a crush on anyone?") until the patient has established a sexual preference.
   D. Assume that they are heterosexual unless they tell you differently.
   E. Use medical terminology.
3. A physical exam after a sexual assault should include which one of the following?
   A. Be performed by a SANE nurse or someone with similar certification.
   B. Be performed by a patient's primary care provider.
   C. Be performed quickly.
   D. Not include a pelvic examination due to patient comfort.

ANSWERS

Question 1: The correct answer is A.
As listed in Table 18.1, gender identity is defined as one's innermost sense of self as male, female, both, or neither.

Question 2: The correct answer is C.
Tips for taking an adolescent's sexual history include use of gender neutral terms (e.g., "do you have a crush on anyone?") until the patient established a sexual preference.

Question 3: The correct answer is A.
Patients reporting sexual assault should be offered the option of sexual assault forensic examination by a SANE or health care provider with similar certification (Fig. 18.2).

REFERENCES

1. Grant RM, Lama JR, Anderson PL, et al. iPrEx Study Team. Preexposure chemoprophylaxis for HIV prevention in men who have sex with men. *N Engl J Med*. 2010;363(27):2587–2599.
2. Baeten JM, Donnell D, Ndase P, et al. Partners PrEP Study Team. Antiretroviral prophylaxis for HIV prevention in heterosexual men and women. *N Engl J Med*. 2012;367(5):399–410.
3. Lindau ST, Schumm LP, Laumann EO, et al. A study of sexuality and health among older adults in the United States. *N Engl J Med*. 2007;357:762–774.
4. Omole F, Fresh EM, Sow C, et al. How to discuss sex with elderly patients. *J Fam Pract*. 2014;63(4):E1–E4.
5. De Giorgi R, Series H. Treatment of inappropriate sexual behavior in dementia. *Curr Treat Options Neurol*. 2016;18(9):41.
6. Alzheimer's Society. Sex and intimate relationships. 2015. Available at: https://www.alzheimers.org.uk/site/scripts/download_info.php?fileID=1801. Accessed October 15, 2016.
7. Copen CE, Daniels K, Vespa J, et al. *First Marriages in the United States: Data From the 2006–2010 National Survey of Family Growth. National Health Statistics Reports; No. 49*. Hyattsville, MD: National Center for Health Statistics; 2012.
8. Copen CE, Daniels K, Mosher WD. *First Premarital Cohabitation in the United States: 2006–2010 National Survey of Family Growth. National Health Statistics Reports; No. 64*. Hyattsville, MD: National Center for Health Statistics; 2013.
9. Dohrenwend BP. Inventorying stressful life events as risk factors for psychopathology: Toward resolution of the problem of intracategory variability. *Psychol Bull*. 2006;132(3):477–495.
10. Segal J, Kemp G, Smith M. Coping with a breakup or divorce. Available at: http://www.helpguide.org/articles/family-divorce/coping-with-a-breakup-or-divorce.htm. Accessed October 15, 2016.
11. Cohen GJ; American Academy of Pediatrics. Committee on Psychosocial Aspects of Child and Family Health. Helping children and families deal with divorce and separation. *Pediatrics*. 2002;110(5):1019–1023.
12. Basile KC, Smith SG, Breiding MJ, et al. *Sexual Violence Surveillance: Uniform Definitions and Recommended Data Elements, Version 2.0*. Atlanta, GA: National Center for Injury Prevention and Control, Centers for Disease Control and Prevention; 2014.
13. Black MD, Basile KC, Breiding MJ, et al. *The National Intimate Partner and Sexual Violence Survey (NISVS): 2010 Summary Report*. Atlanta, GA: National Center for Injury Prevention and Control, Centers for Disease Control and Prevention; 2011.
14. Centers for Disease Control and Prevention. Sexual violence: Consequences. Available at: http://www.cdc.gov/violenceprevention/sexualviolence/consequences.html. Accessed October 15, 2016.
15. Shear MK, Ghesquiere A, Glickman K. Bereavement and complicated grief. *Curr Psychiatry Rep*. 2013;15(11):406.
16. Chentsova Dutton Y, Zisook S. Adaptation to bereavement. *Death Stud*. 2005;29(10):877–903.
17. American Psychiatric Association. *Diagnostic and Statistical Manual of Mental Disorders*. 5th ed. Washington, DC: American Psychiatric Association; 2013.
18. Shear MK, Reynolds CF 3rd, Simon NM, et al. Optimizing treatment of complicated grief: A randomized clinical trial. *JAMA Psychiatry*. 2016;73(7):685–694.

KEY POINTS

1 ▶ The most common types of dermatitis are: atopic dermatitis, seborrheic dermatitis, contact dermatitis, and nummular eczema.

2 ▶ Acne that is predominantly obstructive causes comedones and is referred to as comedonal acne, while acne that becomes inflammatory is referred to as inflammatory acne; the former is best treated with retinoids and the latter with topical or oral antibiotics.

3 ▶ Psoriasis that involves <5% of the body surface area can often be treated with topical steroids and topical vitamin D; with larger areas of involvement or associated psoriatic arthritis, treat with methotrexate or biologic agents.

4 ▶ The most common skin cancers, in their order of prevalence, include basal cell carcinomas, squamous cell carcinomas, and melanomas.

5 ▶ Doing a physical exam of the skin with a dermatoscope in hand allows you to find smaller, less-advanced skin cancers before they become big, deep, and potentially fatal.

MEETING THE PATIENT

While listening to a patient's lungs during a physical exam, you notice a 9-mm pigmented lesion on the back (Fig. 19.1). The lesion has some of the ABCDEs of melanoma (Table 19.1).

Although the USPSTF found insufficient evidence to assess the balance of benefits and harms of visual skin examination to screen for skin cancer in (the general population of)

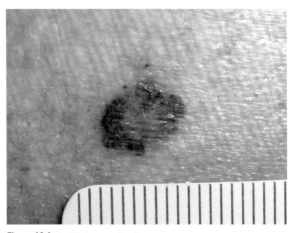

Figure 19.1 ▶ Melanoma in situ.

Table 19.1 ▸ ABCDE of Melanoma

ABCDE	Description
Asymmetry	The lesion is asymmetrical
Border irregularity	Edges of lesion are irregular (ragged, blurred, or notched)
Color	There are variations in color
Diameter	Lesion is larger than 6 mm
Evolution	The lesion is evolving in color, size, or shape

adults, picking up melanoma early saves lives. However, the data suggest that screening for skin cancer does benefit groups at higher risk for skin cancer including those with personal and family history of skin cancer, immunosuppressed individuals, and persons with various high-risk skin conditions.

Dermoscopy permits the trained clinician to find melanomas as small as 2 to 3 mm and ones that are not pigmented (Figs. 19.2 and 19.3).

Your attending looks at the lesion more closely with his dermatoscope, noting areas of regression and other suspicious features (Fig. 19.2). A saucerization biopsy is performed and a diagnosis of melanoma in situ is made on pathology. Surgery is scheduled the following week, and the family physician removes any remaining tumor with 5-mm margins. This should produce over a 99% chance of cure.

PRINCIPLES FOR DIAGNOSIS OF SKIN CONDITIONS

Although we are taught to perform the history before doing the physical exam, this is not the most efficient way to approach the diagnosis of a skin condition. When the patient has a skin

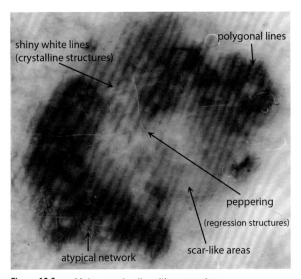

Figure 19.2 ▸ Melanoma in situ with regression.

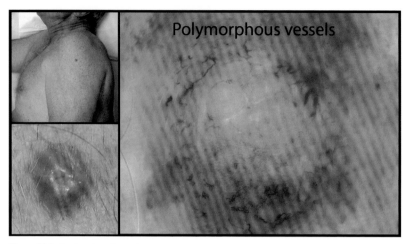

Figure 19.3 ► Amelanotic melanoma.

concern or something is seen on the skin during a physical exam, take a look at the skin right away and ask your questions while you have a look. Had the student in the case above not noticed the skin lesion and brought it to the attention of the attending physician, the lesion may not have been noted until much later, greatly reducing the chances for successful cure.

One new way of looking is to use a dermatoscope as in the case above. In these modern times of innovations in technology, a high-quality skin exam is greatly enhanced by looking into the skin with a dermatoscope.

A dermatoscope uses polarized light and a cross-polarized filter to see deeper into the skin. Dermatoscopes come in all shapes and sizes and are made by a number of companies. The best dermatoscopes attach to a smart phone and a camera to allow you to photograph and then blow up the image 10-fold for greater in-depth views. Dermoscopy increases the sensitivity and specificity of skin cancer diagnosis.[1]

In addition to the benefits listed above, another added benefit is the ability to see the scabies mite with the dermatoscope (Fig. 19.4) to make a firm diagnosis of scabies without having to do a scraping and microscopic exam. For further information on dermoscopy, see the Journal of Family Practice video online (https://www.youtube.com/watch?v=dHXOwNU4tYY&t=2s) and free apps (Dermoscopy: The Two-Step Algorithm and You).

Pattern recognition plays a large role in the learning and practice of dermatology. Experts who have seen countless cases of skin conditions can look at most lesions and make an immediate and accurate diagnosis through pattern recognition. How does the novice get to this point? The first step is to learn the basic patterns of the primary and secondary lesions listed in Table 19.2. This will give you the proper vocabulary and conceptual model to observe and describe what you are seeing. If you combine keen observation, including type and distribution of lesions, with a careful history, you will be able to create an informed differential diagnosis.

The information you acquire from observation and history can be taken to a dermatology atlas, textbook, or consultant to complete the diagnosis. Sometimes further testing such as a biopsy or culture may be needed; however, you need to know enough about the possible diagnoses to appropriately plan a biopsy or laboratory evaluation. The rapid decision to perform a same-day biopsy on the suspicious lesion resulted in expedited, likely-curative, treatment for the melanoma in situ.

• Magnifies the skin ten-fold; uses polarized light
• Attaches to a smart phone or camera
• Allows you to find smaller cancers before they spread
• Allows you to recognize benign skin tumors and avoid unnecessary biopsies

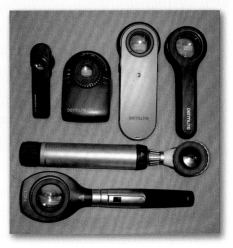

Figure 19.4 ▶ Dermatoscopes.

 Table 19.2 ▶ Primary and Secondary Skin Lesions

Lesions	Description
Primary (Basic) Lesions	
Macule	Circumscribed flat discoloration (up to 10 mm)
Patch	Flat nonpalpable discoloration (>10 mm)
Papule	Elevated solid lesion (up to 10 mm)
Plaque	Elevated solid lesion (>10 mm) (often a confluence of papules)
Nodule	Palpable solid (round) lesion, deeper than a papule
Wheal (hive)	Pink edematous plaque (round or flat), topped and transient
Pustule	Elevated collection of pus
Vesicle	Circumscribed elevated collection of fluid (up to 10 mm in diameter)
Bulla	Circumscribed elevated collection of fluid (>10 mm in diameter)
Secondary (Sequential) Lesions	
Scale (desquamation)	Excess dead epidermal cells
Crusts	Collection of dried serum, blood, or pus
Erosion	Superficial loss of epidermis
Ulcer	Focal loss of epidermis and dermis
Fissure	Linear loss of epidermis and dermis
Atrophy	Depression in skin from thinning of epidermis/dermis
Excoriation	Erosion caused by scratching
Lichenification	Thickened epidermis with prominent skin lines

CLINICAL EVALUATION

Physical Examination

Look and Touch

Try to determine the type of primary lesions and any secondary lesions (see Table 19.2). Use gloves if you think the lesions may be transmissible, as in scabies or herpetic lesions. For some lesions, such as actinic keratosis with scaling or the sandpaper rash of scarlet fever, feeling the skin lightly gives you much information. For deeper lesions, such as nodules and cysts, deep palpation is needed.

Distribution

Are the primary lesions are arranged in groups, rings, lines, or merely scattered over the skin. For example, the vesicles of herpes simplex are usually grouped together because they follow a sensory nerve, whereas chickenpox vesicles are often scattered because the virus is blood-borne. Determine which parts of the skin are affected and which are spared.

Expanded Look

Look at the remainder of the skin, nails, hair, and mucous membranes. Patients often only show you one small area and appear reluctant to show you the rest of their skin. With many skin conditions, it is essential to look beyond the most affected area.

Think of yourself as a detective, collecting clues. For example, it helps to look for nail pitting when considering a diagnosis of psoriasis. Patients may have lesions on their back or feet that they have not observed; for example, a patient may have a hand eruption that is an autoeczematization to a foot fungal infection—if you don't look for the fungus on the feet, you will miss the diagnosis. Some skin diseases (like lichen planus) have manifestations in the mouth; finding white patches on the buccal mucosa may lead you to the correct diagnosis.

Don't be shy about asking patients to remove their shoes and clothing and to show you whatever areas of the body needed to make an accurate diagnosis. A good light source and magnifying glass is helpful to distinguish the morphology of many skin conditions. Alternatively, photographing a skin lesion with a smartphone and blowing it up on the screen can show detail difficult to discern with the naked eye alone.

History

Once you have started to look at the skin, your history will be more focused and directed toward zeroing in on the correct diagnosis. The following information will help you make a diagnosis and plan treatment:

▶ **Onset and duration** of skin lesions—continuous or intermittent?

▶ **Pattern of eruption:** Where did it start? How has it changed?

▶ **Any known precipitants,** such as exposure to medication (prescription and over-the-counter), foods, plants, sun, topical agents, chemicals (occupation and hobbies)?

▶ **Skin symptoms:** Itching, pain

▶ **Systemic symptoms:** Fever, chills, night sweats, fatigue, weakness, weight loss

▶ **Underlying illnesses:** Diabetes, human immunodeficiency virus (HIV)

▶ **Family history:** Acne, atopic dermatitis, psoriasis, skin cancers, dysplastic nevi

Laboratory Tests

In most cases, the laboratory tests are used to confirm your clinical diagnosis based on history and physical exam. The most important laboratory tests in dermatology are:

▶ **Microscopy:** In diagnosing a fungal infection, scrape some of the scale onto a microscope slide, add KOH (with fungal stain or DMSO) and look for the hyphae of dermatophytes or the pseudohyphae of yeast forms of *Candida* or *Pityrosporum* species. How to do a KOH preparation: https://www.youtube.com/watch?v=LUwNQI_0BWU.

▶ **Cultures:** May be useful for some suspected bacterial, viral, or mycologic infections.

▶ **Blood tests:** Rapid plasma reagin and antinuclear antibody are helpful in determining the etiology of unknown lesions that might be syphilis or lupus erythematosus.

▶ **Wood light (ultraviolet) examination:** Helpful in diagnosing tinea capitis and erythrasma. Tinea capitis caused by *Microsporum* species produce green fluorescence, but *Trichophyton* species do not fluoresce. Erythrasma has a coral red fluorescence.

▶ **Surgical biopsy:** Can be used as a diagnostic and treatment tool for skin cancers, benign tumors, or unknown rashes. Having a reasonable differential diagnosis will help you choose the appropriate biopsy type—usually a shave or punch biopsy. In the case of a suspected melanoma, an excisional biopsy (saucerization or ellipse) is recommended to be sure that the deepest thickness of the melanoma is obtained for staging. Saucerization (deep shave) is performed efficiently with a razor blade to obtain breadth and depth of tissue for diagnostic accuracy.

TYPES OF DERMATITIS

Some of the most common types of dermatitis are described Table 19.3.

The most common types of skin conditions (excluding tumors) seen on the face are acne and rosacea (Table 19.4). While lupus is not common, it has a predilection for skin lesions on the face too.

Psoriasis

Psoriasis is a chronic immune-mediated condition characterized by epidermal proliferation and inflammation. The lesions are well-circumscribed, salmon-colored, scaling patches with white or silvery thickened scales (Fig. 19.5) in light-skinned individuals but can be silvery or hyperpigmented in darker-skinned persons. Areas affected can include the scalp, nails, and extensor surfaces of limbs, elbows, knees, the sacral region, and genitalia.

Psoriasis lesions may also be guttate, as in water drops; inverse when found in intertriginous areas such as the inguinal and intergluteal folds; or palmar–plantar when found on the palms or soles. Psoriatic nail changes occur in 20% to 40% of persons with psoriasis.[2] These nail changes include pitting, onycholysis, subungual keratosis. Patients with psoriasis can also have psoriatic arthritis.

Table 19.3 ▶ Common Types of Dermatitis

Type	Characteristics	Treatment	Image
Atopic (aka eczema)	Starts in childhood on the face and then involves flexural areas	Emollients, topical steroids, calcineurin inhibitors	
Contact	Allergic or irritant dermatitis caused by an allergen or an irritant (common triggers are poison ivy and nickel)	Identify and avoid the offending agents, topical steroids	
Seborrheic	Causes dandruff on the scalp and erythematous flaky areas on the face and is a reaction to Malassezia furfur	Anti-dandruff shampoos, topical antifungal agents, topical steroids	
Nummular	Coin-shaped areas of erythema and scale, most often found on extremities	Emollients and topical steroids	

Treatment options for psoriasis are many and varied.[3] Psoriasis that involves less than 5% of the body surface area can often be treated with topical steroids and topical vitamin D. Patients who have larger areas of involvement or have psoriatic arthritis should be treated with methotrexate or biologic agents. Narrowband ultraviolet B light is one option for patients with larger areas of involvement but no psoriatic arthritis. Topical tar and salicylic acid shampoos are useful for scalp psoriasis. Other oral agents for more severe psoriasis include cyclosporin, oral retinoids, and apremilast.

Table 19.4 ▶ Common Facial Skin Conditions

Name	Characteristics	Treatment	Image
Comedonal acne	Open and closed comedones caused by obstruction of the pilosebaceous unit	Topical agents such as benzyl peroxide and retinoids; retinoids are the most beneficial	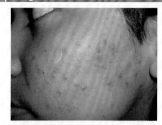
Inflammatory and cystic acne	Occurs when there is disruption of the pilosebaceous unit resulting in papules, pustules, nodules, and cysts. Cystic acne refers to acne with severe inflammatory changes	Start with a topical or oral antibiotic. Add another topical agent such as benzyl peroxide and retinoids. Reserve oral isotretinoin for the most severe recalcitrant cases	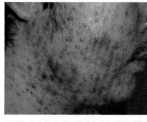
Rosacea	Erythema, telangiectasias, papules, and pustules (no comedones)	Topical metronidazole, topical azelaic acid, oral doxycycline or minocycline	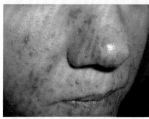
Lupus (discoid or systemic)	Erythema with or without scarring, particularly in a butterfly pattern or malar distribution	Oral hydroxychloroquine and immunosuppressive medicine if needed	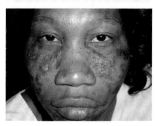

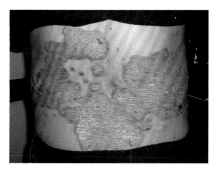

Figure 19.5 ▶ Psoriasis.

Table 19.5 ▸ Potency of Topical Corticosteroids

Potency	Generic Names (Examples by Class)
"Superpotent" (class 1)	Clobetasol
High potency (classes 2 and 3)	Fluocinonide
Mid potency (classes 4 and 5)	Triamcinolone
Low potency (classes 6 and 7)	Hydrocortisone, desonide

The most common treatment of psoriasis involves topical steroids (Table 19.5), with strong ointments being the most effective. Systemic steroids are avoided in psoriasis as they can precipitate severe flares and generalized pustular disease.

Skin Infections

Skin infections can be bacterial, fungal, viral, or infestations. These are shown in Tables 19.6 to 19.9.[4]

Table 19.6 ▸ Bacterial Skin Infections

Diagnosis	Depth	Cause	Treatment	Image
Impetigo	Superficial (epidermis)	GABHS and *S. aureus* (usually MSSA)	Topical mupirocin or oral antibiotics that treat MSSA	
Cellulitis	Deeper (involving dermis too)	Predominantly GABHS, but if purulent, suspect *S. aureus* which could be MRSA	Oral antibiotic to cover MSSA; if purulence noted, use antibiotic to cover MRSA. Hospitalize based on severity and immune status	
Abscess	Subcutaneous pocket of infection with more superficial skin layers involved	Predominantly *S. aureus* (high rate of MRSA)	Incision and drainage is the primary treatment. If surrounding cellulitis, use oral antibiotic to cover MRSA. Hospitalize based on severity and immune status	

Diagnosis	Depth	Cause	Treatment	Image
Necro-tizing fasciitis	Deepest (involving muscle)	GABHS and many other organisms	Admit and consult surgeon for immediate surgery. Intravenous antibiotics administered aggressively based on suspected organisms. Re-evaluate when tissue cultures are available	

GABHS, group A β-hemolytic strep; MRSA, methicillin-resistant Staphylococcus aureus; MSSA, methicillin-sensitive Staphylococcus aureus; S. aureus, Staphylococcus aureus.

Table 19.7 ▸ Superficial Fungal Skin Infections

Diagnosis	Location	Organism	Treatment	Image
Tinea capitis	Scalp	Dermatophytes—microsporum canis (m.c.), *Trichophyton tonsurans,* and others	Oral antifungal	
Tinea corporis Tinea pedis (manus) Tinea cruris	Body Feet (hands) Groin/inguinal	Dermatophytes—m.c., *Trichophyton rubrum*	Topical antifungal for small areas, oral antifungal for larger areas or resistant	

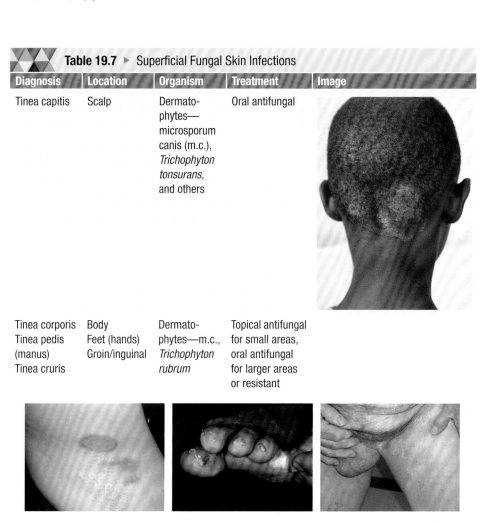

(continued)

Table 19.7 ▶ Superficial Fungal Skin Infections *(Continued)*

Diagnosis	Location	Organism	Treatment	Image
Onychomy-cosis	Nails	Dermato-phytes—m.c., *Trichophyton rubrum*	Oral terbinafine for months; top-ical agents have low effectiveness	
Tinea versi-color	Trunk but can involve neck and arms	*Malassezia furfur* (Pity-rosporum)	Topical azole antifungal or selenium and/or oral fluconazole 400 mg once	
Candida infections (thrush, bala-nitis, vaginitis, and intertrigo)	Mouth, gen-italia, groin, and in skin folds	*Candida albicans* and other Candida species	Topical azole, nystatin, or oral fluconazole (dose based on loca-tion and immune status)	

Skin Cancers

The most common skin cancers are shown in Tables 19.10 and 19.11; they are[5–7]:

▶ Basal cell carcinoma (BCC): The most common
▶ Squamous cell carcinoma (SCC): Next most common (Fig. 19.6)
▶ Melanoma: 4% (least common and the most deadly)

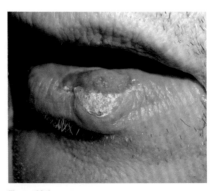

Figure 19.6 ▶ Squamous cell carcinoma in HIV.

Table 19.8 ▶ Viral Skin Infections

Diagnosis	Characteristics	Treatment	Image
Condyloma, warts (human papilloma virus)	Condyloma may have a cauliflower appearance. Warts can be verrucous, flat, or plantar. There is usually no pain but there may be itching	Cryotherapy, topical salicylic acid, topical imiquimod	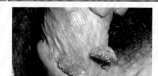
Hand-foot-and-mouth (coxsackieviruses)	Flat top, oblong vesicles on the palms and soles with small ulcers in the mouth. More often in children, and they may have fever and experience discomfort	Supportive therapy only	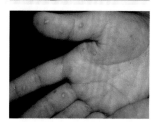
Herpes simplex (HSV-1 and HSV-2)	Groups of vesicles that ulcerate and then crust over. There is significant pain before and during the visible skin manifestations	Oral antiviral therapy including acyclovir and valacyclovir	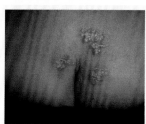
Molluscum contagiosum (poxvirus)	Pearly papules with central umbilication. Not painful but may itch	Cryotherapy, topical salicylic acid, topical imiquimod	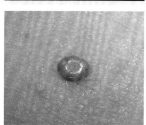
Chickenpox and zoster (varicella zoster virus)	Varicela starts with crops of vesicles that then crust over. These can be distributed from head to toe. Zoster is a reactivation which is usually confined to a single dermatome. Both conditions are painful	Oral antiviral therapy including acyclovir and valacyclovir	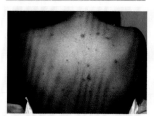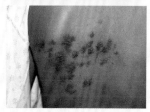

Table 19.9 ▶ Common Infestations

Diagnosis	Treatment	Image
Scabies (*Sarcoptes scabiei*)	Topical permethrin, other topical medicines, oral ivermectin	
Lice (head, body, pubic) (*Pediculosis capitis, Pediculosis corporis, Pediculosis pubis*)	Topical permethrin, other topical medicines, oral ivermectin	
Cutaneous larva migrans (*Ancylostoma*)	Oral albendazole or oral ivermectin	

Table 19.10 ▶ Basal Cell Carcinomas

Type	Characteristics	How Aggressive	Image
Nodular	Elevated, pearly, telangiectasias, ulcers	Moderately aggressive, especially if micronodular	

Type	Characteristics	How Aggressive	Image
Superficial	Relatively flat, thready border, spotted pigmentation	Least aggressive	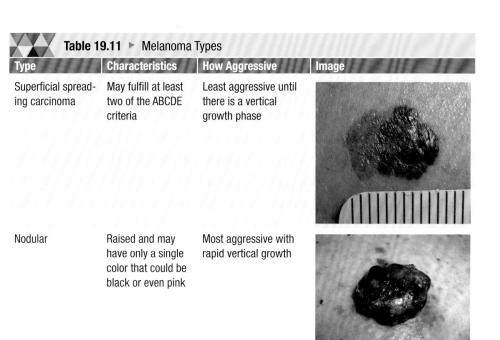
Sclerosing/ infiltrative	Scar-like, indurated, may be elevated or ulcerated	Most aggressive	

Table 19.11 ▶ Melanoma Types

Type	Characteristics	How Aggressive	Image
Superficial spreading carcinoma	May fulfill at least two of the ABCDE criteria	Least aggressive until there is a vertical growth phase	
Nodular	Raised and may have only a single color that could be black or even pink	Most aggressive with rapid vertical growth	

(continued)

Table 19.11 ▶ Melanoma Types (Continued)

Type	Characteristics	How Aggressive	Image
Lentigo maligna	Tends to occur on the face of elderly persons with significant sun exposure, may be flat and slow-growing	Tends to grow horizontally and slowly but can be difficult to treat due to its most common location on the face	
Acral lentiginous	Occurs on the hands and feet including in the nail unit	Can be very aggressive	
Amelanotic	Usually pink- or skin-colored and can be a pink nodule	Can be very aggressive and is not recognized by the ABCDE criteria	

Sun exposure is the most important risk factor; other risk factors include a positive family history and fair skin type. The incidence of these cancers increases with age, probably because of cumulative sun exposure. However, all of these skin cancers can occur in non–sun-exposed areas.

BCC and SCC are most commonly found on the head and neck followed by the trunk and extremities. SCCs occur more often in persons who are immunosuppressed such as patients taking medications to prevent transplant rejection. SCCs occur on the lower lip and also may be found on the hands, genitalia, and perianal regions related to human papilloma virus exposure.

Sun protection is essential for the prevention of skin cancers and photo aging. Sun protection includes:

▶ Sun avoidance, especially during the midday sun
▶ Protective clothing
▶ Protective hats, especially with a broad brim
▶ Sunscreens

QUESTIONS

1. For evaluating patients with skin lesions, which one of the following increases the sensitivity and specificity of skin cancer diagnosis?
   A. History of onset of the lesion.
   B. Reported precipitants of the lesion.
   C. The presence of erosion of the lesion.
   D. Use Wood light examination.
   E. Use of a dermatoscope for examination.

2. A parent brings a 4-year-old to see you who has an itchy papular rash that began on her face and is now located primarily in the flexural areas of her arms and legs. Which one of the following conditions is likely in this patient?
   A. Contact dermatitis.
   B. Eczema (atopic dermatitis).
   C. Seborrheic dermatitis.
   D. Impetigo.
   E. Tinea corporis.

3. You are seeing a teenager with acne that is primarily characterized by open and closed comedones. Nonprescription creams have not been helpful. Which one of the following is most beneficial for this type of acne?
   A. Topical retinoids.
   B. Topical antibiotics.
   C. Oral antibiotics.
   D. Oral isotretinoin.

4. Which one of the following is true of psoriasis?
   A. Lesions are diffuse and papular.
   B. Nail changes are seen in virtually all patients.
   C. Topical steroids and topical vitamin D are often beneficial.
   D. Systemic steroids are used in patients with more severe psoriasis.
   E. Narrowband ultraviolet B light is used if psoriatic arthritis is present.

5. Which one of the following is true of evaluation and treatment of skin cancer?
   A. The ABCDE criteria help determine presence of BCC.
   B. SCC is most common.
   C. Family history is the most important risk factor.
   D. Sun protection is essential for the prevention of skin cancers.
   E. Amelanotic melanoma is the least aggressive.

ANSWERS

Question 1: The correct answer is E.
Dermoscopy increases the sensitivity and specificity of skin cancer diagnosis.

Question 2: The correct answer is B.
As shown in Table 19.3, atopic dermatitis starts in childhood on the face and then involves flexural areas.

Question 3: The correct answer is A.
As shown in Table 19.4, treatment for comedogenic acne includes topical agents such as benzyl peroxide and retinoids; retinoids are the most beneficial.

Question 4: The correct answer is C.
Treatment options for psoriasis are many and varied. Psoriasis that involves less than 5% of the body surface area can often be treated with topical steroids and topical vitamin D. The most common treatment of psoriasis involves topical steroids (see Table 19.5), with strong ointments being the most effective.

Question 5: The correct answer is D.
Sun protection is essential for the prevention of skin cancers and photo aging. Sun protection includes sun avoidance, especially during the midday sun, protective clothing; protective hats, especially with a broad brim; and sunscreens.

REFERENCES

1. Argenziano G, Puig S, Zalaudek I, et al. Dermoscopy improves accuracy of primary care physicians to triage lesions suggestive of skin cancer. *J Clin Oncol.* 2006;24(12):1877–1882.
2. Edwards F, de Berker D. Nail psoriasis: clinical presentation and best practice recommendations. *Drugs.* 2009;69(17):2351–2361.
3. Hsu S, Papp KA, Lebwohl MG, et al. Consensus guidelines for the management of plaque psoriasis. *Arch Dermatol.* 2012;148(1):95–102.
4. Stevens DL, Bisno AL, Chambers HF, et al. Practice guidelines for the diagnosis and management of skin and soft tissue infections: 2014 update by the Infectious Diseases Society of America. *Clin Infect Dis.* 2014;59(2):e10–52.
5. Katalinic A, Kunze U, Schäfer T. Epidemiology of cutaneous melanoma and non-melanoma skin cancer in Schleswig-Holstein, Germany: incidence, clinical subtypes, tumour stages and localization (epidemiology of skin cancer). *Br J Dermatol.* 2003;149(6):1200–1206.
6. Leiter U, Eigentler T, Garbe C. Epidemiology of skin cancer. *Adv Exp Med Biol.* 2014;810:120–140.
7. Rogers HW, Weinstock MA, Feldman SR, et al. Incidence estimate of nonmelanoma skin cancer (keratinocyte carcinomas) in the U.S. *population,* 2012. *JAMA Dermatol.* 2015;151(10):1081–1086. http://jamanetwork.com/journals/jamadermatology/fullarticle/2281227.

Chronic Pain

KEY POINTS

1 ▶ A comprehensive pain evaluation is needed prior to development of a treatment plan.

2 ▶ The management of chronic pain is often best approached from a multidisciplinary perspective.

3 ▶ Pain management includes nonpharmacologic and pharmacologic treatments.

4 ▶ The use of opioids in the management of chronic pain introduces complex issues including appropriate patient selection, abuse and misuse, side effects, and special monitoring procedures

5 ▶ Careful documentation of goals, response to treatment, and revisions of the treatment plan are essential for safe and effective chronic pain management.

6 ▶ Buprenorphine and naloxone are becoming useful adjuncts in managing chronic pain and misuse disorders.

Martha is a 43-year-old woman establishing care at your clinic. She transferred her records to your office and brings a copy of them to this visit. She is employed, smokes, but does not drink more than two alcoholic drinks weekly. Her only documented medical problem is fibromyalgia. Her previous physician was treating her fibromyalgia with hydrocodone/APAP three times daily with an additional dose, as needed, once daily, which she generally takes. She is concerned about her monthly prescription refill (120 tablets) due in 28 days.

Chronic pain is one of the most common problems in primary care, and one of the most difficult to manage.[1] Over 100 million Americans suffer from chronic pain, with an associated economic burden of $560 to $600 billion annually.[2–5] With our aging population, we can expect an increase in the already substantial number of patients with chronic pain-seeking care.

We have witnessed, in the past 10 years, a proliferation of pain guidelines, regulations, specialized clinics, research, pain journals, and specialized training in pain medicine.[6] One of the main drivers for the guidelines, including new recommendations from the Surgeon General, has been the huge number of opiate-related deaths annually in the United States (28,647 in 2014 and 33,091 in 2015), now outstripping annual death rates from automobile accidents.[7]

Despite this, inadequate pain management persists in primary care. This is due, in part, to physician barriers of lack of treatment knowledge, inadequate pain-assessment skills, and fear of regulatory scrutiny, as well as patient factors such as risk for respiratory depression, worsening sleep apnea, overdose and death, increased fracture risk, and opioid-use disorder.[8]

A comprehensive and organized approach is needed to be successful in treating the many pain syndromes that present to primary care. Common pain conditions include chronic neck and low-back pain, migraine and other headache syndromes, osteoarthritis, fibromyalgia, chronic abdominal and pelvic pain, diabetic neuropathy, postherpetic neuralgia, phantom pain secondary to disease or injury of the nervous system, poststroke pain, multiple sclerosis, and mixed pain syndromes.

GENERAL APPROACH TO TREATMENT OF CHRONIC PAIN

A chronic pain treatment plan should be thorough and include a comprehensive evaluation, development of a treatment plan based on diagnosis and pain mechanisms, patient education, and realistic goal setting. The treatment plan includes maintenance and monitoring phases.[6,9] Treatment plans should address the patient's physical, social, functional, and psychological needs,[10] with the **goal to improve quality of life, increase function, and decrease pain.**

Not all three may be achievable. While treatment modalities are recommended in guidelines, actual evidence of the effectiveness of most treatment options is lacking. Successful treatment requires a fine balance between pain relief and improvement in quality of life on the one hand and medication side effects and risks on the other (Fig. 20.1).

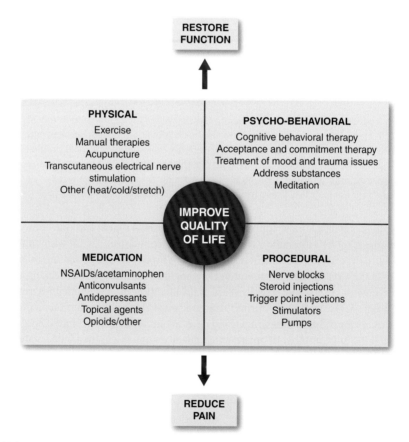

Figure 20.1 ► Treatment options that support goals. Data from Massachusetts Medical Society Webinar "Incorporating the New Opioid Prescribing Guidelines into Practice" by Daniel Alford, MD, MPH, FACP, FASAM. http://www.massmed.org/Patient-Care/Health-Topics/Opioids/Incorporating-the-New-Opioid-Prescribing-Guidelines-Into-Practice-(Webinar)

As a first step, Martha's records should be reviewed to determine if her treatment plan is appropriate.

A comprehensive and organized approach is shown in Table 20.1. This approach is based on the 2013 Federation of State Medical Boards (FSMB) Model Policy on Use of Opioid Analgesics in the Treatment of Chronic Pain.[9] Diversion, addiction and abuse of opioid medications, lack of knowledge, concerns about opioid side effects, and fears of regulatory scrutiny[11,12] are challenges that can be overcome by adherence to this type of structure.

Table 20.1 ▶ Approach to the Use of Opioid Analgesics in the Treatment of Chronic Pain[a]

Patient Evaluation

Perform and document a medical history and physical that includes:
- Nature/intensity of pain
- Current/past treatment for pain
- Underlying/coexisting disease or conditions
- Effect of pain on function (physical/psychological)
- History of substance abuse
- Document if a controlled substance is indicated medically

Treatment Plan

A written treatment plan should:
- State objectives to determine success
- State if further diagnostic tests are indicated
- Address psychosocial as well as physical function
- Adjust therapy to meet patient needs
- Use nonpharmacologic treatment modalities in addition to medication

Informed Consent and Agreement for Treatment
- Discuss risks/benefits of drug therapy with patient or surrogate
- Patient should receive prescriptions from one physician and pharmacy whenever possible
- High-risk patients should have a written agreement that includes:
  a. Urine drug screens when requested
  b. Written documentation of refill numbers and frequency
  c. Reasons for which drug therapy may be discontinued (violations of agreement)

Consultation

Be willing to refer to achieve objectives. Special attention should be given to patients at risk for medication misuse, abuse, or diversion. Consultation may be required in those with:
- Psychiatric disorders
- Substance abuse issues (past or present)

Periodic Review

The clinician should:
- Periodically review the course of pain treatment and any new information about the etiology of the pain
- Evaluate and modify drug treatment based upon:
  a. Patient's response
  b. Objective evidence of improved/diminished function
  c. If progress is unsatisfactory, assess the appropriateness of continuing or modifying therapy

(continued)

Table 20.1 ▶ Approach to the Use of Opioid Analgesics in the Treatment of Chronic Pain[a] *(Continued)*

Medical Records
Documentation should include:
- Medical history and physical
- Diagnostic tests and lab results
- Evaluations and consultations
- Treatment objectives and treatments
- Informed consent and discussion of risks and benefits
- Medication and refill documentation
- Instructions and agreements
- Periodic reviews
Records are to be current and easily assessable for review

Compliance with Controlled Substances Laws and Regulations
- State and Federal Regulations must be met
- Refer to USDEA and state medical boards for relevant documents

[a]Data from Model Policy on the Use of Opioid Analgesics in the Treatment of Chronic Pain. Federation of State Medical Boards of the United States, Inc. Available at http://www.fsmb.org/Media/Default/PDF/FSMB/Advocacy/pain_policy_july2013.pdf. Accessed December 2016.

When psychiatric comorbidities are present, risk of substance abuse is high and specialized treatments, consultation, or referral to a pain management specialist can be helpful and appropriate.[12] Patients, like Martha, who suffer from chronic pain often have accompanying mood disorders, so inquiring about this will be important. Certain types of chronic pain are also more common in those who have suffered trauma, such as adult survivors of physical, psychological, or sexual abuse. A diagnosis of posttraumatic stress disorder (PTSD) similarly increases risk for chronic pain.

TYPES OF CHRONIC PAIN

Chronic pain is characterized as either nociceptive or neuropathic.

▶ **Nociceptive pain** arises from tissue injury and/or inflammation, often from musculoskeletal, inflammatory, or mechanical/compression. Common conditions described as associated with nociceptive pain include osteoarthritis, low-back pain, and posttraumatic pain. Nociceptive pain often responds to NSAIDs and opioid medications, implicating opioid receptors in this type of pain.

▶ **Neuropathic pain** occurs when a pathologic process causes damage or injury to nerve tissue either in the peripheral or central nervous system. Numerous medical disorders are associated with injury or toxic effects on neurons, resulting in alterations of neural processing. Neuropathic pain is often described as "burning, electrical, zinging, lightning, ice-like, shooting, tingling, or lancinating." Common examples include diabetic neuropathy, postherpetic neuralgia, trigeminal neuralgia, and possibly fibromyalgia. Neuropathic pain responds predominantly to nonopioid adjuvant medications such as anticonvulsants and antidepressants.

▶ Most chronic pain syndromes are **mixed pain syndromes**, which have both nociceptive and neuropathic components. For this reason, chronic pain rarely responds to a single pharmacologic intervention. This concept provides the basis for using combinations of medications with different mechanisms.

CLINICAL EVALUATION

History and Physical Examination

A chronic pain evaluation consists of pain history, past medical history, social and psychiatric history, and physical examination. It is important to assess the pain's quality, type, timing, distribution, and relieving and exacerbating factors. In doing so:

▸ Identify the pain as nociceptive (tissue injury), neuropathic (a neurologic response to neural or nonneural injury), or both.

▸ Quantify the pain using visual analog scales such as Faces Pain Scale (http://www.iasp-pain.org/Education/Content.aspx?ItemNumber=1519) and/or the 0 to 10 numeric rating scales. These scales have been validated, are simple to administer, and can be used with young children, cognitively impaired individuals, and patients with language barriers. They are useful for identifying pain and documenting treatment response.[13,14] Martha's pain between doses of medication is sometimes 8 out of 10.

History should include prior evaluations of the painful condition, prior surgical and nonsurgical treatments, all nonpharmacologic and pharmacologic treatments, and any comorbid and psychiatric conditions. Effects of the patient's pain on quality of life, activity, work, sleep, mood, and relationships should be documented.

The physician should review past records and documentation to determine if criteria for resuming and continuing any previous treatments are met. Establishing and confirming a legitimate chronic pain diagnosis is important; consider further investigations if indicated and be watchful for conditions such as malingering, factitious disorder, drug seeking, or other aberrant behavior.

A social and psychiatric history will alert the physician to issues such as current or past substance abuse, depression, anxiety, or other factors that may interfere with achieving pain treatment goals. Current level of functioning and support network is also important.

A patient's risk of opioid abuse should also be evaluated. Chapter 23 contains information about an opioid risk assessment tool. Other tools can be found in this chapter's references.[13,15–18] In addition, state prescription drug monitoring programs (PDMPs) have been enacted or are operational in nearly all states.[19] PDMPs collect prescription data from physicians and pharmacies, and the data are made available to regulatory agencies and health care providers. It is believed that these programs will be useful for identifying, reducing, and possibly eliminating routes of diversion.[20]

By identifying patients at risk for possible opioid misuse, such as those with a history of prior or current substance abuse or those with serious psychiatric issues, you can choose to modify the treatment plan or refer to a pain specialist.

A physical examination provides an opportunity to evaluate objective findings in the area of pain, determine neurologic and musculoskeletal function, and observe any physical disability resulting from the chronic pain condition.

After reviewing Martha's history, it appears she has fought depression but never been formally treated. She had a good medical workup for her symptoms and meets the diagnostic criteria for fibromyalgia. She has no recorded urine drug screens, no red flags for abuse, and no evidence of opioid risk tools being used. Objective diagnostic and physical findings are few in fibromyalgia, which makes treatment more challenging.

Diagnostic Testing

Diagnostic testing may be performed to determine or verify a diagnosis, rule out more ominous disorders, and identify comorbid medical conditions. This could include laboratory studies and radiologic investigations depending on the patient's presenting complaints. Occasionally, an interventional diagnostic test may help clarify the cause of a patient's pain.

Diagnostic interventions include selective spinal nerve root block to determine the level of pathology if an MRI is inconclusive; discography to determine if a disc is the "pain generator"; and nerve blocks prior to radiofrequency lesioning to project treatment efficacy.

MANAGEMENT

You believe that Martha's pain management may need to be changed and updated to reflect some of the new guidelines available that do not recommend use of opioids in the treatment of fibromyalgia.

The general management of chronic pain includes developing and documenting a treatment plan and including setting realistic goals for treatment. The treatment plan should have achievable goals such as improvement of function and quality of life. Treatment options for chronic pain should include nonpharmacologic and pharmacologic modalities. Nonpharmacologic modalities include lifestyle and psychological approaches, complementary and alternative medicine, physical therapy, and interventional medical procedures. Pharmacologic treatments include adjunctive medications and nonopioid and opioid analgesics.

When a choice is made to use opioids, you should follow the guidelines of the FSMB. The FSMB stresses appropriate patient selection by: Assessment of risk factors for medication misuse, use of opioid agreements, choice of opioid medication, periodic review of treatment effectiveness, use of urine drug tests, addressing psychiatric issues, and minimizing medication side effects.

Developing and Documenting a Treatment Plan

The character or mechanism of the patient's pain, the specific pain disorder diagnosis, and the intensity of the pain help determine appropriate treatment choices.[21] Once the pain disorder diagnosis is determined, an individualized treatment plan is developed and documented, and the diagnosis, management options, and goals of treatment are discussed with the patient.

Successful management begins with patient education and setting realistic goals.[21] Completely eliminating pain is rarely a realistic goal; improving quality of life should be the focus. Nonpharmacologic options, with or without medication, are tried initially.[6] Nonpharmacologic treatments such as physical therapy, exercise, yoga, counseling, relaxation,

Table 20.2 ▶ Initial Pharmacologic Choices Based on Pain Type

Nociceptive Pain	Neuropathic Pain	Mixed Pain
First line	First line	First line
• Nonsteroidal anti-inflammatory drugs, high-dose acetaminophen	• Topical lidocaine, tricyclic antidepressants, SNRIs, gabapentin, or pregabalin	• Nonsteroidal anti-inflammatory drugs, high-dose acetaminophen
Second line	Second line	Second line
• Opioids	• Tramadol or opioids	• Antidepressants, anticonvulsants, topical lidocaine
Third line	Third line	Third line
• Adjunctive antidepressants, anticonvulsants, topical lidocaine	• Other opioids, topical capsaicin, anticonvulsants (e.g., carbamazepine, Valproic acid)	• Opioid/nonopioid combinations (limited by maximum dose of nonopioid component)

or cognitive-behavioral therapy require patient participation and motivation. This will take time. While the hope is that these strategies will result in improved physical mobility, fitness, mood, sleep and general health, it may be very difficult for patients who may have avoided engaging in any activity that may exacerbate the pain—the so-called pain-avoidance cycle.

Pharmacologic treatment depends upon the pain disorder diagnosis and whether the underlying pain mechanism is characterized as nociceptive, neuropathic, or mixed (Table 20.2).[1,8,11,21,22]

Initial pharmacologic choices should be nonopioids. If opioids are used, start with weaker opioids in immediate-release formulations with titration upward if needed. Medication combinations target different locations along the pain pathways, and drug side effects and additive effects are often used to treat coexisting complaints.[23]

Opioids have been shown to improve moderate to severe acute pain;[24] however, the evidence to support long-term use of opioids to reduce pain and improve function in patients with chronic pain is, at best, weak.[25] Despite this, consensus remains in favor of opioid use for moderate to severe chronic pain in well-selected patients, with adequate supervision. Martha may fall into this group, but if she has underlying depression, alternative or adjunctive treatments should be considered.

The decision to use opioids should be based on a set of guiding principles, previously reviewed, and justification for their use must be determined and documented. The prescriber should also have a clear understanding of opioid pharmacokinetics and the anticipated and unanticipated consequences of opioid use. These include tolerance, dependence, addiction, pseudoaddiction, abuse, and adverse side effects. Each clinician should also be familiar with the rules and regulations for the use of controlled substances for treatment of pain in each state where they practice.

Misuse or addiction issues arise in 8% to 29% of patients using opioids for pain.[26] The strongest predictors of misuse are personal or family history of substance abuse, younger age, and the presence of psychiatric conditions.[26] Other known risk factors are age <41 years, male sex, unemployed status, psychiatric comorbidity (personality, anxiety, depressive, or bipolar disorder), and social factors such as a history of legal problems or motor vehicle accidents.[27]

High-risk patients can be treated with opioids but may require a more regimented and strict monitoring program, including other disciplines. This may include more frequent visits, increased random urine drug testing (UDT), and the provision of fewer medications at each visit. Advice from an addiction specialist or pain specialist may be necessary when risk of abuse outweighs the benefits of opioid use.

It is essential for the patient to understand that opioids are *one part* of a multimodal treatment plan. Current guidelines suggest that an improvement of 2 to 3 points on the 0 to 10 pain scale is a reasonable expectation.[27] More importantly, setting small but achievable functional goals, such as walking three blocks, going back to work, or increasing outdoor activity, will help the patient remain motivated but realistic. Tobacco use and weight issues also need to be addressed.

Informed consent and agreement for treatment is accomplished through use of "opioid agreements."[28] The agreement provides written documentation of the diagnosis, medications, discussions between physician and patient about opioid use, and anticipated and unanticipated consequences of use. This agreement also includes the conditions that the patient must meet to improve the safety of opioid use and limit the risk of abuse. A sample agreement from the journal *Family Practice Management* is here: https://www.aafp.org/fpm/2010/1100/fpm20101100p22-rt1.pdf.

Prescribing Opioid Medications

Careful prescribing and judicious use are keys to successful use of opioids in managing pain. The CDC has guidelines for prescribing opioids for chronic pain (https://www.cdc.gov/mmwr/volumes/65/rr/rr6501e1.htm#) summarized in Box 20.1, as well as a checklist (https://www.cdc.gov/drugoverdose/pdf/PDO_Checklist-a.pdf).

Methadone, fentanyl, and OxyContin have markedly contributed to fatal drug overdoses, both intentionally and unintentionally,[29,30] and most opioid overdose deaths involve

---

BOX 20.1 GUIDELINES FOR PRESCRIBING OPIOIDS FOR CHRONIC PAIN

► Nonpharmacologic and nonopioid therapies are preferred

► Opioids should be prescribed only after setting clear treatment goals focused on improving function and pain control

► Risks of opioid use should be discussed

► Prefer immediate-release over extended-release opioids, avoiding methadone

► Prescribe lowest effective dose of opioids.[a] Use caution when prescribing opioids in doses that exceed 50 morphine milligram equivalents (MME) daily and avoid prescribing over 90 MME daily.[6]

► Limit opioids to 3 days for acute pain

► Review appropriateness of opioid use in 1–4 weeks and then no less often then every 3 months

► Avoid opioids in high-risk patients or use additional referral resources for comanagement; consider coprescribing naloxone

► Consider urine drug testing before starting opioid therapy and periodically thereafter

► Avoid use of opioid pain medication and benzodiazepine concurrently

► Monitor for opioid use disorder and arrange for treatment if present

[a]The CDC has an MME chart at https://www.cdc.gov/drugoverdose/pdf/calculating_total_daily_dose-a.pdf

more than one drug.[31] Methadone, for example, has enhanced toxicity when combined with benzodiazepines; deaths are believed to be related to systemic accumulation of methadone causing QT interval prolongation and torsade de pointes.[32] Heroin laced with synthetic opioids contributes significantly to drug overdose deaths as well.

Buprenorphine and Naloxone

Buprenorphine is considered safe and effective for the treatment of opioid dependency, especially in combination with counseling and behavioral therapies. Unlike methadone, which must be dispensed in a highly structured clinic, buprenorphine has no special prescribing restrictions, significantly increasing treatment access. Buprenorphine is an opioid partial agonist. Like opioids, it produces effects such as euphoria or respiratory depression, but these effects are weaker than those of full agonists such as heroin or methadone. Buprenorphine has a significantly reduced effect on physical dependency with reduced withdrawal effects and is safer in cases of overdose.

Naloxone is a lifesaving drug that can temporarily stop or reverse overdose by opioids by blocking opioid receptor sites, reversing their effects. Naloxone can be given by intranasal spray, intramuscularly, subcutaneously, or intravenously. Ambulances often carry and dispense naloxone in the field in cases of suspected overdose. New treatment guidelines include recommendations for giving prescriptions for intranasal naloxone to those who use opioids chronically, with instructions for use. Naloxone is also combined with buprenorphine. Links to further information are available in the references.[33,34]

> In considering Martha's situation, you note that opioid treatment has little supporting evidence of success for fibromyalgia. You decide to broach the topic of opioid weaning and tapering. You offer to reschedule her for a more extensive visit to explain your plan. She accepts and returns in 3 days for a longer visit and discussion. You review your clinic chronic pain guidelines (based on the CDC and FSMB guidelines) and explain that opioids may not be the best treatment for her and that counseling and further nonpharmacologic intervention might be more appropriate.

Patient Monitoring

Follow-up visits allow you to monitor treatment effectiveness, side effects, adherence, and patient behaviors that may indicate violation of the opioid agreement or medication misuse. These visits also allow discussion of direction for further treatment and goal revision.

Follow-up chronic pain management tools are available,[35] and increasingly, electronic medical records are integrating them. At a minimum, the PEG scale, a Likert scale that addresses average **P**ain, **E**njoyment of life, and **G**eneral activity should be assessed at follow-up visits,[36] as well as all components of the six As[35]:

▶ **A**nalgesia
▶ **A**ffect (mood)
▶ **A**ctivities (evaluate activities of daily living and function)
▶ **A**djuncts (nonpharmacologic/nonopioid treatments)
▶ **A**dverse effects (side effects of treatment)
▶ **A**berrant behavior (tolerance, dependence, and addiction-like behaviors)

Early in treatment or with treatment plan adjustments, patient return intervals will be relatively frequent. Once stable, follow-up intervals of no less than every 3 months are recommended.

UDT is not legally required but is recommended by many guidelines.[9,35] Appropriately used, UDT can assist in the management of chronic pain with opioids by uncovering illicit drug use and confirming treatment adherence even in the absence of behaviors suggestive of medication misuse. The use of UDT, together with monitoring for aberrant behaviors results in the highest rate of identification of misuse of opioid medication in patients with chronic pain.[37]

Prescribing clinicians should understand which medications are screened in their specific laboratory, as pain panels and opioid screening tests vary between labs. Some patients refrain from illicit substance use prior to office visits and provide misleading UDTs. Random UDT is therefore the preferred method of testing. Clinicians using UDT should be familiar with opiate and opioid metabolites as well.[38] This monograph can help with considerations regarding urine testing: http://www.udtmonograph6.com/view-monograph.html.

Prior to UDT, physicians should anticipate actions that will be prompted by a positive UDT (a test showing nonprescribed or illicit substances or absence of prescribed substances). All positive UDTs must be addressed and should result in some action—dismissal, referral for substance abuse counseling or treatment, or refusal to prescribe further controlled substances.

Monitor and remain vigilant for aberrant behaviors that may suggest medication misuse during follow-up visits. Aberrant behaviors include use of pain medications for reasons other than pain, impaired control (of self or use of medication), compulsive use of medication, continued use of medication despite harm (or lack of benefit), and craving or escalation of medication use.[39] Selling, altering prescriptions, stealing or diverting medications, early refill requests, losing prescriptions, drug-seeking behavior, doctor shopping, or reluctance to try nonpharmacologic interventions are other examples of aberrant behavior.[39]

At Martha's follow-up visit, she acknowledges being depressed and mentions a traumatic event in her life that, at the moment, she prefers not to discuss. This gets you thinking about PTSD and the interplay between her physical pain and her psychological distress. You initiate a discussion about SNRIs, common antidepressants used for chronic pain syndromes. She finds the possibility of addressing these issues and use of an SNRI to help her pain encouraging, and it makes the opioid tapering conversation go a bit smoother.

Psychiatric problems including mood disorders, anxiety, somatoform disorders, substance abuse, and personality disorders are frequent comorbid conditions. An understanding of their diagnosis and treatment is essential.[40]

Medication Side Effects

Medication side effects, especially of opioids, need to be addressed and anticipated. Side effects include respiratory suppression (especially in those with sleep apnea), somnolence, nausea, sedation (tolerance or resolution usually develops within 10 days), and constipation (no tolerance or resolution develops).

Patients starting opioids can take a combination stimulant/softener laxative to prevent constipation. Senna with docusate sodium, for example, is commonly used; an antinausea medication can also be added for 10 days. Avoid use of stool bulking agents as they can worsen constipation in those taking opioids, as constipation is due to slowing of stool transit time.

Chronic use of sustained-release opioids is associated with hypogonadism. Evidence is not sufficient to recommend routine testosterone testing in asymptomatic patients, but if symptoms such as significantly decreased libido, sexual dysfunction, fatigue, or a poor sense of well-being are reported, it may be prudent to check testosterone levels (see Chapter 16). Prolonged administration of opiates is also associated with tolerance and possibly increased pain sensitivity, known as *opiate-induced hypernociception*. This may result in paradoxical pain in regions of the body unrelated to the initial pain stimulus and is thought to be mediated through cytokine dysregulation.[41]

Other potential medication problems encountered in patients with chronic pain include prolonged QT with methadone and NSAID-related peptic ulcer disease, dyspepsia, chronic renal insufficiency, hypertension, renal failure, and congestive heart failure exacerbations. Acetaminophen is associated with liver toxicity in high doses and should be avoided in those with significant liver dysfunction or alcohol use disorders.[27,42,43]

> You explain to Martha that close monitoring no less often than every 3 months, routine and random UDT, and risk tools are part of her opioid agreement. You recommend a slow taper from her opioids. She is very apprehensive about this and you offer to refer her to a pain specialist for a second opinion. She defers and wants more information about tapering as she is beginning to trust you and your judgment.

Referral and Pain Clinics

When chronic pain problems persist despite appropriate multidimensional management and ongoing opioid use, referral to a pain management specialist is suggested.[39,41] Patients with a history of substance abuse or interpersonal dynamics that seem to be complicating pain treatment may benefit from a consultation.[12,40]

Pain specialists may provide suggestions for further evaluation (imaging studies, neurologic testing, surgical or physiatrist consultation) for complex pain problems that are difficult to manage. Psychiatric consultation may be recommended to address psychiatric issues that often arise due to chronic pain or that interfere with successful pain management.

Interventional pain modalities have evolved significantly and include procedures to both further elucidate the etiology of chronic pain and to provide treatment. Diagnostic interventions are used to determine the level of spinal nerve pathology (selective spinal nerve root blocks), to determine if the pain originates from a disc (discography), and to improve radiofrequency lesioning effectiveness (nerve blocks).

Therapeutic interventions include epidural steroid injection for spinal nerve root inflammation, facet joint injection, radiofrequency lesioning, sacroiliac joint injection, sympathetic block (stellate or lumbar blocks) for complex regional pain syndrome, Botox injections for spasm, nucleoplasty or annuloplasty for discogenic pain, and implantation of devices such as spinal cord stimulators and intrathecal drug infusion pumps for refractory pain. Deep brain stimulation has also been attempted for intractable neuropathic pain.[44] Table 20.3 lists treatment efficacy evidence based on the Cochrane Collaboration (www.cochranelibrary.com).

Table 20.3 ▸ Key Therapies for Chronic Pain with Evidence of Effectiveness[a]

Intervention	Evidence	Comments and Cautions
Lifestyle and Psychological Approaches		
Weight loss, tobacco or alcohol cessation, PT, counseling, hypnosis		No reviews of efficacy regarding chronic pain
CBT/BT	Maintained at 6 months for CBT	CBT: Weak effects on improving pain, mood and disability; BT: No effect
Exercise	Low quality	Effective for fibromyalgia symptoms
	High quality	Improves OA hip pain—10 RCTs[b]
	Good	OA—high-quality evidence for reduced knee pain and moderate for improved physical function
	Slight effect	Effective for nonspecific chronic LBP
Manipulation	High quality	As effective as standard care for LBP
Occupational therapy/ back schools	Low quality	Uncertain if back schools are effective for acute and subacute nonspecific LBP
TENS	Studies lack rigor	Insufficient evidence to recommend (4 RCTs)
Drug Therapy		
Salicylates, opioid combinations		No reviews of efficacy regarding chronic pain
Atypical antidepressants (NNT = 3)	Moderate evidence	Venlafaxine effective for neuropathic pain
		Duloxetine (60 and 120 mg) effective for diabetic neuropathy and fibromyalgia
NSAIDs/acetaminophen	Modest effects	Superior to placebo for chronic pain
Opioids, long-term	Weak	Clinically significant pain relief but many discontinue due to adverse side effects
Opioids, noncombination	Very low to moderate quality	Effective for short term (<120 days) pain relief, no placebo-RCTs for chronic LBP effectiveness
	Variable quality	Hydromorphone is as effective as morphine
	Contradictory and equivocal studies	No better than placebo for long-term neuropathic pain
Tramadol	NNT = 3.8, NNH = 8.3	Effective for neuropathic pain and small benefits for OA
Adjunctive Drug Therapy		
Antidepressants	No clear evidence	No evidence for LBP
	NNT = 3	TCAs are effective for neuropathic pain
Anticonvulsants	NNT = 5.9 (DN)	Gabapentin effective for neuropathic pain
		Carbamazepine probably effective for neuropathic pain
		Lamotrigine not effective for neuropathic pain
		Pregabalin effective for neuropathic pain and fibromyalgia

Intervention	Evidence	Comments and Cautions
Topicals	Versus placebo NNT = 6.9–9.8 NNT = 8.8	Salicylate analog not effective Diclofenac and ketoprofen provide relief in OA for some; no evidence for other chronic pain conditions No evidence from high-quality RCTs for topical lidocaine to treat neuropathic pain High concentration for PHN and HIV-neuropathy generates more pain relief than control
Medical Procedures		
Nucleopathy/ annuloplasty Intrathecal infusion		No reviews of efficacy regarding chronic pain
Sympathectomy	Low quality	No evidence to recommend for neuropathic or CRPS pain
Epidural, facet joints, TP injection; Botox injection, Radiofrequency denervation	Heterogeneous studies	Insufficient evidence to support use for LBP or chronic LBP for radiofrequency denervation
Sympathetic block	Low quality	Unable to conclude; scarcity of studies for CRPS
Deep brain stimulation	Heterogeneous	May have small short-term effects on chronic pain
Complementary/Alternative Therapies		
Biofeedback, yoga, stretching, reflexology		No reviews of efficacy regarding chronic pain
Mindfulness meditation	Very low quality	Effectiveness remains unclear for treating fibromyalgia
Relaxation therapy	Low quality	
Movement therapy	Very low quality	
Biofeedback	Low quality	
Acupuncture	Low quality	Chronic low-back pain: More effective than no or sham treatment up to 3 months. As effective as conventional treatment; may be useful adjunct Migraine or TTH: (at least 6 treatment sessions) effective
	Moderate quality Heterogeneous study quality	Fibromyalgia: (at least 6 treatment sessions) improves pain and stiffness
Behavioral: Operant, cognitive, respondent	Low quality	Various minor effects, not much added benefit for treatment of chronic LBP
Herbal and Chinese medication	Moderate quality Low quality Low to moderate quality	Slight to moderate improvement in short-term OA pain Compound Qishe tablet more effective than placebo for chronic neck pain secondary to OA Four herbal medicines may reduce pain in acute and chronic LBP in the short-term and have few side effects

(continued)

Table 20.3 ▸ Key Therapies for Chronic Pain with Evidence of Effectiveness[a] *(Continued)*

Intervention	Evidence	Comments and Cautions
Massage	Low or very low quality	Massage may be effective for pain from acute, subacute, and chronic LBP in short-term follow-up
Music therapy	NNT = 5	Music reduces pain intensity and opioid requirements but magnitude of benefits small. Review withdrawn
Touch therapies: Healing, therapeutic touch, Reiki		Modest effect in pain relief, more studies needed. This review is out of date and has been withdrawn

[a]The Cochrane Collaboration is an international nonprofit, independent organization focused on systemic reviews of health care interventions.
[b]A = consistent, good-quality patient-oriented evidence; B = inconsistent or limited-quality patient-oriented evidence; C = consensus, disease-oriented evidence, usual practice, expert opinion. For information about the SORT evidence rating system, see http://www.aafp.org/afpsort.xml.
CBT/BT, cognitive-behavioral therapy/behavioral therapy; CRPS, complex regional pain syndrome; DN, diabetic neuropathy; LBP, low-back pain; NNH, number needed to harm; NNT, number needed to treat; NSAID, nonsteroidal anti-inflammatory drug; OA, osteoarthritis; PHN, postherpetic neuralgia; PT, physical therapy; RCT, randomized controlled trial; TCA, tricyclic antidepressant; TENS, transcutaneous electrical nerve stimulation; TP, trigger point; TTH, tension-type headache.

QUESTIONS

1. In working with those who suffer chronic pain, the primary goal should be which one of the following?
   A. Eliminate pain.
   B. Improve function.
   C. Reduce harm from opiates.
   D. Prolong life.
   E. Work in teams.

2. First-line treatment for neuropathic pain may include which one of the following?
   A. Tramadol.
   B. Valproic acid.
   C. Tricyclic antidepressants.
   D. Opioids.
   E. Capsaicin.

3. In addition to potential addiction, anticipated consequences of opioid use could include which one of the following?
   A. Hypernociception
   B. Diarrhea.
   C. Tolerance.
   D. Hypergonadism.

4. Which one of the following is true of UDT in the management of patients with chronic pain who use opiates daily?
   A. Testing is mandatory in most states.
   B. Testing is useful for looking for drug side effects.
   C. Testing is best practice for each patient visit.
   D. Testing is best done without having discussed the use of UDT with the patient.
   E. Testing is helpful to confirm treatment adherence to prescribed opiates.

5. All patients who see primary care physicians for the management of chronic pain should be under the care of a pain management specialist.
   A. True.
   B. False.

ANSWERS

Question 1: The correct answer is B.
The primary goal in the care of the patient with chronic pain disorders is to improve quality of life, increase function, and decrease pain. Elimination of all pain is rarely achievable.

Question 2: The correct answer is C.
(Table 20.2) First-line treatment for neuropathic pain includes topical lidocaine, tricyclic antidepressants, SNRIs, gabapentin, and pregabalin.

Question 3: The correct answer is C.
The prescriber should also have a clear understanding of opioid pharmacokinetics and the anticipated and unanticipated consequences of opioid use. These include tolerance, dependence, addiction, pseudo-addiction, abuse, and adverse side effects.

Question 4: The correct answer is E.
UDT is not legally required but is recommended by many guidelines. Appropriately used, UDT can assist in the management of chronic pain with opioids by uncovering illicit drug use and confirming treatment adherence even in the absence of behaviors suggestive of medication misuse.

Question 5: The correct answer is B.
When chronic pain problems persist despite appropriate multidimensional management and ongoing opioid use, referral to a pain management specialist is suggested.

REFERENCES

1. Argoff C. Tailoring chronic pain treatment to the patient: Long-acting, short-acting and rapid-onset opioids. *Medscape Neurology & Neurosurgery.* 2007; Available at: www.medscape.com/viewarticle/554015. Accessed December 2016.
2. Institute of Medicine. *Relieving Pain in America: A Blueprint for Transforming Prevention, Care, Education, and Research.* Washington, DC: The National Academies Press; 2011.
3. Dzau VJ, Pizzo PA. Relieving pain in America: insights from an institute of medicine committee. *JAMA.* 2014;312(15):1507–1508.
4. Reuben DB, Alvanzo AA, Ashikaga T, et al. National Institutes of Health Pathways to Prevention Workshop: the role of opioids in the treatment of chronic pain. *Ann Intern Med.* 2015;162:295–300.
5. Walk D, Poliak-Tunis M. Chronic pain management: an overview of taxonomy, conditions commonly encountered, and assessment. *Med Clin North Am.* 2016;100(1):1–16.
6. Dowell D, Haegerich TM, Chou R. CDC Guideline for prescribing opioids for chronic pain—United States, 2016. *MMWR Recomm Rep.* 2016;65(1):1–49.
7. Rudd RA, Seth P, David F, et al. Increases in drug and opioid-involved overdose deaths—United States, 2010–2015. *MMWR Morb Mortal Wkly Rep.* 2016;65:1445–1452.
8. Glajchen M. Chronic pain: treatment barriers and strategies for clinical practice. *J Am Board Fam Pract.* 2001;14(3): 211–218.
9. Model policy on the use of opioid analgesics in the treatment of chronic pain. Federation of State Medical Boards of the United States, Inc. Available at: http://www.fsmb.org/Media/Default/PDF/FSMB/Advocacy/pain_policy_july2013.pdf. Accessed December 2016.
10. Brookoff D. Chronic pain: 1. A new disease? *Hosp Pract.* 2000;35:45–52.

11. Potter M, Schafer S, Gonzalez-Mendez E, et al. Opioids for chronic non-malignant pain. Attitudes and practices of primary care physicians in the UCSF/Standford Collaborative Network. University of California, San Francisco. *J Fam Pract*. 2001;50:145–151.
12. Gatchel RJ. Psychological disorders and chronic pain: cause-and-effect relationships. In Gatchel RJ, Turk DC, eds. *Psychological approaches to pain management: a practitioner's handbook*. New York: Guilford Press; 1996;36.
13. Jensen MP, Mcfarland CA. Increasing the reliability and validity of pain intensity measurement in chronic pain patients. *Pain*. 1998;55:195–203.
14. Bieri D, Reeve RA, Champion GD, et al. The faces pain scale for the self-assessment of the severity of pain experienced by children: development, initial validation, and preliminary investigation for ratio scale properties. *Pain*. 1990;41:139–150.
15. Webster LR, Webster RM. Predicting aberrant behaviors in opioid-treated patients: preliminary validation of the opioid risk tool. *Pain Med*. 2005;6:432–442.
16. Butler SF, Budman SH, Fernandez K, et al. Validation of a screener and opioid assessment measure for patients with chronic pain. *Pain*. 2007;112:65–75.
17. Passik SD, Kirsh KL, Whitcomb L, et al. A new tool to assess and document pain outcomes in chronic pain patients receiving opioid therapy. *Clin Ther*. 2004;26(4):552–561.
18. Butler SF, Budman SH, Fernandez KC, et al. Development and validation of the current opioid misuse measure. *Pain*. 2007;130(1–2):144–156.
19. Status of state prescription drug monitoring programs, July 2009. Available at: http://www.namsdl.org/library/1810E284-A0D7-D440-C3A9A0560A1115D7/. Accessed March 2017.
20. Wang J, Christo PJ. The influence of prescription monitoring programs on chronic pain management. *Pain Physician*. 2009;12(3):507–515.
21. Institute for Clinical Systems Improvement *Health Care Guidelines: Assessment and Management of Chronic Pain*. 2nd ed.2007:89: NCG 005586.
22. Stanos S. Use of opioid. *J Fam Pract*. 2007;56(2 Suppl Pain):23–32.
23. Fishbain DA. Polypharmacy treatment approaches to the psychiatric and comorbidities found in patients with chronic pain. *Am J Phys Med Rehabil*. 2005;84(suppl):S56–S63.
24. Ballantyne JC. Opioids for chronic nonterminal pain. *South Med J*. 2006;99(11):1245–1255.
25. Kalso E. Edwards JE, Moore RA, et al Opioids in chronic non-cancer pain: systematic review of efficacy and safety. *Pain*. 2004;112:372–380.
26. Vowles KE, McEntee ML, Julnes PS, et al. Rates of opioid misuse, abuse, and addiction in chronic pain: a systematic review and data synthesis. *Pain*. 2015;156(4):569–576.
27. Chou R, Fanciullo GJ, Fine PG; American Pain Society/American Academy of Pain Medicine Opioids Guidelines Panel. Clinical guidelines for the use of chronic opioid therapy in chronic noncancer pain. *J Pain*. 2009;10(2):113–130.
28. Arnold RM, Han PKJ, Deborah Seltzer D. Opioid contracts in chronic nonmalignant pain management: objectives and uncertainties. *Am J Med*. 2006;119:292–296.
29. Warner M, Chen LH, Makuc DM. Increase in fatal poisonings involving opioid analgesics in the United States, 1999–2006. *NCHS Data Brief*. 2009;(22):1–8. Available at: https://www.cdc.gov/nchs/data/databriefs/db22.pdf.htm. Accessed April 2017.
30. Methadone-associated overdose deaths: factors contributing to increased deaths and efforts to prevent them GAO-09-341. 2009. Available at: http://www.gao.gov/new.items/d09341.pdf. Accessed April 2017.
31. Centers for Disease Control and Prevention (CDC). Overdose deaths involving prescription opioids among Medicaid enrollees—Washington, 2004–2007. *MMWR Morb Mortal Wkly Rep*. 2009;58(42):1171–1175.
32. Andrews CM, Krantz MJ, Wedam EF, et al. Methadone-induced mortality in the treatment of chronic pain. *Cardiol J*. 2009;16(3):210–217.
33. Buprenorphine. Available at: https://www.samhsa.gov/medication-assisted-treatment/treatment/buprenorphine. Accessed April 2017.
34. Naloxone. Available at: https://www.samhsa.gov/medication-assisted-treatment/treatment/naloxone. Accessed April 2017.
35. Trescot AM, Boswell MV, Atluri SL, et al. Opioid guidelines in the management of chronic non-cancer pain. *Pain Physician*. 2006;9:1–39.
36. Krebs EE, Lorenz KA, Bair MJ, et al. Development and initial validation of the PEG, a three-item scale assessing pain intensity and interference. *J Gen Intern Med*. 2009;24(6):733–738.
37. Katz NP, Sherburne S, Beach M, et al. Behavioral monitoring and urine toxicology testing in patients receiving long-term opioid therapy. *Anesth Analg*. 2003;97(4):1097–1102.

38. Gourlay D, Heit H, Caplan Y. Urine drug testing in primary care: dispelling the myths and designing strategies. California Academy of Family Physicians Monograph. PharmaCom Group, Inc. 2002;1–25.
39. Portnoy RK, Payne R. Acute and chronic pain. In: Lowinson JH, Ruiz P, Millman RB, eds. *Comprehensive Textbook of Substance Abuse.* 3rd ed. Baltimore, MD: Williams and Wilkins; 1997:564. Table 57.1.
40. Gureje O. Psychiatric aspects of pain. *Curr Opin Psychiatry.* 2007;20(1):42–46.
41. Continuing Medical Education; Pain Management Series. American Medical Association; Physician Resources, Online CME, Pain Management: The Online Series. No longer available.
42. White F, Wilson N. Opiate-induced hypernociception and chemokine receptors. *Neuropharmacology.* 2010;58:35–37.
43. Krantz, MJ, Martin J, Stimmel B, et al. QTc interval screening in methadone treatment. *Ann Intern Med.* 2009;150:387–395.
44. Mao J. Translational pain research: achievements and challenges. *J Pain.* 2009;10(10):1001–1011.

Family Violence

1 ▶ Child abuse, intimate partner violence (IPV), and elder mistreatment commonly occur in the United States and are associated with substantial physical and mental health consequences.

2 ▶ Routine screening for IPV is recommended for women of childbearing age.

3 ▶ Current evidence does not support routine screening for child maltreatment or elder abuse.

4 ▶ All states require physicians to report suspicion of child abuse. Elder mistreatment is required to be reported in most states.

5 ▶ Referral to community-based organizations and enlisting the assistance of a multidisciplinary team of professionals with expertise are key components of managing family violence.

Estimating the true prevalence of family violence is challenging, since it occurs in the privacy of the home and not all cases come to medical or professional attention. All forms of family violence can have serious physical and mental health consequences. It is important that the family physician be alert to signs that might suggest family violence and understand approaches to managing the problem.

CHILD MALTREATMENT

You are a family physician who takes care of Tonya, a 21-year-old woman, Lucas, her 4-year-old son, and Grace, her 1-year-old daughter. You have only met Kevin, Tonya's 35-year-old husband, once. Tonya brings Lucas to your office for evaluation of a rash. During history taking, you note that Lucas does not mind his mother's escalating verbal discipline. She smacks him hard on the bottom. You ask her if discipline has been hard. She reports that he is out of control, even though she started spanking him when he was 6 months old. In examining him, you note scars from a belt or switch across his buttocks. Mom starts to cry when you see those, and admits to using a belt, but she says that when Lucas misbehaves, her husband takes it out on her.

Child maltreatment includes physical abuse, sexual abuse, psychological abuse, and neglect. Child maltreatment often presents with symptoms of inattention, school failure, disruptive symptoms, anxiety, depression, failure to thrive, and a broad range of somatic symptoms (ranging from the physical pain of a broken bone to psychogenic symptoms such as recurrent abdominal pain). Table 21.1 displays risk factors for child maltreatment.[1]

Table 21.1 ▶ Risk Factors for Child Maltreatment

Risk Factor
• Age less than 4 years
• Chronic disease, disability, or mental illness in the child
• Parental substance abuse or mental illness
• Parental history of child abuse victimization
• Young parental age
• Low socioeconomic status
• Nonbiologic caregivers in the home (e.g., step-parents)
• Social isolation

Estimates of child maltreatment rates vary widely, ranging from 10.6 to 17 cases of abuse or neglect per 1,000 children per year in the United States.[2] However, these statistics include only cases of child maltreatment that come to the attention of child protective services or other professionals and likely significantly undercount true cases of abuse or neglect.[3,4] The true incidence of child maltreatment may be much higher.

Physical Abuse

The family physician should suspect physical abuse in cases of childhood injury that are (1) unexplained, (2) not plausible by the explanation offered, (3) in a pattern suspicious for inflicted injury, (4) developmentally inconsistent, or (5) due to punishment with excessive force.[5]

Sexual Abuse

Sexual abuse includes all forms of sexual contact (oral–genital, genital, anal) by or to a child in which there is age or developmental discordance between the child and the perpetrator. It also includes noncontact abuse such as exhibitionism, voyeurism, and use of a child to produce pornography.[6]

Neglect

Child neglect accounts for the vast majority of protective service cases.[7] Neglect alone accounts for over one third of annual child maltreatment fatalities and about 60% of cases substantiated by departments of social services.

Neglect can be thought of as failing to meet the basic needs of a child, including adequate supervision, food, clothing, shelter, medical care, education, and love. Neglect often manifests as a pattern of chronic unmet needs. Some states exclude situations due to poverty from reporting laws. However, the family physician should avoid this judgment if she recognizes inadequate care that may jeopardize the health or development of a child. For example, a poor single father may leave his 2-year-old home alone sleeping at night to work a second shift job. Even though his circumstances drove him to this omission of care, the child is still at risk of significant harm.

Psychological Abuse

Psychological abuse of children is common; however, it is the least often substantiated type of abuse due to social norms and the challenges of proving both intent of the parent and harm to the child. In one survey of parents, 12.8% of parents surveyed endorsed one or more of the following in the last year: (1) threatening to leave or abandon a child, (2) threatening to kick a child out of the home, (3) locking a child out of the house, or (4) calling a name like stupid, ugly, or useless.[8] It is difficult to determine when such behavior is abusive, as it is common, often chronic, and harm is difficult to measure or prove.

Assessment

Physical Abuse

In considering an injury for suspicion of abuse, many physicians use the practical **24-hour rule**. That is, if a mark lasts 24 hours, it is considered a significant injury. Red marks from spanking (with open hand, paddle, or switch) that resolve in less than 24 hours do not rise to the level of concern for injury by protective services in most jurisdictions.[5]

In evaluating any injury to a child, a detailed history should be obtained and carefully documented. Detailed drawings or photographs can be helpful. The injury should be carefully matched to the reported mechanism. Loops, teeth marks, and linear welts (from belts or switches) are common patterns in abusive injuries. Pre-mobile children rarely bruise: fewer than 1% of children not yet cruising have bruises thought to be due to unintentional injury.[9]

Certain skeletal injuries are highly suggestive of abuse. Rib fractures and metaphyseal corner fractures of long bones in children under age 2 years (in the absence of a high impact trauma history or metabolic bone disease) are nearly always due to abuse.[10–13]

Inflicted head injury is the most common cause of death due to child physical abuse. Children under age 2 years with other significant abusive injuries should be evaluated with brain imaging (CT or MR), to identify occult brain injury, and a skeletal survey.[12,14–17]

Clinicians with special training or experience in child abuse can be helpful in clarifying mechanisms in ambiguous injuries and helping search for alternative explanations for disease and injury patterns (e.g., coagulopathy, metabolic bone disease). Table 21.2 lists injuries that should raise suspicion of child abuse.

Table 21.2 ▶ Suspicious Injuries for Child Abuse

Injury
• Bruises in non–weight-bearing child
• Numerous bruises
• Bruises over fleshy body parts (i.e., buttocks, thighs, cheeks)
• Scalds (especially symmetric, perineal, clear margins)
• Rib fractures
• Metaphyseal fractures in children <2 years
• Brain injuries (especially subdural hemorrhage)
• Pattern skin injuries (e.g., iron, stove eye, loop, cigarette burn)
• Oral injuries (especially labial frenulum laceration in non–weight-bearing child)

Sexual Abuse

Child sexual abuse usually presents with child disclosure. However, presentations vary and include acute sexual trauma, sexually transmitted infections, pregnancy, extremes of sexualized behavior, and somatic symptoms such as dysuria and enuresis. Interviewing children for evidence of sexual abuse requires special skill and training. That does not preclude the family physician from taking a thorough medical history of a child, including open-ended and nonleading questions about various types of trauma and the etiology of specific findings, for example, asking, "Is anything bothering you" or "Can you tell me about how this happened?" When possible, medical history documentation of a disclosure should include direct quotations of questions asked by the provider and responses of the victim.

The physical examination for child sexual abuse should include visual inspection of the genitals and anus in supine frog-leg and knee-chest positions. Resources on how to do the exam are available in the literature.[18] The exam may be aided by the use of lighting devices and a colposcope for magnification. Instruments such as probes or specula should never be inserted into a prepubertal vagina without anesthesia or conscious sedation.

Photo documentation can be helpful for legal reference, but accurate pen and paper diagrams can also be used. Routine cultures for sexually transmitted diseases are not necessary in the absence of symptoms. Clinicians unskilled in the physical exam for sexual abuse should seek expert consultation. In the overwhelming majority of cases of chronic or past sexual abuse, physical exam findings will be either normal or nonspecific, making the history critical in determining sexual abuse victimization.[18,19]

Neglect

Neglect may come to the family physician's attention in the form of medical nonadherence, failure or delay in seeking medical care, failure to thrive, unmanaged obesity, behavior problems, school failure, poor hygiene, or homelessness.[20] In identifying suspected neglect, asking nonjudgmental questions about resources can help identify sources of problems and potential solutions. As neglect often manifests as a chronic pattern, the physician must assure follow-up over time. When a pattern of omissions in care (or a single egregious episode) rises to the level of harm or significant risk of harm, the physician is obligated to report the case to protective services.

Psychological Abuse

The diagnosis of psychological abuse is often made only through long-term observation of parent-child interaction, supplemented by querying other adults involved in the life of the child (e.g., teachers, coaches). In the evaluation of children with disorders of behavior and development, clinicians often witness parents belittling children in cruel ways ("he's stupid just like his daddy" or "she drives me crazy"). Discussing destructive behavior and role modeling positive behavior can begin to help a parent identify problem parenting. Table 21.3 lists symptoms of psychological abuse.

Management

All states, districts, and territories in the United States mandate that physicians report suspected child abuse and neglect. These laws include immunity from lawsuits for reports

◢◣ **Table 21.3** ▶ Symptoms of Psychological Abuse	
Symptom	
• Aggressiveness	• Inattention
• Impulsivity	• Disturbances of conduct
• Depression	• Anxiety
• Hyperactivity	• Eating disorders
• School failure	• Somatic symptoms

made in good faith. The parent should be counseled that the report is not placing blame or making judgment, but carrying out a legal responsibility. It is not required by law to inform the parent of the report to be made; however, this can set the stage for an open dialog and continued support of a family.

Attention to careful documentation of history (both questions asked and responses in quotes) and injuries with drawings or photodocumentation is critical. In many cases, a physician caring for a child suspected to be a victim of abuse or neglect may need to make a safety plan in conjunction with social services while the child is in the clinic, emergency room, or hospital.

> Based on your findings when you see Lucas in the office, you inform Tonya that you are going to make a report to Child Protective Services (CPS). You reassure her that you will continue to support her and her family as CPS proceeds with its investigation. Physical abuse is substantiated by CPS, but evaluation reveals no injuries beyond the scars that you noted on exam. Tonya is referred to an Incredible Years parenting class (http://incredibleyears.com/) and has ongoing contact with her CPS caseworker.

INTIMATE PARTNER VIOLENCE

> Three months later, Tonya presents to your office for vaginal discharge. She apologizes for being late for her appointment, stating that her husband, Kevin, tried to prevent her from coming. During your exam, you notice that Tonya has bruising around her left eye. When you ask about how it happened, Tonya doesn't make eye contact and mumbles that she and Kevin got in a fight. You reflect on the missed opportunity to discuss these issues with Tonya at her last visit 3 months prior when she mentioned that when Lucas misbehaves "he (Kevin) takes it out on her" and plan to pay more attention in the future.

Intimate partner violence (IPV), which includes physical, emotional, and sexual harm by a current or former partner or spouse, is a common problem with serious physical and mental health consequences for victims and their children. Although women are most commonly affected, IPV affects both men and women and occurs among married and unmarried couples, affecting both heterosexual and same-sex couples. Full descriptions of the different categories can be found at http://www.cdc.gov/violenceprevention/intimate-partnerviolence/definitions.html.

Common to all forms of IPV is a pervasive pattern of coercion and control. First person accounts from survivors of IPV, such as the TED talk by Leslie Morgan Steiner

(http://www.ted.com/talks/leslie_morgan_steiner_why_domestic_violence_victims_
don_t_leave?language=en), can provide insight into the complex dynamics of relationships affected by IPV.

About 36% of women and 29% of men in the United States have been victims of rape,
physical violence, or stalking by an intimate partner in their lifetimes.[21,22] Although IPV
affects all ages, races, ethnicities and socioeconomic strata, young women and individuals
with low incomes are at greatest risk.[23,24]

Because victims of IPV tend to have high rates of physical and mental health morbidity,
they are frequent users of the health care system. IPV is thus a condition that family physicians will encounter frequently over the course of their careers.

Common Presentations

IPV influences multiple aspects of physical and mental health, affecting victims' health for
many years, even after abuse has ended.

Injuries

The most direct health effect of IPV is injury. Certain patterns of injury, such as injuries
to the head, neck, breast, or abdomen, should raise suspicion of intentional injury. Facial
trauma, for example, an orbital fracture or dental injury, is particularly suggestive,[25,26]
although fractures, sprains, and dislocations of the extremities are also common.[25] Victims of IPV also suffer long-term sequelae of injury, such as symptoms of traumatic brain
injury.[27] Worldwide, more than one third of female victims of homicide were killed by an
intimate partner.[28]

Other Physical Health Effects

Common conditions in victims of IPV include sexual health concerns, such as sexually
transmitted infections and unplanned pregnancy;[27,29] chronic diseases such as cardiovascular disease and stroke;[30] and functional gastrointestinal disorders such as irritable bowel
syndrome.[31] Patients with IPV may present with multiple somatic complaints including
stomach pain, back pain, menstrual problems, headaches, chest pain, dizziness, fainting
spells, palpitations, shortness of breath, constipation, generalized fatigue, and insomnia.[32,33]
IPV may increase risk for such a wide range of conditions due to the direct consequences
of trauma, the long-term accumulated effects of chronic stress, and high prevalence of risky
health behaviors.

Intimate Partner Violence and Pregnancy

IPV often continues throughout pregnancy, increasing risk for complications such as
spontaneous abortion, hypertensive disorders of pregnancy, vaginal bleeding, placental
abruption, severe nausea and vomiting, dehydration, diabetes, urinary tract infection,
and premature rupture of membranes.[27,33] Victims of IPV often delay seeking prenatal
care, and the possibility of IPV should be considered in women who receive late or no
prenatal care.[27] IPV-related homicide is the leading cause of maternal mortality in the
United States.[27] Infants of mothers who experience IPV during pregnancy also are at
risk for medical complications including low birth weight, prematurity, and perinatal
death.[33–38]

Mental Health

Victims of IPV commonly experience depression, suicidal thoughts and attempts, and PTSD.[31,33,39] Tobacco, alcohol, and illicit drug abuse are common,[30,40] and victims of IPV are more likely to engage in risky sexual behaviors.[27,41]

Screening and Assessment

The United States Preventive Services Task Force (USPSTF) recommends screening all women of childbearing age for IPV and referring women who screen positive for intervention services.[42] This recommendation is based on evidence that IPV can be accurately detected using currently available screening instruments, that effective interventions can mitigate the adverse health outcomes of IPV, and that screening causes minimal harm.[43]

Primary care physicians should be aware of the clusters of symptoms that are common in victims of IPV. When patients present with issues consistent with IPV (Table 21.4), clinicians should inquire about IPV because such knowledge could influence the treatment plan or help the clinician understand barriers to treatment. What physicians perceive as poor adherence to medical recommendations may in fact be related to the abuse a patient is experiencing; interference with receipt of health care may be part of the control that abusers exert in their partners' lives.[27] Primary care physicians who diagnose IPV, and therefore begin to understand the barriers that their abused patients face, may be able to form more effective therapeutic relationships. Identifying IPV also provides an important opportunity for providing the patient with empathic support; educating her regarding the dynamics of IPV and the future risks it poses to her and her children; and opening the door to future conversations.

Several questionnaires for assessing for IPV have been validated in a variety of settings and are practical for use in primary care such as HITS, Woman Abuse Screening Tool, and the Ongoing Violence Assessment Tool (https://www.cdc.gov/violenceprevention/pdf/ipv/ipvandsvscreening.pdf).[44]

Physicians should ensure a private setting, without friends or family members present, politely informing others in the exam room that it is standard procedure to examine patients privately. Physicians should assure patients of confidentiality, but notify them of any reporting requirements. It is often helpful to preface questions about IPV with normalizing statements, for example, "Because violence is a common problem, I routinely ask my

Table 21.4 ► Situations That Should Raise Suspicion for IPV

Consider IPV in Patients with
• Injuries to the face or trunk
• Pattern of injury not consistent with explanation given
• Frequent somatic complaints
• Chronic pain syndromes
• Recurrent sexual health concerns
• Late entry into prenatal care
• Frequent late or missed appointments
• Substance abuse
• Frequent mental health complaints

patients about it," or "Many people with [condition] have worse symptoms if they have been physically, emotionally, or sexually abused in the past." If language barriers are present, physicians should use the assistance of an interpreter.[45]

Management

When IPV is detected in the clinical setting, clinicians should respond in a way that builds trust and sets the stage for an ongoing therapeutic relationship.

Key components of an initial interaction should include:

▶ Validation of the patient's concerns

▶ Education regarding the dynamics and consequences of IPV

▶ Safety assessment

▶ Referral to local resources

A growing body of evidence suggests that a variety of counseling and advocacy interventions are effective at reducing violence and mitigating its negative health effects.[46,47] IPV is usually a chronic problem that will not be solved in the one or two visits, but rather can be worked on over time.

An initial response to a disclosure of IPV should include listening to the patient empathically and nonjudgmentally, expressing concern for her health and safety, and affirming a commitment to help her address the problem. Women who have long been subjected to abuse may believe that the abuse is their fault. Physicians can help counter this belief, reassuring patients that although partner violence is common, it is unacceptable and not the fault of the victim. Clinicians should also convey respect for IPV victims' choices regarding how to respond to the violence. Victims of IPV may have a clearer understanding than their physicians about what courses of action may result in increased danger.

Clinicians should educate patients on the dynamics of partner violence and potential effects on victims and their children, helping them understand that once violent dynamics are established in a relationship, the violence generally continues and escalates over time. In a nonjudgmental way, physicians can convey concern to patients regarding the negative physical and mental effects that IPV may have on patients and their children.

Although addressing IPV is usually a long-term process, physicians should be alert to crisis situations that indicate imminent danger (see Red Flags below). Handouts on safety planning can be found at the National Domestic Violence Hotline website (www.thehotline. org), in English and Spanish.

 Clues or "red flags" for increased risks for serious injury of homicide:

▶ Increasing frequency or severity of violence

▶ Recent use of, or threats with, a weapon

▶ Threats of homicide or suicide

▶ Hostage-taking or stalking

▶ Alcohol or drug use

▶ Recent separation from, or threats to leave, partner

Finally, physicians should provide victims of IPV with referral to local resources that can provide advocacy and support. Resources might include community-based advocacy groups, shelters, law enforcement agencies, or social workers. The National Domestic Violence Hotline (800-799-SAFE) can serve as a resource. If immediate concerns for safety exist, the physician can offer the patient an opportunity to contact these resources from the office. A follow-up visit should be scheduled, and IPV should be readdressed at future visits.

> During your visit with Tonya, you learn that Kevin's physical violence has escalated in recent months. You provide contact information for the local IPV agency and offer for Tonya to call from your office. Tonya says that she loves Kevin and would never want to "take my children away from their father." Over the next year, you see Tonya for frequent visits and check in on how things are going with Kevin. At one visit, she tells you that she called the IPV support agency and that she is working on a plan to leave Kevin. Two years later, she, Lucas, and Grace have their own apartment. Tonya continues to attend an IPV support group and a parenting group.

ELDER MISTREATMENT

Elder abuse is defined as (a) "intentional actions that cause harm or create a serious risk of harm (whether or not harm is intended) to a vulnerable elder by a caregiver or other person who stands in a trust relationship to the elder" OR (b) "failure by a caregiver to satisfy the elder's basic needs or to protect the elder from harm."[48] Elder abuse is less well understood than child abuse and IPV. Elder mistreatment includes physical abuse, psychological abuse, sexual abuse, financial exploitation, and neglect. Elder self-neglect, or the failure of an elderly person to meet his or her own basic needs or protect his or her health and safety, is also sometimes considered to be a type of elder mistreatment.

Population-based studies suggest that between 2% and 11% of older adults have been subject to some form of abuse in the last year.[49–51] Neglect is most commonly reported, followed by emotional, physical, and sexual mistreatment.[49] Family caregivers and long-term care staff report even higher levels of abuse than do the elders themselves.[50,52] Elder mistreatment is common enough that family physicians who care for elderly patients in outpatient, inpatient, or long-term care settings will encounter it in clinical practice.

Several patient, caregiver, social, and environmental factors are markers of increased risk for elder mistreatment as shown in Table 21.5. Elder mistreatment is linked to adverse

Table 21.5 ▶ Risk Factors for Elder Mistreatment

Risk Factor
• Social isolation of both elders and their caregivers
• Disruptive behavior or aggression by the elder
• Caregiver mental illness, especially depression
• Caregiver alcohol abuse
• Caregiver financial dependency on the elder
• Inadequate staffing and staff training in long-term care facilities

health outcomes, including increased depression, hospitalizations, nursing home place-ment, and mortality.[51,53,54]

Assessment

The USPSTF states that there is insufficient evidence to recommend for or against rou-tine screening for elder abuse because of lack of evidence that we can accurately identify and effectively intervene upon elder abuse in the clinical setting.[42] The lack of evidence for screening, however, does not obviate the need to remain alert to signs of elder mistreatment and intervene when elder mistreatment is identified.

No clear constellation of symptoms can identify elder mistreatment. Falls and frac-tures, skin injuries, and weight loss are all common in frail older patients. Individuals with cognitive impairment, who are particularly vulnerable, may not be able to give accurate accounts of abuse or neglect.[48,51] Mistrust of caregivers can be part of dementia; it may be difficult to distinguish between financial exploitation and appropriate efforts by caregivers to take control of finances when a loved one cannot manage independently.

Providers should remain alert to bruises or burns in unusual locations such as neck, ears or genitals or injuries that are not consistent with the explanation offered.[55] Injuries to wrists or ankles could be an indication of use of restraints. Dehydration, malnutrition, pres-sure ulcers, poor hygiene, or medical nonadherence should raise suspicion for neglect.[56]

No instruments to assess for elder mistreatment have been well validated, but several principles can guide clinicians assessing for abuse or neglect. The patient should be ques-tioned and examined in private. General questions about home environment and safety can be followed with more direct questions about whether the patient has been hurt or threatened, food or medicines have been denied, the patient has been made to feel guilty about asking for help, personal belongings have been taken away, or unwanted touch has occurred. History and physical findings should be documented carefully. For patients with cognitive impairment, assessment of decision-making capacity will guide an approach to intervention.[51]

Caregivers may also be questioned directly about abuse or neglect, but physicians must be careful to avoid alienating caregivers, who could in turn restrict access to the elderly patient. It may be helpful precede direct inquiries with permissive statements, such as "Car-ing for your father must be stressful. How do you manage?"

Management

There is no good evidence to support specific management of elder mistreatment.[57] The most appropriate strategy will be determined by the nature of the abuse or neglect and the circumstances of the individual patient. In most states, reporting elder abuse and neglect is legally mandated. Adult Protective Services agencies are the point of first contact for reporting suspected elder mistreatment. Each state also has a Long-Term Care Ombuds-man Program that can provide assistance if abuse or neglect in a long-term care facility is suspected. State-level reporting requirements can be found at the National Center on Elder Abuse website (https://ncea.acl.gov/resources/state.html).

Connecting elders with resources for social support is likely to be beneficial. Inter-ventions targeted toward caregivers might include caregiver education regarding what constitutes abuse, referral to respite care resources, connection with social support, and psychotherapy or pharmacotherapy to address mental health concerns.

If abuse is a response to or is perpetrated by an aggressive patient with dementia, interventions to address the aggressive behavior are indicated. For patients who lack capacity for decision-making, pursuing guardianship may be necessary. Ideally, physicians should enlist the assistance of a multidisciplinary team including, nurses, government agencies, social workers, and legal professionals with expertise in various aspects of elder mistreatment.[51]

QUESTIONS

1. The USPSTF recommends that Family Physicians screen which one of the following groups for violence?
   A. Elderly.
   B. Children.
   C. Women of reproductive age.
   D. Teenagers.

2. Physicians are required to report suspected child abuse.
   A. True.
   B. False.

3. Which of the following arc "red flags" for increased risk of serious injury or homicide in a relationship with IPV?
   A. Pregnancy.
   B. Weight gain.
   C. New employment.
   D. Recent attempt to leave partner.
   E. Smoking.

4. Which of the following should be part of a family physician's response when a patient reveals that she is a victim of IPV?
   A. Informing the patient that she should leave her abuser as soon as possible.
   B. Notifying law enforcement so that an investigation of her partner can begin.
   C. Notifying child protective services, if there are any children in the home.
   D. Reassuring the patient that the violence is not her fault.

ANSWERS

Question 1: The correct answer is C.
The USPSTF recommends screening all women of childbearing age for IPV and referring women who screen positive for intervention services.

Question 2: The correct answer is A.
All states, districts, and territories in the United States mandate that physicians report suspected child abuse and neglect. These laws include immunity from lawsuits for reports made in good faith.

Question 3: The correct answer is D.
As shown in the text box, red flags for increased risk of serious injury or homicide in a relationship with IPV are: increasing frequency or severity of violence, recent use of or threats with a weapon, homicide or suicide threats, hostage taking or stalking, alcohol or drug use, and recent separation from or threats to leave partner.

Question 4: The correct answer is D.

An initial response to a disclosure of IPV should include listening to the patient empathically and nonjudgmentally, expressing concern for her health and safety, and affirming a commitment to help her address the problem. Women who have long been subjected to abuse may believe that the abuse is their fault. Physicians can help counter this belief, reassuring patients that although partner violence is common, it is unacceptable and not the fault of the victim.

REFERENCES

1. Child abuse and neglect: risk and protective factors. 2016. Available at: http://www.cdc.gov/violenceprevention/childmaltreatment/riskprotectivefactors.html. Accessed November 23, 2016.
2. Child maltreatment 2014. 2016. Available at: https://www.acf.hhs.gov/sites/default/files/cb/cm2014.pdf. Accessed October 13, 2016.
3. Zolotor AJ, Motsinger BM, Runyan DK, et al. Building an effective child maltreatment surveillance system in North Carolina. *NC Med J.* 2005;66:360–363.
4. Finkelhor D, Turner HA, Shattuck A, et al. Prevalence of childhood exposure to violence, crime, and abuse: results from the National Survey of Children's Exposure to Violence. *JAMA Pediatr.* 2015;169:746–754.
5. Committee on Child Abuse and Neglect. American Academy of Pediatrics. When inflicted skin injuries constitute child abuse. *Pediatrics.* 2002;110:644–645.
6. Kellogg N. The evaluation of sexual abuse in children. *Pediatrics.* 2005;116:506–512.
7. Sedlak AJ, Mettenberg J, Basena M, et al. *Fourth National Incidence Study of Child Abuse and Neglect (NIS-4): Report to Congress.* Washington, DC: US Department of Health and Human Services, Administration for Children and Families; 2010.
8. Zolotor AJ, Runyan DK. Social capital, family violence, and neglect. *Pediatrics.* 2006;117:e1124–e1131.
9. Maguire S, Mann MK, Sibert J, et al. Are there patterns of bruising in childhood which are diagnostic or suggestive of abuse? A systematic review. *Arch Dis Child.* 2005;90:182–186.
10. Bulloch B, Schubert CJ, Brophy PD, et al. Cause and clinical characteristics of rib fractures in infants. *Pediatrics.* 2000;105:E48.
11. Maguire S, Mann M, John N, et al. Does cardiopulmonary resuscitation cause rib fractures in children? A systematic review. *Child Abuse Negl.* 2006;30:739–751.
12. Kemp AM, Dunstan F, Harrison S, et al. Patterns of skeletal fractures in child abuse: systematic review. *BMJ.* 2008;337:a1518.
13. Flaherty EG, Perez-Rossello JM, Levine MA, et al. Evaluating children with fractures for child physical abuse. *Pediatrics.* 2014;133:e477–e489.
14. Rubin DM, Christian CW, Bilaniuk LT, et al. Occult head injury in high-risk abused children. *Pediatrics.* 2003;111:1382–1386.
15. Kemp AM, Rajaram S, Mann M, et al. What neuroimaging should be performed in children in whom inflicted brain injury (iBI) is suspected? A systematic review. *Clin Radiol.* 2009;64:473–483.
16. Christian, Committee on Child Abuse and Neglect. The evaluation of suspected child physical abuse. *Pediatrics.* 2015;135(5):e1337–e1354.
17. Duffy SO, Squires J, Fromkin JB, et al. Use of skeletal surveys to evaluate for physical abuse: analysis of 703 consecutive skeletal surveys. *Pediatrics.* 2011;127:e47–e52.
18. Berkoff MC, Zolotor AJ, Makoroff KL, et al. Has this prepubertal girl been sexually abused?. *JAMA.* 2008;300:2779–2792.
19. Adams JA, Harper K, Knudson S, et al. Examination findings in legally confirmed child sexual abuse: it's normal to be normal. *Pediatrics.* 1994;94:310–317.
20. Dubowitz H, Giardino A, Gustavson E. Child neglect: guidance for pediatricians. *Pediatr Rev.* 2000;21:111–116.
21. Hibbard R, Barlow J, Macmillan H. Psychological maltreatment. *Pediatrics.* 2012;130:372–378.
22. Black MC, Basile KC, Breiding MJ, et al. *National Intimate Partner and Sexual Violence Survey: 2010 Summary Report.* Atlanta, GA: National Center for Injury Prevention and Control, Centers for Disease Control and Prevention; 2011.
23. U.S. Department of Justice, 2012. Intimate Partner Violence, 1993–2010. Available at: http://www.bjs.gov/index.cfm?ty=pbdetail&iid=4536. Accessed August 24, 2016.

24. Capaldi DM, Knoble NB, Shortt JW, et al. A systematic review of risk factors for intimate partner violence. *Partner Abuse*. 2012;3:231–280.

25. Bhandari M, Dosanjh S, Tornetta P, 3rd, et al. Musculoskeletal manifestations of physical abuse after intimate partner violence. *J Trauma*. 2006;61:1473–1479.

26. Allen T, Novak SA, Bench LL. Patterns of injuries: accident or abuse. *Violence Against Women*. 2007;13: 802–816.

27. Plichta SB. Intimate partner violence and physical health consequences: policy and practice implications. *J Interpers Violence*. 2004;19:1296–1323.

28. Stockl H, Devries K, Rotstein A, et al. The global prevalence of intimate partner homicide: a systematic review. *Lancet*. 2013;382:859–865.

29. McFarlane J, Malecha A, Watson K, et al. Intimate partner sexual assault against women: frequency, health consequences, and treatment outcomes. *Obstet Gynecol*. 2005;105:99–108.

30. Breiding MJ, Black MC, Ryan GW. Chronic and health risk behaviors associated with intimate partner violence-18 U.S. states/territories, 2005. *Ann Epidemiol*. 2008;18:538–544.

31. Ellsberg M, Jansen HA, Heise L, et al. Intimate partner violence and women's physical and mental health in the WHO multi-country study on women's health and domestic violence: an observational study. *Lancet*. 2008;371:1165–1172.

32. Eberhard-Gran M, Schei B, Eskild A. Somatic symptoms and diseases are more common in women exposed to violence. *J Gen Intern Med*. 2007;22:1668–1673.

33. Woods SJ. Intimate partner violence and post-traumatic stress disorder symptoms in women: what we know and need to know. *J Interpers Violence*. 2005;20:394–402.

34. Taft CT, Vogt DS, Mechanic MB, et al. Posttraumatic stress disorder and physical health symptoms among women seeking help for relationship aggression. *J Fam Psychol*. 2007;21:354–362.

35. Coker AL, Sanderson M, Dong B. Partner violence during pregnancy and risk of adverse pregnancy outcomes. *Paediatr Perinat Epidemiol*. 2004;18:260–269.

36. Sharps PW, Laughon K, Giangrande SK. Intimate partner violence and the childbearing year: maternal and infant health consequences. *Trauma Violence Abuse*. 2007;8:105–116.

37. Silverman JG, Decker MR, Reed E, et al. Intimate partner violence victimization prior to and during pregnancy among women residing in 26 U.S. states: associations with maternal and neonatal health. *Am J Obstet Gynecol*. 2006;195:140–148.

38. Murphy CC, Schei B, Myhr TL, et al. Abuse: a risk factor for low birth weight? A systematic review and meta-analysis. *CMAJ*. 2001;164:1567–1572.

39. Dutton MA, Green BL, Kaltman SI, et al. Intimate partner violence, PTSD, and adverse health outcomes. *J Interpers Violence*. 2006;21:955–968.

40. Bonomi AE, Anderson ML, Reid RJ, et al. Medical and psychosocial diagnoses in women with a history of intimate partner violence. *Arch Int Med*. 2009;169:1692–1697.

41. Adverse health conditions and health risk behaviors associated with intimate partner violence—United States, 2005. *MMWR Morb Mortal Wkly Rep*. 2008;57:113–117.

42. Moyer VA; USPSTF. Screening for intimate partner violence and abuse of elderly and vulnerable adults: U.S. preventive services task force recommendation statement. *Ann Intern Med*. 2013;158:478–486.

43. Final Update Summary: Intimate partner violence and abuse of elderly and vulnerable adults: screening. 2015. Available at: http://www.uspreventiveservicestaskforce.org/Page/Document/UpdateSummaryFinal/intimate-partner-violence-and-abuse-of-elderly-and-vulnerable-adults-screening. Accessed August 25, 2016.

44. Basile KC, Hertz MF, Back SE. *Intimate Partner Violence and Sexual Violence Victimization Assessment Instruments for Use in Healthcare Settings: Version 1*. Atlanta, GA: Centers for Disease Control and Prevention, National Center for Injury Prevention and Control; 2007.

45. *National Consensus Guidelines on Identifying and Responding to Domestic Violence Victimization*. San Francisco: Family Violence Prevention Fund; 2004.

46. Nelson HD, Bougatsos C, Blazina I. Screening women for intimate partner violence: a systematic review to update the U.S. Preventive Services Task Force recommendation. *Ann Intern Med*. 2012;156:796–808, W-279, W-80, W-81, W-82.

47. Rivas C, Ramsay J, Sadowski L, et al. Advocacy interventions to reduce or eliminate violence and promote the physical and psychosocial well-being of women who experience intimate partner abuse. *Cochrane Database Syst Rev*. 2015;(12):CD005043.

48. Bonnie RJ, Wallace RB, National Research Council (U.S.). Panel to Review Risk and Prevalence of Elder Abuse and Neglect., National Research Council (U.S.). Committee on National Statistics., National Research

Council (U.S.). Committee on Law and Justice. *Elder Mistreatment: Abuse, Neglect, and Exploitation in an Aging America.* Washington, DC: National Academies Press; 2003.

49. Acierno R, Hernandez MA, Amstadter AB, et al. Prevalence and correlates of emotional, physical, sexual, and financial abuse and potential neglect in the United States: the National Elder Mistreatment Study. *Am J Public Health.* 2010;100(2):292–297.

50. Cooper C, Selwood A, Livingston G. The prevalence of elder abuse and neglect: a systematic review. *Age Ageing.* 2008;37:151–160.

51. Lachs MS, Pillemer K. Elder abuse. *Lancet.* 2004;364:1263–1272.

52. Lindbloom EJ, Brandt J, Hough LD, et al. Elder mistreatment in the nursing home: a systematic review. *J Am Med Dir Assoc.* 2007;8:610–616.

53. Dong X, Simon M, Mendes de Leon C, et al. Elder self-neglect and abuse and mortality risk in a community-dwelling population. *JAMA.* 2009;302:517–526.

54. Dong X, Simon MA. Elder abuse as a risk factor for hospitalization in older persons. *JAMA Intern Med.* 2013;173:911–917.

55. Gibbs LM. Understanding the medical markers of elder abuse and neglect: physical examination findings. *Clin Geriatr Med.* 2014;30:687–712.

56. del Carmen T, LoFaso VM. Elder neglect. *Clin Geriatr Med.* 2014;30:769–777.

57. Baker PR, Francis DP, Hairi NN, et al. Interventions for preventing abuse in the elderly. *Cochrane Database Syst Rev.* 2016;(8):CD010321.

Common Psychosocial Problems

KEY POINTS

1 ▸ Depression and anxiety are common conditions presenting in primary care settings.

2 ▸ Primary care clinicians can use brief screening tools to assess depression and anxiety.

3 ▸ A wide array of pharmacotherapy options can be used to treat patients presenting with depression or anxiety.

4 ▸ Primary care clinicians can use brief, evidence-based behavioral interventions to help reduce depressive or anxious symptomatology for patients.

5 ▸ Collaboration with behavioral health can greatly enhance the quality of care for psychosocial problems at the primary care level.

Jessica is a 37-year-old Latina who is being seen for frequent yeast vaginitis. She is married, employed, and has two children. As part of your workup of her frequent yeast vaginitis, you ordered a hemoglobin A1c which has returned with a value of 7.9, establishing a diagnosis of type 2 diabetes mellitus (DM). Jessica has a strongly positive family history of DM and witnessed many of their struggles with the disease. She is very distressed about going down that same path.

During the visit, you explore her concerns and offer support, emphasizing the team approach that your office provides. You prescribe metformin and schedule a follow-up visit for her with yourself in 2 weeks and an initial visit with your care manager to discuss self-management. Jessica appears reassured and expresses hope for successful management.

Two weeks later, Jessica returns for her follow-up appointment. Your care manager was able to connect with her by phone in the interim, and her note indicates that Jessica sounded overwhelmed with her new diagnosis. As you enter the exam room, it is apparent that she is distressed. After a brief conversation exploring how things have gone over the past 2 weeks, you ask Jessica to complete a new Patient Health Questionnaire (PHQ)-9 and General Anxiety Disorder (GAD)-7 screen which shows scores of 13 and 12, respectively. Recognizing these as being positive, you also ask her to complete a Diabetes Distress Scale, which is positive.

The case of Jessica, who has depression and anxiety while managing a chronic disease, is a common one in family medicine settings. Primary care providers furnish over half of mental health treatment in the United States, and about 25% of all primary care patients have diagnosable mental health disorders (most commonly, depression and anxiety).[1] More than half of outpatient medical visits in primary care are for somatic complaints, which are often associated with depression and anxiety.[2] Latino individuals such as Jessica as well as members of other ethnic groups may present with culturally-bound manifestations of mental health conditions that may pose challenges for successful screening for these conditions.[3]

Depression and anxiety can complicate other medical conditions and increase the costs of care. In addition, 68% of adults with mental illness have one or more chronic physical conditions.[4] In fact, people with mental illness die earlier than the general population, perhaps because they have more co-occurring health conditions.[5]

According to the World Health Organization (WHO), a person's mental health and many common mental disorders are shaped by social, economic, and risk factors.[6] Family physicians are in a unique position to learn about social inequalities for patients, including housing, finances, and education and can potentially connect patients to resources to help reduce the burden of these inequalities on patients. It is important for family physicians and their staff to be knowledgeable and, where possible, have active referral relationships with community service organizations and resources that can help individuals in need. Chapter 24 discusses these issues.

COMMON MENTAL HEALTH DISORDERS IN PRIMARY CARE

Mood Disorders	Anxiety Disorders
▶ National Comorbidity Survey Replication: 12-month prevalence of depression 6.6% and lifetime rate 16.2%[7]	▶ In one survey, 19.5% of primary care patients had at least one anxiety disorder[10]
▶ 70–80% of antidepressants are prescribed in primary care[8]	▶ Numerous medical conditions can mimic anxiety symptoms including cardiac, endocrine, respiratory, neurologic, and gynecologic disorders
▶ U.S. Preventive Services Task Force recommends depression screening for the general adult population and postpartum women[9]	▶ Individuals with depression are at higher risk for comorbid anxiety and there is considerable symptom overlap[11]

MOOD AND ANXIETY DISORDERS IN PRIMARY CARE

Mood disorders that present in primary care settings include major depressive disorder (MDD), dysthymic disorder, adjustment disorder with depressed mood, mood disorders due to a general medical condition (or substance), and bipolar disorder type I and type II. MDD is a common comorbidity seen with many chronic diseases such as stroke, diabetes, chronic obstructive pulmonary disease (COPD), heart disease, and Parkinson disease.

Anxiety is one of the most common psychiatric conditions presenting in primary care after depression. Up to 20% of patients in primary care settings may present with an anxiety disorder.[10] Specific anxiety disorders (and their prevalence) in primary care settings include generalized anxiety disorder (7.6%), panic disorder with or without agoraphobia (6.8%), obsessive compulsive disorder (unknown), posttraumatic stress disorder (8.6%), and social anxiety disorder (6.2%).[10] Although increasing attention has been paid to anxiety, it still lags far behind depression in terms of research as well as clinical and public health efforts in screening, diagnosis, and treating affected individuals.

SCREENING FOR PSYCHIATRIC CONDITIONS IN PRIMARY CARE

Physicians working in primary care settings have a unique opportunity to assess and initiate treatment for a wide array of psychiatric conditions. Although screening for depression is

Table 22.1 ▶ Screening Tools for Depression and Anxiety in Primary Care

Tool	Description	Comments
Patient Health Questionnaire (PHQ)-9	Nine-item self-report measure for depression	Simple to administer High sensitivity for MD (92%) and reasonable specificity (82%)
General Anxiety Disorder Questionnaire (GAD)-7	Seven-item self-report generalized anxiety disorder measure	Simple to administer Sensitivity 82% and specificity 89%
Primary Care Post-Traumatic Stress Disorder Scale (PC-PTSD)	Four-item self-report questionnaire	Sensitivity 78% and specificity of 87%
Mood Disorder Questionnaire (MDQ)	Seventeen-item self-report on symptoms, family history, and previous diagnoses	Sensitivity 61.3% and specificity 87.5% for psychiatric outpatients
Bipolar Spectrum Disorder Scale (BSDS)	Nineteen statements describing symptoms which patients check, if applicable; each counts for one point	Sensitivity 76% and specificity 85–93%

recommended by the US Preventive Services Task Force (USPSTF),[12] systems must be in place to ensure proper diagnosis, treatment, and follow-up. Therefore, physicians must be realistic about the time they have available to assess psychiatric conditions. Using screening tools designed for primary care settings can assist in this process (Table 22.1).

Screening for Depression

One of the best and most practical tools for physicians to use to screen for depression is the PHQ-9 (http://www.phqscreeners.com).[13,14] Positive results on the PHQ-9 do not equal a diagnosis of depression, however, and require further evaluation to confirm that a patient meets the Diagnostic and Statistical Manual of Mental Disorders (DSM)-5 criteria for MDD. Patients can be given the PHQ-9 by a medical assistant, for example, who can then score the form and provide results to the medical provider to complete the assessment.

If a patient screens positive for suicidal ideation, the SAD PERSONS scale can be administered to assess the likelihood of a suicide attempt (https://www.qxmd.com/calculate/calculator_201/modified-sad-persons-scale). We recommend adding the letter A to the scale to (SAD PERSONAS) to assess **A**vailability of lethal means.[15] Patients presenting with comorbid medical conditions such as diabetes, COPD, and coronary artery disease may also benefit from depression screening or specific screening measures to assess for condition-related distress (e.g., Diabetes Distress Scale; http://www.diabetesed.net/page/_files/diabetes-distress.pdf).

Screening for Anxiety

GAD-7 (https://www.mdcalc.com/gad-7-general-anxiety-disorder-7) was developed for use in the primary care setting.[16] Although this tool is designed to assess for generalized anxiety disorder, one of the most common anxiety disorders seen in primary care,[16] it also is moderately good at screening for panic disorder (sensitivity 74%, specificity 81%), social anxiety disorder (sensitivity 72%, specificity 80%), and PTSD (sensitivity 66%, specificity 81%).[17] A brief screening tool for PTSD, entitled the PC-PTSD, is also available.[18]

Positive results on either screening tool warrants further assessment using the DSM-5 criteria for GAD and PTSD. Additional assessment should be considered to rule out medical conditions that are associated with anxiety symptoms (e.g., hyperthyroidism, respiratory disorders such as COPD and asthma, and drug abuse or withdrawal) and understand the role of comorbid medical conditions.

Screening for Bipolar Disorder

When assessing patients in primary care settings for depression and anxiety, it is important to consider other comorbid psychiatric conditions such as bipolar disorder. Two bipolar disorder screening tools intended for primary care settings, the MDQ and BSDS are shown in Table 22.1.[19,20] A positive screen for either tool warrants further assessment as well as additional medical screening to rule out medical causes.

Substance Dependence in Primary Care

In the United States, 22.5 million persons older than 12 years meet criteria for substance abuse or dependence.[21] Patients presenting in primary care setting with depression, anxiety, or bipolar disorder may be at a higher risk for substance dependence and alcohol misuse. Further information on substance dependence screening and treatment can be found in Chapter 23.

DIAGNOSING DEPRESSION AND ANXIETY

In order to establish a diagnosis for MDD or GAD, we encourage providers to confirm the diagnosis using the diagnostic criteria from the DSM-5.[22] **For MDD**, the patient must have five (or more) of the symptoms listed below, present during the same 2-week period and representing a change from previous functioning; at least one of the symptoms is either (1) depressed mood or (2) loss of interest or pleasure. *Note:* Do not include symptoms that are clearly attributable to another medical condition.

▶ Depressed mood most of the day, nearly every day, as indicated by either subjective report (e.g., feels sad, empty, hopeless) or observation made by others (e.g., appears tearful). (*Note:* In children and adolescents, can be irritable mood.)

▶ Markedly diminished interest or pleasure in all, or almost all, activities most of the day, nearly every day (as indicated by either subjective account or observation.)

▶ Significant weight loss when not dieting or weight gain (e.g., a change of more than 5% of body weight in a month), or decrease or increase in appetite nearly every day. (*Note:* In children, consider failure to make expected weight gain.)

▶ Insomnia or hypersomnia nearly every day.

▶ Psychomotor agitation or retardation nearly every day (observable by others, not merely subjective feelings of restlessness or being slowed down).

▶ Fatigue or loss of energy nearly every day.

▶ Feelings of worthlessness or excessive or inappropriate guilt (which may be delusional) nearly every day (not merely self-reproach or guilt about being sick).

▶ Diminished ability to think or concentrate, or indecisiveness, nearly every day (either by subjective account or as observed by others).

▶ Recurrent thoughts of death (not just fear of dying), recurrent suicidal ideation without a specific plan, or a suicide attempt or a specific plan for committing suicide.

Importantly, to diagnose depressive symptoms as MDD, the symptoms must cause clinically significant distress or impairment in social, occupational, or other important areas of functioning. Further, the episode of depression should not be attributable to the physiologic effects of a substance or another medical condition.

Responses to a significant loss (e.g., bereavement, financial ruin, losses from a natural disaster, a serious medical illness, or disability) may include the feelings of intense sadness, rumination about the loss, insomnia, poor appetite, and weight loss noted above which may resemble a depressive episode. Although such symptoms may be understandable or considered appropriate to the loss, the presence of a major depressive episode in addition to the normal response to a significant loss should also be carefully considered. Finally, the episode of depression should not be better explained by another disorder (e.g., schizoaffective disorder, schizophrenia, or other psychotic disorders) and there should not be a history of a manic or hypomanic episode.

With respect to GAD, DSM-5 requires that the patients have excessive anxiety and worry (apprehensive expectation) occurring more days than not for at least 6 months and about a number of events or activities (such as work or school performance).[22] Further, the individual finds it difficult to control the worry. The anxiety and worry are associated with three (or more) of the following six symptoms (with at least some symptoms having been present for more days than not for the past 6 months): *Note:* Only one item required in children.

▶ Restlessness, feeling keyed up, or on edge.

▶ Being easily fatigued.

▶ Difficulty concentrating or mind going blank.

▶ Irritability.

▶ Muscle tension.

▶ Sleep disturbance (difficulty falling or staying asleep, or restless, unsatisfying sleep).

Similar to MDD, to diagnose GAD, the anxiety, worry, or physical symptoms must cause clinically significant distress or impairment in social, occupational, or other important areas of functioning. In addition, the disturbance should not be attributable to the physiologic effects of a substance (e.g., a drug of abuse, a medication) or another medical condition (e.g., hyperthyroidism), and is not better explained by another medical disorder (e.g., panic disorder, social phobia, or the content of delusional beliefs in schizophrenia or delusional disorder).

TREATMENT FOR DEPRESSION AND ANXIETY

A positive score on either the PHQ-9 or GAD-7 with confirmation from the DSM-5 can lead to several treatment strategies. We strongly recommend checking several symptoms with the patient to verify the validity of the PHQ-9 (e.g., patient reports recent situational stressors that may be elevating symptoms versus a true MDD).

Patients with depression or anxiety may feel stigmatized by having symptoms of a psychiatric condition and it is crucial for the provider to provide an explanation for the disorder,

Table 22.2 ▶ Treatment Actions Based on Score and Depression Severity

PHQ-9 Score	Severity	Treatment Actions
0–4	None–minimal	None
5–9	Mild	Watchful waiting; repeat PHQ-9 at 2–4 weeks follow-up
10–14	Moderate	Treatment plan, consider psychotherapy, follow-up, and/or pharmacotherapy
15–19	Moderately severe	Active treatment with pharmacotherapy and/or psychotherapy
20–27	Severe	Immediate initiation and, if severe impairment or poor response to therapy, expedited referral to a mental health specialist for psychotherapy and/or collaborative management

noting that it is a biologic condition and does not mean that the patient is a "weak" person. It can be helpful to let patients know that depression is a common condition and affects up to 6.7% of the US population (1 out of every 15 people). Another important component of this discussion is to give the patient hope that their mood disorder is treatable and can be treated with pharmacotherapy, behavioral interventions, and/or formal psychotherapy.

One explanation that we have employed for several years is the following:

"People experiencing depression (or anxiety) can often feel like they are drowning in the storm of their symptoms. Medication can act as a life preserver, helping to float you above the stormy waters. Psychotherapy can give you the skills to swim back to shore."[23]

Table 22.2 can be used to help guide treatment decisions based upon the PHQ-9 score.[24] Please note that for any level of severity, behavioral activation, exercise, and education are recommended.

Behavioral Interventions for Depression and Anxiety in Primary Care

There is ample evidence supporting the use of behavioral interventions in primary care. Behavioral interventions can help to build skills for patients while also leading to symptom reduction. Furthermore, behavioral interventions may be the treatment of choice for mild depression or anxiety symptoms.

Behavioral activation is an evidence-based treatment shown to reduce depression symptoms.[25] Patients with depression are at a greater risk for engaging in avoiding and isolation, which can worsen their symptoms. The goal of behavioral activation is to help patients reduce their avoidance and isolation by gradually increasing activities that can bring them joy or pleasure. Patients are also encouraged to monitor their activity level and mood daily. This effort can be facilitated using a chart like the one shown in Figure 22.1.

Deep breathing and relaxation exercises can be helpful for patients to reduce symptoms of depression and anxiety. A popular breathing exercise is the 4-7-8 breath. Below are instructions for initiating this exercise (http://www.drweil.com/health-wellness/body-mind-spirit/stress-anxiety/breathing-three-exercises/):

1. Exhale completely through your mouth, making a whoosh sound.
2. Close your mouth and inhale quietly through your nose to a mental count of **four**.
3. Hold your breath for a count of **seven**.
4. Exhale completely through your mouth, making a whoosh sound to a count of **eight**.
5. This is one breath. Now inhale again and repeat the cycle three more times for a total of four breaths.

Time	Planned positive activity (see reference list)*	Complete (Yes/No)	Mood rating (0-100, 0=worst, 100=best) before and after activity
Before 8 am			
8 am to 12 noon			
12 noon to 4 pm			
4 pm to 8 pm			
After 8 pm			
Total # of activities			
*Providers can also offer patients a list of potential activities to consider. Available at: http://www.cci.health.wa.gov.au/docs/Fun%20Activities%20Catalogue.pdf			

Figure 22.1 ▶ This form is for planning and tracking your positive planned activities. Write down what you plan to do for the day, either the night before or in the morning.

Exercise has some benefit for depression and anxiety. Investigators have found that exercise improves symptoms in people with depression compared with control treatment or no intervention.[26] Providers can counsel patients to begin exercise slowly and choose an enjoyable mode of exercise which can result in a more positive exercise experience for the patient and increase the likelihood of maintained exercise involvement.[27]

Brief cognitive disputation is a specific cognitive behavioral tool to help patients with depressed or anxious thoughts change the way they think. Patients can learn to question their thoughts by asking themselves a question when they are experiencing depressed or anxious thoughts such as, "If my best friend or someone I love had this thought, what would I tell them?" or "If you were to ask or tell yourself that, how do you think that would be helpful?"[28] Questions such as these can allow patients to respond in ways that are consistent with their values (e.g., being friendly) instead of reacting to their initial thoughts.

Pharmacotherapy for Depression

Pharmacotherapy is an important treatment option for patients presenting with depression symptoms in primary care settings. Specific antidepressant treatment guidelines have been developed from the TMAP and STAR*D trials.[29,30] In STAR*D, roughly half of patients responded to initial treatment and a third reached remission within 6 weeks.[31] The ARTIST trial showed recovery rates around 80% at 9 months in patients randomized to either fluoxetine, sertraline, or paroxetine.[32] However, the particular drug or drugs used are not as important as following a rational plan:[28]

▶ Giving antidepressant medications in adequate doses.
▶ Monitoring the patient's symptoms and side effects and adjusting the regimen accordingly.
▶ Switching drugs or adding new drugs to the regimen only after an adequate trial.

Table 22.3 lists treatment guidelines based upon the STAR*D trials that also include behavioral health interventions and other issues that can influence symptoms and treatment

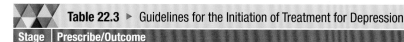

Table 22.3 ▶ Guidelines for the Initiation of Treatment for Depression

Stage	Prescribe/Outcome
1	SSRI, behavioral health interventions, 2-week follow-up, readminister PHQ-9 • If >50% improvement, follow-up in 4 weeks • If 25–49% improvement, increase dose, 2-week follow-up (repeat 2 times, then go to next stage)
2	Different SSRI, bupropion, or SNRI, behavioral health interventions, 2-week follow-up, readminister PHQ-9 • If >50% improvement, follow-up in 4 weeks • If 25–49% improvement, increase dose, 2-week follow-up (repeat 2 times, then go to next stage)
3	SNRI or add bupropion to SSRI, behavioral health interventions, refer to psychiatry

PHQ, Patient Health Questionnaire; SNRI, serotonin-norepinephrine reuptake inhibitor; SSRI, selective serotonin reuptake inhibitor.

adherence. Providers use Table 22.3 as a guide for the initiation of treatment (stage 1) and can adjust treatment based upon response (stages 2 and 3). At each stage, consider adherence, past/current suicidal ideation, history of response, comorbid conditions, and cultural factors that influence treatment and response.

Several medication options are available for treatment of depression (Table 22.4).

Table 22.4 ▶ Side Effects of Antidepressant Medications

Drug	Anti-cholinergic	Drowsi-ness	Insomnia/Agitation	Orthostatic Hyperten-sion	Pro-longed QTc	GI	Weight Gain	Sexual Dys-function
Selective Serotonin Reuptake Inhibitors								
Citalopram	0	0	1+	1+	1+	1+	1+	3+
Escitalo-pram	0	0	1+	1+	1+	1+	1+	3+
Fluoxetine	0	0	2+	1+	1+	1+	1+	3+
Paroxetine	1+	1+	1+	2+	0–1+	1+	2+	4+
Sertraline	0	0	2+	1+	0–1+	2+	1+	3+
Serotonin-Norepinephrine Reuptake Inhibitors								
Desvenla-faxine	0	1+	2+	0	0	1–2+	0	3+
Duloxetine	0	0	2+	0	0	2+	0	3+
Venlafaxine	0	1+	2+	0	1+	1–2+	0	3+
Atypical Agents								
Bupropion	0	0	1–2+	0	1+	1+	0	0
Mirtazapine	1+	4+	0	0	1+	0	4+	1+

0 = none; 1+ = slight; 2+ = low; 3+ = moderate; 4+ = high.

▶ **Selective serotonergic reuptake inhibitors** (SSRIs) are typically the first-line pharmacotherapy treatment for depression in primary care. Treatment with SSRIs is usually well tolerated, although side effects such as jitteriness, restlessness, insomnia, and increased anxiety that occur within the first 5 to 7 days can affect treatment compliance. It is important, however, to ensure that no bipolar symptoms are present as SSRIs can unmask and potentiate an underlying bipolar disorder presenting with depressive symptoms.

▶ **Serotonin norepinephrine reuptake inhibitors** (SNRIs) are a second option for treatment of anxiety disorders in primary care. Like SSRIs, side effects such as nausea, insomnia, and headaches can affect medication adherence.

▶ **Tetracyclic noradrenaline and specific antidepressants**, specifically mirtazapine, are another option, with benefits including improved sleep duration and fewer sexual side effects. However, weight gain can be more significant, which can make these a good option in older adults suffering from decreased appetite and weight loss as a part of their depression.

▶ **Norepinephrine dopamine reuptake inhibitors**, specifically bupropion, are antidepressants that have fewer sexual side effects and can be activating for patients. However, patients with comorbid anxiety disorders may be at risk for increased activation and agitation. Bupropion is also used for smoking cessation.

▶ **The atypical antipsychotic aripiprazole** has shown efficacy as an augmentation option with standard antidepressant therapy for patients who have failed to achieve remission with initial treatment and has been approved by the FDA as adjunctive therapy for MDD. However, their use remains controversial mostly due to the frequency of significant side effects. The most common side effect reported for this medication has been akathisia and weight gain.[33] Other options for treatment-resistant depression should be explored first.

Treatment for Anxiety

Table 22.5 lists treatment recommendations based on GAD-7 scores. We recommend behavioral interventions including behavioral activation, exercise, and education for patients at any level of severity.

Table 22.5 ▶ Treatment Actions Based on Score and Depression Severity

GAD-7 Score	Severity	Treatment Actions
0–4	None–minimal	None
5–9	Mild	Watchful waiting; repeat GAD-7 at 2–4 weeks follow-up
10–14	Moderate	Treatment plan, consider psychotherapy, follow-up, and/or pharmacotherapy
15–19	Moderately severe	Active treatment with pharmacotherapy and/or psychotherapy
20–27	Severe	Immediate initiation and, if severe impairment or poor response to therapy, expedited referral to a mental health specialist for psychotherapy and/or collaborative management

Pharmacotherapy for Anxiety

Several pharmacotherapy options are available for the treatment of anxiety.

▶ **SSRIs** are typically first-line pharmacotherapy treatment for anxiety in primary care. Treatment is usually well tolerated, although side effects as noted above can affect treatment adherence.[31] Reducing the starting dosage may help reduce initial side effects.

▶ **SNRIs** are a second option for treatment of anxiety disorders in primary care. Like SSRIs side effect can affect adherence (see Table 22.4).

▶ **Pregabalin** can be a useful medication for GAD symptoms in that the onset of efficacy occurs typically within the first few days of treatment.[34]

▶ **Benzodiazepines** provide reduction of anxiety symptoms, although benzodiazepine treatment may be associated with sedation, dizziness, and prolonged reaction time as well as negative effects on cognitive function and driving skills. Risks include dependency after a few weeks or months of continuous treatment. Longer-acting agents are preferable to short-acting agents to help reduce risk of dependency. Patients with a history of alcohol or substance dependence are not candidates for benzodiazepine treatment due to heightened risks for dependency. Benzodiazepines may also be useful during the first few weeks of initiating a serotonergic medication to help reduce the accompanying anxiety with these medications.[34]

▶ **Antihistamines** such as hydroxyzine can be an alternative to benzodiazepines. Side effects include sedation, anticholinergic effects at high doses, blurred vision, confusion, delirium, and others.[34]

▶ **Beta blockers** such as propranolol have been used to help reduce anxiety symptoms. Authors of a systematic review reported that the evidence for efficacy of propranolol is insufficient to support its routine use in the treatment of anxiety disorders.[32] It has been proposed that propranolol's anxiolytic properties may result from its peripheral (autonomic) rather than its central activity. Beta blockers may work better for performance anxiety rather than general anxiety.[35]

▶ **Azapirones** such as buspirone are an option for patients suffering from anxiety disorders such as GAD. Authors of a systematic review found that azapirones appear to be superior to placebo in the short term (4 to 9 weeks) but may not be superior to benzodiazepines and may not be as acceptable by patients as benzodiazepines.[36]

Bipolar Disorder Treatment in Primary Care

A positive MDQ or BSDS warrants further evaluation to confirm a diagnosis of bipolar disorder. Treatment options include the use of agents such as mood stabilizers (lithium), atypical antipsychotics, and anticonvulsants. Consultation with psychiatry can be useful to help guide treatment initiation depending on the symptom presentation.

Psychotherapy

The most widely studied formal psychotherapy for both depression and anxiety disorders is cognitive behavioral therapy (CBT). CBT is a time-sensitive, structured, present-oriented psychotherapy directed toward solving problems and teaching patients skills to modify thinking and behavior.[37] CBT has been shown to be an effective treatment for depression and anxiety.[38,39] We recommended referring patients to licensed psychologists, social workers, or counselors who have received appropriate training in CBT to provide these services.[39] For information on CBT see https://www.beckinstitute.org/get-informed/what-is-cognitive-therapy.

QUESTIONS

1. Mental health disorders are common problems in primary care. Which one of the following is true of these disorders among primary care patients?
   A. Lifetime prevalence of depression is about 50%.
   B. Individuals with depression are at the same risk for anxiety as nondepressed individuals.
   C. Most patients with mental illness have one or more chronic physical conditions.
   D. Posttraumatic stress disorder is the least common anxiety disorder.

2. Which one of the following is true of screening for depression and anxiety in primary care settings?
   A. Depression screening is recommended for adults provided that systems are in place to ensure proper diagnosis, treatment, and follow-up.
   B. A positive screen on the PHQ-9 is diagnostic of depression.
   C. Patients who screen positive for suicidal ideation should be hospitalized.
   D. The GAD Questionnaire is only helpful for screening for generalized anxiety disorder.
   E. Screening tools are unavailable for detecting bipolar disorder.

3. A patient with newly diagnosed depression is seen in the clinic to discuss possible treatment options. Which one of the following is true of depression management?
   A. Symptoms reported on the screening questionnaire do not require verification
   B. Providing a biologic explanation for the disorder is helpful
   C. Exercise and breathing exercises are not useful for depression symptoms
   D. Medication is more effective for patients with mild depression than behavioral interventions

4. Which one of the following is typically a first-line medication for generalized anxiety disorder?
   A. Beta blocker
   B. Serotonergic norepinephrine reuptake inhibitor
   C. Benzodiazepine
   D. Selective serotonergic reuptake inhibitor
   E. Norepinephrine dopamine reuptake inhibitor

5. CBT, a psychotherapy directed toward solving problems and teaching skills to modify thinking and behavior, is an effective treatment for both depression and anxiety.
   A. True
   B. False

ANSWERS

Question 1: The correct answer is C.
In addition, 68% of adults with mental illness have one or more chronic physical conditions. In fact, people with mental illness die earlier than the general population, perhaps because they have more co-occurring health conditions.

Question 2: The correct answer is A.

Although screening for depression is recommended by the USPSTF, systems must be in place to ensure proper diagnosis, treatment, and follow-up.

Question 3: The correct answer is B.

Patients with depression or anxiety may feel stigmatized by having symptoms of a psychiatric condition and it is crucial for the provider to provide an explanation for the disorder, noting that it is a biologic condition and does not mean that the patient is a "weak" person.

Question 4: The correct answer is D.

SSRIs are typically first-line pharmacotherapy treatment for anxiety in primary care. Treatment is usually well tolerated, although side effects as noted above can affect treatment adherence.

Question 5: The correct answer is A.

CBT is a time-sensitive, structured, present-oriented psychotherapy directed toward solving problems and teaching patients skills to modify thinking and behavior. CBT has been shown to be an effective treatment for depression and anxiety.

REFERENCES

1. Reiger D, Narrow W, Rae D, et al. The de facto US mental and addictive disorders service system: Epidemiologic Catchment Area prospective 1-year prevalence rates of disorders and services. *Arch Gen Psychiatry*. 1993;50:85–94.
2. U.S. Department of Health and Human Services. *Report of a Surgeon General's Working Meeting on The Integration of Mental Health Services and Primary Health Care*. Rockville, MD: 2001. Available at: www.surgeongeneral.gov/library/mentalhealthservices/mentalhealthservices.PDF4. Accessed December 15, 2016.
3. Office of the Surgeon General (US); Center for Mental Health Services (US); National Institute of Mental Health (US). *Mental Health: Culture, Race and Ethnicity: A Supplement to Mental Health: A Report of the Surgeon General*. Rockville, MD: Substance Abuse and Mental Health Services Administration (US); 2001.
4. Kroenke K. The interface between physical and psychological symptoms. *Prim Care Companion J Clin Psychiatry*. 2003;5(suppl 7):11–18.
5. Substance Abuse and Mental Health Services Administration/ Health Resources Services Administration. Back to basics: what you need to know about primary and behavioral health care integration. Available at: http://www.integration.samhsa.gov/about-us/CIHS_Integration_101_FINAL.pdf. Accessed November 14, 2016.
6. World Health Organization. Social determinants of mental health. 2014. Available at: http://apps.who.int/iris/bitstream/10665/112828/1/9789241506809_eng.pdf. Accessed November 10, 2016.
7. Kessler RC, Berglund P, Demler O, et al. The epidemiology of major depressive disorder: results from the National Comorbidity Survey Replication. *JAMA*. 2003;289:3095–3105.
8. Mojtabai R, Olfson M. National patterns in antidepressant treatment by psychiatrists and general medical providers: results from the national comorbidity survey replication. *J Clin Psychiatry*. 2008;69(7):1064–1074.
9. United States Preventative Services Task Force. Depression in Adults: Screening. Available at: https://www.uspreventiveservicestaskforce.org/Page/Document/UpdateSummaryFinal/depression-in-adults-screening1?ds=1&s=depression screening adults. Accessed on November 14, 2016.
10. Kroenke K, Spitzer RL, Williams J, et al. Anxiety disorders in primary care: prevalence, impairment, comorbidity, and detection. *Ann Intern Med*. 2007;146(5):317–325.
11. Nease DE, Aikens JE. DSM depression and anxiety criteria and severity of symptoms in primary care: cross sectional study. *BMJ*. 2003;327(7422):1030–1031.
12. Siu AL, Bibbins-Domingo K, Grossman DC, et al. Screening for depression in adults: US Preventive Services Task Force recommendation statement. *JAMA*. 2016;315(4):380–387.
13. Gilbody S, Richards D, Brealey S, et al. Screening for depression in medical settings with the patient health questionnaire (PHQ): a diagnostic meta-analysis. *J Gen Intern Med*. 2007;22(11):1596–1602.
14. Nease DE, Maloin JM. Depression screening: a practical strategy. *J Fam Practice*. 2003;52(2):118–124.

15. Campbell, W. Revised SAD PERSONS helps assess suicide risk. 2004. Available at: https://www.qxmd.com/calculate/calculator_201/modified-sad-persons-scale. Accessed January 6, 2017.

16. Spitzer RL, Kroenke K, Williams JB, et al. A brief measure for assessing generalized anxiety disorder: The GAD-7. *Arch Intern Med.* 2006;166(10):1092–1097.

17. Psychiatric times. GAD-7. Available at: http://www.psychiatrictimes.com/clinical-scales-gad-7/clinical-scales-gad-7/gad-7. Accessed November 16, 2016.

18. U.S. Department of Veterans Affairs. Primary care PTSD screen (PC-PTSD). Available at: http://www.ptsd.va.gov/professional/assessment/screens/pc-ptsd.asp. Accessed November 16, 2016.

19. Zimmerman M, Galione JN. Screening for bipolar disorder with the Mood Disorders Questionnaire: A review. *Harv Rev Psychiatry.* 2011;19(5):219–228.

20. Nassir GS, Miller CJ, Berv DA, et al. Sensitivity and specificity of a new bipolar disorder spectrum diagnostic scale. *J Affect Disord.* 2005;84(2-3):273–277.

21. U.S. Department. of Health and Human Services, Substance Abuse and Mental Health Services Administration. Results from the 2009 National Survey on Drug Use and Health: Volume I. Summary of national findings. Available at: http://oas.samhsa.gov/nsduh/2k9nsduh/2k9resultsp.pdf. Accessed November 16, 2016.

22. American Psychiatric Association. *Diagnostic and Statistical Manual of Mental Disorders.* 5th ed. 2013.

23. Ingeborg Van Pelt. "Where is the hurt? How do we help?" *Clin Psychiatry News.* 2009;37(6):10.

24. Instruction manual for Patient Health Questionnaire (PHQ) and GAD-7 measures. Available at: https://phqscreeners.pfizer.edrupalgardens.com/sites/g/files/g10016261/f/201412/instructions.pdf. Accessed November 16, 2016.

25. Dimidjian S, Dobson K, Kohlenberg RJ, et al. Randomized trial of behavioral activation, cognitive therapy and antidepressant medication in the acute treatment of adults with major depression. *J Consult Clin Psychol.* 2006;74(4):658–670.

26. Cooney GM, Dwan K, Greig CA, et al. Exercise for depression. *Cochrane Database Syst Rev.* 2013;(9):CD004366.

27. Craft L, Perna F. The benefits of exercise for the clinically depressed. *Primary Care Companion to J Clin Psychiatry.* 2004;6(3):104–111.

28. Hunter CL, Goodie JL, Oordt MS, et al. *Integrated Behavioral Health in Primary Care.* Washington, DC: American Psychological Association; 2009.

29. Trivedi MH, Rush AJ, Crismon ML, et al. Clinical results for patients with major depressive disorder in the Texas Medication Algorithm Project. *Arch Gen Psychiatry.* 2004;61(7):669–680.

30. Trivedi MH, Rush AJ, Wisniewski SR, et al. Evaluation of outcomes with citalopram for depression using measurement-based care in STAR*D: Implications for clinical practice. *Am J Psychiatry.* 2006;163(1):28–40.

31. Gaynes BN, Rush AJ, Trivedi MH, et al. The STAR*D study: Treating depression in the real world. *Clev Clin J Med.* 2008;75:57–66.

32. Kroenke K, West S, Swindle R, et al. Similar effectiveness of paroxetine, fluoxetine, and sertraline in primary care a randomized trial. *JAMA.* 2001;286(23):2947–2955.

33. Nelson JC, Pikalov A, Berman R. Augmentation treatment in major depressive disorder: Focus on aripiprazole. *Neuropsychiatr Dis Treat.* 2008;4(5):937–948.

34. Bandelow B, Sher L, Bunevicius R, et al.; WFSBP Task Force on Mental Disorders in Primary Care. WFSBP Task Force on Anxiety Disorders. *Int J Psychiatry Clin Pract.* 2012;16:77–84.

35. Steenen SA, Wijk AJ, van der Heijden G, et al. Propranolol for the treatment of anxiety disorders: Systematic review and meta-analysis. *J Psychopharmacol.* 2016;30(2):128–139.

36. Chessick CA, Allen MH, Thase M, et al. Azapirones for generalized anxiety disorder. *Cochrane Database Syst Rev.* 2006;(3):CD006115.

37. The Beck Institute. What is cognitive behavioral therapy? Available at: https://www.beckinstitute.org/get-informed/what-is-cognitive-therapy. Accessed November 10, 2016.

38. Hoffman SG, Asnaani A, Vonk IJ, et al. The efficacy of cognitive behavioral therapy: A review of meta-analyses. *Cognit Ther Res.* 2012;36(5):427–444.

39. Cape J, Whittington C, Buszewicz M, et al. Brief psychological therapies for anxiety and depression in primary care: Meta-analysis and meta-regression. *BMC Med.* 2010;8:38.

Substance Use Disorders

KEY POINTS

1 ▶ In the primary care setting, substance use disorders are rarely the patient's presenting problem, although they are common contributors to patient's medical problems.

2 ▶ Substance abuse and dependence are similar to many other chronic illnesses such as type II diabetes and cardiovascular disease with respect to their course and patient adherence and should be considered as chronic medical diseases.

3 ▶ There are established interview instruments that can be administered efficiently in the primary care setting and have adequate sensitivity and specificity to assist in the care of patients with substance use disorders.

4 ▶ Psychosocial issues are common "red flags" in the early detection of substance use disorders.

5 ▶ While medications can be very useful in treating substance use disorders, particularly opioid addiction, pharmacotherapy is more effective when combined with counseling.

Recent societal problems with opioids have highlighted challenges that many of our patients struggle with in their daily lives—that of substance use disorders. The 2016 "Facing Addiction in America: The Surgeon General's Report on Alcohol, Drugs and Health"[1] chronicles this well and is worth reviewing. Addiction is a chronic disease and not a character flaw. As with any other chronic medical condition, a combination of patient willingness to take responsibility and work hard to learn about caring for this disease together with an understanding that it will take more than just willpower to heal serves patients best.

While there are unique features of each misused substance and differences in health risks associated with each, there are some common shared features.

PREVALENCE AND DIAGNOSIS

▶ In adult and pediatric primary care settings, the prevalence of drug or alcohol use disorders is 10%.[2]

▶ Most patients with active substance use problems do not report this issue as their reason for seeking care.[3] The physician should be knowledgeable about types of presenting symptoms and syndromes associated with substance misuse as well as the epidemiology of these disorders in the population they serve and should ask appropriate questions about substance misuse if the situation warrants.

▶ Relapse rates for substance use disorders (40% to 60%) are comparable to those for other chronic illnesses, including type II diabetes (20% to 50%) and hypertension (50% to 70%).[1]

▶ The presence of a substance use disorder doubles the likelihood of multiple chronic illnesses, including arthritis, chronic pain syndromes, stroke, hypertension, diabetes, and asthma.[1]

▶ The Diagnostic and Statistical Manual of Mental Disorders, fifth edition (DSM-5), now uses the term "Substance Use Disorders" with the modifiers *mild, moderate,* and *severe* rather than "Substance Abuse" and "Substance Dependence" disorders. This better aligns with the spectrum of use disorders seen in primary care.[4]

▶ Despite changes in DSM-5, the clinical determination of abuse versus dependence is still useful, especially with issues of drug tolerance and withdrawal and problems associated with drug dependence.

- Tolerance occurs when more of the same drug is needed to achieve the desired effect and typically develops among daily users of many drugs and alcohol.
- Withdrawal is a pattern of symptoms specific to a particular habitually used drug when withdrawn.

Patient Engagement and Treatment of Substance Use Disorders—General Guidelines

Asking about drug and alcohol use should be a standard part of a comprehensive history and physical for adults and adolescents. Traditionally, questions about alcohol and drug use have been discussed later in medical history gathering, after rapport has been established, because these topics are often sensitive and patients with problems are often defensive. The use of patient-completed comprehensive review of systems forms that include questions about alcohol and recreational drug use, changes how and when this conversation might begin, but regardless of the approach taken, it should not change how you should respond to the information provided and ask additional questions. You should do so in a frank and nonconfrontational way—the same way you would ask other medical history questions.

The Substance Abuse and Mental Health Services Administration, or SAMHSA, has promoted **SBIRT** (https://www.samhsa.gov/sbirt), or **S**creening, **B**rief **I**ntervention, and **R**eferral to **T**reatment to aid clinicians in identifying and initiating engagement with patients with substance use disorders. **An annual survey of patients to screen for substance use disorders is encouraged** and consists of two steps.

Step 1: Ask About Alcohol and Drug Use

Alcohol use:

▶ Do you sometimes drink beer, wine, or other alcoholic beverages?

▶ How many times in the past year have you had five or more drinks (four or more for women and men over age 65 years) in a day? (*See details of what is a drink below. **One or more is considered positive.** If positive, patient is at risk for acute consequences, e.g., trauma and accidents.*)

▶ If the score is greater than zero, ask:

- On average, how many alcoholic drinks do you have per week?
- On a typical drinking day, how many drinks do you have? (If average exceeds 14 drinks per week for healthy men up to age 65 years or 7 drinks per week for all healthy women and healthy men over age 65 years, patient is at risk for chronic health problems.)

Drug use:

▶ How many times in the past year have you used an illegal drug or used a prescription medication for nonmedical reasons? *(If asked what nonmedical reasons means, you can say because of the experience or feeling the drug caused. One or more is considered positive.)*

If the answers to the alcohol or drug use screening tools are positive, then go to Step 2. Your patient at least shows evidence of risky alcohol and/or drug use. If answers are negative, then reinforce good health habits.

Step 2: Assess for Alcohol and/or Drug Severity Using the CAGE–AID Questionnaire

For each question below a 'yes' = 1 point. A score of >1 suggests the need for further diagnostics, discussion, and/or referral. For more information, go to http://www.integration.samhsa.gov/images/res/CAGEAID.pdf.

▶ Have you ever felt that you ought to **CUT** down on your drinking or drug use?

▶ Have people ever **ANNOYED** you by criticizing your drinking or drug use?

▶ Have you ever felt bad or **GUILTY** about your drinking or drug use?

▶ Have you ever had a drink or used drugs first thing in the morning (**EYE-OPENER**) to steady your nerves or get rid of a hangover?

WHAT NOW?

The next step is usually to consider how you can help/levels of intervention. Primary care clinicians are often involved in the screening/brief intervention, working toward treatment engagement and referral for treatment levels noted in Table 23.1 below. Inpatient and intensive day programs/residential programs are most commonly run by specialists in those areas.

Counseling Techniques

With some modifications, Motivational Interviewing, Counseling based upon the Stages of Change (both described in Chapter 5), and FRAMES (Table 23.2), a technique in which specific medical findings are used to initiate the discussion of substance use, are applicable to patients with multiple specific types of substance use problems.

Support

Twelve-step programs or other peer-based groups that originated with Alcoholics Anonymous have been modified for other types of substance use disorders. While their structure makes it difficult to draw firm conclusions about their effectiveness, these programs appear to be beneficial adjuncts to treatment. Sites that allow patients to search for meetings in their area by day, time, and location:

▶ Alcoholics Anonymous: http://www.aa.org/pages/en_US/find-local-aa

▶ Narcotics Anonymous: http://www.naws.org/meetingsearch/

▶ Marijuana: https://www.marijuana-anonymous.org/meetings/find

Table 23.1 ▶ Treatment Levels of Intervention for Substance Use Disorders

Level of Intervention[1]	Action	Notes
Screening and brief intervention	Patient assessment followed by brief informationally oriented counseling (FRAMES, see Table 23.2)	Effective for alcohol abuse, less consistent evidence for other drugs of abuse
Working toward treatment engagement	Working with patients who are reluctant to enter formal treatment	Motivational interviewing is a common communication strategy
Referral for treatment	This usually involves linking the patient to self-help and/or outpatient services.	Knowledge of local outpatient community resources is essential. Primary care clinician continues to follow the patient and treat comorbid conditions and/or provide pharmacotherapy
Inpatient treatment	Used primarily for short-term detoxification and to reduce the risk of drug withdrawal. Up to 70% of those undergoing detox refuse subsequent treatment[1]	Knowledge of local inpatient services within the community are important
Intensive day and/or residential programs	Provide individual and group counseling, psychoeducation, and 12-step programs for 14, 21, 30, 60, or 90 days	Often initiated by specialists or in transitions from inpatient detox or other programs

Pharmacotherapy

Medication directed at helping your patient reduce problematic drinking or substance misuse is most effective when combined with psychosocial treatment, particularly those that involve family members. Specific psychopharmacology options for various substance use disorders are discussed below.

Comorbid Conditions

▶ Substance misuse often coexists with psychiatric conditions[7] and patients with both problems are often said to have "dual-diagnosis." Major depressive disorder (MDD) is commonly comorbid with substance misuse; it is often difficult to distinguish the neurovegetative, cognitive, and behavioral symptoms of substance use disorders from MDD. It is a common practice to delay formally diagnosing a primary psychiatric disorder until at least 30 days after the last substance use episode, unless the history suggests that mood disorder symptoms preceded the substance misuse.

▶ Cigarette smoking is more common in people with alcohol or other substance use disorders. Traditionally, the alcohol or other substance use disorder is addressed first and then, once under control, smoking cessation is addressed. However, recent studies conducted in residential/inpatient substance abuse treatment programs suggest that both conditions can be effectively treated simultaneously.[1]

Harm Reduction

This is an evolving approach to substance use disorders in which the goal is not abstinence but on reducing the harmful consequences of drugs and drug use. It challenges the

▲ Table 23.2 ▶ FRAMES

Dimension	Description	Example
Feedback	When possible, begin with specific feedback including objective medical data (e.g., physical signs, lab results, BP). Describe how these data relate to substance use	"Chronic cough and frequent respiratory infections often go along with daily marijuana use." "More than 3–4 drinks per day has been associated with increased BP"
Responsibility	State clearly that the responsibility for change rests with the patient	"Reducing alcohol use is ultimately your decision." "If you decide to stop smoking marijuana, I will be glad to assist—but the choice is yours"
Advice	Cleary state your recommendation with specific parameters	"I recommend that you reduce your use of alcohol to no more than two glasses of wine daily." "I recommend that you stop taking oxycodone for your back pain"
Menu of options	Patients are more likely to modify behavior if given several options for achieving a substance use reduction/abstinence goal. By providing patients with control, they can select options most compatible with their circumstances	"Here are some approaches that patients have found useful." "Some patients take medication to reduce their craving for opioids; others have found self-help groups like Narcotics Anonymous to be most helpful"
Empathy	Make empathic statements to your patient to convey your appreciation of their ambivalence about change and the accompanying challenge in reducing or eliminating substance use	"I hear you saying that drinking alcohol is the major way that you relax after work but you are feeling more hung over for the past several months and feel like it might be time to stop drinking. It sounds like quitting will be worth it but it will be challenging"
Self-efficacy	Express confidence that patient can be successful; it is often useful to ask patients about life challenges that they have overcome in the past and how they overcame them	"I am impressed with your desire to quit drinking. It takes courage to recognize how alcohol is disrupting your life. I remember several years ago, that you quit smoking on your own. The same skills and determination you used to stop smoking can be used to beat alcohol"

BP, blood pressure.
Data from: Miller WR, Hester RK. Treating alcohol problems: toward an informed eclecticism. In Hester R, Miller W, Eds. *Handbook of Alcoholism Treatment Approaches: Effective Alternatives*. Elmsford, NY: Pergamon Press; 1989:pp 3–13;[5] Searight HR. Efficient counseling techniques for the primary care physician. *Prim Care Clin Office Pract*. 2007;34(3):551–570.[6]

long-held approach of zero tolerance around which most approaches to substance use disorders have traditionally been based. Examples include:

▶ Brief, one-time counseling has been found to reduce patients' alcohol consumption while not achieving abstinence.[8]

▶ With marijuana use, reducing THC exposure by reducing quantity smoked or by conscious reductions in inhalation.[9]

▶ Methadone maintenance therapy for heroin and prescription opioid addiction.

▶ For injection drug users, needle exchange programs reduce risk of HIV and other needle-borne illnesses. Naloxone given to injection users as well as for daily opiate users to use in case of emergency/overdose are also seeing more use.

SPECIFIC DRUGS

Alcohol

Allen is a 50-year-old white man whom you have been treating for hypertension for the past 7 years. His chart indicates that he is seeing you today for suture removal as a follow-up from an emergency department (ED) visit 7 days ago. The note from the ED indicates that Allen was seen after an auto accident in which he hit his head on the dashboard and sustained a laceration. The ED note also mentions that Allen smelled of alcohol. While Allen's blood pressure has generally been well controlled, today it is 156/90 mm Hg.

What is a Drink?

Each of the beverages in the quantity depicted in Figure 23.1 is ONE drink or 14 g of alcohol.

How Much Alcohol is Too Much?

Most US adults have consumed an alcoholic drink in the past month. One of the differences between many illicit drugs such as cocaine or heroin and alcohol is that some level of alcohol consumption is not considered problematic and may even have health benefits. For example, among drinkers consuming under two drinks per day, bone density is greater and risk of cardiovascular disease is reduced.[1]

▶ While there is no specific cut-off for "normal" drinking, low-risk drinking is:
  • For men: No more than 4 drinks per day; no more than 14 drinks per week
  • For women: No more than three drinks per day; no more than seven drinks per week

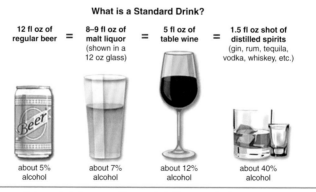

What is a Standard Drink?

| 12 fl oz of regular beer | 8–9 fl oz of malt liquor (shown in a 12 oz glass) | 5 fl oz of table wine | 1.5 fl oz shot of distilled spirits (gin, rum, tequila, vodka, whiskey, etc.) |

about 5% alcohol = about 7% alcohol = about 12% alcohol = about 40% alcohol

The percent of pure alcohol, expressed here as alcohol by volume (alc/vol), varies by beverage.

From What Is A Standard Drink? National Institute of Alcohol Abuse and Alcoholism,
https://www.niaaa.nih.gov/alcohol-health/overview-alcohol-consumption/what-standard-drink

Figure 23.1 ▶ Defining a Standard Drink.

▶ Binge drinking: The number of drinks in one sitting required to attain a blood alcohol level of 0.08 g/dL:

- For women: typically, four drinks in 2 hours
- For men: typically, five drinks in 2 hours

What are Early Clinical Indicators of Alcohol Use Problems?

Early stages of problem drinking are typically associated with predominantly psychosocial problems. These include arrests for driving under the influence or disorderly conduct, relationship problems, marital separation, domestic violence, job loss, and fights. Earlier screening for alcohol use or questioning Allen about psychosocial issues during prior visits may have helped prevent his accident. Medical problems from binge use are more likely to result from injuries sustained while under the influence, such as head trauma, broken bones, burns, or other injuries. Suicide attempts are also more likely while under the influence of alcohol. In primary care patient populations, additional problems, signs or symptoms that should raise concern about a possible alcohol use disorder are listed in Table 23.3.

What are the Medical Consequences of Excessive Alcohol Use?

Most significant medical conditions associated with habitual moderate or severe alcohol use disorder stem from long-term consumption. While the physiologic effects manifest in many organ systems, common ones include:

▶ Liver disease: 90% of those consuming an average of more than 60 g of alcohol daily will develop fatty liver disease. Of this group of heavy drinkers, 10% to 35% will develop alcoholic hepatitis and 5% to 15% will develop cirrhosis.[1] Approximately one-fifth of liver transplants are associated with alcohol-related liver disease.

▶ Pancreatitis: 35% of patients with acute pancreatitis and 75% of patients with chronic pancreatitis have a history of significant alcohol use. The combination of cigarette smoking with heavy alcohol use elevates the risk of pancreatitis.

▶ Neurocognitive disorders: Long-term alcohol use is associated with dementia syndromes which may not always be reversible after drinking cessation.

- Wernicke encephalopathy: Results from vitamin B1 (thiamine) deficiency. Usually seen in patients with multi-year histories of severe alcohol use disorder. Symptoms include ataxia, confusion, hypothermia, and vision problems. Proper nutrition, hydration, thiamine replacement usually addresses symptoms.

Table 23.3 ▶ Signs and Symptoms of a Possible Alcohol Use Disorder

Problems, Signs, or Symptoms	
Fatigue	Dyspepsia
Insomnia	Nausea and vomiting
Episodes of high blood pressure	Diarrhea
Numbness and tingling in the limbs	Erectile dysfunction
Problems with short-term memory and concentration	Decreased libido

- Korsakoff syndrome: Often follows Wernicke encephalopathy. Characterized by amnesia, tremor, and disorientation. Improvement can occur with alcohol cessation and vitamin replacement, but the patient may still have enduring short-term memory deficits.

> Allen indicates that he has been drinking 4 to 5 beers daily on weekdays and 24 from Friday through Sunday nights. He states that this pattern has been present for about 6 months. He dates his increased alcohol use to his wife moving out and filing for divorce. "I have been a mess ever since she left me; I don't know what to do with myself. I feel like I should cut down and I often feel guilty, especially when I'm doing poorly at work."

Laboratory Tests

Except for blood alcohol levels, most lab tests are not specific to alcohol use and are not sensitive for detecting problem drinking in its earlier stages.[3]

▶ Mean corpuscular volume (MCV) and gamma-glutamyl transferase (GGT) are often elevated in patients with significant alcohol use histories.

▶ Carbohydrate deficient transferrin (CDT) elevations are found among patients consuming five or more drinks daily over an 8-week period.[1]

Pharmacotherapy for Alcohol Use Disorders[10]

While a detailed discussion of outpatient alcohol treatment use disorders is beyond the scope of this text, there are a few medications, displayed in Table 23.4, that can be helpful for some patients.

CANNABIS

> Ricky is a 22-year-old university student who presents with a cough. He also wonders if he might have attention-deficit hyperactivity disorder (ADHD) because he has difficulty focusing and concentrating on school work. Review of his record indicates that he has been into the office several times in the past 18 months with respiratory symptoms.

Before recent state marijuana legalization, approximately 40% to 45% of the US population reported having used marijuana at least once, and close to 25% of the population reported

Table 23.4 ▶ Medications Useful for Alcohol Disorder Treatment

Medication	Mode of Action
Disulfiram	Inhibits acetaldehyde dehydrogenase. Ten to 30 minutes after alcohol ingestion, the patient will feel ill with symptoms of hyperventilation, nausea, chest pain, tachycardia, and flushing of the chest and face. Used as an alcohol use deterrent
Naltrexone (oral and injectable forms)	Initially developed for heroin addiction, this agent reduces the reinforcing effects and craving for alcohol
Acamprosate	Initiated 5 days after last drink; reduces symptoms of withdrawal and helps maintain abstinence

using the drug in the past month.[11] While federal law states that possessing, growing, and distributing marijuana is illegal unless for research purposes, at the time of this writing, most states have laws that allow cannabis use for medical conditions including chronic pain, muscle spasms, seizure disorders, and nausea from chemotherapy, and a growing number of states and the District of Columbia have passed laws legalizing marijuana for recreational use.

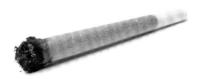

Courtesy of Picturepartners/Shutterstock.com.

Distinguishing High-Risk from Low-Risk Cannabis Use

It is often challenging to determine the boundary between recreational use and problem use of marijuana. Some guidelines:

▶ **Quantity:** While number of grams or joints smoked daily provides some rough estimate of use, quantity is often more difficult to establish with marijuana compared with alcohol. Several factors account for this and include variable tetrahydrocannabinol (THC) levels, size of joints, whether they are shared, and the various other forms in which cannabis can be found.[12] Since edibles take longer to have an effect, overuse in noninhaled forms has been a growing concern.

▶ **Frequency:** Daily or almost daily use is suggestive of a problem, particularly if this pattern has been present for multiple months.

▶ **Mood Effects:** More problematic use is associated with patients who report that they need cannabis to level out their mood.[12]

▶ **Withdrawal:** Abrupt cessation is associated with rebound anxiety and insomnia in habitual users.

▶ **Signs of Excessive Use:** Symptoms and syndromes associated with excessive use of cannabis include[12]:

- Cognitive problems—deficits in attention, concentration, and short-term memory.
- Anxiety—this is a common reported reason for chronic cannabis use; rebound anxiety is also common when habitual users suddenly stop.
- Chronic cough and recurrent respiratory infections.
- Nausea and vomiting (cannabis hyperemesis syndrome).
- Schizophrenia—while NOT caused by cannabis use, people genetically predisposed to schizophrenia are very likely to use cannabis extensively and begin use at a younger age. Cannabis use predicts the appearance of clear psychotic symptoms within 5 to 10 years.

Screening for Drug Dependence

There are many instruments used to assess the degree of psychological dependence on drugs. One of these is the Severity of Dependence Use Scale or SDS (Table 23.5) (https://ncpic.org.au/media/1590/severity-of-dependence-scale-1.pdf). The SDS was developed to assess dependence on heroin, cocaine, cannabis, and other substances and can be useful to review with patients who are trying to assess their level of psychological dependence on any of these substances.[13,14] While higher point scores clearly indicate higher levels of

Table 23.5 ▸ Severity of Dependence Use Scale: Adapted for Cannabis

Please answer each question on a 0–3 scale:
0 = never or almost never
1 = sometimes
2 = often
3 = always or nearly always
   1. Did you ever think your use off cannabis was out of control?
   2. Did the prospect of missing a dose of cannabis make you very anxious or worried?
   3. Did you ever worry about your use of cannabis?
   4. Did you wish you could stop the use of cannabis?
   5. How difficult would you find it to stop or go without?

dependence, there is still some disagreement about what constitutes a positive screening cutoff for different populations screened. **A commonly used cutoff is a score of 3 or higher**.

Ricky indicates that he smokes approximately three large joints daily, usually by himself. He typically will have his first joint within an hour of waking, and he has difficulty relaxing if he does not smoke. He reports age of first use at 13 years and regular use at age 17 years. On the SDS, he receives a score of 1 on item 3 and a score of 3 on items 2 and 5 for a total score of 7.

Note: His established pattern of use as well as initial use of cannabis under the age of 16 years, together with his SDS score, makes it very likely that he is cannabis dependent. With respect to his concern about ADHD, he should abstain from cannabis for 30 days and then undergo neurocognitive testing.

If total abstinence from cannabis is not an option, then a possible **harm reduction strategy** could include[14]:

▸ Keep a record of consumption on a calendar.

▸ Roll smaller joints.

▸ Wait slightly longer between each inhalation.

▸ Try to confine use to weekends.

OPIOIDS

Helen is a new patient to your practice. She is 37 years. The MA note indicates that her presenting concern is "I need my pain meds refilled." In speaking with Helen, you learn that she recently moved to the area. She has been taking oxycodone several times daily since she slipped and fell in one of the bathrooms while on the job as a hotel housekeeper, injuring her back. Since then she has needed pain medication just to be able to function. The remainder of her health has been excellent. She does not smoke cigarettes or use other recreational drugs.

On physical exam, she appears well and has normal vital signs. She grimaces when asked to bend over at the waist. On straight leg raise, she reports pain with slight leg elevation. She has no lateralizing findings on neurologic exam nor signs of cauda equina syndrome.

Many physicians have lived through aggressive pain management marketing in the 1980s, 90s, and early 2000s, as pain assessment became the "fifth vital sign." Pain level assessment continues in most primary care offices to this day. While this has undoubtedly allowed us to see a problem that we had not fully appreciated, our response to that problem in the form of prescription opiates did not serve many well and laid the foundation for much of the reason that we have an opiate epidemic in the United States today.

Opioids are substances that act on opioid receptors in the body. They consist of:

▶ Opiates: Substances like morphine and codeine that occur naturally within the poppy plant.

▶ Semisynthetic opioids: Include heroin, hydrocodone, hydromorphone, and oxycodone.

▶ Synthetic opioids: Include fentanyl, buprenorphine, and methadone.

Since 1999, the number of opioid prescriptions has increased by a factor of four,[15] and it is estimated that about 25% of patients receiving long-term opioid treatment in primary care settings are at risk for abuse and dependence on these substances.

Pain management strategies are reviewed in Chapter 20, Chronic Pain. If you consider prescribing opioids for acute or chronic pain, it is helpful to consider who may be at risk for opioid abuse before you begin. The Opioid Risk Assessment Tool, shown in Table 23.6, can help you with this.[16]

Table 23.6 ▶ Opioid Risk Assessment Tool

These screening questions are intended to be used to assess a patient's risk for future opioid abuse. It is recommended that this questionnaire be verbally administered immediately before initiating opioid therapy

Mark Each Box that Applies	Female	Male
Family history of substance abuse		
• Alcohol	1	3
• Illegal drugs (including cannabis)	2	3
• Prescription drugs	4	4
Personal history of substance abuse		
• Alcohol	3	3
• Illegal drugs (including cannabis)	4	4
• Prescription drugs	5	5
Age between 16 and 45	1	1
History of preadolescent sexual abuse	3	0
Psychological disease		
• ADD, OCD, bipolar, schizophrenia	2	2
• Depression	1	1
Scoring totals:	26	26

Interpretation:

≤3—low risk for opiate abuse, 4–7—moderate risk, ≥8—high risk

Helen's father is an alcoholic (1 point). She describes a period between ages 20 and 25 years when she "got kind of wild" and used alcohol excessively resulting in a DUI violation (3 points). She also smoked considerable amounts of marijuana during this period of her life (4 points). She was not sexually abused as a child (0 points). Three years ago, she was diagnosed with depression and was prescribed fluoxetine (1 point), which she no longer takes. Total score is 9, placing her at high risk of abuse.

The CDC guideline for prescribing opioids for chronic pain states that "Clinicians should offer or arrange evidence-based treatment for patients with opioid use disorder."[17] This usually takes the form of medication use, counseling, and supportive assistance from family and friends.

While the treatment of opiate abuse and addiction is beyond the scope of this chapter, it is not beyond the scope of care for many primary care clinicians. All clinicians should recognize and treat pain appropriately and judiciously. In addition, we should learn to recognize when patients are impaired with a substance use disorder, including that of opiate addiction, and should learn how to approach these problems with care and empathy. It is helpful to know about medications that are used to treat this disease (Table 23.7), although most primary care physicians do not incorporate the pharmacotherapy of substance use disorder treatment into their practices.

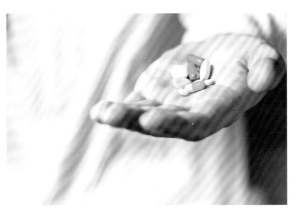

Table 23.7 ▶ Pharmacotherapy for Opioid Abuse

Medication	Mode of Action
Methadone[a] (Methadose, Dolophine)	Opioid agonist; effects similar to morphine
Buprenorphine[b] (Subutex, Buprenex, Butrans, Suboxone if combined with naloxone)	Attaches to opiate receptors, blocks opioid effects, reduces opiate-related euphoria
Naltrexone (Vivitrol, Revia, others)	Binds the *mu* opioid receptor, blocks euphoric effects of opioids

[a]Can only be dispensed by specialized opioid treatment programs; minimum treatment period of 3 months. Well established as effective for heroin and other opiate addictions.[18]
[b]Can only be prescribed by physicians with specialized training and certification; a physician can treat a limited number of patients per year.
Data from: Webster LR, Webster RM. Predicting aberrant behaviors in opioid-treated patients: preliminary validation of the Opioid Risk Tool. *Pain Med.* 2005;6(6):432–442. Available at: https://academic.oup.com/painmedicine/article-lookup/doi/10.1111/j.1526-4637.2005.00072.x

RESOURCES

▶ Facing Addiction in America: The Surgeon General's Report on Alcohol, Drugs, and Health. https://addiction.surgeongeneral.gov/

▶ NIDA—National Institute on Drug Abuse: Centers of Excellence for Physician Information https://www.drugabuse.gov/nidamed-medical-health-professionals/centers-excellence-coe-physician-information. Here are useful video clips of interviews with primary care patients with substance abuse issues; includes counseling techniques.

▶ NIAAA—National Institute on Alcohol Abuse and Alcoholism. https://www.niaaa.nih.gov/

▶ SAMHSA—Substance Abuse and Mental Health Services Administration. https://www.samhsa.gov/

QUESTIONS

1. You are working with a 34-year-old woman who is a longstanding cannabis user. She asks if you think she is addicted. You administer the Severity of Dependence Use Scale (SDS), and she scores a 2. Which response to the results do you think would be most appropriate?
   A. This test shows that you are not psychologically dependent on cannabis, and at this point, there is nothing further to do.
   B. The results show that you have a moderate problem with cannabis and should consider stopping.
   C. The results show a severe dependence on cannabis, and I strongly recommend you stop now.
   D. While this test shows that you are not very dependent on cannabis psychologically, we should consider other elements of your cannabis use to determine the degree to which it may be a problem.

2. Mary is a 32-year-old woman with chronic back pain. You are considering opioids as part of a comprehensive management plan and are assessing her risk for opioid abuse by using the Opioid Risk Assessment Tool. Of the risk factors noted in this tool, which one carries the greatest weighted risk?
   A. Family history of prescription drug abuse.
   B. Age.
   C. Previous personal history of alcohol abuse.
   D. History of preadolescent sexual abuse.
   E. Bipolar disorder.

3. Your patient, Afshin, reports recent difficulties and arguments with family members about many things. He has also had recurrent chest pain, mild constipation, and mild weight gain. He does not smoke cigarettes. His exam is normal and labs show an MCV of 89 and normal AST and ALT. What is the strongest early indicator that he may have an alcohol use disorder?
   A. Relationship problems.
   B. MCV and liver enzymes.
   C. Chest pain.
   D. Weight gain.

4. Samantha is an 18-year-old African-American high school senior whom you have seen since she was a preschooler. You screen her for alcohol and drug use. She states that she has not used any recreational drugs, but she does drink alcohol, on average 10 to 12 drinks per week. She last had four or more drinks this past weekend at a party. At this point, the best next step would be which one of the following?

A. Refer her to Dr. Bacchus who works with people who have alcohol use disorders.

B. Inpatient treatment.

C. Administer the CAGE-AID questionnaire to determine severity of alcohol use.

D. "Thank you for sharing this with me. If you haven't had any problems with your drinking so far, then please just be careful."

5. Jordy would like a prescription for Vivitrol to help him get clean from heroin that he has been using for the last 2 years, after years of oxycodone use. He lives alone, is unemployed, and has been depressed for about 1 year or so. Which one of the following would be your best response to this request?

A. I am delighted you want to get clean. We need to refer you out for this treatment.

B. I cannot prescribe this for you because it requires a special certification.

C. Vivitrol has no role in the treatment of heroin but can be useful for alcohol.

D. I would be willing to consider this request. We will also want to review the need for treatment of depression as well.

ANSWERS

Question 1: The correct answer is D.
The Severity of Dependence Use Scale was developed to assess dependence on heroin, cocaine, cannabis, and other substances… higher point scores clearly indicate higher levels of dependence, although there is still some disagreement about what constitutes a positive screening cut-off for different populations screened. A commonly used cut-off is a score of 3 or higher.

Question 2: The correct answer is A.
(Table 23.6) The Opioid Risk Assessment Tool gives a weight of 4 points to a family history of prescription drug abuse, 3 points to a previous personal history of alcohol abuse, 3 points to a history of preadolescent sexual abuse, 2 points to a diagnosis of bipolar disorder, and 1 point to age 16 to 45 years.

Question 3: The correct answer is A.
Early stages of problem drinking are typically associated with predominantly psychosocial problems. These include arrests for driving under the influence or disorderly conduct, relationship problems, marital separation, domestic violence, job loss, and fights.

Question 4: The correct answer is C.
In the section on Patient Engagement and Treatment of Substance Use Disorders—General Guidelines, it is stated that for patients who show evidence of risky alcohol and/or drug use follow Step 2 of SBIRT—to assess for alcohol and/or drug severity using the CAGE-AID questionnaire.

Question 5: The correct answer is D.
In the general section on pharmacotherapy, it is mentioned that in patients with dual-diagnoses, a formal diagnosis of MDD may need to wait until at least 30 days from the last substance use. The section on pharmacotherapy for opioid abuse notes that Vivitrol has an indication for opioid abuse and does not require a special certification.

REFERENCES

1. U.S. Department of Health and Human Services (HHS). *Office of the Surgeon General, Facing Addiction in America: The Surgeon General's Report on Alcohol, Drugs, and Health.* Washington, DC: HHS; 2016.
2. Bowman S, Eiserman J, Beletsky L, et al. Reducing the health consequences of opioid addiction in primary care. *Am J Med.* 2013;126(7):565–571.
3. Searight HR. Screening for alcohol abuse in primary care: current status and research needs. *Fam Pract Res J.* 1992;12(2):193–204.
4. American Psychiatric Association. *DSM 5.* American Psychiatric Association; 2013.
5. Miller WR, Hester RK. Treating alcohol problems: toward an informed eclecticism. In Hester R, Miller W, Eds. *Handbook of Alcoholism Treatment Approaches: Effective Alternatives.* Elmsford, NY: Pergamon Press; 1989:3–13.
6. Searight HR. Efficient counseling techniques for the primary care physician. *Prim Care Clin Office Pract.* 2007;34(3):551–570.
7. Nunes EV, Levin FR. Treatment of depression in patients with alcohol or other drug dependence: a meta-analysis. *JAMA.* 2004;291(15):1887–1896.
8. Bertholet N, Daeppen JB, Wietlisbach V, et al. Reduction of alcohol consumption by brief alcohol intervention in primary care: systematic review and meta-analysis. *Arch Intern Med.* 2005;165(9):986–995.
9. Winstock AR, Ford C, Witton J. Assessment and management of cannabis use disorders in primary care. *BMJ.* 2010;340;1571.
10. Lee J, Kresina TF, Campopiano M, et al. Use of pharmacotherapies in the treatment of alcohol use disorders and opioid dependence in primary care. *BioMed Res International.* 2015:137020. http://dx.doi.org/10.1155/2015/137020.
11. Azofeifa A, Mattson ME, Schauer G, et al. National estimates of marijuana use and related indicators—National Survey on Drug Use and Health, United States, 2002–2014. *MMWR Surveill Summ.* 2016;65(11):1–28.
12. Turner SD, Spithoff S, Kahan M. Approach to cannabis use disorder in primary care: focus on youth and other high-risk users. *Can Fam Physician.* 2014;60(9):801–808.
13. Gossop M, Darke S, Griffiths P, et al. The Severity of Dependence Scale (SDS): psychometric properties of the SDS in English and Australian samples of heroin, cocaine and amphetamine users. *Addiction.* 1995;90:607–614.
14. Piontek D, Kraus L, Klempova D. Short scales to assess cannabis-related problems: a review of psychometric properties. *Subst Abuse Treat Prev Policy.* 2008;3:25–34.
15. Boscarino JA, Rukstalis M, Hoffman SN, et al. Risk factors for drug dependence among outpatients on opioid therapy in a large US healthcare system. *Addiction.* 2010;105(10):1776–1782.
16. Webster LR, Webster R. Predicting aberrant behaviors in opioid-treated patients: preliminary validation of the opioid risk tool. *Pain Med.* 2005;6(6):432–442.
17. Dowell D, Haegerich TM, Chou R. CDC Guideline for prescribing opioids for chronic pain—United States, 2016. *MMWR Recomm Rep.* 2016;65(No. RR-1):1–49.
18. Schuckit MA. Treatment of opioid-use disorders. *N Engl J Med.* 2016;375(4):357–368.

Community Engagement, Health Equity, and Advocacy

KEY POINTS

1 ▶ Students have the power to make a difference in their communities

2 ▶ Asset-Based Community Development is an approach for identifying resources and making change

3 ▶ There are many levels of advocacy; pick your target carefully

4 ▶ Assess projects for feasibility and sustainability

5 ▶ Identify a support network to sustain and inform your ongoing advocacy work/practice

Health care providers can play instrumental roles in advocacy for their patients and communities. This can occur at every stage of our careers, starting as premedical and medical students. To be advocates is an unwritten detail of our job description as physicians.

"Medical education does not exist to teach individuals how to make a living, but to empower them to protect the health of the public."[1]

An advocate is, "a person who argues for or supports a cause or policy."[2] To argue for a cause, community, or patient, a physician must understand the social determinants of health, know the assets and needs of their community, and let those needs guide their advocacy.[3]

Despite spending the most money per person on health care, the United States has worse outcomes than most developed nations (see Chapter 1). Promoting health equity by addressing the social determinants of health may help achieve the triple aim of improving the patient care experience, reducing cost, and improving population health and guide our advocacy.[3]

THE POWER OF STUDENTS AND SOCIAL DETERMINANTS OF HEALTH

STUDENT VIGNETTE

▶ Student Impact: Creation of a Community Advisory Board

One medical student Williams served in a clinic that wanted to know how to best serve the community's needs. He met with patients, staff, and community organizations. Common threads from these conversations were a need for increased cultural sensitivity and improved communication with community members. Based on this information, this student helped the clinic start a community advisory board that was organized and staffed by subsequent students. The community board has become an integral part of the clinic's functioning, identity, and service development.

Assessing social determinants of health is critical to addressing patient's health concerns and a powerful area for students to influence patient health. Consider the child with severe asthma who fails to improve despite controller and rescue medications. What else could be going on?

Obtaining affordable medications and knowing how to use them correctly are important, but so is addressing the child's exposure to mold, smoke, and cockroaches. Here is where you

Smokers at home	Mold in the home	Cockroaches

hold immense power. Students often have time to obtain a complete social history and discover barriers and promoters to good health and successful treatment.

In the case of the child with asthma described above, students participating in her care identified these triggers in the child's home and worked with a tenant's rights organization to advocate for the patient to address the mold and cockroaches. Students also helped connect the family to community programs supporting smoking cessation.

Many opportunities exist; a student could also consider the broader community and write an op-ed piece to alert everyone to environmental health hazards and tenants' rights. In this case, students started a postcard campaign to help bring their patients' voices and needs to local government leaders, which eventually led to changes in policies and tenants' rights.

You can play a critical role as an advocate for your patients by assessing social determinants of health even within a limited time span. As health professionals hear patient's stories, they can become aware of the social contexts in which their patients live. Creating an Eco Map[4] for a patient's social context can help guide next advocacy steps. Some projects may be difficult to complete in a 4- to 8-week rotation. Consider instead completing one step within a project—like the Eco Map itself—and initiating a project, or contributing to an ongoing project, that will be continued by subsequent students rotating through the clinic.

HEALTH EQUITY MATTERS

Health equity is the ideal that everyone should be able to achieve the highest possible level of health. Unfortunately, health inequities, or differences in health status that are avoidable and unfair, are commonplace both within and between countries, and between different social, racial, ethnic, and geographic groups. For instance, institutionalized, interpersonally mediated, and internalized structures of privilege and racism and their effect on health equity are well described in Camara Jones' *Gardener's Tale,* in which Jones uses a garden metaphor to illustrate the compounding effects of context and privilege (quality soil, water, and attention) on health.[5] Health inequities are strongly influenced by social and economic conditions.

STUDENT VIGNETTE

▶ **Development of a Community-Engaged Project**

MK Brown was curious about the impact of poverty on health and decided to focus his community project on early childhood education. Working with a local school that served children from low-income backgrounds, he conducted a needs assessment and designed and introduced a program on mindfulness-based stress reduction for teachers and students. The program has grown and now reaches children, teachers, and the parents of school-aged children.

Health Equity[6]**:** Attainment of the highest level of health for all people

Health Inequities: Differences in health status that are avoidable, unfair, and unjust

Health Disparities: Differences in health status among groups of people

Information from UW ICTR, Collaborative Center for Health Equity. Community Based Participatory Research (CBPR) 101. Available at: https://ictr.wisc.edu/files/CBPR101onCCHE.pdf. Accessed September 2016.

The early 21st century is an exciting time with great potential to promote health equity. During the last two centuries, humans have achieved greater progress in improving their quality and length of life than at any previous time in history. These gains are beautifully described in Dr. Hans Rosling's *200 countries, 200 years, 4 minutes* (https://www.youtube.com/watch?v=jbkSRLYSojo).

Models of Health

The socioecologic model of health (www.cdc.gov/violenceprevention/overview/social-ecologicalmodel.html) is a set of inclusive circles beginning with the individual and surrounded by interpersonal, community, and societal circles. This model shows that the health status of an individual is strongly influenced by social determinants including history, location, culture, and the people around them, including family, friends, and community. For example, in the case of an adolescent who is overweight, his condition is strongly influenced by family eating patterns; community and economic access to healthy foods; options for exercise; and societal and cultural norms of food choices, serving sizes, and consumption of sugary beverages.

Epidemiologic and demographic data confirm that an individual's health is more strongly linked to their zip code than their genetic code. The County Health Rankings' determinants of health model shows the relative percentages of various factors' influence on quality and length of life for most people in the United States (Fig. 24.1).

As shown, social and economic factors have the greatest influence on health (40%); these factors in turn influence health behaviors and choices (30%). Clinical care exerts a smaller influence (20%) followed by influence from the physical environment (10%). The relative influence of these factors varies by situation. For example, it is easy to understand that people living in a war zone are far more likely to be influenced by social factors and the physical environment.

Poverty, one of the strongest contributors to health disparities, has complex influences on health and disease. People living in poverty are less likely to have high-quality education and health literacy, nutritious food, and opportunities for regular exercise; they are more likely to suffer from chronic stress, live in substandard housing, and be exposed to environmental toxins. This has become known as **toxic stress**.[7] This complex web of interrelated social and economic factors requires multifaceted solutions. Physicians can work with others to identify and address these factors when they act as advocates for their patients.

▶ Toxic stress is a consequence of interactions between environmental, social, and genetic factors that stress an individual or population and lead to alterations in biochemical pathways affecting learning, behavior, and health.[7]

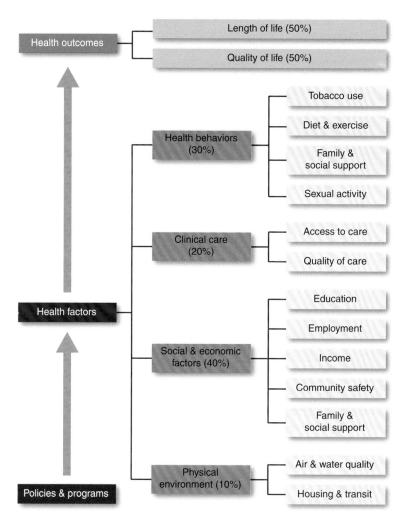

Figure 24.1 ▶ Health components. (University of Wisconsin Population Health Institute. County Health Rankings & Roadmaps 2017. www.countyhealthrankings.org)

▶ Adverse childhood experiences are toxic stressors that influence brain and child development with consequences often extending through adulthood.[8]

Ethical Responsibility

Health professionals' duty to treat and promote health for all, regardless of a patient's circumstances, is central to physicians' ethical responsibilities.

The Flexner report, a study of North American medical education published by Abraham Flexner in 1910, called for reforms of medical education based on a strong foundation of biomedical sciences. One hundred years after the Flexner report, a new movement called Beyond Flexner is promoting another widespread reform of medical education to embrace the social mission of medicine and to train health professionals to become agents of more equitable health care (http://www.ncbi.nlm.nih.gov/pmc/articles/PMC3178858/; http://beyondflexner.org/).

Taking Action

Delivery of primary and comprehensive health care services by health care professionals to those who need it is critical to addressing health equity. Yet most countries are facing serious current and future projected shortages of human resources for health. The US government defines and tracks rural and urban health professional shortage areas. The World Health Organization has developed global strategies to recruit, train, and retain health professionals.[9]

▶ **Insurance coverage** is a major factor that determines whether or not people will seek care. Despite recent progress through the Affordable Care Act, more than 29 million Americans remained uninsured in 2015.[10] Many more have difficulty affording health care due to high copayments, deductibles, and medication costs. Ultimately the future of coverage under the Affordable Care Act, Medicare, and Medicaid remains to be determined following the 2016 presidential and congressional elections.

▶ **Improving access through collaboration:** Many examples of public health, clinical, educational, and community health collaborations can be seen such as the Multnomah County Health Department (https://multco.us/health/public-health-practice/health-equity-initiative), the City of Milwaukee Health Department (http://city.milwaukee.gov/health/wisconsin-Center-for-Health-Equity#.WDOG_VxuNHR), and the University of Wisconsin Training in Urban Medicine and Public Health (TRIUMPH) program (https://www.med.wisc.edu/education/md-program/triumph/). Table 24.1 gives some examples of what health professionals can do to promote health equity.

Table 24.1 ▶ What Can Health Professionals Do to Promote Health Equity?

Clinical Activities
• Recognize, avoid, and address bias[a] (e.g., cultural, racial, sex, age)
• Express compassion—don't blame victims
• Screen for socioeconomic factors
• Coordinate care with interdisciplinary teams
• Refer patients to community resources

Public Activities
• Advocate for prohealth policies
• Promote health system changes
• Work collectively with others outside the health system
• Address structural violence
• VOTE!

[a]For a discussion of bias in clinical care, see https://www.ncbi.nlm.nih.gov/pmc/articles/PMC3140753/
Information from https://www.wisconsinmedicalsociety.org/_WMS/publications/wmj/pdf/113/6/218.pdf

Since physicians are respected as experts, they can serve as powerful advocates for health equity. Advocacy can be pursued on many levels: personally, professionally, within health systems, and with the public.

COMMUNITY ENGAGEMENT

STUDENT VIGNETTE

▶ **Common Purpose**

AJ Bryant observed that there were several strong community organizations serving the clinic population with the same goals as the clinic itself. To align interests and build wellness of the clinic population, she coordinated mutual site visits by community and clinic representatives.

Since then, these organizations are working to formalize referral pathways to best connect community members with needed resources.

The Centers for Disease Control (CDC) defines community engagement in the first edition of *Principles of Community Engagement* as: "the process of working collaboratively with and through groups of people affiliated by geographic proximity, special interest, or similar situations to address issues affecting the well-being of those people... It often involves partnerships and coalitions that help mobilize resources and influence systems, change relationships among partners, and serve as catalysts for changing policies, programs, and practices."[11]

Effective community engagement requires the practice and implementation of several key skills. Primary are the skills of presence; listening; asset assessment; developing relationships, networks, and teams; assessing community readiness to engage or change; and consistency. Several key questions are useful in guiding engagement and are outlined in Table 24.2.

▶ **Presence:** The first step is showing up. Talk *with* people versus *to* people. A community survey, sometimes referred to as asset mapping or a "windshield survey" can be used to initiate conversations. In this exercise a student walks, bikes, and/or drives the neighborhood or community in which they wish to invest and reflects on what they see, engaging people in conversations about the area.

▶ **Listening:** A student's first job in a new area is active listening and seeking to understand and appreciate. This can be accomplished through informal conversation and/or formal surveying. Asking clarifying questions will help you gain more historical context and communicate your desire to learn.

▶ **Assess Assets:** Asset-based community development is a widely-adopted approach to successful community engagement.[12] Using this approach, a community is examined for its resources. This exercise can involve the literal creation of a community map or resource lists and is an alternative to historically paternalistic, deficit-based approaches to communities that have resulted in many well-intentioned projects failing. (Examples of tools for community mapping can be found at http://www.abcdinstitute.org/toolkit/.)

Table 24.2 ▸ Key Questions for Community Engagement

Steps of Engagement	Key Questions to Ask Yourself
Presence	• What do you see, hear, feel? • Who do you meet? • What is the history of the neighborhood? • Does their telling of the history differ from your observations?
Listening	• What do community members value and identify as their hopes, goals, and aspirations? • What has been tried in the past or is underway now? • Are there literary/published resources that can help you?
Assess Assets	• What assets exist in the community that can be built on for positive improvement? • What is the physical space? Are there empty buildings or lots that can be repurposed? • What knowledge and experiences do people living in the community bring? • What organizations already exist whether public, private, or religious? • What relationship structures already exist? • Who are the unofficial as well as official community leaders?
Connection/Team Development	• Who is available to help? How much time can they offer? • What expertise do you need? Is anyone missing?
Summarize Understanding and Community Readiness to Change[a]	• What are the resources? • What are the needs? • How ready is a community to change? • How able is your team to Mobilize Assets?
Consistency/Reliability	• What time do you have to give? • What energy do you have to give? • Does the scope of the project or a well-defined piece of the project match your availability?

[a]Tri-Ethnic Center, College of Natural Sciences, Colorado State University. Community Readiness Model. Available at: http://triethniccenter.
colostate.edu/communityReadiness_home.htm

▸ **Connection/Team Development:** Work to develop relationships and build a team of people with similar interests and goals. Remember that local residents are experts in their own lives and communities and are crucial to engagement. The CDC refers to developing connections and team development as coalition building (http://www.atsdr.cdc.gov/communityengagement/pdf/PCE_Report_508_FINAL.pdf). Use the Multnomah County Health Equity Lens to help identify which team members you may need.[13]

▸ **Readiness to Change:** Similar to motivational interviewing in a clinical context, a systematic analysis of the community can reveal the stage of community readiness with regard to a particular issue (no awareness, denial/resistance, vague awareness, preplanning, preparation, initiation, stabilization confirmation/expansion, and high level of community ownership). This strategy will allow you to invest your efforts fruitfully and to avoid selecting an intervention that is not likely to be sustained after your departure.

▸ **Consistency/Reliability:** Commit to activities that are feasible with resources available. Follow through on commitments. Avoid the common pitfall of agreeing to something you *want* to do, but will not be able to follow to completion or hand off to another. This is a key step in trust and relationship building. This requires an accurate, honest assessment of your availability and resources while setting aside whatever the ideal may be.

EFFECTIVE ADVOCACY

▶ Educational Advocacy

Dr. KK Kelley was engaged in many community outreach and extracurricular activities as a medical student, but her residency program did not provide these opportunities. She worked with colleagues to develop and implement a new community health curriculum to learn about the context where they live, work, and serve; to promote interdisciplinary care; and to help family physicians identify and respond to social factors influencing their patients' health and illness.

Effective advocacy requires several steps shown in Table 24.3. Initially investing organizational time to plan your advocacy will allow you to be most effective.

Reaching out to the Target Population

Once your target population has been selected consider how you will reach that population. Advocacy can happen in person "on the ground" whether joining local groups to create green space or in individual meetings with governmental or institutional representatives. Writing to newspapers, journals, political representatives, or internal organization leadership or publications (and encouraging others to do the same) are other ways to improve the visibility of issues that you are passionate about changing.

Levels of advocacy are shown in Table 24.4.

Table 24.3 ▶ Steps to Effective Advocacy

Step	Methods
1. Select project	Combine assets, windshield survey, needs assessment, and readiness assessments. May be one piece of a larger project (e.g., literature review, interviews, recruitment, or project design)
2. Target audience identification and methodology	Be specific about goals, feasibility, and target audience: these could include patients, local institutions, a local geographic area/neighborhood, state-wide, national, or global audience
3. Build your team	Identify team members and assign clear roles and responsibilities. Champions are essential to start, grow, and sustain a movement
4. Mobilize community resources	Identify which assets to mobilize and what it will take to mobilize these, including recruitment of new team members
5. Establish SMART goals[a]	Agree to SMART goals as a team
6. Determine timeline	Agree to a timeline as a team. Be clear about roles and responsibilities
7. Design and evaluate for sustainability	Plan hand-offs and transitions using a team-based approach

[a]SMART, specific, measurable, achievable, realistic, and time bound.

Table 24.4 ▶ Levels of Advocacy	
A	**Action**
Personal	Reflect on your internal values and watch out for implicit or explicit bias toward particular patients or groups
Professional	Examine your language, practices, and treatment of other members of the health professional team and their patients
System	Influence policies, structures, and standards to improve access to health care for all and examine these through a health equity lens[a]
Public	Bring your experience to vote and advocate for policy changes

[a]As an example, see https://multco.us/diversity-equity/equity-and-empowerment-lens

Sustainability

Plan hand-offs and approach the project as a team-based endeavor. Timelines may not always align with your schedule, so look for opportunities to move the project forward with the team. Identify how the project will continue following initial investments and who will sustain momentum for long lasting benefits. The following "Do's" and "Don'ts" may be helpful in creating engagement and supporting advocacy.

DOS AND DON'TS OF COMMUNITY ENGAGEMENT AND STEPS OF ADVOCACY

DO	DON'T
▶ Establish trusting relationships	▶ Assume the community is homogeneous
▶ Listen and learn from the community	▶ Go to a community with a defined project and expect participation
▶ Plan longer timeframes for advocacy steps	
▶ Remain flexible and open to new ideas and approaches	▶ Assume your participation is always the best option
▶ Be present and visible; communicate regularly	▶ Use "academic language"
	▶ Overestimate what one project can accomplish
▶ Learn to manage different or competing priorities	▶ Underestimate the impact of past project experiences
▶ Use shared decision making	▶ Ignore community dynamics and different spheres of power/decision making
▶ Return results to the community and collaboratively interpret outcomes	
▶ Prepare an "exit strategy"	▶ Make decisions "behind closed doors," but do respect information shared in confidence
	▶ Make promises you cannot keep
	▶ Fail to communicate about issues that can affect project timelines

Data from UW ICTR, Collaborative Center for Health Equity. Community Based Participatory Research (CBPR) 101. Available at: https://ictr.wisc.edu/files/CBPR101onCCHE.pdf. Accessed September 2016.

RESILIENCE AND COMMUNITY BUILDING

Take a moment, close your eyes, and imagine a stressful day. It is your first day on rotation at a new hospital, you are expected to round on a number of patients, you don't know where their rooms are or how to log into the computer system. Besides that, you don't know where the bathrooms are, when you are ever going to eat again, and you slept poorly the night before. This doesn't even begin to describe the stress at home or with your family. Sound familiar? In order to provide the best care for your patients, you must also be proactive for your own well-being.

Being a health care professional can be difficult, but being an advocate has its own set of challenges. Think about you, at the center, surrounded by self-care, professional care, and your community. Use each part of Figure 24.2 to consider aspects of your health.

Health care professionals are leaders in their clinics, their communities, and in their advocacy.[14] As advocates, health care professionals will be more effective and self-sustaining if they have a clear sense of self-purpose.

Finding Your Passion

Consider what you are passionate about. If you are unsure, start by writing your own autobiography. It doesn't have to be long, but consider writing what makes you, you. Write it

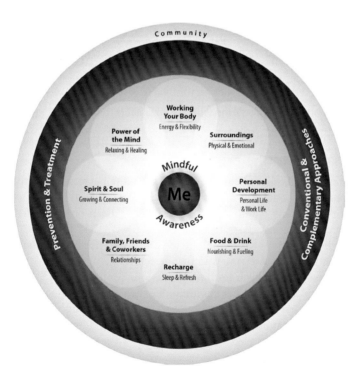

Figure 24.2 ▶ Approaching health holistically. (From Milovani C, Rindfleisch JA. *Whole Health: Changing the Conversation. Advancing Skills in the Delivery of Personalized, Proactive, Patient-Driven Care.* Veterans Health Administration Office of Patient Centered Care and Cultural Transformation. http://projects.hsl.wisc.edu/SERVICE/modules/10/M10_EO_Family_Friends_and_Coworkers.pdf)

for yourself or think about sharing it with your fellow classmates or in your clinic. This will help you focus and realize what type of work you value and gives you meaning, and why.

Self-Care

Find a quiet time and place where you can focus on your self-care plan. Think about setting aside 10 minutes each day to create an individual plan. The information in Figure 24.2 may help you conceptualize this in the context of your spirit and soul, family, surroundings, personal development, food, rest, and relaxation. Caring for yourself also allows you to be present and aware of the needs of others, such as colleagues, patients, family, and friends. The link below may help guide you through questions about which aspects of your self-care plan are lacking and can be shared with others: http://projects.hsl.wisc.edu/SERVICE/modules/13/M13_CT_Healing_The_Healer_Writing_Your_Own_Health_Plan.pdf.

The following resources can also help address areas of need:

▶ University of Wisconsin Madison Integrative Medicine website. While it is designed for patient handouts, you will find guided meditations and ways to explore self-care techniques: http://www.fammed.wisc.edu/integrative/.

▶ Reflective Practice is a website with many modules designed around self-improvement through introspection: http://reflectivepractice.net/.

▶ *"Just One Thing: Developing a Buddha brain one simple practice at a time"* Rick Hanson, PhD. An excellent book to guide you through simple mindfulness activities.

▶ *"The Zen Leader"* by Ginny Whitelaw.[15] This book guides individuals to reframe the challenges of their workplace and their leadership to promote rejuvenation and better leaders.

▶ *"The Upside of Stress: Why stress is good for you, and How to get Good at it"* by Kelly McGonigal.

▶ Consider cell phone apps, YouTube videos, or websites that can lead you in guided meditation.

Building Professional Support

Health care professionals should consider if they have the personal and professional support team necessary to be healthy and successful. For example, are you up to date on your own preventative screening examinations including Pap smears or immunizations? Do you have a physician or someone who you could see if you were sick? Have you explored complementary medicine options as appropriate to your health needs and interests? These are all things to consider when assessing your own needs.

Figure 24.2 also prompts you to think about your community. This can be your professional community as well as other communities such as your neighborhood, the people you like to exercise with, the places you volunteer, and spiritual groups. Take time and make space to nurture these relationships in addition to your professional responsibilities.

Flourishing: Advocacy and You

Throughout your career, you may need to periodically reassess which aspects of your life might need more attention. Identifying your core values will help you select personal and professional priorities and set appropriate limits so you can be an effective advocate for your patients and enjoy a long and satisfying career.

QUESTIONS

1. You are assessing a child with uncontrolled asthma. Which of the following is an important social determinant of health that may be influencing the child's lack of control?
   A. The child's history of asthma exacerbation.
   B. The child's exposure to mold and passive smoke.
   C. The parent's history of asthma.
   D. The lack of the child's knowledge about use of her inhaler.
   E. The lack of regular use of controller medication.

2. Health inequity refers to differences in health status among groups of people that could be prevented.
   A. True
   B. False

3. Which of the following factors has the greatest influence on or contributes most to health outcomes for most people in the United States?
   A. Clinical care
   B. The physical environment
   C. Health behaviors
   D. Social and economic factors
   E. Genetic factors

4. You and your faculty preceptor are meeting with the clinic's community advisory committee about the next quality improvement project for the clinic. Which of the following are the most important skills to use in this initial encounter?
   A. Your ability to listen to, communicate with, and demonstrate respect for others
   B. Your knowledge of key health indicators
   C. Your experiences with patients through medical school
   D. Your understanding of community resources
   E. Your ability to assess the communities' readiness to change

5. You are working on a project to increase immunizations in the family medicine clinic. It is nearing the end of the rotation. Which of the following should you consider to sustain this important effort?
   A. Find ways to continue your participation after the rotation ends
   B. Try harder to finish the project before you leave
   C. Identify a clinic member or incoming student to continue the work
   D. Assume that the preceptor will continue what you are doing

ANSWERS

Question 1: The correct answer is B.
Assessing social determinants of health is critical to addressing patient's health concerns and a powerful area for students to influence patient health. Consider a child with severe asthma who fails to improve despite controller and rescue medications. What else could be going on—smokers at home, mold in the home, or cockroaches.

Question 2: The correct answer is A.

Text box: health inequities are differences in health status that are avoidable, unfair, and unjust.

Question 3: The correct answer is D.

As shown in Figure 24.1, social and economic factors have the greatest influence on health (40%); these factors in turn influence health behaviors and choices (30%).

Question 4: The correct answer is A.

Effective community engagement requires the practice and implementation of several key skills. Primary are the skills of presence; listening; asset assessment; developing relationships, networks, and teams; assessing community readiness to engage or change; and consistency. The first step is showing up. Talk with people versus to people.

Question 5: The correct answer is C.

For sustainability, plan hand-offs and approach the project as a team-based endeavor. Identify how the project will continue following initial investments and who will sustain momentum for long-lasting benefits.

REFERENCES

1. Ehlinger E. (2016, March 30). Entry post. Available at: http://www.commissionerblog.health.state.mn.us/2016/03/national-doctors-day.html. Accessed September 10, 2016.
2. Merriam Webster internet. Accessed August 10, 2016.
3. Garg A, Boynton-Jarrett R, Dworkin PH. Avoiding the unintended consequences of screening for social determinants of health. *JAMA.* 2016;316(8):813–814.
4. Romain AM. The Patient in Context: Teaching Core Psychosocial Assessment Skills Through the Use of Ecomaps. Sparrow/MSU Family Medicine Residency Program; shared with permission through the Society of Teachers of Family Medicine Digital Resource Library. Available at: http://www.fmdrl.org/index.cfm?event=c.AccessResource&rid=3275. Accessed October 2016.
5. Jones CP. Levels of racism: a theoretic framework and a gardener's tale. *Am J Pub Health.* 2000;90(8):1212–1215.
6. Health Equity Institute, San Francisco State University. Available at: http://healthequity.sfsu.edu/. Accessed September 2016.
7. Garner AS, Shonkoff JP. Policy statement: early childhood adversity, toxic stress, and the role of the pediatrician: translating developmental science into lifelong health. *Pediatrics.* 2012;129(1):e224–e231.
8. Centers for Disease Control and Prevention. Available at: https://www.cdc.gov/violenceprevention/acestudy/. Accessed November 2016.
9. World Health Organization. Available at: http://www.who.int/hdp/poverty/en/ and http://www.who.int/social_determinants/thecommission/finalreport/en/. Accessed September 2016.
10. Health Resources and Service Administration. Available at: https://www.census.gov/content/dam/Census/library/publications/2016/demo/p60-257.pdf. Accessed December 2016.
11. Centers for Disease Control and Prevention. *Principles of Community Engagement.* 1st ed. Atlanta, GA: CDC/ATSDR Committee on Community Engagement; 1997.
12. Kretzmann JP, McKnight JL. *Building Communities from the Inside Out: A Path Toward Finding and Mobilizing a Community's Assets.* Skokie, IL: ACTA Publications; 1993.
13. Multnomah County Office of Diversity and Equity. Available at: https://multco.us/diversity-equity/equity-and-empowerment-lens. Accessed September 2016.
14. Schmitz P. *Everyone Leads.* San Francisco, CA: Jossey-Bass; 2012:246.
15. Whitelaw G. *The Zen Leader.* Pompton Plains, NJ: Career Press; 2012:31.

Note: Page number followed by b, f, and t indicates text in box, figure and table respectively.

A

AAO. *See* American Academy of Ophthalmology
AAP. *See* American Academy of Pediatrics
ABCDEs, of melanoma, 393t
Abdominal fat, 293
Abdominal pain, 171–175
  causes of
    by location, 173f
    by referral pattern, 174f
  evaluation, steps in, 173–174
  female patient of childbearing age with, approach
    to, 175f
  management of, 174–175
  red flags for serious conditions, 173
Abnormal uterine bleeding (AUB), 323, 330, 331t
  anovulatory causes of, 331t
  management of, 330, 331t
  ovulatory causes of, 331t
  PALM-COEIN categorization system for, 323, 323f
  terminology related to, 323t
Abortion, 317
Abscess, 400t
Abstinence violation effect, 63
Abuse
  alcohol, 337, 458–460
  child, 426–430
  elder, 434–436
  opioids, 462–464, 464t
  physical, 427, 428
  sexual, 427, 429
ACA. *See* Affordable Care Act
Acamprosate, 460t
Access to care, 5, 6, 7t
AC joint. *See* Acromioclavicular (AC) joint
Acne, 397, 399t
ACOG. *See* American College of Obstetricians and
  Gynecologists
ACR. *See* American College of Radiology
Acromioclavicular (AC) joint
  arthritis, 367t
  sprain, 367t
Action in Diabetes and Vascular Disease: Preterax
  and Diamicron Modified Release Controlled
  Evaluation (ADVANCE), 256
Action to Control Cardiovascular Risk in Diabetes
  (ACCORD), 256
Active life expectancy (ALE), 139

Acute appendicitis, in older adults, 145t
Acute care units (ACE) for elders, 148t
Acute otitis media (AOM), 220, 221t
Acute problems, approach to
  case presentation, 169–170
  diagnostic tests, 165–168
    clinical decision rules for, 166–167
    national organizations publish guidelines for,
     167
    probabilities, understanding of, 166
    risks and benefits of, 167
    where to begin, 168
  differential diagnosis, 168
  documentation (and coding), 171
  emergency, recognization of, 164
  history and physical examinations, 164–165
  meeting and greeting patient
    introductions, 162
    patient's concerns, listening to, 163
  monitoring and follow-up, 171
  treatment options, identifying and ranking of,
    168–169
Acute problems, treatment recommendations for
  abdominal pain, 171–175
  chest pain in adults, 181–185
  dizziness, 185–188
  dysuria, 188–191
  edema, 207–212
  fever, 192–197
  gastrointestinal bleeding, 197–201
  headache, 201–207
  nausea, 212–216
  shortness of breath, 176–181
  upper respiratory tract symptoms, 216–223
  vomiting, 212–216
Acute/sick visit, 52–53, 53t
ADA. *See* American Diabetes Association
Adhesive capsulitis, 370t
Adolescent sexuality, 385–386
Adolescents, well-child care for, 129
  confidentiality, 129
  education for, 131
  immunization for, 131
  parental concerns for, 131
  personal safety, 131
  risk assessment and harm reduction for, 130–131,
    132t

Adolescents, well-child care for (*Continued*)
  screening, 129, 133t
    for depression, 130
    for puberty, 130
    for sexual health, 130
    sports preparticipation, 130
Adult daycare, 149t
Adult Protective Services agencies, 435
Advance directives
  for health care, 385
  older adults and, 156, 156t
Adverse event, 73, 74f
Advocacy, 475–476
  engagement and supporting of, 476
  levels of, 476t
  reaching out to target population, 475
  steps to, 475t
Affirmations, 68
Affordable Care Act (ACA), 4, 10, 20, 22, 54
Agency for Healthcare Research and Quality
    (AHRQ), 54
Agenda setting, patient concerns, 163
Age-related hypogonadism, 346–347
AHRQ. *See* Agency for Healthcare Research
    and Quality
Alcohol, during pregnancy, 101
Alcoholics Anonymous, 455
Alcohol use disorder, 458–460
  laboratory tests, 460
  medical conditions with, 459–460
  pharmacotherapy for, 460, 460t
  signs and symptoms, 459, 459t
ALE. *See* Active life expectancy
Alternative Sexualities Health Research Alliance,
    383
Alzheimer disease, 152–153, 152t
Ambulatory BP monitoring (ABPM), 342
Ambulatory care, 45
  functioning in, 49
    case presentations, 50, 50b
    documentation, 50–51
    every day, 50
    first day, 49
    responsibility, opportunities for, 51, 52t
  general approach to, 51–56
    acute/sick visit, 52–53, 53t
    chronic disease follow-up visit, 53–54
    procedure visits, 55, 56f
    wellness visit, 54–55, 55t
  inpatient *versus* ambulatory setting, 46t
  primary care physician, 46–49
American Academy of Family Physicians (AAFP),
    20, 324
American Academy of Ophthalmology (AAO), 95
American Association of Clinical Endocrinologists
    (AACE), 254

American College of Radiology (ACR), 167
American College of Obstetricians and
    Gynecologists (ACOG), 106, 110
American Diabetes Association (ADA), 254
American Family Physician Podcast, 39
Andropause, 346–347
Anemia, retesting for, 109
Angina, 246, 246t
  Canadian Cardiovascular Society Classification
    System for, 247t
  risk stratification for, 248t
Ankle pain, 354–359
  ankle anatomy, 355–356, 355f, 356f
  differential diagnosis, 358t
  imaging for, 357–358
  initial evaluation, 356, 357t
  injury management, 358–359
    ankle sprain, 358
    chronic ankle instability, 359
    fractures, 359, 359t
    syndesmosis injury, 359
    tendonitis, 359
  Ottawa ankle rules, 357
Anorexia nervosa, 301t
Anterior cruciate ligament (ACL), 360, 360f
Anterior drawer test, 357t
Antidepressant medications, 446–448, 447t
Antihistamines, for anxiety, 449
Anti-inflammatory diet, 299t
Antiviral agents, for influenza, 222t
Anxiety
  diagnosis of, 444
  psychotherapy for, 449–450
  screening for, 442–443
  treatment for, 444–446, 448–449, 448t
    behavioral interventions, 445–446
    pharmacotherapy, 449
AOM. *See* Acute otitis media
Appendicitis, in older adults, 145t
Apprehension test, 366t
Aripiprazole, for depression, 448
Asset-based community development, 473
Assisted living community (ALC) for elders, 148t
Asthma, 233
  ACT for, 236, 236b
  Childhood ACT and, 236, 236b
  classification in adults and children, 234t
  diagnostic evaluation of, 236–237, 237t
  etiology, 233
  home management of, algorithm for, 235f
  monitoring/case management, 240–241
  peak expiratory flow (PEF) for, 236
  physical findings, 233–234
  pulmonary function testing for, 236
  risk factors for, 233
  secondary prevention for, 239–240

severity/control assessment, 233, 235f, 236
treatment
    approach for, 240f
    goals, 237
    options, 238–239
    pharmacotherapy for, 238t–239t
Asthma Control Test (ACT), 236, 236b
Atkins diet, 299t
Atopic dermatitis, 398t
Atrophic vaginitis, 329t
Atrophy, 395t
Attention deficit hyperactivity disorder, for middle
    childhood, 128
Atypical angina, 246t
Atypical presentation of illness, in older adults,
    145, 145t
AUB. *See* Abnormal uterine bleeding
Availability errors, 79
Azapirones, for anxiety, 449

B
Background questions, 29, 29b
    resources for, 34, 35t
Back pain, 112t, 370–377. *See also* Lower back
    pain (LBP)
Bacterial skin infections, 400t–401t
Bacterial vaginosis (BV), 106, 329t
Balanitis, 402t
Basal cell carcinoma (BCC), 402, 404t–405t
    nodular, 404t
    sclerosing/infiltrative, 405t
    superficial, 405t
BATHE technique, 60–62
    elements of, 61–62
    questions, 61–62
BCC. *See* Basal cell carcinoma
Behavior change, 60
    BATHE technique and, 60–62
    motivational interviewing in, 65–70
    stages of, 62–63, 64t
Benign prostatic hypertrophy (BPH), 344–345
    American Urological Association Symptom
        Score Index Questionnaire, 345t
    medications for, 346t
    in older adults, 143t
Benzodiazepines, for anxiety, 449
Bereavement and grief, 388–390
Beta blockers, 31t, 199, 263t
    for anxiety, 449
Beta human chorionic gonadotropin (β-HCG),
    102–103
Beyond Flexner, 471
β-HCG. *See* Beta human chorionic gonadotropin
Bias affecting illness scripts, types of, 48t
Billing requirements, for outpatient office visits, 172t
Binge drinking, 101

Binge-eating disorder, 302t
Biopsychosocial model, 46–47
Bipolar disorder
    screening for, 443
    treatment for, 449
Bipolar Spectrum Disorder Scale (BSDS), 442t
Blood pressure (BP), 269
    measurement technique, 270
Blood tests, in dermatology, 397
Body mass index (BMI), 105, 105t, 293
    adults, categories for, 293t
    BMI-for-age calculator, 293
    BMI-for-age percentiles, 294t
Botox injections, 419
Bowel movements, newborns, 123
BP. *See* Blood pressure
BPH. *See* Benign prostatic hypertrophy
Breast examination, 324–326
    breast pain, 326
    nipple discharge, 326
    red flags for breast cancer, 326
    screening recommendations, 325t
Breathing exercises, 445
Brief cognitive disputation, 446
Bright Futures Pocket Guide, 122
Bulimia nervosa, 301t
Bulla, 395t
Bullying, 126
Buprenorphine, 417, 464t
BV. *See* Bacterial vaginosis

C
CABG. *See* Coronary artery bypass grafting
CAD. *See* Coronary artery disease
CADReS. *See* Clinical Assessment of Driving
    Related Skills
Canadian Cardiovascular Society Classification
    System grades angina, 246t
Candida infections, 402t
Candidiasis, 329t
Cannabis use, 460–462
    harm reduction strategy, 462
    severity of dependence use scale, 461, 462t
Cardiac stress testing, 248f, 249t
Care in lifecycle, 7t
Care sites, for older adults, 146–147, 148t–150t,
    150
Carrier testing, 99
Car seats safety, 126
CAT. *See* COPD Assessment Test
Cellulitis, 400t
Centers for Disease Control and Prevention, 23,
    324, 473
CF. *See* Cystic fibrosis
Chemoprevention. *See* Chemoprophylaxis
Chemoprophylaxis, 93, 93t

Chest pain (CP) in adults, 181–185
  causes of, 182t
  clues/red flags about seriousness of, 183
  evaluation, steps in, 181, 183
  history and physical examination of, 184t–185t
  from ischemia, decision rule for, 183t
  management of, 184f, 185
  types and features of, 246t
Chest radiography, for shortness of breath, 180
Chickenpox, 403t
Childhood ACT, asthma and, 236, 236b
Child maltreatment, 426–430
  assessment, 428–429
  incidence of, 427
  management, 429–430
  neglect, 427
  physical abuse, 427
  psychological abuse, 428
  risk factors for, 427t
  sexual abuse, 427
Child neglect, 427, 429
Children
  abusive injuries, 428, 428t
  dietary patterns for, 300
  obesity in, 303–304
    management of, 303t
Chlamydia trachomatis, 329t
CHNA. *See* Community Health Needs Assessment
ChoosingWisely campaign, 346
Chorionic villus sampling (CVS), 108
Chronic care model, 230, 231t
Chronic disease
  asthma, 233–241
  care, 231t
  chronic obstructive pulmonary disease,
    241–245
  coronary artery disease, 246–252
  diabetes mellitus, 252–257
  facts about, 230
  follow-up visit, 53–54, 230–231
  general approach to visit for, 230–232
  heart failure, 258–264
  hyperlipidemia, 264–268
  hypertension, 268–273
  management, 47, 231t, 232
  obesity, 273–279
  osteoporosis, 279–283
Chronic obstructive pulmonary disease (COPD),
    241
  diagnostics for, 242
  differential diagnosis of, 242
  hospital assessment/admission for patients with,
    244–245
  monitoring, 245
  prevalence of, 241
  secondary prevention from, 245

severity/control assessment, 241–242
  tests for, 243t
  treatment
    acute exacerbation, 244
    goals, 242
    medications, 244
    options, 243–244, 243t
    surgery, 244
Chronic pain, 409–422
  approach to treatment of, 410–412
  clinical evaluation
    diagnostic testing, 414
    history and physical examination, 413–414
  management of, 414
    interventional pain modalities, 419
    medication side effects, 418–419
    nonpharmacologic modalities, 414
    opioid medications, 416–417, 416b
    patient monitoring, 417–418
    pharmacologic treatment, 415, 415t
    referral and pain clinics, 419
    therapeutic interventions, 419
    treatment efficacy evidence, 420t–422t
    treatment plan, development and
      documentation of, 414–416
  types of, 412
    mixed pain syndromes, 412–413
    neuropathic pain, 412
    nociceptive pain, 412
Churning, 22
City of Milwaukee Health Department, 472
Clinical Assessment of Driving Related Skills
    (CADReS), 155
Clinical decision rules, 166–167
Clinical microsystem, 78
Cochrane Database of Systematic Reviews, 38
Cochrane Library, 38
Cognitive behavioral therapy (CBT), for anxiety and
    depression, 449–450
Cohen-Mansfield Agitation Inventory, 151
Colic, 123–124
Colitis, 201t
Colonic cleansing, 304
Colonoscopy, 90
Comedonal acne, 399t
Community advisory board, 468
Community engagement, 473–474
  definition of, 473
  key questions for, 474t
  steps for, 473
    assess assets, 473
    connection/team development, 474
    consistency/reliability, 474
    listening, 473
    presence, 473
    readiness to change, 474

Community focus, 7t
Community Guide, 24, 24t
Community Health Needs Assessment (CHNA) process, 20, 21t
Community Health Resource Navigator, tool, 20
Community-level population health data, 20
Complementary/alternative therapies, for pain management, 421t–422t
Complex regional pain syndrome, 419
Comprehensiveness of care, 5
Condom use, 338
Condyloma, 403t
Consensus guidelines, 37
Consent, 386
Constipation, in newborns, 123
Contact dermatitis, 398t
Context errors, 79
Continuing care retirement community (CCRC) for elders, 149t
Continuity of care, 5, 6, 7t
Contraception, 308–318
    emergency, 316
    methods for, 311t
    options and counseling, 308–310, 315
    permanent, 318
    postpartum, 318t
    unprotected intercourse and, 316
    when to start, 310–312
    WHO medical eligibility criteria, 312
Contraception counseling, 309
    patient-centered, 310
    shared decision making in, 309
Contraceptive methods, 311t
    switching between, 314t, 316
Contraceptive options, 308–309
Contraceptive patch, 315
Contraceptive ring (NuvaRing), 315, 317
Coordination of care, 5, 7t
COPD. *See* Chronic obstructive pulmonary disease
COPD Assessment Test (CAT), 245
Copper IUD, 316
Coronary artery bypass grafting (CABG), 252t
Coronary artery disease (CAD), 246
    diagnosis of, 247–249
        cardiac stress testing, 248f, 249t
        history and physical examination, 247
        laboratory and imaging testing, 247
    prevalence of, 246
    revascularization for, 251, 252t
    severity/control assessment, 246–247
    treatment, 249–250
        pharmacotherapy for, 251t
        strategies for, 250t
Counseling, as preventive care plan, 93. *See also* Motivational interviewing
Crash cart, 164, 164f

Crusts, 395t
Culture test, in dermatology, 397
Current Procedural Terminology (CPT) code, 171
Cutaneous larva migrans, 404t
CVS. *See* Chorionic villus sampling
Cystic fibrosis (CF), 100t

D
DALYs. *See* Disability adjusted life years
DASH diet, 298, 299t
Deciphering research, 39–41
Deep brain stimulation, 419
Degenerative disk, 374t
Degenerative facet joint, 374t
Dehydration, 214
Dementia, 150–153, 151t, 152t
Depression, 441
    diagnosis of, 443–444
    in older adults, 145t
    psychotherapy for, 449–450
    screening for, 130, 442
        tools for, 442t
    treatment for, 444–448, 445t
        behavioral interventions, 445–446
        guidelines for initiation of, 447t
        pharmacotherapy, 446–448, 447t
Dermatitis, 397, 398t
Dermatoscopes, 394, 395f
Developmental delays and disabilities screening, for newborns, 121–122
DEXA. *See* Dual energy x-ray absorptiometry
Diabetes mellitus (DM), 252–257
    complications, prevention efforts for, 257t
    diagnostics, 253–254
    incidence of, 252–253
    monitoring/case management, 255t, 257, 257t
    risk factors for, 254, 255t
    screening, 99, 254
    secondary prevention from, 257
    severity/control assessment, 253
        comorbidities, 253
        hyperglycemia, 253
    testing recommended for, 254t
    treatment
        goals, 254–255
        options, 255–256
    type 1, 252
    type 2, 252
Diagnostic and Statistical Manual of Mental Disorders, fifth edition (DSM-5), 442, 454
Diagnostic errors, 78–80
Diet
    fads, 298
    healthy, 298
    popular, 299t–300t

Diet and dietary supplements, of pregnant women, 110
Dietary diary software applications, 292, 293t
Dietary recall, 292t
Differential diagnosis
acute problems, approach to, 168
bias affecting illness scripts, types of, 48t
of chronic obstructive pulmonary disease, 242
of dysuria, 189t, 191
of fever, 193t
of headache, 202t–203t
resources for, 48t
of shortness of breath, 176t
of undifferentiated complaint, 48
Disability adjusted life years (DALYs), 87
Discipline, for middle childhood, 128
Disclosure of medication errors, 80–82
Discrepancy, 66
Disease, 46
Disease-oriented evidence (DOE), 30–31
versus patient-oriented evidence that matters (POEM), 31t
Disequilibrium, 185, 186t, 188t
Disordered eating, 302t
Disulfiram, 460t
Diuresis, 261
Diuretics, for heart failure, 261
Diverticulitis, 201t
Diverticulosis, 197
Divorce, 387–388
Dix–Hallpike maneuver, 186
Dizziness, 185–188
causes of, 186t
clues/"red flags" in patients with, 187
evaluation, steps in, 187
management of, 187, 187f, 188f
in older adults, 144t
physical examination for, 186
types of, 185
DM. *See* Diabetes mellitus
DOE. *See* Disease-oriented evidence
Down syndrome, 108
Driving rehabilitation specialist (DRS), 155
Drop arm test, 366t
DRS. *See* Driving rehabilitation specialist
Dual energy x-ray absorptiometry (DEXA), 279, 280, 281f, 294
DynaMed Topic Alerts, 39
Dysmenorrhea, 323t
Dyspnea. *See* Shortness of breath
Dysuria, 188–191
causes of, 189, 189t
clues/"red flags" in patients with, 189
differential diagnosis of, 189t, 191
evaluation, steps in, 189–191
initial approach to patient with, 190f
management of, 191–192
physical examination for, 189
urinalysis for, 189, 190f

E

Early pregnancy loss and ectopic pregnancy, 103
Eating disorders, 300, 301t–302t. *See also specific disorder*
in older adults, 144t
Eating pattern, healthy, 298
EBM. *See* Evidence-based medicine
Eco Map, 469
Ectopic pregnancy, 103
ED. *See* Erectile dysfunction
EDD. *See* Estimated date of delivery
Edema, 207–212
causes of, 207–208, 208f, 208t–209t
clues/"red flags" in patients with, 209
evaluation, steps in, 209–211, 210f, 211f
management of, 212
EHR. *See* Electronic health record
Elderly man, 343. *See also* Older adults
benign prostatic hypertrophy (BPH), 344–345, 345t, 346t
lower urinary tract symptoms, 344–345, 344b
preventive services for medicare-covered men, 348
prioritizing care of, 343
prostate cancer screening, 346, 347t
sexuality in, 386–387
testosterone and andropause, 346–347, 348t
Elder mistreatment, 434–436
assessment, 435
management of, 435–436
risk factors for, 434, 434t
Electronic health record (EHR), 19, 50–51
Electronic Preventive Services Selector (ePSS), 54–55
Emancipated minors, 129
Emergency contraception (EC), 316
Emotional wellbeing, older adults, 153
Empathy, 66
Empty can testing, 366t
End-of-life care, for older adults, 157t, 158
Epilepsy screening, 100–101
ePSS. *See* Electronic Preventive Services Selector
Erectile dysfunction (ED), 340–341, 341t
causes, 340
evaluation of, 340, 341t
five-item International Index of Erectile Function (IIEF-5), 341t
testosterone deficiency, testing for, 340
treatment of, 341, 341t
Erosion, 395t
Errors of commission, 76
Errors of omission, 76
Escherichia coli (*E. coli*), 110
Esophagitis, 200t

Estimated date of delivery (EDD), 102
Evidence-based community interventions, 23–24, 24t
Evidence-based medicine (EBM), 27
    systems-based approach to, 38–39
Evidence-based practice, 7t
Excoriation, 395t
Expert opinion, 37

F
Faces Pain Scale, 413
Failure to thrive, 121
Fair Housing Act, 149t
Falls, older adults, 142t
Family medicine
    career options for physicians in, 10–12, 11f
    future role of, 10–12
    principles of, 6, 7t
    quality monitoring in, 6, 8f–9f
Family physicians
    approach to maternity care, 98
    and obstetric consultants, 114, 114t–115t
Family relationships, 7t
Family violence, 426
    child maltreatment, 426–430
    intimate partner violence, 430–434
Fecal immunochemical test (FIT), 90
Feelings of dissociation, 185
Fever
    causes of, 192
    definitions, 192
    differential diagnosis for, 193t
    evaluation, steps in, 192, 194–197
    management of, 196f, 197
Fever of unknown origin (FUO), 192
Fever without source (FWS), 192
FIF. See Finding information framework
FIFE mnemonic, 163
Finding information framework (FIF), 29, 30f
First trimester, prenatal care, 105
    genetic screening, 106, 108
    immunization, 106
    laboratory testing, 106, 107t
    physical examination, 105–106
    ultrasound, 106, 108t
Fissure, 395t
FIT. See Fecal immunochemical test
"Five As" approach, 93
Flexner report, 471
Folic acid supplementation, United States recommendations for, 99, 99b
Food diary, 292, 293t
Food Frequency Questionnaire (FFQ), 292
Foreground questions, 29, 29b
    resources for, 34–36
    structuring, 30, 31b

Fractures, ankle, 359, 359t
Frailty, in older adults, 142t
Framingham criteria (modified), for diagnosis of heart failure, 260t
FRAX, 281
Fundal height, 109
Fungal skin infections, 401t–402t
FUO. See Fever of unknown origin
Fussy baby, parental concerns for, 123–124
FWS. See Fever without source

G
Gabapentin, for hot flashes, 333
GABS. See Group A β-hemolytic strep
Galactorrhea, 326, 327t
Gastritis, 200t
Gastrointestinal (GI) bleeding, 197–201
    causes of, 198t–199t
    clues/"red flags" in patients with, 199
    evaluation, steps in, 199–200
    management of, 200, 200t–201t
    risk factors, 197
GBS. See Group B streptococcus
GDM. See Gestational diabetes
Gender identity, 382t
General Anxiety Disorder Questionnaire (GAD)-7, 442–443, 442t
Genetic screening and counseling, 99, 100t
Genital physical exam, 384
Genital warts, 327
Genograms, 2f
Geriatric syndromes, in older adults, 141t–142t
Gestational diabetes (GDM), 108–109
Gestational hypertension, 105
Ginger, 111
Glenohumeral joint arthritis, 367t
Glucose tolerance test (GTT), 109
Glutamic acid decarboxylase (GAD65), 252
Gluten-free diet, 299t
Glycemic control, 256f
Gonorrhea, 109, 329t
Group A β-hemolytic strep (GABS), 219
Group B streptococcus (GBS), 110
Growth screening, for newborns, 121
GTT. See Glucose tolerance test

H
Hand-foot-and mouth disease, 403t
Hawkins test, 366t
HD. See Heart disease
Headache, 201–207
    American College of Radiology imaging recommendations for, 204t
    clues/"red flags" in patients with, 203
    differential diagnosis for, 202t–203t
    evaluation, steps in, 203–204

Headache (*Continued*)
management of, 204, 205t–206t, 207
risk factors for, 203
therapies for, 205t–206t
triggers, 205t
Health care
men's, 335–349
women's, 321–333
Health care power of attorney, 385
Healthcare proxy, 156, 156t
Health disparities, 16, 470
Health equity, 15–16, 16f, 469–473
ethical responsibilities, 471–472
model of health, 470–471, 471f
taking action, 472–473, 472t
Health habits, improving, 104
Health outcomes, social determinants and,
16–17, 17f
Healthy diet, 298, 299t–300t
Hearing impairment, in older adults, 143t
Hearing screening, for newborns, 121
Heartburn, 112t
Heart disease (HD), 265
Heart failure (HF), 258
ACCF/AHA stages of, 259f
algorithm for evaluation and diagnosis of,
261f
causes of, 258, 258f
diagnosis of, 259–260, 260t
diuretics for, 261
echocardiography for, 259
Framingham criteria (modified) for diagnosis of,
260t
laboratory tests for, 259–260
nonpharmacologic therapies for, 262
NYHA functional classes of, 259f
patient education for, 262
pharmacologic therapy for, 261–262, 263t
prevalence of, 258
risk factors for, 258
secondary prevention of, 262
self-care for, 262
severity/control assessment, 258
stages in development of, 264f
terms, abbreviations and definitions of, 259t
treatment for
goals of, 260
options of, 261–262
Heckerling Clinical Decision Tool for community-
acquired pneumonia, 219, 220
HEEADSSS interview, 126
Hematemesis, 197
Hematochezia, 197
Hemorrhoids, 112t, 201t
Hepatitis B, 109
Herd immunity, 92

Herniated disk, 374t
Herpes simplex, 329t, 403t
Herpes simplex infection (HSV), 109–110
Heterogeneity, of older adults, 138–139, 138t
HF. *See* Heart failure
High risk behaviors, in young adult men, 335
alcohol and substance use, 337
screening for, 336t, 337
sexual health counseling, 338
sexually transmitted infection, 337–338
Hip fracture, 280
HIV. *See* Human immunodeficiency virus
Home care/home healthcare, 149t
Home safety, for older adults, 154
Home Safety Self-Assessment Tool (HSSAT),
154
Hop test, 357t
Hospice care, 150t
Hospitalization hazards, older adults and,
146, 147f
Hot flashes, 331–332
gabapentin for, 333
hormone therapy for, 332–333
HSSAT. *See* Home Safety Self-Assessment Tool
HSV. *See* Herpes simplex infection
Human immunodeficiency virus (HIV), 106
Human papilloma virus (HPV), 329t
Huntington disease, 95
Hyperglycemia, 253
Hyperkyphosis, in older adults, 141t
Hyperlipidemia, 255t, 264
diagnosis of, 265–266, 266t
heart disease, 265
monitoring for, 268
prevalence of, 265
statin therapy for, 266–267, 266t, 267t
treatment
goal, 267
nonstatin pharmacologic therapy for, 268t
options, 267, 268t
primary prevention to reduce CVD risk,
267t
statins and recommendations for, 268t
USPSTF recommendations on screening for,
266t
Hypermenorrhea, 323t
Hyperpyrexia, 192
Hypertension, 255t, 268–269
consequences of, 269
diagnostics for, 270, 271f
monitoring for, 272
patient education for, 272–273
prevalence of, 269
risk factors for, 270t
secondary causes of, 270t
self-care for, 272–273

treatment
  goals, 271
  Joint National Committee medication
    recommendations for, 272t
  nonpharmacologic options for, 272t
  options, 271
Hyperthermia, 192
Hypoglycemia, 256
Hypomenorrhea, 323t

I

I-HOPE, 154
Iliotibial band (ITB), 363t, 364
Illicit substance use, 337
Illness, 46
Illness presentations, in older adults, 145t
Immunizations, 91–92, 91t, 92t, 106
  for adolescent (ages 12 to 18 years), 131
  antibody screen for, 109
  for middle childhood (ages 2 to 11 years), 128
  for newborns (ages 0 to 2 years), 124
  status, 101
Impetigo, 400t
Infant weight, 120
Infections
  in older adults, 145t
  sexually transmitted, 329t, 337–338
  skin, 400, 400t–404t
  vaginal, 329t
Inflammatory and cystic acne, 399t
Influenza, 221
  antiviral agents for, 222t
  antiviral treatment for, 222
  websites about, 222
InfoPOEMs podcast, 39
Information management, 28–29
  background questions, 29, 29b
  finding information framework, 29, 30f
  foreground questions, 29, 29b
Information mastery, 29–32
  deciphering research, 39–41
  EBM, systems-based approach to, 38–39
    clinical practice design, 39
    literature, keeping up with, 38–39
  evidence hierarchy, in clinical medicine, 36–38,
    36f
    expert opinion, 37
    meta-analyses, 37–38
    pathophysiologic reasoning, 36–37
    practice guidelines, 37
    systematic reviews, 37–38
  resources, 33–36
    for background questions, 34, 35t
    for foreground questions, 34–36
    internet, 18
    transparency, 36

usefulness, 27–28, 32, 41–42
  relevance, 32
  validity, 33
  work, 33
Inpatient rehabilitation facility (IRF) for elders, 148t
Insomnia, in older adults, 143t
Insurance churning, on population health, 22
Insurance coverage, 472
Integrated community health, 93–94
International Statistical Classification of Diseases
  and Related Health Problems, version 10
  (ICD-10), 171
Internet safety, 126
Intertrigo, 402t
Intimate partner violence (IPV), 111, 430–434
  management, 433–434
  pattern of coercion and control in, 430
  during pregnancy, 431
  presentations, 431
    injuries, 431
    mental Health, 432
    physical health effects, 431
  red flags for imminent danger, 433
  screening and assessment, 324, 432–433, 432t
Intrathecal drug infusion pumps, 419
Intrauterine device (IUD), 311t, 313
  hormonal progestin-only, 313
  myths vs, facts, 313t
  nonhormonal/copper IUD, 313
IPV. *See* Intimate partner violence
Ischemic heart disease (IHD). *See* Coronary artery
  disease (CAD)
IUD. *See* Intrauterine device

J

Jaundice, in newborns, 119
Joint physical exam, 354
Juice cleanses, 299t

K

Knee pain, 359–364
  anatomy related to, 360–361, 360f
  differential diagnosis, 363t
  examination in, 361–362, 361t, 362t
  imaging in, 361
  management, 362–364
    anterior cruciate ligament tear, 363
    iliotibial band (ITB), 364
    lateral collateral ligament tear, 363
    medial collateral ligament tear, 362
    mensicus tear, 363–364
    osteoarthritis (OA), 364
    patellofemoral pain syndrome/chondromalacia
      patella, 364
    posterior cruciate ligament tear, 362
    rest, ice, compression, and elevation (RICE), 362

Knee pain (*Continued*)
mechanism of injury, 363t
Ottawa knee rules, 361
physical exam findings, 363t
risk factors for, 360
tests in evaluation of, 362t
Korsakoff syndrome, 460
Kwashiorkor, 297t

L

Lachman's test, 362t
Lateral collateral ligament (LCL), 360, 360f
LBW. *See* Low birth weight
Lead-time bias, 94–95, 94f
Leg swelling. *See* Edema
Length-time bias, 95
Leukorrhea, 112t
Lice infestation, 404t
Lichenification, 395t
Life care facility for elders, 149t
Life expectancy, of older adults, 138t, 139, 140f
Lifestyle topics, of pregnant women, 110–111
Lift off test, 366t
Lightheadedness, 188t
Likelihood ratios (LRs), 41, 41f, 166
Lipid levels, normal, 265t
Listeriosis, 110
Liver disease, alcohol use and, 459
Living wills, 156, 156t
Long-term acute care hospital (LTACH) for elders, 148t
Long-term care (LTC) facility for elders, 148t
Long-Term Care Ombudsman Program, 435
Low birth weight (LBW), 102
Lower back pain (LBP), 370–377
acute, 371, 376
back examination and tests, 373t
neurologic findings in, 373t
chronic, 371, 376–377
differential diagnosis, 371
differential diagnosis of, 374t–375t
imaging in, 376, 376t
initial evaluation, 371
management of, 376–377
algorithm for, 375f
non-spine causes, 372–373
red flags for early imaging, 371
referral, indications for, 377
spine anatomy, 371, 372f
Lower urinary tract symptoms (LUTS), 344–345, 344b
benign prostatic hypertrophy and, 344, 345t
causes of, 344, 344b
evaluation and management of, 345
LRs. *See* Likelihood ratios
Lupus, 399t

M

Macule, 395t
Major depressive disorder (MDD), 441, 443. *See also* Depression
and substance misuse, 456
Mallory–Weiss tear, 200t
Malnutrition, in older adults, 141t
Mammography, 168f
Marasmus, 297t
Mature minors, 129
MCI. *See* Mild cognitive impairment
McMurray's test, 362t
Medial collateral ligament (MCL), 360, 360f
Medicaid, 5
Medication errors, 73, 74, 74f, 75–77, 76f
disclosure of, 80–82
prevention from, 76–77
5 Whys analysis for, 76, 76f
Medication reconciliation, 146
Medication use, during pregnancy, 111
Medicine practice, in information age, 28
Mediterranean diet, 298, 299t
Melanoma, 392f, 402, 405t–406t
ABCDE of, 393t
acral lentiginous, 406t
amelanotic, 394f, 406t
lentigo maligna, 406t
melanoma in situ with regression, 393f
nodular, 405t
superficial spreading carcinoma, 405t
Melena, 197
Memory loss, 152t
Menometrorrhagia, 323t
Menopause, 331–333
diagnosis, 331
genitourinary syndrome of, 332
mean age for, 331
menopausal symptoms, 331–332
hormone therapy for, 332–333
management of, 332–333
Women's Health Initiative (WHI) study, 332, 332t
serum markers of, 331
Menorrhagia, 323t
Men's health care, 335–349
elderly man, 343
benign prostatic hypertrophy (BPH), 344–345, 345t, 346t
lower urinary tract symptoms, 344–345, 344b
preventive services for medicare-covered men, 348
prioritizing care of, 343
prostate cancer screening, 346, 347t
testosterone and andropause, 346–347, 348t
middle-aged man, 339, 340b
cardiovascular disease screening, 342
CDC guidelines for physical activity, 342t

erectile dysfunction, 340–341, 341t
hypertension screening, 342
lipid measurement, 342
overweight/obesity, 342
prioritizing care for, 339
suicide in, 342–343
young adult man, 335
  alcohol and substance use, screening for, 337
  cancer screening, 338–339
  mortality in, 335, 336f, 336t
  physical examination, 338
  prioritizing care for, 335
  sexual health counseling, 338
  sexually transmitted infection screening, 337–338
Menstrual cycle, 321–323
abnormal menstrual flow, terminology related to, 323t
normal, 322f
Mental health disorders, 440–450. *See also* Anxiety; Depression
Men who have sex with men (MSM), 338
Meta-analyses, 37–38
Metacognition, 80
Methadone, 416–417, 464t
Metrorrhagia, 323t
Microscopy, in dermatology, 397
Middle childhood, well-child care for, 124–125
education for, 127, 127t
immunization for, 128
parental concerns for, 127–128
  attention deficit hyperactivity disorder, 128
  discipline, 128
  school readiness, 128
  sleep, 127–128
prepuberty of, 126
puberty of, 126
risk assessment and harm reduction for, 126
screening for, 125, 133t
Mild cognitive impairment (MCI), 150–151
Mirtazapine, for depression, 448
Molluscum contagiosum, 403t
Mood and anxiety disorders, in primary care, 441
screening for, 441–442, 442t
  anxiety, 442–443
  bipolar disorder, 443
  depression, 442
  substance dependence, 443
Mood Disorder Questionnaire (MDQ), 442t
Morning sickness, 102
Mortality, in young adult man, 335, 336f, 336t
Motivational interviewing, 65–70. *See also* Counseling, as preventive care plan
basic assumptions of, 65
counseling principles
  discrepancy, 66
  empathy, 66

roll with resistance, 67
self-efficacy enhancement, 67
information presentation within, 68–69
OARS techniques for, 67–68
"rolling with" resistance, 69–70
spirit of, 65–66
MRC dyspnea scale, 245
Multnomah County Health Department, 472
Musculoskeletal problems
ankle pain, 354–359
knee pain, 359–364
lower back pain, 370–377
shoulder pain, 364–370
Myocardial infarction, in older adults, 145t

N
Naegele's rule, for EDD, 102
Naloxone, 417
Naltrexone, 460t, 464t
Narcotics Anonymous, 455
National Center on Elder Abuse website, 435
National Domestic Violence Hotline, 434
National Guideline Clearinghouse, 37, 167
Nausea, 212–216
causes for, 213t
clues/red flags in patients with, 214
dehydration and, 214
evaluation, steps in, 212, 214
initial testing for, 213t
key features for, 213t
management of, 214, 215t–216t
medications for, 215t–216t
Near misses, 74
Necrotizing fasciitis, 401t
Neer's test, 366t
Negative predictive value (NPV), 41
Nephropathy, 257t
Neural tube defects (NTDs), 99
Neuropathic pain, 412
Newborns, well-child care for
immunizations for, 124
issues, 119, 120t
  jaundice, 119
  weight, 120
parental concerns for, 123t
  bowel movements, 123
  fussy baby, 123–124
  sleep, 122–123, 123t
  tantrums, 124
parental education for, 122
risks assessment and harm reduction, 122
screening, 121
  for developmental delays and disabilities, 121–122
  of growth, 121
  for hearing, 121
Nipple discharge, 326

NIPT. *See* Noninvasive prenatal testing
NNH. *See* Number needed to harm
NNT. *See* Number needed to treat
Nociceptive pain, 412
Nodule, 395t
Nomogram, 166, 166f
Noncardiac chest pain, 246t
Noninvasive prenatal testing (NIPT), 108
NPV. *See* Negative predictive value
NTDs. *See* Neural tube defects
Number needed to harm (NNH), 39, 41
Number needed to treat (NNT), 39, 40f, 40t, 41
Nummular dermatitis, 398t
Nutrient deficiencies, 295t
Nutrigenomics, 305
Nutritional ecology, 304–305
Nutrition and weight loss applications, 293t
Nutrition and weight management
  eating disorders and, 300, 301t–302t
  future directions, 304–305
    intestinal microbiome, influence of, 305
    nutrigenomics, 305
    nutritional ecology, 304–305
    role of fat type in energy balance, 305
  healthy eating pattern, 298
  myths and trends, 304
  nutrient deficiencies, physical signs of, 294–300,
    295t, 296t
    photographs of, 297t
    specific nutrient deficiencies, 295t
    vitamin deficiencies, 296t
  nutrition assessment, 291–294
    dietary history, 291–292, 293t
    office-based assessment, approach to, 292t
    physical exam, 293–294, 293t, 294f, 294t
  overweight and obesity, 300, 303–304

O

OARS techniques, for motivational interviewing, 67–68
  affirmations, 68
  open-ended questions, 68
  reflections, 68
  summarizing, 68
Ober test, 362t
Obesity, 300, 303–304. *See also* Weight management
    and nutrition
  in adults, 342
  approach to patients with, 274, 275f
  in children, 303–304
    management of, 303t
  future directions in, 304–305
  guideline recommendations, 275
  incidence of, 273
  monitoring for, 279
  resources for patients, 279
  risk factor for, 273

secondary prevention from, 278
  severity assessment of, 273–274
  treatment
    bariatric surgery, 276–277
    devices, 277–278
    diet, 275–276
    exercise, 276
    gastric banding and bypass procedures, 278t
    goals, 274–275
    medication options for, 276, 277t
O'Brien's test, 366t
Obstetric history, 103, 104t
Occupational risks, 99
Office of Dietary Supplements at the National
    Institutes of Health, 296, 298
OGTT. *See* Oral glucose tolerance test
OLDCARTS mnemonic, 53, 53t
Older adults
  atypical presentation in, 145, 145t
  care sites for, 146–147, 148t–150t, 150
  domains of care, 139, 140f
  environmental assessment for, 153–154
  geriatric syndromes in, 141t–142t
  heterogeneity of, 138–139, 138t
  home safety and evaluation for, 154
  hospitalization hazards and, 146, 147f
  illness presentations in, 145t
  life expectancy of, 138t, 139, 140f
  mental health of, 150
    cognitive screening, 150–153, 151t, 152t
    emotional wellbeing, 153
  morbidity and mortality, causes of, 139–140, 141t
  physical assessment of, 154–156, 155f
  preventive care, 137–139
  problems common in, 143t–144t
  social assessment for
    advance directives, 156, 156t
    end-of-life, 157t, 158
    palliative care, 158
  transitions of care for, 146–147
Oligomenorrhea, 323t
OME. *See* Otitis media with effusion
Ongoing Violence Assessment Tool, 432
Onychomycosis, 402t
OP. *See* Osteoporosis
Open-ended questions, 68
Opiate-induced hypernociception, 419
Opioid Risk Assessment Tool, 463t
Opioids, 463
  abuse, 462–464, 464t
  for chronic pain, 411, 411t–412t, 415–416
    buprenorphine, 417
    methadone, 416–417
    naloxone, 417
    prescribing, guidelines for, 416, 416t
  opiates, 463

semisynthetic, 463
synthetic, 463
OPQRST (mnemonic), 354
Oral glucose tolerance test (OGTT), 254
Orlistat, 304
Osteoarthritis (OA), knee, 363t, 364
Osteopenia, 279–280
Osteoporosis (OP), 279–280, 279f, 281f
    bone density measurement with DEXA, 281f
    causes of secondary, 280t
    consequences of, 280
    diagnostics for, 280–282
    monitoring for, 282–283
    in older adults, 143t
    patient education for, 283
    prevalence of, 280
    risk factors for, 280t
    self-care for, 283
    treatment
        goals, 282
        medications for, 283t
        options, 282
Otitis media with effusion (OME), 220, 221t
Ottawa ankle rules, 357
Ottawa knee rules, 361
Outpatient primary care settings, common errors
    in, 75–80
Overdiagnosis, 95
Overweight, 300, 303–304, 303t. *See also* Weight
    management and nutrition
    in children, 303–304
    myths about, 300, 303–304, 303t

P
Pain, chronic, 409–422. *See also* Chronic pain
Palliative care, 149t
Pancreatitis, alcohol use and, 459
Papule, 395t
Paroxetine (Brisdelle), 333
PASTE mnemonic, 131
Patch, 395t
Patellar compression test, 362t
Pathophysiologic reasoning, 36–37
Patient care, clinical questions during, 32
Patient education, 170
    for heart failure, 262
    for hypertension, 272–273
    for osteoporosis, 283
    for prenatal care, 110
Patient Health Questionnaire (PHQ)-9, 442t
Patient-oriented evidence (POE), 30
Patient-oriented evidence that matters (POEM), 30
    versus disease-oriented evidence (DOE), 31t
Patient safety, in primary care, 73–82
    definition, 74
    diagnostic errors and, 78–80

medication errors and, 75–77, 76f
outpatient primary care settings, common errors
    in, 75–80
    communication factor for, 75
    contributing factors, 75
    system factor for, 75
    thinking errors and bias factor for, 75
    testing process errors and, 77–78, 77f
Patient-team partnership, 5, 7t
PCPs. *See* Primary care physicians
PE. *See* Pulmonary embolism
Peak expiratory flow (PEF), for asthma, 236
Pediatric well-child check, 119
    adolescent (ages 12 to 18 years), 129
        confidentiality, 129
        education for, 131
        immunization for, 131
        parental concerns for, 131
        risk assessment and harm reduction for,
            130–131, 132t
        screening of, 129–130, 133t
    middle childhood (ages 2 to 11 years),
        124–125
        education for, 127, 127t
        immunization for, 128
        parental concerns for, 127–128
        prepuberty of, 126
        puberty of, 126
        risk assessment and harm reduction for,
            126
        screening for, 125
    newborns (ages 0 to 2 years)
        immunizations for, 124
        issues, 119–120, 120t
        parental concerns for, 122–124, 123t
        parental education for, 122
        risks assessment and harm reduction, 122
        screening, 121–122
Pelvic examination, 326–327, 328t
Peptic ulcer disease (PUD), 197
PERC. *See* Pulmonary Embolism Rule-out Criteria
Peritoneal inflammation, tests for, 173
Personal safety, for adolescents, 131
Physical abuse, of children, 427
    assessment of, 428, 428t
Physical activity, in adults, 342, 342t
Physician–patient communication, 47
PICO, 30, 31b
Plaque, 395t
PLLR. *See* Pregnancy and Lactation Labeling
    Rule
Pneumonia, in older adults, 145t
POE. *See* Patient-oriented evidence
Point-of-care resource, 34
Polyethylene glycol, 123
Polymenorrhea, 323t

Population health, 15–17
  insurance churning on, 22
  for patients, 18, 18f
    Community Health Needs Assessment (CHNA)
      process, 20, 21t
    community-level population health data, 20
    individual care, 21
    practice-level population health data, 19
    social history, 18–19
  policy interventions for
    evidence-based community interventions,
      23–24, 24t
    hospitals and accountable care organizations
      investing in communities, 22–23, 23f
Population management, 7t
Positive predictive value (PPV), 41
Postdate pregnancy, 113, 113t
Posterior cruciate ligament (PCL), 360, 360f
Posterior drawer test, 362t
Posterior sag test, 362t
Postpartum contraception, 318t
PPV. See Positive predictive value
Practice guidelines, 37
Practice-level population health data, 19
Preconception visit, 98–101
  alcohol, 101
  folic acid, 99
  genetic screening and counseling, 99, 100t
  immunization status, 101
  medical conditions, 99–101
  medication history, 101
  occupational risks, 99
  tobacco, 101
Pregabalin, for anxiety, 449
Pregnancy
  abdominal pain during, 175f
  alcohol during, 101
  backache during, 112t
  body mass index, 105, 105t
  common problems in, 111–112, 112t
  diagnosing and dating, 102–103
  early loss, 103
  ectopic, 103
  heartburn during, 112t
  hemorrhoids during, 112t
  intimate partner violence in, 431
  leukorrhea during, 112t
  nutrition during, 104
  postdate, 113, 113t
  round ligament pain during, 112t
  stress urinary incontinence during, 112t
  symptoms of, 102
  tests, 102–103
  tobacco during, 101
  unplanned, 317
  urinary frequency during, 112t

Pregnancy and Lactation Labeling Rule (PLLR), 101
Pregnancy test, 330
Pregnant women. See also Pregnancy
  diet and dietary supplements, 110
  intimate partner violence, 111
  lifestyle topics, 110–111
  medication use, 111
Premature closure, 79–80
Prenatal care, 54, 98, 102
  diagnosing and dating pregnancy, 102–103
  early pregnancy loss and ectopic pregnancy, 103
  family physicians
    approach to maternity care, 98
    and obstetric consultants, 114, 114t–115t
  first trimester visit, 105
    genetic screening, 106, 108
    immunization, 106
    laboratory testing, 106, 107t
    physical examination, 105–106
    ultrasound, 106, 108t
  patient education and psychosocial support, 110
    common problems, 111–112, 112t
    diet and dietary supplements, 110
    intimate partner violence, 111
    lifestyle topics, 110–111
    medication use, 111
    postdate pregnancy, 113, 113t
    TOLAC/VBAC, 112–113
  preconception visit, 98–101
    alcohol, 101
    folic acid, 99
    genetic screening and counseling, 99, 100t
    immunization status, 101
    medical conditions, 99–101
    medication history, 101
    occupational risks, 99
    tobacco, 101
  prenatal visits, 104–105
  risk assessment
    current medical and past surgical history,
      104
    health habits, 104
    nutrition, 104
    obstetric history, 103, 104t
  second and third trimester visit, 108
    laboratory testing, 109–110
    physical examination, 108–109
Prenatal visits, 104–105
Prepuberty, 126
Pressure ulcer, in older adults, 142t
Presyncope, 185, 186t, 188t
Preterm delivery, rates of, 102
Prevention focus, 4, 7t
Preventive care plan, 85–86
  benefits assessment, criteria for, 87–88
  chemoprophylaxis, 93, 93t

counseling as, 93
evidence for, 94–95
guidelines for, 95–96
immunizations, 91–92, 91t, 92t
integrated community health, 93–94
levels of, 86–87, 86t
resources for, 95–96
systems of, 96
Primary care
career options for physicians in, 10–12, 11f
errors in, 75–80
family medicine
principles of, 6, 7t
quality monitoring in, 6, 8f–9f
future role of, 10–12
healthcare organization and, 2–5
healthcare systems in developed nations,
comparison of, 3t
improvement, 6–7
issues, 2–5
patient safety in, 73–82
role of, 5–6
US healthcare system, 2, 4–5, 4f
Primary care physicians (PCPs), 5, 46
biopsychosocial model and, 46–47
calibration, 49
chronic disease management and, 47
disease *versus* illness and, 46
physician–patient communication, 47
undifferentiated complaint, differential diagnosis
of, 48, 48t
Primary Care Post-Traumatic Stress Disorder Scale
(PC-PTSD), 442t
Procedure visits, 55, 56f
Prostate cancer, screening for, 346, 347t
Prostate-specific antigen (PSA), 345
PSNet, 80, 82
Psoriasis, 397–400
lesions, 397, 399f
scalp, 398
topical steroids in, 400t
treatment options, 398
Psoriatic nail changes, 397
Psychological abuse, of children, 428, 429
symptoms of, 430t
Psychosocial problems, 440–450. *See also* Anxiety;
Depression
Psychotherapy, for anxiety and depression, 449–450
Puberty, 126, 130
PUD. *See* Peptic ulcer disease
Pulmonary embolism (PE), 177
Wells criteria for, 179t
Pulmonary Embolism Rule-out Criteria (PERC), 177
Pulmonary function testing, for asthma, 236
Pulmonary rehabilitation, 244
Pustule, 395t

Q
qSOFA. *See* Quick Sequential Organ Failure
Assessment
Quadruple Aim approach, 6
Quick Sequential Organ Failure Assessment
(qSOFA), 194

R
Randomized clinical trials (RCTs), 105
Raspberry leaf, 111
Raw food diet, 299t
RCA. *See* Root cause analysis
RCTs. *See* Randomized clinical trials
Reactive airway disease, 233. *See also* Asthma
Reflections, OARS techniques, 68
Relationships, 387
bereavement and grief, 388–390
separation and divorce, 387–388
sexual assault, 388
Relaxation exercises, 445
Relevance, information, 32
Remaining life expectancy, 139
Resilience and community building, 477–478
Resource stewardship, 7t
Retinopathy, 257t
Review articles, 35t
Righting reflex, 65–66
RISE mnemonic, 96
Root cause analysis (RCA), 76
Rosacea, 399t
Rotator cuff tears, 370t
Round ligament pain, 112t
Roux-en-Y gastric bypass, 278f

S
SAD PERSONS scale, 442
SAFER-HOME v3, 154
Salicylic acid shampoos, 398
Sarcopenia, 304
Scabies, 404t
Scale (desquamation), 395t
School readiness, for middle childhood, 128
Screening tests, 88–90
acceptability to patients, 90
benefits *versus* harms of, 89
evidence for, 94–95
goal of, 88
guidelines for, 95–96
performance of, 89–90
preclinical phase, detectable, 89, 90f
programs, 88, 88t
resources for, 95–96
sources of bias in, 94–95, 94f
Seborrheic dermatitis, 398t
Second and third trimester visit, prenatal care, 108
laboratory testing, 109–110
physical examination, 108–109

Selective serotonergic reuptake inhibitors (SSRIs)
  for anxiety, 449
  for depression, 448
Self-care plan, 478
Self-efficacy, enhancement of, 67
Self-empowerment, 7t
Self-management, 7t
Senior housing for elders, 149t
Sepsis, 194, 194f
  clues/red flags in patients with, 194–195
Septic shock, 194, 194f
Serotonin norepinephrine reuptake inhibitors
    (SNRIs)
  for anxiety, 449
  for depression, 448
Severe sepsis, 194, 194f
Sexual abstinence, 338
Sexual abuse, of children, 427
  medical history, 429
  noncontact abuse, 427
  physical examination, 429
  presentations, 429
  sexual contact, 427
Sexual Assault Nurse Examiner (SANE), 388, 389f
Sexual behaviors, high-risk, 338
Sexual dysfunction, 324
Sexual health screening, for adolescents, 130
Sexual history, taking of, 323–324, 381–382
  approach to, 382f
  5 Ps approach, 383b
  of transgender patients, 383
Sexuality, 381
  adolescent, 385–386
  and gender terminology, 382t
  in older adults, 386–387
  screening and prevention, 384
Sexually transmitted infections (STIs), 329t
  preventive measures against, 338
  screening for men, 337–338
Sexual orientation, 382t
Sexual violence, 388
Shared decision-making, 170
Shortness of breath, 176–181
  causes of, 178t–179t
  chest radiography for, 180
  complete blood count for, 180
  differential diagnosis of, 176t
  ECG findings for, 180t
  emergent findings of, 178t–179t
  evaluation of patients with, 177, 178t–180t, 180
  management of, 180–181
  office management of, 178t–179t
  pulmonary embolism, Wells criteria for, 179t
  spirometry for, 180t
Shoulder pain, 364–370
  approach to patient with, 368f

differential diagnosis, 367t
  examination and tests, 366t
  joint anatomy, 365, 365f
  management of
    adhesive capsulitis, 370t
    anterior shoulder dislocation, 367–368
    arthritis, 370t
    posterior shoulder dislocation, 369
    sprains and tears, 370t
Shoulder stability, 365
Sickle cell anemia, 100t
SIRS. See Systemic inflammatory response syndrome
Skilled nursing facility (SNF) for elders, 148t
Skin fold thickness, 294
Skin problems, 392–393
  dermatitis, 397, 398t
  diagnosis of, principles for, 392–395
    dermatoscope, use of, 394, 395f
    pattern recognition, 394, 395t
    primary and secondary lesions, 395t
  facial skin conditions, 399t
  history taking, 396–397
  laboratory tests, 397
  physical examination
    distribution, 396
    expanded look, 396
    look and touch, 395t, 396
  psoriasis, 397–400, 399f, 400t
  skin cancers, 402, 404t–406t, 406–407
    basal cell carcinoma (BCC), 402, 404t–405t
    melanoma, 402, 405t–406t
    risk factor, 406
    squamous cell carcinoma (SCC), 402, 402f
    sun protection for prevention of, 407
  skin infections, 400
    bacterial, 400t–401t
    common Infestations, 404t
    fungal, 401t–402t
    viral, 403t
Sleep
  for middle childhood, 127–128
  newborns, 122–123, 123t
SMA. See Spinal muscular atrophy
Smoking, 101, 255t
SNAPPS, 50, 50b
SOAP format, 171
SOR. See Strength of recommendation
SORT. See Strength of Recommendation Taxonomy
South Beach diet, 299t
Spinal cord stimulators, 419
Spinal muscular atrophy (SMA), 100t
Spinal stenosis, 374t
Spirit of motivational interviewing, 65–66
Spirometry, for shortness of breath, 180t
Spondylolisthesis, 374t
Spondylolysis, 374t

Sports preparticipation screening, for adolescents, 130
Squamous cell carcinoma (SCC), of skin, 402, 402f
Squeeze test, 357t
State prescription drug monitoring programs (PDMPs), 413
Sterilization
  female, 318
  male, 318
Stool, newborns, 123
Stork test, 373t
Straight leg raise test, 373t
Strength of recommendation (SOR), 169
Strength of Recommendation Taxonomy (SORT), 34, 35t
Stress tests, algorithm for selection of, 248t
Stress urinary incontinence, 112t
Substance Abuse and Mental Health Services Administration (SAMHSA), 454
Substance dependence, in primary care, 443
Substance use disorders, 453
  alcohol use, 458–460
  cannabis use, 460–462
  comorbid conditions, 456
  counseling techniques, 455
    FRAMES, 455, 457t
  harm reduction, 456–458
  opioids abuse, 462–464
  patient engagement and treatment, 454–455
  pharmacotherapy, 456
  prevalence and diagnosis, 453–454
  resources related to, 465
  screening for, 454–455
  support and peer-based groups, 455
  treatment levels of intervention for, 456t
Suicide, in middle-aged men, 342–343
Summarizing, OARS techniques, 68
Surgical biopsy, 397
Swimming/floating sensations, 185
Syncope, in older adults, 144t
Syphilis, 109, 329t
Systematic reviews, 37–38
Systemic inflammatory response syndrome (SIRS), 194, 194f

T
Talar tilt test, 357t
Tantrums, parental concerns for, 124
Task Force on Community Preventive Services, 24
Tay–Sachs disease, 100t
Team-based care, 5, 7t
Testicular cancer, 338–339
Testing process errors, 77–78, 77f
Testosterone deficiency, 340–341
Testosterone replacement therapy (TST), 347, 348t

Tetracyclic noradrenaline, for depression, 448
Thalassemia alpha type, 100t
Thalassemia beta type, 100t
Thompson test, 357t
Thrush, 402t
Thyrotoxicosis, in older adults, 145t
Tinea capitis, 401t
Tinea corporis, 401t
Tinea cruris, 401t
Tinea pedis, 401t
Tinea versicolor, 402t
Tobacco, during pregnancy, 101
TOLAC. *See* Trial of labor after cesarean
Toxic stress, 470–471
Transgender, 382t, 383
  physical exam of, considerations in, 384
Transitions of care, for older adults, 146–147
Trans-theoretical model, 62–63, 64t
Transvaginal ultrasound, 103
Trial of labor after cesarean (TOLAC), 112–113
Trichomoniasis, 329t
Triple Aim approach, 6–7
T-score, 281
TST. *See* Testosterone replacement therapy
Tumor/polyp, 201t
Type 1 diabetes mellitus, 252
Type 2 diabetes mellitus, 252
  testing recommended for, 254t
Typical angina, 246t

U
Ulcer, 395t
Ulipristal acetate (UPA), 316
Ultrasound, 106
Underwater weighing, 294
Undifferentiated complaint, differential diagnosis of, 48, 48t
United Kingdom Prospective Diabetes Study (UKPDS), 256
United States Preventive Services Task Force (USPSTF), 54, 95–96, 106, 270
University of Wisconsin Training in Urban Medicine and Public Health (TRIUMPH) program, 472
Unmarried people, caring for, 385
Upper respiratory tract symptoms, 216–223
  causes of, 217
  clues/"red flags" in patients with, 217t
  evaluation, steps in, 217–220
  management of, 220–223, 220t–221t
Urinary frequency, 112t
Urinary incontinence (UI), in older adults, 142t
Urinary tract infection, in older adults, 145t
Urine drug testing (UDT), 416, 418
Usefulness equation, 32, 34
Usefulness of information, 27–28, 32–33

US healthcare system, 2, 4–5, 4f
  future role of, 10–12
  improvement in, 6–7
US Preventive Services Task Force (USPSTF), 442t
  on breast examination, 325, 325t
USPSTF. *See* United States Preventive Services Task
    Force

V

Vaccination, 91
  for adolescent, 131
  for middle childhood, 128
  misconceptions about, 92t
  for newborns, 124
  preventable diseases, 91t
Vaginal birth after cesarean (VBAC), 98, 112–113
Vaginal candidiasis, 329t
Vaginal discharge and lesions, 327–329, 329t
  sexually transmitted infections, 329t
  vaginal infections, 329t
  wet prep, 327, 328t
Vaginitis, 402t
Vague light-headedness, 185
Valgus test, 362t
Validity, of research, 33
Varices, 200t
Varus test, 362t
Vasectomy, 318
Vasomotor (hot flashes), 331–332
VBAC. *See* Vaginal birth after cesarean
Vegan diet, 299t
Vegetarian diet, 300t
Venlafaxine, 333
Vertebral compression fractures, 280
Vertical banded gastroplasty, 278f
Vertigo, 185, 186t, 188t
Vesicle, 395t
Veterans Administration Diabetes Trial (VADT), 256
Vibrio cholera, 110
Vibrio parahaemolyticus, 110
Viral skin infections, 403t
Visual impairment, in older adults, 143t
Vitamin B_2 deficiency, 296t, 297t
Vitamin B_6 deficiency, 296t, 297t
Vitamin C deficiency, 296t, 297t
Vitamin D deficiency, 296t, 297t
Vitamin deficiencies, 296t
Vomiting, 212–216
  causes for, 213t
  clues/"red flags" in patients with, 214
  dehydration and, 214
  evaluation, steps in, 212, 214
  initial testing for, 213t
  key features for, 213t
  management of, 214, 215t–216t
  medications for, 215t–216t

W

Waist circumference, 293, 294
  measurement of, 294f
Warts, 403t
Weight gain, medications for, 274t
Weight loss
  devices for, 227–228
  in older adults, 141t
Weight management and nutrition
  eating disorders and, 300, 301t–302t
  future directions, 304–305
    intestinal microbiome, influence of, 305
    mutritional ecology, 304–305
    nutrigenomics, 305
    role of fat type in energy balance, 305
  healthy eating pattern, 298
  myths and trends, 304
  nutrient deficiencies, physical signs of, 294–300,
      295t, 296t
    photographs of, 297t
    specific nutrient deficiencies, 295t
    vitamin deficiencies, 296t
  nutrition assessment, 291–294
    dietary history, 291–292, 293t
    office-based assessment, approach to, 292t
    physical exam, 293–294, 293t, 294f, 294t
  overweight and obesity, 300, 303–304
Weight Watchers Plan, 300t
Well-child care for adolescents, 129
  confidentiality, 129
  education for, 131
  immunization for, 131
  parental concerns for, 131
  personal safety, 131
  risk assessment and harm reduction for,
      130–131, 132t
  screening, 129, 133t
    for depression, 130
    for puberty, 130
    for sexual health, 130
    sports preparticipation, 130
Well-child care for middle childhood, 124–125
  education for, 127, 127t
  immunization for, 128
  parental concerns for, 127–128
    attention deficit hyperactivity disorder, 128
    discipline, 128
    school readiness, 128
    sleep, 127–128
  prepuberty of, 126
  puberty of, 126
  risk assessment and harm reduction for, 126
  screening for, 125, 133t
Well-child care for newborns
  immunizations for, 124
  issues, 119, 120t

jaundice, 119
  weight, 120
parental concerns for, 123t
  bowel movements, 123
  fussy baby, 123–124
  sleep, 122–123, 123t
  tantrums, 124
parental education for, 122
risks assessment and harm reduction, 122
screening, 121
  for developmental delays and disabilities,
    121–122
  of growth, 121
  for hearing, 121
Wellness visit, 54–55, 55t
Wells criteria for pulmonary embolism, 179t
Wernicke encephalopathy, 459
Wheal (hive), 395t
Wheezing, 236–237
  cause of, 237t

5 Whys analysis, for medication errors, 76, 76f
Windshield survey, 473
Woman Abuse Screening Tool, 432
Women's health care, 321, 322f
  abnormal uterine bleeding, 330, 331t
  breast examination, 324–326, 325t
  intimate partner violence, screening for, 324
  menopause and menopausal symptoms,
    331–333
  menstrual cycle, 321–323, 322f, 323f
  pelvic examination, 326–327, 328t
  sexual history, taking of, 323–324
  vaginal discharge and lesions, 327–329, 329t
Wood light examination, 397
Work, idea of, 33
World Health Organization (WHO), 441, 472

Z
Zone Diet, 300t
Z-score, 281